Language
Disorders and
Language
Development

Language Disorders and Language Development

Margaret Lahey
Emerson College

MACMILLAN PUBLISHING COMPANY
New York
COLLIER MACMILLAN PUBLISHERS
London

Copyright © 1988, Macmillan Publishing Company,
a division of Macmillan, Inc.

Printed in the United States of America

Revised from *Language Development and Language Disorders*, by Lois Bloom and Margaret Lahey, copyright © 1978 by Macmillan Publishing Company.

Macmillan Publishing Company
866 Third Avenue, New York, New York 10022

Collier Macmillan Canada, Inc.

Library of Congress Cataloging-in-Publication Data

Lahey, Margaret.
  Language disorders and language development.

  Rev. ed. of: Language development and language disorders/Lois Bloom, Margaret Lahey. 1978.
  Bibliography: p.
  Includes indexes.
  1. Language disorders in children. 2. Children—Language. I. Bloom, Lois. Language development and language disorders. II. Title. [DNLM: 1. Language Development. 2. Language Disorders—in infancy & childhood. WS 105.5.C8 L183L]
RJ496.L35L34 1988   618.92′855   87-22059
ISBN 0-02-367130-0

Printing: 5 6 7   Year: 1 2 3 4

To my husband, Hank,
my daughters, Denise and Diane,
and in memory of my parents, Jeannette and George Malloy

Preface

In 1978 a book entitled *Language Development and Language Disorders* was published; it was coauthored by Lois Bloom and myself. Our intent was to revise that book in a similar format, and we began that task a few years ago. In the meantime, other commitments made it impossible for Lois Bloom to continue with the revision of the language development chapters. We both thought, however, that the revision of the language disorders chapters should continue. What follows is a revision and expansion of the second half of the original text (Chapters 10 through 21, as well as Chapter 1).

The book is intended as a text for courses in childhood language disorders and as a resource book for professionals working with these children. In addition, it can serve as a supplementary book in classes dealing with assessment strategies, intervention strategies, or any aspect of developmental disorders including learning disabilities, mental retardation, emotional disturbance, and deafness. Although Chapters 9, 10, and 11 are about the sequence of normal language development, the book is not intended as a primary text for courses in language development. It presumes that students have had some introductory course work in language development.

As before, three fundamental assumptions underlie the view presented here of language learning in children with language disorders. The first assumption is that language is a means of representing information. Thus, children with language disorders need to learn how the linguistic forms of sounds, words, and phrases encode elements of content that have to do with knowledge of objects and events in the world. Linguistic forms and elements of content come together so that one aspect of messages cannot be considered apart from the other; the form of language always relates to content.

The second assumption is that the use of language is a social act, and that children learn language in the context of and as a means for obtaining, maintaining, and regulating contact with other persons. Thus, children with language disorders need to learn language in interaction with other people and they need to learn how to use messages to inquire, converse, direct, and otherwise enjoy social interaction with others. The form of a message and the content that is represented in the message are influenced by how individuals use their messages in communicative contexts; the form and content of language always relate to language use. Language assessment and language intervention need to be concerned with the interactions of language content, language form, and language use.

The third assumption is that normal developmental sequences provide the best hypotheses about the sequence in which the language-disordered child will learn language. Information on normal development is presented as a hypothesis for a plan for language learning. As in the plan presented in the original text, the material presented is limited to empirical data about development in children's oral-language productions.

Some changes will be found in the plan since 1978—changes that reflect new information about language development. In particular, information on complex sentences has been revised and expanded to include a number of new studies. The major portion of the Plan is still derived from longitudinal analyses of the children (Allison, Eric, Gia, Kathryn, & Peter) studied by Bloom and her colleagues; it also reflects similar findings reported by other researchers in both longitudinal and cross-sectional research. In addition, narrative development is now presented in the framework of content/form/use goals based on the cross-sectional data of a number of researchers. It is expected that the plan will continue to evolve as we come to learn more about the development of content/form/use interactions and about the application of such plans to children with language disorders.

Language Disorders and Language Development begins with a revision, by Lois Bloom, of the first chapter in the original text; a definition of language is provided using the format of content/form/use interactions. This is followed by a definition of language disorders using the same format. The next three chapters concern some general information on developmental language disorders, including prevalence and orientations (or models) for describing and explaining such disorders. The information on categorical and specific-abilities orientations has been updated and expanded.

The last two-thirds of the book is oriented toward those who work with children who, for whatever reason, are having difficulty learning a first language. Chapter 6 is an overview of assessment, while Chapter 7 is concerned with identifying children with a language disorder. Following these two chapters are four chapters that present a Content/Form/Use (C/F/U) Goal Plan for Language Learning based on information that is known about the sequence of normal language development. Chapter 8 presents the plan and discusses alternative plans. Chapters 9–11 elaborate on the information presented in the C/F/U Goal Plan; they present more detailed descriptions and examples of behaviors that were sequenced within the plan. Implementation of this plan (i.e., how to use it to determine goals of language intervention for a particular child) is the focus of Chapters 12 and 13; Chapter

12 is concerned with analysis of a language sample while Chapter 13 is concerned with eliciting information. Finally Chapters 14 and 15 are devoted to general principles and specific techniques for facilitating the learning of the interactions among language content, language form, and language use.

A number of possible sequences could have been used in organizing the information in the text and a number of possible sequences can be employed in using the text. For example, some may wish to use Chapters 9–11 as a review of language development at the beginning of the course. In this case, Chapters 9–11 (and possibly 8) might be presented after Chapter 1, but before the remainder of the text. Others may wish to hold Chapters 4 and 5 until after information has been presented on language assessment—that is after Chapter 13 (as was the organization in the original text). If, as a part of the course, students are required to do a language sample analysis, then Appendix G should probably be assigned along with Chapter 12. Thus, a number of the chapters can be assigned and discussed in a different order from that presented here.

Many persons have influenced the revision of this book. Feedback from the original text has been most helpful—feedback from students, from professors who have used the book as a text, and from professionals who are working daily with language-disordered children. It is because of the positive manner in which the original text was received that this revision was attempted. Within this supportive framework, many of you have also challenged some of the applications, questioned procedures, or added innovative touches. You may find the influence of your suggestions included; they were all taken seriously and were appreciated. Another important source of feedback has come more subtly from the children with whom I have worked on facilitating language learning; each has taught me something and has made me continually aware of how much we have to learn.

My thanks to my colleagues and students at City University of New York where I was a member of the faculty (at Hunter College and the Graduate Center) during the preparation of part of this book. In addition my semester as post-doctoral fellow at the Child Language Laboratory, University of Arizona enabled me to complete the research for a number of chapters within a supportive environment. I have benefited from sharing many of the ideas presented in this book from colleagues at these institutions as well as from other colleagues throughout the country.

Many have read and reacted to portions of this revision: in particular, I would like to acknowledge the contributions of Carol Alpern, Pat Launer, Linda Swisher, Naomi Schiff-Myers, Elaine Silliman, Elaine Geller, Sima Gerber, and Rene Toueg. A number of reviewers reacted to the entire manuscript and their thoughtful reactions were most helpful. In the final stages of preparation the assistance of Marta Kazandjian, Lisa Wolter,

Micaela CornisPop and of Barbara Chernow and her associates was invaluable.

Furthermore, I want to acknowledge the enormous impact that Lois Bloom has had on this book and on the fields of language development and language disorders. Although, she is no longer a coauthor, her influence is found in almost every chapter. She served as a mentor in my early explorations about how children learn language; she has been a special friend and colleague ever since.

There is my family—the ones who make it all worthwhile and to whom this book is dedicated. My *very* special thanks to my husband, Hank, who has not only provided important information, advice, and assistance, but who has had to do without me for so many months. Without his tolerance and support the revision would not have been completed.

M. L.

Acknowledgments

Ablex Publishing Company. Figure 1, p. 11 from J. Martin "The development of register" in J. Fine and R. Freedle (Eds.), *Developmental issues in discourse*, 1983. Reprinted by permission.

American Guidance Service, Inc. Excerpt from the Test Record of the *Peabody Picture Vocabulary Test-Revised*, by L. Dunn and L. Dunn, 1981. Reprinted by permission.

American Psychological Association. Figure 2, p. 46 from "Perception of the speech code," by A. Liberman, F. Cooper, D. Shankweiler, and M. Studdert-Kennedy, *Psychological Review*, 74, 1967. Reprinted by permission.

American Speech and Hearing Association. Figure 1, p. 334 and Figure 2 p. 336 from "Signed English: A manual approach to English language development," by H. Bornstein, *Journal of Speech and Hearing Disorders*, 39, 1974; Figure 1 p. 513 from "Nonspeech noun usage training with severely and profoundly retarded children," by J. Carrier, *Journal of Speech and Hearing Research*, 17, 1974; Table 1, p. 433 from "What is deviant language?" by L. Leonard, *Journal of Speech and Hearing Disorders*, 37, 1972; Table 3, p. 158, from "Research Note: The relation between age and mean length of utterance in morphemes" by J. Miller and R. Chapman; Figure 2, p. 326, from "Studies in aphasia: Background and theoretical formulations," by J. Wepman, L. Jones, R. D. Bock, and D. Van Pelt, *Journal of Speech and Hearing Disorders*, 25, 1960; Figure 1, p. 95, from "Speech style modifications of language-impaired children" by M. Fey, L. Leonard, and J. Wilcox, *Journal of Speech and Hearing Disorders*, 46, 1981; Table 1, p. 381, from "An examination of the semantic relations reflected in the language usage of normal and language-disordered children," by L. Leonard, J. Bolders, and J. Miller in *Journal of Speech and Hearing Research*, 19, 1976. All reprinted by permission.

Blackwell Scientific Publications, Ltd. Table 1, p. 57 from "A study of the oral vocabularies of severely sub-normal patients" by R. Mein in *Journal of Mental Deficiency Research*, 5, 1961. Reprinted by permission.

Cambridge University Press. Figure 1, p. 327 from "Prediction of production: Elicited imitation and spontaneous speech productions of language disordered children" by M. Lahey, P. Launer, N. Schiff-Myers, *Applied Psycholinguistics*, 4, 1983. Reprinted by permission.

Harcourt Brace Jovanovich, Inc. Figure 5 from "Grammars of speech and language" by A. Lieberman, *Cognitive Psychology*, 1970, p. 309. Reprinted by permission. Excerpts from pages 11–13 from *Language* by E. Sapir, copyright 1921 by Harcourt, Brace Jovanovich, Inc., revised by J. V. Sapir in 1949. Reprinted by permission.

Harvard University Press. Table 7, p. 54 from *A first language* by R. Brown, 1973. Reprinted by permission.

National Association of the Deaf. Figures from pages 17–18 of *A basic course in manual communication* by the Communication Skills Program, 1970. Reprinted by permission.

Pergamon Journals Inc. Table 5, p. 306 from "A developmental study of language behavior in retarded children" by J. Lackner published in *Neuropsychologia* 6, 1968. Reprinted by permission.

Prentice-Hall, Inc. Excerpts from pages 21 and 31–32 from *The wild boy of Aveyron* by J. Itard, translation by G. and M. Humphry, 1962. Reprinted by permission.

Pro-ED, Austin, Texas. Tables 1 and 5 from "The use of grammatical morphemes by children with communication disorders" by J. Johnston and T. Schery, published in D. Morehead and A. Morehead (Eds.), *Normal and deficient child language*, 1976. Reprinted by permission.

The Psychological Corporation. The normal curve chart from Test Service Bulletin No. 48. Reprinted by permission.

University of Illinois Press. Figure 2-1, p. 20, in *Psycholinguistic learning disabilities*, by S. Kirk and W. Kirk, 1971. Reprinted by permission.

University of Minnesota Press. Table on p. 116 from *Certain language skills in children*, by M. Templin, 1957. Reprinted by permission.

University of Pennsylvania Press. Excerpts from *The folkstories of children*, by B. Sutton-Smith, 1981. Reprinted by permission.

Contents

13 Determining Goals of Language Learning From Elicited Information   334

14 General Considerations of Language Intervention   350

15 Facilitating the Induction of Content/Form /Use Interactions   377

APPENDICES

REFERENCES

AUTHOR INDEX

SUBJECT INDEX

1

What Is Language?*

Watch and listen to a young child talk! You may be amused, impressed, puzzled, or curious, and you are bound to learn something. You will learn that when young children talk, they interact with and influence other persons; they talk about what they are doing, or are about to do, or want someone else to do; they say sounds, or words, or phrases. And having noticed these things, you will also have learned something about language.

The definition of language in this chapter will provide a frame of reference for describing language development, and a plan for language disorders, in the chapters that follow. Three basic dimensions of language will emerge from this definition. The first is language *content,* what individuals talk about or understand in messages. The second is language *form,* the shape or sound of the units, and their combination, in the message. The third dimension is language *use.* One aspect of language use has to do with the reasons why individuals speak. The second concerns the ways in which individuals construct conversations, and in

* This chapter was contributed by Lois Bloom.

doing so, choose different forms of messages depending upon what they know about the listener and the context.

Defining Language

The answer to the question "What is language?" depends on who is asking the question and why (Halliday, 1975). You may be interested in language in art, as poetry and drama; or the history of language and how words change from one century to another; or language in culture and how languages are used in different societies; or the formal, logical properties of language. In this book, however, we are interested in what children learn about language and how they learn language. To begin with, then, the answer to the question "What is language?" will come from what is most relevant to the descriptions of language development that will follow.

> A language is a code whereby ideas about the world are expressed through a conventional system of arbitrary signals for communication.

The key words in the definition are *communication, ideas, code, system,* and *conventional.* Let's consider what each means and what each contributes to defining language and to understanding how languages work.

Language Is Used to Communicate

We communicate in many ways (for example, through facial expressions, tone of voice, gesture); however, language is our prime means of intentional communication, and speech is the most common expression of language. Language is used for many and varied purposes, most of which involve interactions with other persons. As people interact in different circumstances in the course of a day, they use language to establish and maintain contact, to gain and give information, and, in general, to influence the beliefs and the actions of themselves and other persons. Knowing what can be done with language is an important part of knowing language. Children learn language for the purposes that it serves; they learn to communicate.

In addition to the purposes or functions of language, communication also depends upon the ways in which the speakers vary what they say according to whom they are talking to and what else is happening when they talk. People can say the same thing, but in different ways, to achieve the same purpose. For example, you can talk about objects by referring to them by name: "Here comes the bus," or you can use a pronoun: "Here it comes." If you want a drink of water, you can ask a question: "Do you have water?" Or you can make a statement: "I'm thirsty." Or you can give a directive: "Get me a glass of water" (with or without a "please").

Whether you use a noun or a pronoun, or ask a question or make a statement, depends on many things. At the least, you need to make inferences about what the listener already knows and what the listener needs to know. If the listener is standing at the bus stop, then you can safely say "Here it comes," and you can assume that the listener knows that "it" is the bus. But imagine the reaction if you

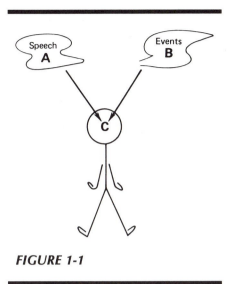

FIGURE 1-1

made the same announcement to a group of strangers sitting with you *on* the bus. How well the speaker knows the listener, and the status relations between speaker and listener, will also influence which alternative message to use for accomplishing the same purpose. For example, you would most likely ask "Do you have any water?" or "May I have some water?" if you were a guest in the home of your great aunt or your professor, and you are more likely to say "Get me a glass of water" if you were calling out to your roommate or spouse who was already in the kitchen. The use of language has to do with how people vary what they say according to the needs of different listeners in different situations, and according to individual goals and purposes.

Language Expresses Ideas

Language expresses what individuals have in mind—their beliefs and desires. The contents of these mental states, the thoughts we express in language, result, in part, from our perceptions—that is, from aspects of what we see, hear, and feel at the moment. But, in large part, the content of these thoughts comes from the knowledge we have stored in memory about objects, events, and relations in the world. What this means is that the *ideas* that people have about events, rather than the events themselves, are expressed with language. The figure in Figure 1-1 shows this relationship. A speech event (A), such as a word or a sentence, does not represent (or map onto) an actual event in the world (B), such as an object or happening. Instead, what people say, and how they interpret what others say, depends on an intervening mental state (indicated by C in the figure) which is derived from previous knowledge as well as present perceptions.

Even a concrete noun such as *cookie* or *house* expresses an idea, and that idea depends upon a concept in memory that somehow organizes what we know about cookies or about houses. This point is basic in linguistic as well as psychological views of language. For example, the linguist Edward Sapir (1921) pointed out that:

> the word "house" is not a linguistic fact if by it is meant merely the acoustic effect produced on the ear by its constituent consonants and vowels, pronounced in a certain order; nor the motor processes and tactile feelings which make up the articulation of the word; nor the visual perception on the part of the hearer of this articulation . . . nor the memory of any or all of these experiences. It is only when these, and possibly still other, associated experiences are automatically associated with the image of a house that they begin to take on the nature of a symbol, a word, an element of language. . . . The elements of language [are] associated with whole groups, delimited classes, of experience rather than with the single experiences themselves. . . . The single experience lodges in an individual consciousness and is, strictly speaking, incommunicable. . . . Thus, the single impression which I have had of a particular house must be identified with all my other impressions of it. Further, my generalized memory or my "notion" of this house must be merged with the notions that all other individuals who have seen the house have formed of it . . . [and ultimately] this house and that house and thousands of other phenomena of like character are thought of as having enough in common, in spite of great and obvious differences of detail, to be classed under the same heading. In other words, the speech element "house" is the symbol, first and foremost, not of a single perception, nor even of the notion of a particular object, but of a "concept," in other words, of a *convenient capsule of thought that embraces thousands of distinct experiences and that is ready to take in thousands more.* (emphasis added, pp. 11–13)

Children learn language in order to express their thoughts and to interpret the speech of others so as to attribute thoughts to them (Bloom & Beckwith, 1986). But expressing an idea about a cookie depends upon knowing what cookies are. And knowing about cookies and what they are depends upon experience. Experience consists of numerous encounters with many different objects (such as houses, cups, apples, raisins, books, and cookies). Cookies may differ from one another in shape, size, and texture, but they share the similarities that distinguish them from other objects, such as houses, cups, apples, or books. Children perceive regularities in the environment. For example, all cookies are basically similar in shape, size, and function (to be eaten). And books are different from cookies, but books are similar to one another in their relative size, shape, and function. Furthermore, some objects can be moved (such as cookies and books), but others (such as refrigerators) usually cannot be (Gibson, 1966).

Children also have many encounters with persons and objects: persons doing things to objects, objects being affected by certain actions, persons habitually associated with objects, and other such person-object relations. Children make a mental record of the regularities in these relations, so that when they come upon a relationship again, they will recognize it. Words or signs take on meaning by themselves, or in relation to one another, only in connection with underlying mental representations of objects and person-object relations such as these.

In sum, knowing just the sounds in the word *cookie* is meaningless unless you also know what cookies are. Similarly, knowing that some nouns precede verbs and other nouns follow verbs in sentences is meaningless unless you also know about the relationships between the objects and actions that such nouns and verbs represent. You cannot know about sentences and the relations between the parts of the sentence unless you also know about relations between persons, actions, and objects. For example, nouns can mean different things in relation to different verbs. A noun such as *boy* can be the agent of an action (as in "The boy ate the cookie"); a noun such as *key* can be the instrument of an action (as in "The key opened the door"); and a noun such as *girl* can be the object affected by some state (as in "The girl felt sad"). The content of language has to do with the knowledge that individuals have about persons, objects, events, and the relations among them.

Language Is a Code

A code is a means of representing one thing by another, and language is a means of representation. Given an object, event, or relationship, one can represent it schematically—with a picture, a map, a graph, a word, or a sentence—so that it is possible to consider it, to preserve it, and to share it. In this way, the picture, map, graph, word, or sentence can be said to stand for, or represent, the object, event, or relationship.

As an example, a cookie is an object that can be baked, eaten, dropped, moved, or broken. A picture of a cookie would have to represent both its characteristic shape, usually roundness and flatness, and its texture, smoothness or lumpiness. A picture of the event of a person eating a cookie would represent the action relation between a person (the eater) and an object (the cookie). A picture of the event of a person taking a cookie would represent the action relations between a person (the taker), an object (the cookie), and the place the cookie is taken from (a surface or a container). And, conceivably, although not likely, a graph could be constructed to represent such information as the sizes of different cookies in relation to the number of bites it takes to eat each one.

Representations such as pictures, maps, and graphs are fairly direct. They reproduce and preserve the proportions and relations of whatever is being represented. Such reproductions are not independent of the objects, events, and relations that they represent. In contrast, sounds, words and sentences differ in that they represent what an individual knows about an object or event *indirectly*. When speakers and hearers use a linguistic code to construct words and sentences and conversations, they represent information about objects and events, but the words and sentences and conversations themselves do not reproduce the objects and events. In encoding, a speaker recalls and combines the units of the code to represent information in a message; in decoding, a listener recognizes and segments the units of the code to extract information from a message. The code provides ways in which essentially arbitrary elements (either the sounds of spoken languages or the movements of signed languages) combine with one another to stand for any and all possible objects and events that the individual knows or will ever know. The code provides the form of language.

The Code Is a System

The ways in which sounds combine to form words, words combine to form sentences, and sentences combine to form conversations are predictable because they are systematic. In the construction of words, we follow certain rules that specify which sounds can combine with one another and which sounds cannot be combined. For example, in English, a word cannot consist of only consonants but must also include a vowel; nasal consonants such as /n/ or /m/ can precede other consonants at the ends of words (such as in *dump* and *drink*), but nasal consonants cannot precede other consonants at the beginning of a word (e.g., **nkup* and **mkup* would not be acceptable words in English).

The rules for sentences make up a grammar, and grammatical rules specify how linguistic units are combined to code meaning. One rule in English is that a word that represents the agent of an action, such as *girl*, must occur before the word that represents the object affected by the action, such as *cookie*, as, for example, in the simple sentence "The girl is eating the cookie." But if the focus of attention in the action is the cookie rather than the girl, another rule allows *cookie* to precede the verb. The rule reverses the order in which the words *cookie* and *girl* are mentioned in a sentence, but only if we also change or add other parts to the sentence; for example, "The cookie is being eaten by the girl," or "It is a cookie that the girl is eating."

Given a group of sentences, we can make predictions about other possible sentences. For example, given the group of sentences—"The boy baked the pie," "The girl climbed the tree," "The man carried the bag"—we could predict that the words *woman, the, tower,* and *built* would combine to form the sentence "The woman built the tower." Our prediction would follow from our noticing that in the given set of sentences (1) names of persons that act precede the name of an action, (2) names of objects that are affected by an action follow the name of the action, (3) a word *the* precedes the names for persons and objects but not actions, and so on.

The sounds of a language make up its alphabet. The words of a language make up its dictionary (or lexicon). The rules for combining sounds to form words and for combining words to form sentences make up a grammar. The number of sounds, the number of words, and the number of rules in a language system are limited and finite. This means that an alphabet contains a fixed number of sounds; one can count the number of words in a dictionary; and a grammar for forming sentences consists of a fixed number of rules.

However, the number of possible combinations of elements, the number of possible sentences in a language, is unlimited. Indeed, while certain familiar routines and formulas have become frozen forms in the language (such as "Hi, how are ya?" and "How much does this cost?"), the great majority of the utterances that you might say or hear on any given day will be utterances that you have neither seen nor heard before. Yet, despite their novelty, you will ordinarily not have any difficulty in saying and understanding new sentences. The speakers and hearers of a language can readily say and understand sentences that they have never said or heard before because they know the units of the language and the rules for combining them.

This use of finite means (units and rules for combining units) to produce an endless number of expressions, most of which have not been said or understood before, is the property of language known as *linguistic creativity*. The linguistic creativity of speakers and hearers is evidence that they know the rules that are related to one another to form a system. Noam Chomsky (1972) made this relationship between linguistic behavior and linguistic knowledge explicit:

Having mastered a language, one is able to understand an indefinite number of expressions that are new to one's experience . . . to produce such expressions on an appropriate occasion, despite their novelty . . . and to be understood by others who share this still mysterious ability. . . . A person who knows a language has mastered a system of rules. . . . Of course, the person who knows the language has no consciousness of having mastered these rules or of putting them to use, nor is there any reason to suppose that this knowledge of the rules of language can be brought to consciousness. (pp. 100–104)

Thus, a speaker can express and a hearer can interpret an infinite number of possible sentences. Moreover, a speaker can say and a hearer can understand new sentences that neither one has ever said or heard before. This linguistic creativity comes from knowing the system of grammatical rules for the language.

The Code Is a Convention

Just as new words can be introduced and accepted by members of a speech community, any of the facts about language can be changed—although it may be highly inconvenient and a nuisance to do so. For example, a 5-year-old child announced one day that from that moment on she intended to call apples "peaches" and to call peaches "apples." We pointed out to her that she would have a hard time at the market, because when she asked for apples she would be given peaches. She immediately understood the dilemma and said that she would then have to tell the people at the market, who would then have to tell the truckers who bring the fruit, who would then have to tell the farmers who grow the fruit, who would then have to tell all the other farmers as well as the scientists who grow the seeds for planting the trees, and many others besides. Although hardly worth the effort, the important fact is that it could be done, which is an essential fact about language. Words and sentences are used as they are only because the speakers in a language community agree on such matters. The community norms, principles, strategies, and values that guide the use of speech are the "community ground rules for speaking" (Bauman and Sherzer, 1974, p. 7). They are the conventional facts about language, and they exist for social reasons rather than logical or empirical reasons (Fodor, Bever, and Garrett, 1974).

The elements of the system and the way in which the system works have been agreed on and accepted by the members of a particular community. Thus, a language represents shared knowledge. The fact that any group of speakers (a linguistic community of any size) recognizes and accepts a particular word, or accepts a sentence as grammatical or a conversation as appropriate, is evidence enough for including the word in the dictionary and the rules for the sentence and the conversation in the language of that community. Of course, in this context, agreement and acceptance of an aspect of language are always implicit and understood among the speakers of the language without their having to talk about it or, indeed, without their even being able to talk about it. Most adult speakers of a language would find it hard to describe or explain their language—or even explain how language works. Nonetheless, we know what we can and cannot say. We also know that unless we share the same knowledge about words and possible combinations of words with other persons, we cannot use the language. We are especially aware of the social conventions of language when we enter a foreign community and cannot share the language.

In order to define language, we have had to consider what people do and what they say, together with what they mean. Children that are learning language need to learn about persons, objects, events, and the relations among them, for the *content* of language. They need to learn to recognize the different contexts that require different kinds of language *use*. And children need to learn the *forms* of the linguistic code for representing language content, in different contexts, and for many purposes. Thus, language has three major dimensions: content, form, and use. *Content* is the meaning (or semantics) of language. *Form* is the shape of language. *Use* is the function of language and its relations to the everyday contexts (or pragmatics).

Language Content

Language content consists of topics but is broader than topics. A topic is the particular idea represented in a particular message. When a 2-year-old says, "This is a truck," the topic of the message is the truck. When a teenager says, "I need a new dress," the topic of the message is the dress. When someone tells you, "Eat your dinner," the topic of the message is the action relation between you and the dinner. Thus, one can talk about a truck or about a new dress, or one can talk about eating dinner or riding a bike or buying a new pair of shoes. The number of topics or things in the world that can be talked about is probably limitless.

However, all the different topics of messages can be categorized according to the general kinds of meaning that they share. One category of topics is about objects in general (including trucks, new dresses, mommy, daddy, cookies, plants, etc.). Another category is about actions in general (eating, throwing, hitting, etc.); still another category is the relations in general that exist between objects (e.g., the possessive relation between mommy and her coat, daddy and his chair, or baby and the doll), or between events (e.g., the causal relation between walking in the rain and getting wet). Thus, mommy's coat may be the topic of the message, but the content represented in the message has to do with the possession relation— the same content category that also includes daddy's chair and baby's doll. Language content is the categorization of the topics of messages. Language content has to do with the meaning (the semantics) represented by language.

The difference between language topic and language content (schematized in Figure 1-2), then, is the difference between the particular idea in a message, such as a particular object (the topic), and the broader, more general categorization of topics in many messages, such as objects in general (content). Virtually all children can be alike in the content of their messages. For example, all children learn to talk about objects, actions, and relations such as possession and location. At the same time, children can also differ in the topics that they can understand and talk about. Thus, while all children talk about animate objects (a category of content), children from middle-class urban homes in the United States talk about their pet fish, dogs, or cats, while children from farm homes talk about cows and chickens (different topics). Children in the United States talk about eating ice cream, cookies, and hamburgers; children in New Guinea talk about eating sugarcane and pan-

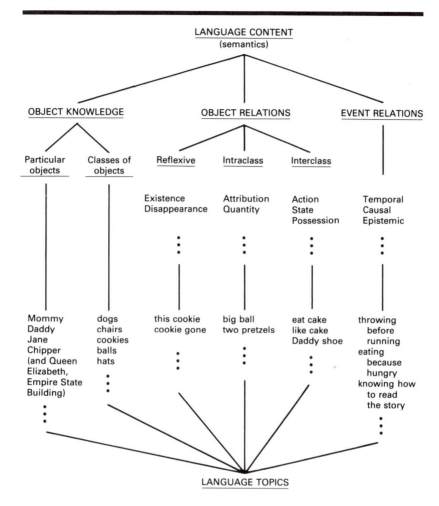

FIGURE 1-2 *Language Content and Language Topics*

danus. But children everywhere learn to talk about objects that can be eaten and action relationships between persons and objects, regardless of what the particular objects are and even though the particular actions between persons and objects may differ. As a result, the vocabularies of children from different cultures are different, because the topics they talk about are different, but the content of their language is the same.

Language content is continuous over the life span, from earliest child language to later and eventually mature language. Two-year-olds, 5-year-olds, and adults all talk about the same content; they talk about objects, actions, and relations. But whereas the content of language is continuous as it evolves in the course of development, the topics of language are variable and change with age as well as culture. Two-year-olds might talk about bouncing balls, five-year-olds about baseballs, and adults about golf balls. Thus, the topics of language are varied and probably indefinitely many in number, but the content of language is defined by categorization.

The distinction between language content and language topic is analogous to the distinction in cognitive psychology between semantic memory and episodic memory, a distinction that was introduced originally by Tulving (1972). Episodic memory is a person's store of individual experiences, such memories as, for example, watching the 1986 Super Bowl game between the New York Giants and the Denver Broncos. Semantic memory is general knowledge, such knowledge as, for example, the procedures for deciding which football teams end the season at the Super Bowl. Obviously, knowledge is derived from the individualized and personal experiences we have had, for example, with each football game we have watched or perhaps even played. However, memories of these particular events become depersonalized and separated from their original context to form more global categories of knowledge, such as our knowledge of football. Such global knowledge is more broadly useful than the separate and specific, personal, context-bound experiences (Kintsch, 1974).

Similarly, whereas language topic is particular, personal, and contextual, language content is general, depersonalized, and independent of particular context. We could add that language topic can be more or less idiosyncratic with individual societies or cultures, whereas language content is shared by common human experience and may well be universal.

Three primary categories of language content are schematized in Box 1-2. They are (1) objects, (2) relations between objects, and (3) relations between events. In the first category, the two kinds of objects are particular objects and classes of objects. Particular objects are unique instances like mommy, daddy, Chipper (the family dog), Queen Elizabeth, and the Statue of Liberty. Classes of objects are categories of topics such as dogs, chairs, cookies, balls, and boxes.

The second category is relations between objects. Certain object relations have to do with the relation of one object to itself, or the relation of one object to another object just like (e.g., reflexive). Thus, an object can simply exist ("This is a cookie") or disappear ("Cookie gone"), or the same object or one just like it can reappear ("More cookie"). Other object relations have to do with the ways that objects from the same class are different from one another. For example, take the general class of dogs. Some dogs are small and some are large; there are black and brown dogs, long-haired and short-haired dogs, and so forth. Such attributes and properties as these distinguish among the objects from the same class of objects, for example, according to their relative size ("the big ball" and "the little ball") or their color ("the red shirt" and "the yellow shirt").

Still other object relations have to do with the way that objects from different classes relate to one another. Such object relations involve locations, action, and possession relations between persons and objects and between different kinds of objects. A *locative* relation is the relation between objects according to their places in space; for example, one object can be *in*, *on*, or *above* another object. An *action* relation entails movement. The movement of a single person, such as a girl dancing, and the movement of a single object, such as a ball rolling, are one kind of action relations, called intransitive relations. Other kinds of object relations involve either two objects or a person and an object and are called transitive relations. For example, one object can be *eaten*, or *pushed*, by some other object like a dog or person. A *possession* relation has to do with the connection between persons and the objects with which they are typically associated.

Event relations include relations between two different events, or relations within a single event. For example, two events can be related to one another according to the time each occurs ("You take a walk and then come back"—in this instance, one thing happens before the other). Two events also have a relation between them when one thing happens *because* something else happened ("I don't have a cookie because I ate it"). Relations within the same event have to do with the time that the event occurs ("I went home last week"), the mood of the speaker toward the event ("I might go home"), or what the speaker knows or thinks about the event ("I think I'm on my way home").

In sum, language content is what people talk about: the linguistic expression of what we have in mind, which depends upon what we know about the world of objects, events, and relations. Our ideas about objects and events, and the way in which objects relate to themselves and to one another in different events, can be expressed by different sorts of words or signs and by the linguistic relations between words or signs. Such linguistic representation depends on the conventional, arbitrary units that give language its form.

Language Form

When we describe form, we describe the shape or contour of the surface features of what is actually said or signed. (See Figure 1–3.) Spoken messages can be described in terms of their sounds, and signed messages can be described in terms of movements and hand configurations. Sounds and signs form segments of an utterance. We also describe spoken and signed messages in terms of features of stress and intonation which provide the rhythm of sequences of segments.

Just as with language content, there is a difference between the particular forms of language on one level and the categories of forms on a more general and abstract level. Three broad categories of language form are schematized in Figure 1-3: the phonology, the morphology, and the syntax of language. Together, these three categories contribute to the underlying rule system, or the grammar, of a language. Each represents a categorization of the superficial forms of language that persons actually say and hear, or sign and see.

Phonology

The phonology of a language is the categorization of the sounds of the language. The sound categories of the language are the separate phonemes, such as /b/, /p/, and /o/, and the minimum combinations of phonemes, such as /ba/, /po/, /pa/, that form syllables. Syllables are the segments of language. When segments are combined in words and phrases, the rhythmic contour of combinations of segments make up the prosody of language. Features of prosody include the relative stress on one or another syllable in a string, the melodic rise and fall of the intonation of syllables as they are spoken, and the pattern of pause time that occurs between segments. Prosodic features of sound (such as stress, intonation, and pause) are

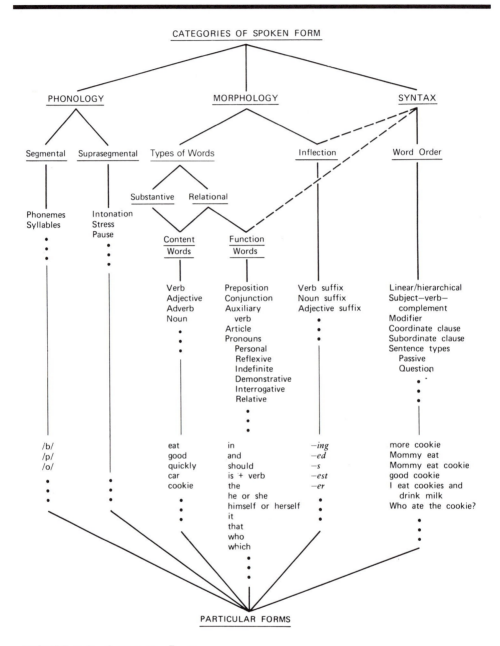

FIGURE 1-3   Language Form

superimposed on the sound segments—the sounds and syllables—and so are called the suprasegmental aspect of phonology.

When we change the intonation contour of a sentence from falling, ↘, to rising, ↗, we change the sentence from a statement, "She's coming to the party," to a question, "She's coming to the party?" We can convey different information about the content of a sentence by changing the pattern of stress. For example, "Shé rode the gray horse," with the emphatic stress on "she," indicates that some other person rode a different horse. "She rode the gráy horse," with the stress on "gray," indicates that the rider had a choice among horses to ride.

Morphology

A morpheme is the smallest segment of speech that carries meaning. The individual phonemes or sounds, such as /p/ and /b/, do not carry meaning by themselves. Many syllables—such as the *ta-* or the *-ble* syllables in *table*—also do not carry meaning by themselves. But other syllables and combinations of syllables do carry meaning. These meaningful segments are morphological units and include the words (*table*) and grammatical inflections (the *-s* in *tables* or the *-ing* in *running*) of the language. The morphology of the language, then, consists of the words and the inflections of the language.

Two broad classes of words in a lexicon are content words and function words. Content words are the nouns, verbs, adjectives, and adverbs. They are the "major building blocks" (Brown, 1973) that carry meaning in sentences. Each content word can stand alone and still convey some meaning. Some content words refer to objects and can be called substantive words, while others refer to relationships (e.g., verbs and adjectives) and can be called relational words. We are continually adding new content words to our language (think, for example, of the new words that have been added that pertain to computers), and so content words are often referred to as open-class words. In contrast, we rarely add function words to our language; this class of words has been referred to as a closed class.

Function words are the "little words" that provide the glue for holding the building blocks of a sentence together. Function words are also separate words and prepositions (*to, in, on*), articles (*a, the*), conjunctions (*and, so, because*), and pronouns (*that, what, who*). The meaning of function words depends on the relations between the content words that they connect.

The morphological inflections are not separate; they are bound to the nouns, verbs, and adjectives, and they mark different kinds of meaning. The phoneme /s/ is also a morpheme *-s*; in fact, *-s* is really three different morphemes in English. When *-s* is added to count nouns such as *dog, cat, bed,* or *glass,* the meaning that results is "more than one," or plurality. When *-s* is added to an animate noun such as *mommy, baby,* or *dog, -s* can indicate possession. And when *-s* is added to a verb such as *go* or *fit* the resulting meaning has to do with present or habitual action (e.g., The bed goes in the bedroom).

Morphological inflections modulate the meaning of a sentence (Brown, 1973). They provide, for example, indicators of time (present *-s* or past *-ed,* etc.) or number (for example, with nouns, to indicate plurality—*cat/cats;* or with verbs, to indicate one actor versus more than one actor—for instance, "she sits," but "they sit"). Meanings such as time and number have to do with the relations within an event. Their corresponding inflections modulate the major meanings of sentences that come from the relations between nouns, verbs, and adjectives. The relations between nouns, verbs, and adjectives, together with the morphological inflections, are formalized by the syntax of sentences.

Syntax

The syntax of a sentence is the arrangement of words according to the meaning relations among them. Two kinds of syntactic relations between words are linear structure and hierarchical structure. A linear relationship is formed when two (or more) words in combination do not mean anything more than each of the words alone. For example, the word *more* by itself means "recurrence." When a 2-year-old child finishes a cookie, reaches for another cookie, and says "More cookie," the meaning relation between *more* and *cookie* is the same as the meaning of *more* and the meaning of *cookie* added together. The meaning of the relation between the words is "recurrence," and that meaning is the same as the meaning of *more.* When a meaning relation between words is the same as the meaning of one of the words, the syntactic structure can be described as a linear one.

Linear relations can be formalized with the formula $f(x)$: a fixed value, f, which doesn't change, is combined with a variable (x), which can assume many values (Brown, 1973). In this formulation the meaning of the relation $f(x)$ is determined by the meaning of the constant f. No new meaning is added to f or to (x) when they are combined. For example, in the phrases "More cookie," "More airplane," and "More cheese," *more* is the constant f, and the variable (x) is represented by *cookie, airplane,* and *cheese,* respectively. The meaning relation between the words is the same meaning, "recurrence," which is also the meaning of *more.*

When word combinations are linear and additive, the cumulative meanings of the two separate words, when they are joined together, do not produce a new meaning. In the above phrases, the meaning relation between the words is "recurrence," the meaning of *more* is "recurrence," and the meaning of *cookie* is unchanged. Similarly, in the phrase "Cookie gone," the relational meaning between the words is "disappearance" and the meaning of *gone* is "disappearance." The meaning of *cookie* is the same in both phrases, "More cookie" and "Cookie gone." We describe the structural relationship between words as linear when the words in the phrase are joined together and the meanings are added, without a new meaning resulting from their combination.

As was indicated in Figure 1-3, syntax is not independent of either the morphological inflections or the function words in the lexicon. Function words such as *on, in,* and *above* also have relational meanings that combine with other words in linear syntactic structures, for example, "on the table" and "in the box." Similarly, adding the morpheme *-ing* to words like *run* and *eat* results in linear relationships.

On the other hand, other combinations of words do have meaning that is independent of the dictionary meanings of the individual words themselves. When the meaning relation of words in combination with one another is something more than the meanings of the separate words, the syntactic structure can be described as hierarchical. The meaning of such sentences is not simply additive. When a noun and a verb are combined in a sentence, the result is some larger (superordinate) meaning that is more than only the individual meanings of the separate words. Take the nouns *mommy, daddy, baby, dog,* and *Jane,* for instance. Each of these nouns has an inherent, lexical meaning. But they also assume the relational meaning "agent" when we combine them with verbs such as *eat, throw,* and *push* ("Dog eat," "Daddy throw," "Jane push"). By itself, the word *mommy* or the word *dog* does not have the meaning "agent." These words take on the relational meaning "agent" when they are combined with verbs in sentences.

Certain other nouns, for example, *toast, horse, ball,* and *bridge,* assume a different relational meaning in combinations with verbs ("Ride horse," "Eat toast," "Build bridge"). Here their meaning is also a grammatical meaning, "affected object," although their lexical meaning remains the same. Thus, nouns that share the same grammatical meaning in their relation to verbs form categories such as *agent* or *affected object.* In the example above, the nouns *mommy, daddy, baby,* and others form the category *agent* in relation to verbs; the nouns *horse, toast,* and *bridge* form another category, *affected object.* Such nouns, then, have their lexical meanings, but they can also take on grammatical meanings when they occur in relation to verbs in sentences.

Similarly, two nouns, such as *daddy* and *shoe,* can take on a superordinate meaning in relation to each other, as when "daddy shoe" means "possession." "Possession," then, is a superordinate meaning that is separate from the meaning of the word *daddy* or the meaning of the word *shoe,* but comes from the relationship between the two words. A hierarchical structure is a syntactic relation between words, where the meaning relation between the words is different from the lexical meaning of the words themselves.

In summary, the forms that are used by the language can be described in several ways. However, regardless of the ways in which we describe linguistic form, form in language is the means for connecting sound with meaning. The form of language consists of an inventory of linguistic units and the system of rules for their combination. The combination of forms depends only in part upon the meaning relations we express; the purpose of the utterance and the context of the utterance—language use—will also help to determine the form of the utterance.

Language Use

The three major aspects of language use (or pragmatics) are (1) the use of language for different goals or functions, (2) the use of information from the context to determine what we say in order to achieve the goals, and (3) the use of the interaction between persons to initiate, maintain, and terminate conversations. (See Figure 1-4.)

The functions of language are the reasons why we speak and listen to one another. Traditionally, the functions of language were described in linguistic terms referring to the grammatical mood of the sentence. The different grammatical moods are named declarative (making a statement), interrogative (asking a question), imperative (giving a command), and exclamative (exclaiming) (e.g., Lyons, 1968). More recently, the functions of language have been described in terms of both personal and social goals that involve interaction, regulation, and the balance of control between speakers and hearers. Personal functions (sometimes referred to as intrapersonal or mathetic functions) have to do with the speaker's

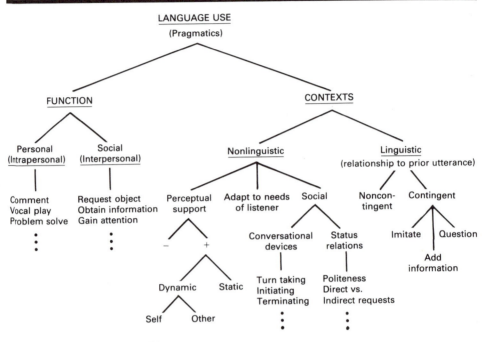

FIGURE 1-4   Language Use

using language to achieve goals which do not involve other persons. Personal goals are served when we comment to ourselves, solve a problem, or ask a question to gain information. Social functions (sometimes referred to as interpersonal or pragmatic functions) have to do with getting things done in the world. Socially mediated goals are served when we seek and maintain the attention of others, or give a direction for someone to act (Halliday, 1975). One part of language use, then, is language function: the use of messages according to the goals of the speaker and the intended effect of the message on the hearer.

Speech does not occur in a vacumn—speech occurs in relation to some context, and the context most often includes other persons. The second aspect of language use has to do with context and the rules that we use for deciding which *form* of the message will serve the *function* of the message in different contexts. Some part of the context of the message is nonlinguistic, and includes the listener as well as the objects, events, relations, and other circumstances in the situation. We all know certain routine formulas to use in everyday situations such as answering the telephone ("Hello") and greeting an acquaintance ("How are you?"). Far more often, however, we formulate new and different messages that require judgments about the state of affairs and the listener.

Speakers need to infer what the listener already knows and does not know in order to formulate messages (i.e., adapt to the listener). Consider the difference between telling and asking. When we have some information and have reason to believe that our hearer does not have the same information, we will ordinarily make a statement, for example, tell the listener that "The cookies are on the table." But when we need to know something that we believe the hearer already knows, we will ordinarily ask a question, for example, "Where are the cookies?" or "Are the cookies on the table?" The form of the message also depends on whether what we are talking about is already present in the situation. For example, the difference between saying "The book is on the table" and saying "It is over there" will depend on whether the hearer knows already that the book and table are in the situation.

When engaged in social exchanges with other persons, another set of skills is required. For example, one must know how to initiate, maintain, and terminate a conversation. To start a conversation, one must alert the listener so as to have the listener's attention in the first place. To maintain the conversation requires skill in taking turns and knowing how to assert, respond, or react to what the listener has, in turn, asserted or responded. And, finally, to end the conversation requires that each of the participants knows how to sign off so that neither of them is left dangling. Furthermore, the form of utterances changes depending upon the status relations between speaker and hearer. Indirect forms of request (e.g., "Are there any more cookies?") and politeness markers (e.g., "Could you please pass me a cookie") are required when speaking to persons of higher status or to persons who are not well known.

Some part of the context is linguistic. The form of a message may or may not be influenced by what is said—either by the speaker or by the listener. On the one hand, when we introduce a new topic and say something that is not related to what has just been said, our message is *noncontingent*. Certain noncontingent messages open a conversation; for example, someone walks into a room and announces, "I think I'll shovel the sidewalk." Other noncontingent messages change the topic of an ongoing conversation; for example, a man and wife are discussing the candidates in an election and one of them asks, "What's for dinner?"

On the other hand, certain messages that occur in sequence after someone says something share the same topic; these are *contingent* messages. Contingency can take several forms. Some part or perhaps even all of a message might be repeated; for example, a grocer tells you, "The bananas cost 59 cents a pound," and you repeat "59 cents a pound?" New information might be added to the original message; for example, you could have said, "But they were 49 cents a pound last week."

All of these factors about situations and speakers and hearers contribute to both the form and the content of messages, to how people do things with words, and to how languages work.

The Integration of Content, Form, and Use

We have presented three components: content, form, and use, as a framework for defining language. One might inquire what else is left to consider. The necessity of the interaction of these three components in language development, and their disruption in language disorders, may well be obvious. The same or similar distinctions have certainly been made by others (see Cherry's 1957 review of similar categorizations). Nevertheless, linguistic theory in the years before the 1970s

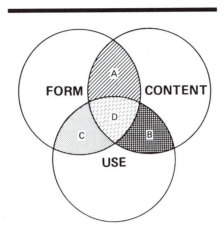

FIGURE 1-5 The Interaction of Content, Form, and Use in Language

considered the *form* of language as the only object of study, and the goal of description could not include an account of meaning in messages. Accounting for meaning was not a reasonable goal for linguistic inquiry because the realm of meaning embraced all possible events in the world (Bloomfield, 1933). In contrast, Skinner's (1957) psychological explanation of verbal behavior centered on language use alone and ignored form and content almost entirely. As a result, accounts of child language before the 1970s described form most often and use less often, but did not consider their interaction with meaning or with one another in any systematic way. By the same token, accounts of language disorders in children were concerned almost exclusively with descriptions of form or use, but rarely both, and almost never in systematic relation to content or meaning.

For individuals using language and for children learning language, the components of content, form, and use come together in understanding and saying messages. Their intersection is schematized in Figure 1-5, Where the overlap of the three components, in the center of the Venn diagram, represents knowledge of language. Our purpose in defining language, to begin with, was to understand what children learn and how they learn about language. We have defined language, for these purposes, as the necessary integration of the three components.

The integration of content, form, and use is knowledge of language. Knowledge of language is language "competence" (Chomsky, 1966), and such competence or knowledge guides the actions of speaking and interpreting messages. Knowledge of language, or competence, can be conceived of as a "plan" in the sense of Miller, Galanter, and Pribram (1960). The mental plan that the child acquires for language is a system of rules and procedures. Certain of the rules pair sound (or movements) with meaning in messages. Certain other rules pair sound-meaning or movement-meaning connections with different expectancies in different situations.

Thus, to know language is to have a plan and to use that plan when we act, that is, when we speak and interpret messages. Because language can be defined in terms of the plan that underlies actions, something about an individual's knowledge of language can be learned by studying the individual's actions. Learning language in the first place, and learning what someone else knows about language in the second place, requires evidence. Children obtain evidence about language, for acquiring language, by acting in certain ways and by observing the actions of others. The evidence that children obtain contributes to acquiring a plan for language. Similarly, the researcher, clinician, or teacher can obtain evidence about what children know about language by listening and watching what children do. This book is about the evidence of language development and how such evidence can be used with children for whom learning language is difficult.

Suggested Readings

Akmajian, A., Demers, R. A., and Harnish, R. M. (1985). *Linguistics: An introduction to language and communication.* Second Edition. Cambridge, MA.: The MIT Press.

Chomsky, N. *Language and mind.* (1972). New York: Harcourt, Brace, Jovanovich.

Halliday, M. A. K. (1973). *Explorations in the functions of language.* London: Edward Arnold.

Lyons, J. (1968). *Introduction to theoretical linguistics.* London: Cambridge University Press.

Sapir, E. (1921). *Language.* New York: Harcourt, Brace, & World.

2

What Is a Language Disorder?

Although most children learn their native language in a relatively short period of time and without instruction, there are other children who have considerable difficulty; they learn language only with much help, or they never learn language at all. These children are the concern of their parents and of specialists in the fields of speech pathology, audiology, education, psychology, and medicine. While much can be done to help these children, many remain a challenging puzzle to all professionals. The solution to the puzzle may eventually help us better understand normal language development, reduce the occurrence of childhood language disorders, and increase our effectiveness in facilitating language learning in the language-disordered child. The next few chapters present a review of general information currently available on childhood language disorders.

A language disorder is often identified by persons who encounter the child interacting in many situations that demand talking and understanding. The different behaviors that might be noticed are varied and include little or no talking, little or no understanding of instructions, unusual use of words or phrases, or grammatical mistakes that interfere with communication. Thus we can use the term *language disorder* to refer to *any disruption in the learning or use of one's native language as evidenced by language behaviors that are different from* (but not superior to) *those expected given a child's chronological age.*

Different Uses of Terminology

No consensus exists on the terminology used to describe the children or the language of the children who are not learning language normally. In addition to the term *language disorder*, the terminology currently used includes *deviant language, delayed language, language disability,* and *language impairment.*

Some professionals use these terms to refer only to children who are having difficulty learning language although there are no intellectual, sensory, or emotional problems. Etiology is either unknown or presumed to be neurological (see Johnston, 1982b; Kleffner, 1973; Leonard, 1981; Morehead, 1975). Another means of describing this subgroup of language-disordered children is to prefix some of the above terms with words such as *specific*—in this text we will use the terms *specific-language disorder* and *specific-language impairment* to refer to this subgroup.

The terms *deviant, disordered, disabled,* and *impaired* are used by others as descriptive terms to refer to language development that is unlike that of normal development in terms of the actual behaviors learned and the sequence in which they are learned. Thus, the terms are used to infer that the language system of these children is qualitatively different from the language system of normal language learners and not just that it develops later. This is a complicated issue. It is not always easy to determine whether a child's system is qualitatively different from that of any non-language-impaired child at some point in development. In this text the above terms will not be used to differentiate qualitative differences from quantitative differences; differences will be specifically described.

It is useful to have a label that serves as an overall descriptive term and refers to both quantitative and qualitative differences in language development. The terms *disordered, deviant,* and *impaired* suggest difference or upset from normal function and have been used frequently in recent textbooks concerned with children who are having difficulty learning their native language (e.g., Aram & Nation, 1982; Bloom & Lahey, 1978; Carrow-Woolfolk & Lynch, 1982; P. Cole, 1982; Hubbell, 1981). They will be used here interchangeably as overall descriptive terms with no implications regarding etiology (in the way such terms as *dysarthria* or *acquired aphasia* would explain or otherwise account for other kinds of behavior) or qualitative differences in the language system of such children. That is, the use of the terms here will only mean that children's language behaviors, or lack of language behaviors, are different from those expected given their chronological age.

Patterns of Deviant Language Development

Language involves the interactions among content, form, and use schematized in the Venn diagram in Figure 2-1 and described in Chapter 1. *Form* refers to the

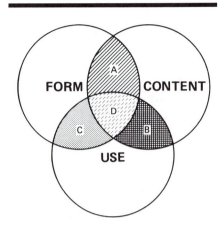

FIGURE 2-1   The Interaction of Content/Form/Use in Language

conventional system of signals—the dictionary of sounds and words, along with the rules for combining the dictionary items so as to form phrases and sentences. *Content* refers to the ideas about objects and events in the world that are coded by language. *Use* refers to the contexts in which language can be used and functions for which it is used. Normal language development has been described as the successful development within and interaction among the three, as represented in Area D (see Chapter 1 and Bloom & Lahey, 1978). *Disordered, or deviant, language development can be described as any disruption in the learning or use of language content, form, or use or in the interaction among these components.*

The disruption could be in the learning or use of the conventional system of arbitrary signals—the form of language; the disruption could be in learning or using these forms as a code for representing ideas about the world—the content of language; the disruption could be in using the code for the purpose of communication—the use of language.

The key words that were elaborated for defining language in Chapter 1 also represent the key elements in defining a language disorder: *ideas, code, conventional system,* and *communication.* Children with a language disorder may have a problem in formulating ideas or conceptualizing information about the world; they may learn a code that does not match the conventional system used in the linguistic community; they may have learned something about the world and something about the conventional code, but are unable to use the code in certain contexts or for certain purposes; or they may develop ideas, the conventional code, and the use of the code, but do so later than their peers, or with dysfunction in the interactions among the components.

Difference from normal development can be described according to the way in which these components interact with one another. It is possible to focus on disruption within individual components and among components, but it should be kept in mind that these disruptions are not themselves diagnostic categories; they are simply broad characterizations that are helpful in emphasizing the way language functions as a system and the ways in which that system can be disrupted. As such, they serve to remind us that language learning by any child involves more than learning form—words and sentences—and that children with language disorders are not homogeneous even in terms of their language. These descriptions are not specific enough to lead directly to intervention, because they do not specify the particular kinds of behaviors within each of the components and the interactions among components that need to be learned. It is neither necessary nor sufficient to use these categories in clinical assessment. Do not think that children should be categorized in this way. Rather, as you read, think about the complexity of language learning and the variety of ways that language learning can go astray; in particular, think about the heterogeneity within the group of children classified as language-disordered.

Developmental Delay

In the description of a language disorder, Area D in Figure 2-1 can represent language development that is normal in all ways except that it begins later than expected or proceeds more slowly than expected. That is, the child uses the same forms to talk of the same ideas in the same contexts and for the same purposes as the child with normal development. The only difference would be the age at which language begins and the rate at which it develops. Although such problems are included under the broad descriptive label of *language disorder,* a more specific descriptive label, such as *language delay* or *maturational lag,* is often used.

Other patterns that can be described as a language disorder differ in the extent to which a component may be disrupted, or in the extent to which there is disruption in the interaction among the components. In the following discussion, some of these possible disruptions will be explored and schematized to show the result of separation of one or another of the components or of their weak interaction. While the other components or interactions may not be entirely intact and well functioning, they represent more intact skills than are available in the separated or weakest component.

Disruptions of Content

Content, as discussed in Chapter 1, refers to the expression of an individual's knowledge of objects, relations between and among objects, and relations between and among events. In some instances, children have been reported to have fairly well developed form/use interactions in contrast to poorly developed content, as illustrated by Figure 2-2.

For example, some young blind children exhibit development of form/use interactions that far exceeds their development of content. Without visual input, certain sensorimotor concepts develop more slowly than the ability to develop social interactions and concepts of form. This slower development may interfere with the development of ideas of the world that language codes (i.e., the content of language). Such blind children are often echolalic and speak in grammatically well-formed sentences that appear in advance of their ideas. Children with visual impairments may well use form as a means of learning about the content of language. (See the discussion of the "original word game" in R. Brown, 1956).

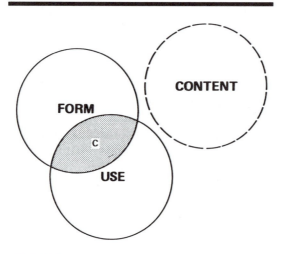

FIGURE 2-2   Disruption of Content

While most children with low cognitive skills exhibit a disruption in all aspects of language, in rare instances children with very low cognitive ability have been reported to have fairly well developed form/use interactions in contrast to poorly developed *content* (Cromer, 1986; Curtiss, 1981). These children produce very complex syntactic and morphological structures, are fluent and articulate, and often produce contingent responses during a conversation. The problem is that their utterances often are inappropriate, or do not make any sense (see Box 2-1). Such behavior has been used as evidence of a dissociation between language and cognition; it suggests, however, a close association between language *content* and cognition.

BOX 2-1   An Example of a Disruption in Content From a Mentally Retarded Girl

Marta, 1 16-year-old mentally retarded girl with an IQ of 44, demonstrates weak content but well-developed form and use (e.g., contingent responses).

Q. How many nights did you stay there?

M. Oh, about four out of one.

Q. His cousin flied in?

M. It's flying in between ours . . . / So now it's between mine/ He's my third prinicipal/ He will by my second principal/

Q. When you mean your time's up, you mean it's your time to get a haircut?

M. No, my mother took me in when the last time I've ever been in when, we came home/

From Curtiss, 1981, p. 25.

**BOX 2-2 An Example of a Disruption in Content
From a 6-Year-Old Hydrocephalic Child**

(Shown a button and asked to tell about it)

this is a button/ it has two holes in it/ it's like a lady has/ it has a shape/ it is round/ this is a button/ you put it on your blouse or an apron. in case an apron has a button/ that's big like this/ you can roll it and throw it but you never smash a window/ because if you have a button or a shape that goes on the wall or if you take it and hang it on the dress that would be very nice/ would you do that for me?/ if you have a dress or a coat you can hang it on or you can keep it out to take it to the store/

Note: From E. Schwartz, 1974, pp. 466–477.

The language behaviors of many hydrocephalic children may also be represented by Figure 2-2. These children have been characterized as hyperverbal, with "cocktail party speech" (E. Schwartz, 1974; Swisher & Pinsker, 1971). Cocktail party speech is an example of well-developed form (with well-developed articulation, intonation, and stress patterns) that is used for social interactions but has weak conceptual underpinnings. According to Schwartz, the language of the hydrocephalic child follows normal developmental milestones in terms of form but is superficial and irrelevant in content. It often appears that the children do not know the meaning of what they say. (For an example, see Box 2-2.) Unlike the

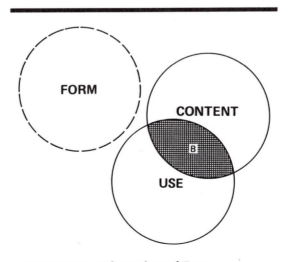

FIGURE 2-3 Disruption of Form

children to be discussed later (Figure 2-4), such children do use form as a means of social interaction and to refer to present contexts; unlike the children to be discussed next (Figure 2-3), such children know about form and the creation of complex sentences. Hydrocephalic children reportedly give many commands, ask many questions, and are extremely sociable. The language used seems to serve interpersonal functions; in fact, some have been described as verbally aggressive. This is not to say that use is entirely appropriate, but that language use and form appear more intact that language content.

Thus, we occasionally see children for whom content is the weakest interaction, and although these children may have some forms and may use them to communicate, they, too, may be described as having a language disorder if the content of their utterances is different from that expected on the basis of their knowledge of form and use, and that expected for their chronological age. Parents, educators, and clinicians are interested in studying and in facilitating the language development of such children.

Disruptions of Form

Form refers to the conventional linguistic system used to code the content of language. It includes the sounds and rules for combining sounds in a spoken language (or the hand configurations, movements and place, as well as the rules for combining in sign language), the description of different types of lexical items that can appear in a language (e.g., nouns and verbs), the rules for combining lexical items into simple and complex sentences, as well as the inflections that can be added to words. In Figure 2-3, the partial overlay of content and use, Area B, with

---

BOX 2-3   Dialogue With Frank, 6 Years Old. An Example of a Disruption Having To Do With Language Form

(Frank walks into the clinician's office)	hi/ doing
I'm typing	help
No, thank you, I'm all through/ I have to teach now	
	teach
yes	
	where
Over in that white building	oh
(Points to pencil sharpener)	that
You know/ what's it for?	
	pencil/ sharp
Right, it's a pencil sharpener.	
(Walks out door)	bye

Frank communicates well but generally with only one- and two-word utterances.

the separation of form, represents children whose ideas about the world of objects and events and whose abilities to communicate these ideas are more intact than their knowledge of the linguistic system for representing and communicating these ideas.

Such children may use gestures or primitive forms for communicating ideas, but they have difficulty learning the conventional system of arbitrary signals for coding and communicating. Boxes 2-3 and 2-4 present dialogues that illustrate a primary weakness in knowledge of linguistic form for coding ideas of the world, but well-developed ideas of the world that are communicated in many contexts for many functions.

Word-finding difficulty that is occasionally observed in children and often reported in adult aphasia is another disruption in the interaction between form and *content*. Such children circumlocute, or talk around the idea they are trying to communicate, having difficulty in recalling the form that represents the content that they wish to express.

Few would quarrel with labeling children such as Frank and Cindy (illustrated in Boxes 2-3 and 2-4) as having a language disorder. Their problem is with the linguistic dimension of language; both the conceptual and interactional dimensions are more intact.

BOX 2-4   Dialogue With Cindy, 7 Years Old. Examples of a Disruption Having To Do With Language Form

Cindy reported to her clinician an incident that happened at home the previous day.

(Cindy points to the tape recorder)	uh/ uh
(Points over shoulder)	home
	Buh (her name for her brother)
(Cindy slides arm over table and down toward floor; points to tape recorder and then to floor; frowns; wags finger)	Mama/ Mama

Cindy communicated an event that had happened in the past by using gestures and a limited number of single words. On another occasion, Cindy met her clinician in the hall.

	hi
(Cindy points to self; then points down hall)	milk

In this latter example, Cindy communicated about an event in the immediate future; she was on her way to obtain milk for lunch. In both examples, it is evident that Cindy was communicating ideas, but only through gestures and limited linguistic form. Cindy is a child who knows about many objects and events in the world, and readily attempts to communicate her ideas, but she has difficulty learning the necessary words and combinations of words to represent what she knows more fully.

Disruptions of Use

Language use refers to the use of language for different goals or functions, the use of information from the context to determine what we say in order to reach goals, and the use of language in the initiation, termination, and maintenance of interactions with people. Some children give evidence of *content/form* interactions that are more intact than use, as schematized by Figure 2-4. With these children, learning the system to code ideas appears to be less of a problem than using the system for communication. The overlay of form *and* content (A in Figure 2-4) represents knowledge of the conventional system as a code for meanings. This interaction is more intact than the interactions of use—either use in various contexts or use for various functions. In some cases, it is just that the children are less responsive to the conversational bids of others or are less assertive in initiating conversation (Fey, 1986). Some rarely verbalize even if questioned or prodded. When they do speak, their productions indicate a greater knowledge of the code than their general use would suggest. A few have a narrower range of functions, or less frequent use of certain functions, than other children with similar mean length of utterance (see, for examples, Donahue, Pearl, & Bryan, 1980; Geller & Wollner, 1976; Schuler, 1980).

In other cases, the disruption of use is quite apparent, as when children use language for primarily intrapersonal functions rather than interpersonal functions. Examples are presented in Boxes 2-5 and 2-6;; be aware that these behaviors must be considered in terms of the frequency with which they appear in the children's daily behavior. Although similar isolated examples can occur with all children (indeed with all of us), the repeated occurrence of such behaviors causes these

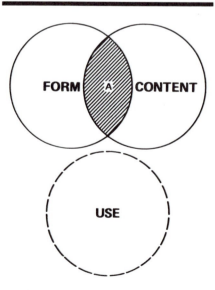

FIGURE 2-4   Disruption in the Use of Language

children to stand out from their peers. Children like George (Box 2-5) use language more frequently for intrapersonal than interpersonal functions; they talk about something that is out of context and either ramble repetitively or tangentially associate ideas without regard for the listener. Again, other components may also be weak, but use appears to be most disrupted. (See also Blank, Gessner, & Esposito, 1979, for a case study of such a child.)

Distorted Interactions of Content, Form, and Use

Certain children use conventional forms to communicate ideas, but the forms are inappropriate both to the context and to the meaning they apparently intend to convey. Interactions among the components are distorted. Such children may produce complex sentences with sophisticated grammatical markings, but produce few utterances that are appropriate (except in a very gross way) to the situation.

BOX 2-5 Dialogue With George, 10 Years Old. An Example of a Disruption in the Use of Language

(George and clinician enter clinic room and look out at falling snow)

Look at that snow. It's all on the grass

> you're not going outside

No, I'm not going outside/ are you going outside?

> no

(George no longer directs gaze toward therapist)

> that's okay/ yeah/ I can stay inside with Joe/ yeah/ okay I can stay inside with Joe/ okay/ I do some work with Joe/ Joe big Joe gonna stay inside/ Jane gonna go outside/ he gone yeah/ I can stay inside with Joe/ okay/ I'll do some work with Joe cut-color-create[a] inside/ okay/ Jane's gonna go out

Who are you talking to? (Pause) George?

> to (---) self

> you can stay inside with Joe/ yeah/ Jane's got boots/ gonna stay inside with Joe

Are you talking to me?

> okay I can stay inside with Joe/ okay

Note: I am indebted to R. Connelly for providing this example.

[a] Cut-color-create is the name of one of the classroom activities. Joe is a student aide. Jane is the teacher.

BOX 2-6 Dialogue With Mark, 10 Years Old. An Example of a Disruption in the Use of Language

(Mark and his teacher are talking)

Mom used to take me to McDonald's February 1974/ she used to put me up in the --- at 1:30/ and I went to the doctor's office at 2:45

What kind of things do you eat when you go to McDonald's?

a hamburger/ a Big Mac/ quarter pounder/ soft drinks/ and french fries/ I never go to McDonald's for breakfast you know

Why not?

Why well you know/ I used to sleep in New York/ in the Catskill Mountains/ I used to go to a motel/ I don't know where I ate breakfast/ you know RD's roast beef sandwich/ that restaurant was in Pennsylvania but it's in New Jersey/ it's now in New York on the way to New York City/ Manhattan.

Note: I am indebted to L. Weber for providing this example.

Although use is limited, the utterances can be a means of getting attention, making requests, or responding to another's utterance. Thus, they are used for communication. In an unconventional way, these children may often be communicating an idea, suggesting some interaction of content with use. Note, for example, in Box 2-7 that Thomas does want some ice cream and uses language as a means of expressing that desire. He has communicated an idea using conventional forms of language. However, the interactions among the components are distorted—these are not the forms used to request ice cream in that context. Thomas, like many of these children, seemed to have learned complete utterances in response to certain situations or ideas without knowing the semantic-syntactic relations that are represented within the sentences uttered.

Messages are well formed and are used for specific purposes in the situation. While some element of content relates the message to the situation in which it occurs, a contradiction exists between the content of the message and its use and between the content of the message and its form. Thus, unlike the children described by Figure 2-4, the children characterized by Figure 2-5 use forms for interpersonal interaction. Such children also produce sophisticated examples of the conventional signal system, and may have complex ideas of the world although

---

BOX 2-7 Examples of Distorted Interactions
of Content, Form, and Use

From M. Cunningham 1968, p. 231.

A child, named Thomas, using words spoken at some prior time by an adult, requests ice cream by saying:

you want some ice cream, Thomas?/
yes, you may.

Another boy, repeating what had been said by a housemother when dinner was demanded at the wrong time, requests dinner by saying:

daresay she'd throw me
out if I gave it to you now.

In each of these examples, forms were used for the purpose of obtaining something. Each child had an idea he attempted to communicate, and the forms used were grammatically correct. However, there was a mismatch between the content of the form that was used, the *content* of the idea being expressed, and the function of the utterance. These children had apparently remembered large segments of form (i.e., one or two complete sentences) associated with an idea or situation, and had learned that such forms could be used to interact with the environment. Further examples support the idea that form and content are globally associated with some function.

From Kanner (1973, p. 165)

(A child, Fred, given a gift)　　　　**you say thank you**

From Rutter (1966, p. 60)

(When wanting someone to go away)　　**see you in a fortnight**

(When meaning no)　　　　　　　　**don't you want it**

From M. Cunningham (1968, p. 237)

(Hitting the interviewer)　　　　　**be a good boy**

(Eating plasticine chips)　　　　　**you mustn't eat the chips**

All these utterances appear to have been associated with a similar situation in some past experience.

---

they do not code these ideas appropriately. (Note that where the circles overlap, the lines are dotted, to suggest that probably all components are somewhat disrupted.)

Separation of Content, Form, and Use

The linguistic behavior of other children suggests a fragmentation of content, form, and use such that none of the components appears to interact with another. For example, these children may recite radio and television commercials or news and sports broadcasts. Such recitations occur without apparent connection to external stimuli in the situation and with no obvious function other than perhaps to establish or maintain contact with others. In these situations, content, form, and

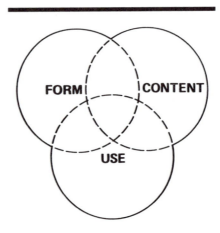

**FIGURE 2-5   *Distorted
Interactions of Content/Form/
Use***

use appear separated from one another, as represented in Figure 2-6. The utterances in Box 2-8 provide an example; the utterances seem unrelated to the watch that the child is gazing at and were not provoked by prior linguistic context. It may be that in such instances of nonstereotypic utterances, content and form are, in fact, interacting. The content, however, is so unrelated to the external environment that any interactions among content, form, and use are not apparent to the listener.

Some apparently irrelevant utterances can be traced to an earlier experience and are, in an idiosyncratic way, associated with the present context (Kanner, 1946). In one example Kanner describes Paul, who, while standing in a clinic room, says, "Don't throw the dog off the balcony," when there is no dog or balcony in view. The utterance had been spoken to him three years before by his mother, who was tired of retrieving a toy dog that Paul had repeatedly thrown from a hotel balcony. According to Kanner, Paul uttered the expression whenever he was tempted to throw anything. Such associations may be true for other utterances that are not stereotypic but appear to have no interaction among the three dimensions of content, form, and use. Again, it is the prevalence of such behaviors that mark them as different from the language behaviors of similar age peers.

Comprehension Versus Production Deficits

Since childhood language disorders were first described, there has been mention of differences between the comprehension and the production skills of various children. These early descriptions have been supported by recent studies (e.g., Aram & Nation, 1975; Silva, 1980; R. Stark & Tallal, 1981; B. Wilson & Risucci, 1986; Wolfus, Moscovitch, & Kinsbourne, 1980) that have described subgroups of language-disordered children who differ in terms of their relative performance on

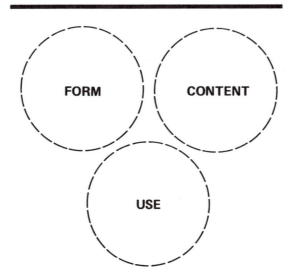

FIGURE 2-6   Separation of Content, Form and Use

production and comprehension tests. Some children scored better on comprehension than production, other children scored better on production than comprehension, and others scored the same on both measures of language (see also Chapter 3). If a discrepancy occurs, the more prevalent pattern is one where comprehension scores are higher than production scores (e.g., R. Stark & Tallal, 1981).

It has been suggested that comprehension and production of language represent mutually dependent but different underlying processes in the acquisition of language (Bloom & Lahey, 1978). If comprehension and production are mutually dependent, how can considerable differences be found between them?

A number of explanations are possible. First, most studies have compared comprehension and production on standardized tests (e.g., R. Stark & Tallal, 1981). As will be discussed in Chapter 7, it is difficult to use norm-referenced test scores to make comparisons between different tests. In many cases the tests are normed on different populations. Comparisons between tests, as well as interpretation of

---

BOX 2-8   An Example of Separation of the Components of Content, Form, and Use

(Looking at a watch)   there's the doors/ make the doors/
                                                          there's the east

From M. Cunningham, 1968, p. 237.

individual tests, should take into account the standard error of measurement (see Chapter 7, McCauley & Swisher, 1984a, or any textbook on measurement). It is quite possible that the differences reportedly found between comprehension and production scores do not represent "real" differences when measurement error is taken into account.

Furthermore, standardized tests do not usually compare comprehension and production on similar structures; they rarely give multiple examples of similar structures. In a number of research studies, differences have been reported in individual children's comprehension and comprehension of particular structures (see Bloom, 1974, and Bloom & Lahey, 1978, for a review). These differences occur both at the lexical level and at the level of grammatical structure (Bates, Bretherton, & Snyder, in press).

An alternative possibility is that the process of production involves a somewhat different knowledge base than the process of comprehension. The variations we see in language-disordered children may reflect variations in the "different" information required for each. For example, to produce a word one needs a well-developed phonetic representation of that word stored in memory. But when comprehending a word spoken by another, a less complete phonetic representation may be adequate as long as that representation differentiates the word from others within the child's vocabulary (see R. Brown & McNeill, 1966). Incomplete phonetic representations may thus manifest themselves in production problems but not in comprehension problems.

Rather than differences in the knowledge base, it may be that some language-disordered children differ in their ability to access language knowledge. For example, subtle motor problems that may not be detectable in a normal oral-peripheral examination could possibly interfere with production but not with comprehension. Further study is needed to clarify these issues, but in the meantime discrepancies in comprehension and production skills are at least apparent differences among children with a language disorder.

Summary

The term *language disorders* is used in this chapter to describe language behaviors that are different from those expected considering a child's chronological age. The various patterns presented here emphasize that language disorders encompass many different kinds of disruption in the integration of content, form, and use. Thus, the term not only describes children who have difficulty learning the form of language (a disruption of form), but also describes children who can talk easily and readily but who say nothing (a disruption of content), or who talk alot but rarely direct their speech to others (a disruption of use), as well as children who use forms to communicate ideas but not in the conventional manner (a distortion of the interactions among content, form, and use) or who utter forms with no apparent meaning or purpose (a separation of content, form, and use). In addition to the behaviors that are described here, there are other behaviors that cannot be so neatly schematized, but that stand out as different from expected behaviors.

This definition of language disorders has resulted in an emphasis on the need to describe what children do, and what they have difficulty in doing, in order to understand possible disruptions in the development of the system and to eventually understand etiological factors and prognosis. It leads to an emphasis on communication and language skills, rather than on etiological considerations, in planning the goals of an effective program for intervention and education. Thus, it differs in emphasis from (but is not incompatible with) other orientations that try to group children according to pathology or etiology or that focus on cognitive abilities and the processes that may be interfering with language learning.

Other orientations as well as information on prevalence and prognosis are presented in the following chapter. The communication-language orientation used in this chapter will be used later in the book to suggest goals of intervention, to assess children (including identifying children with a language disorder, refining descriptions of their language development, and placing these descriptions within a framework that specifies the sequence of goals for intervention), and to facilitate communication and language skills.

3

Language Disorders: Prevalence, Prognosis, and Orientations

Having decided that the term *language disorder* will be used to refer to a heterogeneous group of children whose language behaviors are not like (nor superior to) the language behaviors of similar age peers, you might then ask about the number of children who have such problems with language learning and about what eventually happens to them. Unfortunately, information about numbers (i.e., the prevalence of the problem) and information about outcome (i.e., the prognosis for these children) are limited and quickly outdated as our means of describing children and of facilitating language learning change. But given this caveat we can look at the available data. Later in the chapter we will consider what is perhaps the most intriguing question of all: Why do some children have trouble learning language? But first let's look at information on the prevalence of language disorders in children.

Prevalence

One source of information on prevalence comes from the number of children receiving special services in the schools. According to a 1983 U.S. Department of

Education report (see Karr & Punch, 1984), slightly under 10% of the 3- to 21-year-old population has been served under Public Law 94-142 (the Education of All Handicapped Children Act) as handicapped.[1] This group includes children whose primary handicapping condition was diagnosed as speech impairment, hearing loss, deafness, learning disability, mental retardation, visual impairment, emotional disturbance, orthopedic impairment, deaf-blind, multiple handicap, and other health impairment. Since most of these categories include children who have a language disorder, it is impossible to sort out the prevalence of language disorders from this statistic. The data do suggest, however, that the number of language-disordered children should be under 10% (even considering that some children may not be receiving special services under Public Law 94-142).

In actuality, estimates of the prevalence of language disorders in children have run even higher than 10%; they range from less than 1% to over 12% (see Table 3-1). This wide range reflects a number of factors that must be considered when interpreting prevalence data—for example, the ages sampled, the way in which the sample of children was obtained, and the way in which a language disorder was determined. Some of the results reported in Table 3-1 were based on the number of children referred to speech-language pathologists, while others used random sampling; some included only 3-year-old children, while others included only 5- or 7-year-olds. Finally, there are marked differences in the evidence used to determine which children would be considered language-disordered—differences in the type of information (e.g., type of test, or aspect of language measured) and differences in the degree of difference that was considered evidence of a disorder. Note, for example, that in the study by Beitchmann, Nair, Clegg, and Patel (1986), the percentage of 5-year-old children identified as language-impaired using a cutoff score of 1 standard deviation below the mean was 8.04, while only 1.70% were identified using a cutoff score that was 2 standard deviations below the mean. (See Chapter 6 for further discussion of these and other criteria for identification of children with a language disorder.)

Two of the more recent studies involving large numbers of 3-year-old children are presented below as the best estimates currently available for this age range. There were some differences between the studies, and so there are some differences in the resulting prevalence figures.

The prevalence of language disorders in a random sample of over 700 3-year-old children from an outer-London borough in England was determined by Stevenson and Richman (1976). Using the language age derived from the expressive section of the *Reynell Developmental Language Scales* (1969), the researchers found that 3% of the children scored 6 months below age level and 2% of the children scored one year below age level. These low language scores rarely existed without some other concurrent problem. For example, half of the children with low scores on this language scale were also identified, on the basis of a Behavior Screening Questionnaire, as being at risk for behavior problems (Richman & Graham, 1971). Furthermore, half of the children (but not necessarily the same half) with low language scores were also retarded in their performance of nonlanguage tasks on the *Griffiths Mental Development Scale* (1970). The prevalence of children who had language ages that were 1 year or more below their chronological age and who also had essentially normal IQ scores (i.e., mental ages that were no

---

[1] According to a recent article in *Asha* (July, 1987, p. 9), this figure rose to 11.9% in 1984–1985 and was 10.97% in 1985–1986.

TABLE 3-1 Summary of Studies Reporting Prevalence of Language Disorders

Source	Definition of a Language Disorder	Population Sampled	Sample Size	Age (Years: months)	Prevalence (%)
Morley (1965)	Limited or poor use of language	Unknown	114	3:9	0.80
	Immature sentences	Unknown	114	6:0	5.30
Rutter, Graham and Yule (1970)	Specific language disorder	Referrals to speech pathologists	?	5–14	0.08
Sheridan (1973)	Marked speech defect with normal hearing	National child development study	15,496	7:0	1.38
Randall et al. (1974)	−2 SD in both comprehension and production[a]	Normal population	160	3:0	0.62
	−2 SD comprehension				0.62
	−2 SD production				1.25
Stevenson and Richman (1976)	Production LA = 30 mo	Random sample	705	3:0	3.10
	Production LA = 26 mo				2.30
Silva (1980)	−2 SD production only	All children born in 1 year at a hospital in New Zealand	1,037	3:0	2.50
	−2 SD comprehension only				3.00
	−2 SD both production and comprehension				3.00
	Total for 3 year-olds				8.50
Silva (1980)	−2 SD production		937	5:0	2.70
	−2 SD comprehension				2.50
Beitchman et al. (1986)	−1 SD on language test only[b]	All kindergarten children in a region of Canada	1,655	5:0	8.04
	−1 SD on language and speech tests				4.56
	−2 SD on language test only				1.70
	−2 SD on language and speech tests				1.80

Note: (Adapted from Beitchman et al. (1986), and Stevenson and Richman (1976).

[a] −2 SD = Scores that are equal to or greater than 2 standard deviations below the mean for the child's age.

[b] −1 SD = Scores that are equal to or greater than 1 standard deviation below the mean for a child's age, but less than −2 standard deviations.

LA = language age

more than 6 months below their chronological age) was only 0.06%. All the prevalence figures for language disorders were considered conservative by the authors since they excluded children who were deaf and those identified as having Down's syndrome.

In fact, the prevalence reported by Stevenson and Richman was low in comparison with that found in a sample of 1037 3-year-old children from New Zealand (Silva, 1980). The New Zealand sample represented all surviving infants born in one maternity hospital in a 1-year period; none of the children were excluded. In contrast to the previous study, *both* the receptive and expressive scales of the Reynell were used as measures of language. Over 8% of the children scored 2 standard deviations or more below the mean for their age on one or both of the scales (note here that deviation scores are reported rather than language ages— see Chapter 7). There were three groups of children with low language scores— those with only comprehension deficits (3%), those with only production deficits (2.5%), and those with both comprehension and production deficits (another 3%).

A large percentage of the children who had low scores on both comprehension and production measures also had low scores on an IQ test (*Stanford Binet Intelligence Scale*, Terman & Merrill, 1960); this was not so for the children who had low scores on only comprehension *or* production. While these data suggest that few children with low language scores on both comprehension and production measures have normal intelligence, the data need to be interpreted with caution. The intelligence test used has many language-related items (e.g., vocabulary) and probably overestimated the relation between language disorder and intelligence in this population.

Both studies provide evidence that at least some children have language deficits without accompanying intellectual deficits. Both studies also reported that, at the age of 3, language disorders are more prevalent among boys than girls by a ratio of approximately 2 to 1.

The influence of criterion in estimating prevalence is evident in the results of Beitchman et al. (1986). They reported prevalence of language disorders for 5-year-old kindergarten children in the Ottowa-Carleton region of Canada, using two different criteria. On a battery of language tests, over 12% of the children received scores that fell between 1 and 2 standard deviations below the mean, while only 3.5% of the children received scores that were equal to or greater than 2 standard deviations below the mean. The choice of which criterion will define a language disorder can, therefore, make a marked difference in prevalence figures.

Prognosis

Most of the information we have on prognosis is based on retrospective data—that is, children once labeled as having a language disorder are reassessed at some later point in time. In general, the follow-up studies indicate that 40 to 60% of the children described as having a language disorder in the preschool years have continued difficulty during the school years (e.g., Aram & Nation, 1980; Hall & Tomblin, 1978; King, Jones, & Lasky, 1982). Most of the children had difficulty with school learning; some continued to have difficulty with verbal communication. Of course, the same problem mentioned earlier is present here—how was a language disorder determined? Often the description is taken from old clinic records when standardized tests of language (other than vocabulary comprehension) were not yet available (e.g., Hall & Tomblin, 1978). There is further difficulty with the interpretation of these data. Since control groups were not used, we do not know how many children with similar nonlanguage characteristics (e.g., IQ or socioeconomic status) have difficulty in school. However, even when IQ was within normal limits, the percentage of continued difficulty remained the same (e.g., Hall & Tomblin, 1978). An additional problem with some of the above studies was the use of reported information for follow-up rather than direct observation and testing. Despite these problems, there is little doubt that children with a language disorder in the preschool years are at a high risk for academic failure in the school years (see also National Joint Committee on Learning Disabilities, 1987).

One recent retrospective study included direct observation and test scores for both initial and follow-up data (Aram, Ekelman, & Nation, 1984). Twenty children diagnosed as having language problems without concomitant hearing, neurological, or craniofacial abnormalities were identified during their preschool years (age range 3:5 to 6:11) and were reassessed 10 years later. Despite the fact that 16 of these 20 had, as adolescents, IQ scores that were above 80 on either performance or verbal subtests, 14 of the 20 children had continued problems with language. These 14 children scored approximately 2 standard deviations below the mean on the *Test of Adolescent Language* (Hammill, Brown, Larsen, & Wiederholt, 1980). Only five of the children were progressing in regular classes without supportive services; the remainder were in special classes, were receiving tutoring, or had repeated a grade. For over half of the children, achievement test scores on the *Wide Range Achievement Test* (Jastak & Jastak, 1978) were at or below the 25th percentile. Thus, 70 to 75% of the children diagnosed as having a language disorder in the preschool years were still having academic and/or language difficulties 10 years later. This proportion is even higher than that of the studies noted above that used reported information. This higher proportion is, however, more in line with the report by Cooper and Griffiths (1978). They reported on a follow-up of 49 "severely-language-impaired" children who had received special schooling, for about 2 years, when they were 5 to 9 years of age. While a third of them were able to function in regular classrooms, and in many cases had apparently normal spoken language, they all had difficulty with reading and writing.

To see whether any of the assessment measures given during the preschool years were predictive of status 10 years later, Aram et al. (1984) compared scores on preschool measures (which included both comprehension and production measures of vocabulary and syntax as well as a measure of nonverbal intelligence) with scores on the measures given in adolescence. The best predictor of language scores, of IQ scores, of class placement, and of reading achievement in adolescence was the initial measure of nonverbal intelligence—the Arthur Adaptation of the *Leiter International Performance Scale* (Arthur, 1952). Another weaker predictor of language scores in adolescence was the preschool score on the expressive section of the *Northwestern Syntax Screening Test* (Lee, 1969) (suggesting that expressive measures of syntax may predict later language skills better than comprehension measures or measures of vocabulary).

In an attempt to define some of the factors that might predict the future course of language development and school achievement, Silva (1980, in the study discussed above in the section on Prevalence) followed 931 children for a period of 2 years. He found that those children with both comprehension and production deficits at age 3 had a higher prevalence of low IQ, poor motor coordination, and language problems at age 5 than the children who had only comprehension or only production problems at age 3. In fact, less risk was associated with "comprehension-only" problems (at age 3) than with "production-only" problems. Only a few (3.6%) of the children who had comprehension-only deficits at age 3 still had a comprehension deficit at age 5; none of them had deficits in production. A larger proportion (13%) of the children with production-only deficits at age 3 still had a production deficit at age 5, and a few (4.3%) now had comprehension deficits in addition to their production deficits. In contrast, 50% of the children who had *both* comprehension and production deficits at age 3 still had such deficits at age 5. Thus, this study also reports that poor scores on measures of language production are more predictive of later language problems than poor scores on measures of comprehension. Such findings suggest that screening at age 3 should focus on production measures and that comprehension measures may only be necessary if a child does poorly on production.

This study also points out the problems we have with our ability to answer questions about prognosis. Assessment at age 3 not only overestimated problems at age 5, but did not detect all children who were at risk for language deficits at age 5. Approximately 1% of the children identified as having a deficit in language at age 5 had not been so identified at age 3. This difference may be related to testing error (i.e., this 1% actually had poor language skills at age 3 but were not identified) or may reflect different language skills needed by the 5-year old that are not predicted by measures of language at 3.

We still have a great deal to learn about assessment procedures that will enable us to predict future language and academic learning. Studies like the ones by Silva and by Aram et al. are important beginnings. Most likely, finer descriptions of the children's language behaviors will be needed. As noted in Chapter 2, a language disorder can be reflected in many different patterns of language behaviors. Attempts at prognosis have so far relied only on global scores of comprehension and production; finer descriptions of these areas as well as of language use and other means of communication may be needed. In addition, other information about the child with deviant language development is important to the eventual understanding of the nature of language disorders and to the prediction of success in language learning. When nonlinguistic correlates of language disorders vary, describing differences among children may improve our ability to determine prognosis. In addition, the type of language intervention in which the child has participated needs to be considered as well as any factors that may be maintaining the disorder. Finally, different precipitating factors may lead to similar symptoms at one point in time but not necessarily at all points in time; precipitating factors most likely influence prognosis in ways we have yet to understand.

Orientations to Language Disorders

Descriptions of children with language disorders and hypotheses about explanations of these disorders have been in the literature since the 19th century (for a historical overview of the 19th century see J. E. McLean, 1983, and Weiner, 1984; for a review of more recent history see Aram & Nation, 1982). In the past few decades a number of different approaches have influenced the ways in which children with language disorders have been most typically characterized for research and clinical purposes. Each of these orientations has contributed important information, each has had its limitations, and each appears to serve a different function. These approaches can be grouped according to their focus: (1) a categorical orientation, (2) a specific-abilities orientation, and (3) a communication-language orientation.

A Categorical Orientation

A categorical orientation to language disorders in children concentrates on categorizing individuals on the basis of a number of behavioral manifestations (i.e., syndromes of behavior). The approach focuses on how certain groups of children are like each other in ways that differentiate them from other children. While the behaviors considered include language, the focus is primarily on nonlanguage behaviors such as social interactions, response to sound, and general intellectual behavior. The clinical categories formed are based on factors considered necessary for language learning, such as emotional stability, an intact central nervous system, sensory acuity, and intelligence. Deficits in any of these areas is often presumed to be the factor that precipitates the language disorder. The categories related to these deficits include emotional disturbance, neurological impairment, hearing impairment, and mental retardation.

This categorical orientation dominated the consideration of language disorders in children by speech-language pathologists, educators, and physicians in the 1950s and early 1960s. The orientation still dominates the medical view of language disorders; it is, in fact, derived from the "medical model," which attempts to move from symptoms to pathology, to etiology, to therapy. The categorical orientation continues to have an impact on research and intervention with the language-disordered child. In some localities the categorical label determines what services will be provided to a child and what funding is available for such services. While the behaviors focused on within the orientation and the search for subgroups of homogeneous children are important for understanding language impairment, the usefulness of the current categories for *clinical management* is questionable. This orientation and its usefulness are further discussed in Chapter 4 along with a review of the syndromes and information available on the language behaviors of children who fit these categories.

Specific-Abilities Orientation

In contrast to the categorical orientation, other approaches have categorized behaviors instead of individuals. Some of these approaches have attempted to identify and describe the abilities or processes that are necessary for the learning and use of language—such as memory, attention, discrimination, and association. The child with a language disorder has been described in terms of the relative strengths and weaknesses of certain processes or abilities. Intervention has been geared to remediating or strengthening the abilities or processes that are considered defective or weak. The assumption is that such strengthening will ultimately improve language skills. In this sense, weaknesses in specific abilities are considered as causally related to the language-learning difficulty. This orientation had considerable impact in the 1960s on the clinical description of children with language and learning problems; descriptions and definitions of language disorders focused on a profile of abilities. In the late 1970s and early 1980s some aspects of this orientation (such as auditory processing) have again impacted the field. The consideration of processes involved in language learning and use is certainly important for the understanding of language disorders and for the forming of subgroups for research purposes; its importance for *clinical management* is questionable. The orientation, referred to in this text as a *specific-abilities* orientation, and its usefulness are discussed further in Chapter 5 along with information about the processing skills of children with a language disorder.

A Communication-Language Orientation

Another approach that categorized particular behaviors has concentrated on the *communication* and *language* patterns of children with a language disorder—that is on aspects of content, form, and use and on nonlinguistic communicative behaviors. These categories describe the behaviors of individuals instead of grouping individuals. The description of language disorders within this approach has been based on descriptions of nonlinguistic communicative behaviors and on aspects of language knowledge and use; intervention has concentrated on facilitating language content/form/use interactions and/or on facilitating nonlinguistic communication. Since the behaviors to be changed are the focus of description and intervention, this orientation has a symptomatic, rather than an etiological, focus. It assumes that language will not be learned unless intervention includes measures to facilitate language learning; that is, intervention geared to presumed precipitating factors will not alone improve language knowledge and use. It also assumes that careful description of the child's communication behavior is necessary to the eventual understanding of etiology and that grouping of children for research should consider similarities and differences in communicative behaviors. This approach had a major impact on the field in the 1970s and changed its focus throughout the 1970s and 1980s. The early consideration was primarily one aspect of language form (syntax); next, the primary consideration was the content of language; and more recently, the major emphasis has been on language use and on nonlinguistic communicative behaviors. This communication-language orientation has been considerably influenced by the study of normal language development.

The approach by itself is not likely to lead to explanations of a language disorder, but it is probably a necessary accompaniment to any approach that does look for explanations. At our current state of knowledge about childhood language disorders, it appears that accurate descriptions of deviant language development are important for an eventual understanding of etiological factors. A communication-language orientation provides the framework for future chapters in this text —chapters that deal with identifying the language-disordered child, with describing deviant language development, and with facilitating language in the language-disordered child (see Chapters 6 to 16).

Can The Question "Why?" Be Answered?

When children do not develop facility with their native language, one is most likely to ask "why?" Indeed, "why?" is often the first question asked by both parents and clinicians. Most hypotheses about the etiology of developmental language disorders begin with the premise that something is wrong with the child— something that has interfered with language learning. Certainly this view is implicit in the specific-abilities orientation that searches for weak processing skills in the child. It is also implicit in much, but not all, of the literature based on the categorical orientation. Areas of deficit postulated include sensory channels (such as deafness and blindness), motor skills, cognitive skills (such as low general intellectual level, auditory processing problems, and difficulties with symbolic thinking or with pattern abstraction), and social relations (such as inability to establish relationships, withdrawal, and hostility). Such deficits often co-occur with a language disorder; also in non-language-disordered children measures of cognitive and social development correlate highly with measures of language development. Deficits in social or cognitive skills have been interpreted by some as the cause of the language-learning difficulty. Others point out, however, that occasionally there are dissociations between some aspects of language and cognition (see, for example, Chapter 2) and between some aspects of language and social relations. Such dissociations (which usually involve language form) suggest possible independence of at least morphological and syntactic learning from cognitive and social skills and support the notion that there may be specific language-learning mechanisms that can be impaired or remain intact independent of other cognitive and social skills (e.g., Curtiss, 1981; Gleitman, 1986). Nonetheless, most of the research and models that try to explain language-learning problems focus on cognitive and social behaviors.

Certainly developmental problems related to language, social, motor, or cognitive development could well influence development in another area, and thus be a factor that interferes with language learning. But each of these problems can also be related to another level of cause (e.g., what caused the social or the cognitive problems?). In line with the view that something is wrong with the child, subtle neurological deficits have often been postulated. Language and associated cognitive and social deficits are most often attributed to some level of neurological impairment—impairment that is often undetectable by standard neurological assessment procedures, but that is inferred from deviant behavior.

Even further back in the line of causal explanations one can look for the etiology of any presumed neurological deficit. Some earlier views were that these children had suffered brain damage some time around birth. However, research has not been able to support this view (Ludlow & Cooper, 1983). Other hypotheses have suggested a genetic basis either alone or coupled with neonatal or natal stress factors. While supportive data do exist for some groups of language-disordered children, the data are not compelling, and considerable research is needed (see Ludlow & Cooper, 1983, for further discussion). Part of the problem is defining particular subgroups (a problem mentioned earlier and again discussed in the next two chapters).

Other hypotheses about the etiology of developmental language impairment focus on the role of the environment as a causal explanation. There are a number of suggested sources of difficulty—the linguistic input, the reinforcement of the child's communicative efforts, and the affective relationship established with the care givers. This view taken to its extreme suggests that there is little different about this child at birth. Considerable evidence, however, suggests that the environment of the language-disordered child is not grossly different from that of the non-language-disordered child (see Chapters 4 and 14).

The two views—something wrong with the child and something wrong with the environment—are, of course, not incompatible. It is quite possible that certain genetic predispositions coupled with stress factors at critical times could affect how the environment influences learning. It is the complexity of these interactions in a developing organism that makes answering the "why" question so complex.

Thus, the question about the cause (or causes) of a language-learning problem in a particular child remains an intriguing and usually an unanswerable question. If we understood how the non-language-disordered child learns language and the relative role of, for example, cognitive, social, and environmental factors, we would have clearer hypotheses about why some children do not learn language easily. Clearly, the lack of an agreed-upon theory of language development hinders our search for an understanding of developmental language disorders. On the other hand, a better understanding of language disorders may aid in developing theories of normal language development. Language-disordered children vary in terms of their language, as noted in Chapter 1. They also differ in terms of other areas of development (e.g., social, cognitive, motor). Thus, careful study of these children may provide an opportunity for us to sort out the relative importance of these areas to language learning.

Summary

A number of problems have made it difficult to determine the prevalence of language disorders in children living in the United States. In addition to the dearth of this type of research in the states, there is a lack of agreement on the criteria used to define a language disorder (e.g., scores of approximately −1 standard deviation versus −2 standard deviations), a limited range of language skills tested by standardized measures of language, and, until recently, a limited variety of standardized instruments with adequate normative populations. Most recent epidemiological studies have been done in New Zealand and Canada. These studies suggest that 3 to 8.5% of 3-year-olds and approximately 5% of 5-year-old children score at least 2 standard deviations below the mean on the tests that were used. Certainly, more research is needed to determine both prevalence (the number of children with language disorders that currently exist in the United States) and incidence (the number of new cases that emerge in defined time spans).

Follow-up studies suggest that 40 to 75% of the preschool children diagnosed as having a language disorder continue to have learning or communication problems in the school years. Some evidence suggests that measures of nonverbal intelligence and productive syntax at age 3 correlate with later language and learning achievement. However, the data were on a limited number of children, and considerable variance was not accounted for. While more research has been devoted to determining prognostic indicators than has been devoted to determining prevalence or incidence, no definitive prognostic indicators have been identified. Progress has been hampered by the measurement instruments available. Further research is needed in this area as well. No doubt, we are going to need more complete descriptions of the children's language and nonlanguage behaviors if we are ever to determine prognosis on the basis of empirical data rather than clinical intuition. The population classified as language-disordered is heterogeneous in symptom as well as cause.

Hypotheses about the cause of childhood language disorders focus on problems within the child, on problems within the environment, or occasionally on interactions of the child with the environment. These hypotheses are influenced by the orientations used to characterize the child with a language disorder. Three orientations were described. A categorical orientation attempts to group children according to behaviors that they share with each other but that differentiate them from non-language-impaired children. A specific-abilities orientation focuses on describing and remediating cognitive abilities or the processes that may be interfering with language learning. A communication-language orientation emphasizes the need to describe the child's linguistic and nonlinguistic communicative behaviors in order to understand possible disruptions in the development of the system and to eventually understand etiological factors and prognosis. While there are differences in emphasis that influence descriptions and intervention, the orientations are not incompatible with each other, and each has a role in our eventual understanding of childhood language disorders. The categorizations used by these orientations are important to understand since they are frequently used in research and they are often used to determine funding and placement for educational programs. The next two chapters describe and evaluate these approaches.

Suggested Readings

Aram, D., & Nation, J. (1982). Historical heritage of child language disorders. In *Child language disorders* (Chap. 2). St. Louis: Mosby.

Ludlow, C. L., & Cooper, J. (Eds.) (1983). *Genetic aspects of speech and language disorders.* New York: Academic Press.

Weiner, P. (1984). The study of childhood language disorders in the nineteenth century. *Asha, 26,* 35–38.

4

A Categorical Orientation: Clinical Syndromes Associated With Childhood Language Disorders

Clinical categories of language-disordered children are based upon syndromes of behavior. A syndrome is simply a group of behaviors that differentiates a number of individuals from other individuals. For example, behaviors in social situations, or responses to problem solving or auditory stimuli, might differentiate some children from others. When similar clusters of behaviors—behaviors that are not expected given a child's age—are found in a number of children, these aggregate behaviors form a *syndrome*. The use of syndromes to label, and thus categorize, children for research or clinical purposes is referred to here as a *categorical orientation*.

The clinical categories that are commonly associated with language disorders in children include mental retardation, hearing impairment (including deafness), autism, and specific language impairment (called by many different names including *developmental aphasia*). Clinicians traditionally have been involved in determining the best categorical labels for children on the basis of certain behavioral manifestations; this task has been referred to as *differential diagnosis*. A categorical label emphasizes the similarities among children within a category and the differences between the children given a label and the children who are not so labeled. Within-category differences are not emphasized and are often lost in the search for syndrome of "best fit."

Although clinical categories associated with a language disorder have been considered by some as representing etiologies of a language disorder, this may not be so. The language disorder is simply one of the behavioral manifestations that composes the syndrome. There are other factors that precipitate or otherwise underlie the syndromes of behaviors labeled as *hearing impairment, mental retardation,* and so forth. While these other factors, rather than the retardation, hearing impairment, or emotional disturbance, may be the direct cause of a language disorder, it is the clinical categories that have dominated the thinking about etiology of childhood language disorders. In this chapter, a number of categories frequently associated with language disorders will be described, and the usefulness of these categories both for facilitating language learning and for eventually understanding language development and language disorders will be discussed.

The clinical categories are discussed below both in terms of the general behavioral syndromes that define them and in terms of the language behaviors of the children who fit the syndromes. The language behaviors that have been associated with a category will be presented, when possible, within the paradigm used throughout this textbook to describe language—content/form/use interactions.

Specific Language Impairment

Children who appear to develop normally in all respects except language are often referred to as having a specific language impairment. These children score within normal limits on standard measures of nonverbal intelligence, have normal hearing acuity, and demonstrate no evidence of severe emotional or behavioral problems that could explain their difficulty with language learning. The syndrome is rare. Estimates suggest that only 1 child in every 1000 to 2000 children may fit this description (American Psychiatric Association, 1980; Stevenson & Richman, 1976; also see Chapter 3). Despite the rarity, such children have baffled and intrigued professionals from many disciplines for over a century (see, for example, Gall, 1835; Vaisse, 1866). This intrigue has generated more research on specific language impairment than one would expect given the number of such children.

The syndrome has been described by the American Psychiatric Association (see Box 4-1) in a broad manner. A more detailed and operational description of the syndrome was derived for the purpose of research by R. Stark and Tallal (1981) and is summarized in Box 4-2. Of the 132 children referred to Stark and Tallal as having specific language impairment, only 39 were able to meet the criteria in Box 4-2, suggesting that the clinical use of the label is probably not based on such stringent criteria. More often the criteria are language productions that are below that expected for age-matched peers and that occur concomitant with the impression of normal development in other areas. Many of the children referred to Stark and Tallal did not achieve an IQ score at or above 85—again pointing up the correlation that was mentioned in the prior chapter between language disorders and low intelligence scores. In addition, many of the children did not exhibit a receptive language problem. However, the presence of *both* receptive and expressive language deficits is not generally considered necessary for inclusion in the syndrome (see, for example, the DSM III criteria in Box 4-1). In fact, traditionally it has been recognized that there were three subcategories—children with primarily expressive deficits, children with primarily receptive deficits, and children with deficits in both areas. Thus, in requiring some degree of receptive and expressive delay, the criteria of Stark and Tallal are different from the more traditional definition and that of the American Psychiatric Association.

Terminology

Terminology used to describe these children continues to vary. The early labels were those originally used to describe adults whose loss of language was due to cerebral injury (i.e., aphasia). For years the terms *childhood aphasia, congenital aphasia,* and *developmental aphasia* have been used to differentiate the childhood developmental syndrome from that of acquired aphasia in children and adults. The terminology used implies, as with the adult, that the language disorder is a result of dysfunction in the central nervous system and can be described as receptive (a sensory or auditory aphasia reflected in poor comprehension); expressive (a motor aphasia suggesting a child who understands but cannot talk); and mixed or global

---

BOX 4-1 DSM III Diagnostic Criteria for Specific Developmental Language Disorders [315.31]

1. Difficulty with language learning
   a. Expressive type—failure to develop expressive language despite intact comprehension
   b. Receptive type—failure to develop expressive and receptive language
2. Presence of age-appropriate concepts, such as understanding the use and function of common objects
3. Language-learning difficulty not related to mental retardation, hearing impairment, or a pervasive developmental disorder such as autism.

Adapted from American Psychiatric Association, 1980, pp. 96–97

---

aphasia, which involves both comprehension and expression (Barry, 1961). Since there is rarely direct evidence of central nervous system impairment, the terms *minimal brain damage* and *minimal brain dysfunction* were often applied (Birch, 1964; Strauss & Lehtinen, 1947). More recently, the use of terminology such as

---

BOX 4-2 Criteria for Selection of Children Who Are Specifically Language-Impaired

1. Hearing—Hearing must be at least 25 decibels at frequencies from 250 to 6,000 hertz.
2. Intelligence—IQ must be at least 85 on the Performance Scale of the WISC-R or WPPSI.
3. Neurological—There must be no "frank" neurological signs on exam and no history of head trauma or epilepsy.
4. Emotional—There should be no "severe" behavior or adjustment problems, as reported by parents and teachers.
5. Speech—Exam should show no "obvious" peripheral oral-motor abnormalities, and child must pass two-point discrimination on the tongue.
   Score on the *Templin-Darley Test of Articulation* must be within 6 months[a] of expressive language test scores.
6. Reading—If 7 years of age or older, reading test scores must be within 6 months of overall language age.[a]
7. Language—Overall language age,[a] based on a battery of standardized tests, should be at least 12 months below chronological age *and* mental age* on performance IQ test.
   Receptive language age should be[a] at least 6 months below mental age[a] on performance IQ.
   Expressive language age[a] must be at least 12 months below mental age* on performance IQ.

[a] See Chapter 7 for a critique of age-equivalent scores.
Adapted from Stark and Tallal, 1981

---

childhood aphasia and *minimal brain dysfunction* has given way to less etiologically oriented and more descriptive terms such as *specific-language-impaired* (SLI). This more behavioral designation, SLI, will be used throughout the rest of the text to refer to this syndrome.

The label *learning-disabled* is sometimes applied to this syndrome. Originally, children were considered learning-disabled only after they failed to learn academic subjects in the school setting. Thus, they were school-age and had attended at least the first grade. However, the similarity in the definition of a learning disability (see later in the chapter) and of a specific language impairment plus the growing awareness of the relationship between early language-learning problems and later academic problems (see report of the National Joint Committee on Learning Disabilities, 1987) has often resulted in confusion of terminology. Preschool children are now often referred to as learning-disabled when, in fact, the major presenting symptom is a language disorder. The National Joint Committee on Learning Disabilities (1987) considers a language disorder in the preschool years to be an early manifestation of a learning disability. Throughout this text, the term *learning disability* will be reserved for children who have failed to learn academic subjects normally taught in school (such as reading and writing) despite what appears to be normal intelligence, hearing acuity, and emotional development. However, it should be kept in mind that children must "learn" language— that a language disorder is, in fact, evidence of a problem in learning that will no doubt also be reflected when the child attempts to learn school subjects, particularly when they too involve language.

Associated Factors and Explanations

While the general description of the syndrome suggests that these children have developed normally in all areas except language, finer descriptions indicate a number of areas of deficits that do not show up on traditional tests of intelligence, hearing, or motor development. Such children also evidence perseveration, inconsistent responses, emotional lability, and auditory-perceptual and intellectual inefficiencies—functioning that is easily impaired by fatigue, noise, or other distraction (Eisenson, 1972; Myklebust, 1954; see Box 4-3).

A search for a better understanding of these deficits has concentrated primarily on cognitive abilities with a focus on two areas—representational thinking and auditory perception.

Piaget has suggested that language is but one means of symbolization. Manifestations of the symbolic function include not only language, but also symbolic or pretend play, drawing, and mental imagery. Considerable evidence has accrued suggesting a relation between the normal child's development of representational thinking and language (e.g., Bates, 1976; Bloom, 1973; Lifter & Bloom, 1986; Rocissano, 1979). It is possible that the language deficits may reflect a more general deficit in symbolization rather than a deficit that is only linguistic (Morehead & Ingram, 1973).

A number of studies have provided evidence to support such hypothesis. Compared with their age peers, children with SLI spend less time in symbolic, or pretend, play, and the organization of that play is not as complicated—that is, less decontextualized, fewer sequences, less other-directed, less symbolic substitution,

> ## BOX 4-3 Characteristics of Specific Language Impairment or Childhood Aphasia
>
> 1. Auditory responses—inconsistent and erratic.
> 2. Mental capacity—inconsistent with scatter; perceptual disturbances are evident.
> 3. Social maturity—retarded in communication, socialization, and motor areas.
> 4. Motor—slightly delayed in sitting and walking, with generalized incoordination.
> 5. Communicative behavior—little use of gesture; child does not project voice and may echo.
> 6. Emotional—emotional expression lacks intensity, but child is not bizarre nor oblivious to people.
> 7. Other behavior—disinhibited and hyperactive and does not use other sensory avenues in a compensatory way.
>
> Adapted from Myklebust, 1954, pp. 353–354.

etc. (e.g., J. Brown, Redmond, Bass, Liebergott, & Swope, 1975; Lovell, Hoyle, & Siddall, 1968; Luria & Yudovich, 1979; Rescorla, 1986; Rom & Bliss, 1983; Roth & Clark, 1987; Skarakis, 1982; Terrell, Schwartz, Prelock, & Messick, 1984). Furthermore, children with SLI have some difficulty with tasks requiring mental imagery (Inhelder, 1976; Johnston & Ramsted, 1977; Johnston & Weismer, 1983; Kamhi, 1981; Kamhi, Catts, Koenig, & Lewis, 1984; Savich, 1984) and with some of the Piagetian-based sensorimotor scales (Snyder, 1975). More recently, it has been suggested that deficits in sociocognitive knowledge can also be observed in some SLI children—that is, their social nonlinguistic interactions are less well developed than those of their peers (e.g., Constable & Lahey, 1984). However, there is considerable variability among the children in these studies when individual data are examined (see, for example, Skarakis, 1982). Sorting out this variability will no doubt lead us to a better understanding of possible etiological factors in SLI.

How can it be that any SLI child with normal intelligence test scores can have cognitive deficits involving representational thinking? One answer may be in the measures used to estimate intelligence. For example, the *Arthur Adaptation of the Leiter International Performance Scales* (Arthur, 1952) is a nonverbal intelligence test that is often given to the preschool language-impaired child. It contains many items that require perceptual skills (e.g., the child must match items according to their physical characteristics) rather than more conceptual skills (such as interpreting or transforming data) (Johnston, 1982a). Cognition appears to involve many skills. Measures of the child's cognitive level that are currently in use may be too narrow to detect certain types of cognitive deficiencies.

Similarly, it has been argued that traditional tests of hearing may not be sensitive to certain types of auditory problems that are not peripheral but central in nature—problems in auditory perception, integration, storage, and association. Children with SLI are described as being able to hear but not understand; as having a short auditory memory span; and as having difficulty with temporal sequencing, the repetition of auditory patterns, and rhythm (deHirsch & Jansky, 1977; Kracke, 1975; Masland & Case, 1968; J. Stark, Poppen, & May, 1967). Such children have been found to have difficulty in reporting the order of auditory stimuli and discriminating stimuli unless the duration between stimuli is extremely long (Lowe & Campbell, 1965; Rosenthal, 1972; Schnur, 1971; Tallal & Piercy, 1973a, 1973b, 1974, 1975), more difficulty in discriminating sounds presented in syllables than in isolation (McReynolds, 1966), and, in general, more difficulty in processing rapid successive or simultaneously presented information in a number of modalities (Tallal, Stark, & Mellits, 1985a).

This evidence has been interpreted in different ways. According to some (e.g., Benton, 1964; Eisenson & Ingram, 1972; Lubert, 1981; Tallal & Piercy, 1973a, 1978), auditory-perceptual problems are the bases of the language difficulty; according to others (e.g., Bloom & Lahey, 1978, and Chapter 5 of this text; Johnston, 1982b; Leonard, 1979, in press; Mahecha & Lahey, in preparation; Rees, 1973b, 1981), these problems may well reflect difficulties with language learning. (See Chapter 5 for further discussion of auditory-perceptual abilities in relation to specific language impairment and learning disabilities.) A third alternative is offered by Cromer (1978). He points out that both language and rhythm are hierarchically, not sequentially, organized and that SLI children may have a hierarchical structuring deficit; they are able to learn simple sequencing rules, but not complex syntactic transformations.

Finally, two studies have reported a higher prevalence of difficulties in fine and gross motor skills in language-impaired children (Affolter, Brubaker, & Bischofberger, 1974, as cited in Swisher, 1985; King, Jones, & Lasky, 1982), but it is not clear that these were all SLI children. SLI children are, however, frequently described as clumsy and awkward although they may well score within normal limits on tests of motor coordination (see, e.g., Lahey, Flax, & Schlisselberg, 1985). Moreover, oral-motor problems have been reported for over 20% of preschool children with SLI and considered suggestive for an additional 39% (Schery, 1985), and SLI children are slower and less accurate in repeating multisyllabic words and nonsense syllables than non-language-impaired (NLI) children (Kamhi & Catts, 1986; Tallal, Stark, and Mellits, 1985a). Further information is still needed on the possible role of subtle speech-motor problems on language learning in SLI children, particularly in those children with expressive but not receptive language-learning problems (Lahey & Edwards, in preparation; Lahey, Flax, & Schlisselberg, 1985). Unfortunately, most studies examining correlated factors have not differentiated among children according to different patterns of language (e.g., even level of comprehension in relation to production, or vocabulary versus syntactic and/or phonological levels).

Thus, we see the picture of a child who appears like other children of the same age on gross measures of development in all areas except language, but who, on closer examination, seems to have some deficits in certain areas, such as cognition. The explanation for the language-learning problem may be, then, that these deficits in cognition, motor, and/or perceptual development are responsible for the language-learning problems. However, nonlinguistic deficits reported tend to be subtle. In many studies the SLI child does less well than NLI children of the same age but does slightly better than NLI children with similar language skills. Consequently, it is not clear that such subtle deficits could, alone, be responsible for language-learning difficulties. It is possible that interactions among such deficits could result in language-learning difficulties. Alternatively, some, or all, of these deficits could be the result of the language disorder (see Chapter 5 for further discussion) or could be the result of some other problem that also interferes with language learning.

If deficits cannot be found within the child to fully explain language-learning problems, one can look at differences in the environment of these children. In pursuit of environmental factors that might explain the language-learning difficulties, many have studied the language input that caregivers provide to the SLI child. When SLI and NLI children have been matched for age, considerable differences have been reported (e.g., Bondurant, Romeo, & Kretschmer, 1983; Cramblit & Siegel, 1977; Wulbert, Inglis, Kriegsmann, & Mills, 1975). However, these differences could have been accounted for by the differences in language level; in fact, the patterns observed in the SLI group were more like those observed between caregivers and younger NLI children. When studies attempted to equate SLI and NLI children in terms of level of language development (usually in terms of mean length of utterance), fewer differences have been reported, but some differences remain (e.g., Conti-Ramsded & Friel-Patti, 1983; Johnson, 1985; Lasky & Klopp, 1982; Schodorf & Edwards, 1983). The remaining differences have not, however, always been replicated in other studies (for further information see Leonard, in press, and Chapter 15 on maintaining factors). Combining this lack of replication with our current lack of agreement on what aspects of input influence language development in any child, the case for environmental factors as an explanation of SLI is weak.

If neither differences within the child nor differences within the environment can clearly account for SLI, what are we to conclude? For some (e.g., Leonard, in press), this suggests that SLI may not represent a "disorder." A similar position has been taken in regard to learning disabilities (McGuiness, 1985, as cited in Henig, 1986). In this view, it is because language skills are so highly valued by our society that difficulties in learning such skills are considered a "disorder." These authors point out that poor ability in drawing or poor musical ability is not considered evidence of a disorder, but of normal variation. Given this view, these SLI children are simply weak in language-related skills as other children might be weak in athletic or other aspects of development. While the view does not preclude assessment or intervention with such children (since improved skills may be necessary for success in school and employment), it does suggest that searching for an explanation is not necessary and that the children should not be classified as handicapped.

While the point is well taken (i.e., that variation in skills is not the unusual, but the usual, and that we are too often apt to classify differences as a "disorder"), many are not ready to apply this to all children classified as SLI. Some children who fit this syndrome have such severe difficulties with language learning that if this same degree of difficulty were apparent in motor development, for example, they might well be classified as having a disorder or disability. A number of factors may account for our lack of success in finding an explanation for SLI. Most likely there is not *one* explanation. Interactional factors are no doubt at work. For example, a child could have subtle motor problems that alone might not cause language-learning problems but when combined with weak representational skills result in late language learning, which in turn could trigger unfavorable environmental conditions. Perhaps one of the major drawbacks to understanding this syndrome is the grouping of data. SLI children are often studied as a group if they fit one of the definitions presented earlier. But there is a wide range of abilities that fall within the criteria set, for example, by R. Stark and Tallal (1981). For instance, should we expect similar explanations for children who demonstrate problems in both comprehension and production as for children who have more severe problems in one than the other? Clearly further data are needed before we know best how to subdivide children with SLI and before we understand some, if not all, of the reasons why such children might be having difficulty learning language.

But what about language—is the child's eventual development of language similar to that of other children, or does it differ?

Language

This section reviews some of the available data on the language of SLI children. The findings are reported in terms of form, content, and use as defined in Chapters 1 and 2.

Form. When compared with age-matched peers, differences have been found in the number of SLI children who produced particular structures (Menyuk, 1964) and in the frequency with which certain structures were used (Leonard, 1972). SLI children have more difficulty with grammatical morphemes and complex syntactic constructions than NLI or retarded children matched by mental age (Kamhi & Johnston, 1982). More similarities appear when SLI children are compared with NLI children at a similar level of language learning, as evidenced by the average length of their utterances (Johnston & Schery, 1976; Morehead & Ingram, 1973). Differences that still exist include less frequent use of certain structures (such as copula, auxiliary, grammatical morphemes, and questions) by SLI children (Cromer, 1978; Ingram, 1972a, 1972b; Morehead & Ingram, 1973; Steckol & Leonard, 1979) and more frequent errors in the use of grammatical markers (Johnston & Kamhi, 1980).

Within the category of SLI, difficulties in learning syntax often co-occur with difficulties in speech production. Most children with SLI also have phonological difficulties (e.g., Aram & Nation, 1975; DeBaryshe, Whitehurst, & Fischel, 1986), and children with severe articulatory problems generally have syntactic problems (e.g., Ekelman & Aram, 1983; Paul & Shriberg, 1982; Shriner, Holloway, & Daniloff, 1969). Imitation of polysyllabic nonsense words for these children is less accurate than for age-matched peers (Kamhi & Catts, 1986), and older SLI children frequently omit final consonants (Panagos, 1978; Renfrew, 1966). The phonological deficits of this population have been considered by some (e.g., Leonard, 1982) as a reflection of a general language-learning problem since at the single-word-utterance stage phonological productions of SLI children are similar to those of NLI children (Leonard, 1982; Schwartz, Leonard, Folger, & Wilcox, 1980). Others argue that the production problems are related to auditory-perceptual or motor limitations (e.g., Tallal, Stark, & Curtiss, 1976). Differences are found among SLI as well as NLI children in the use of particular phonological processes.

For example, some children reduplicate syllables in their early utterances more than others, and this use of reduplication has been related to slower language development in both NLI and SLI children (e.g., Ferguson, Peizer, & Weeks, 1973; Lahey, et al., 1985). Differences among SLI children in phonological productions may help in differentiating underlying factors responsible for the language-learning difficulty.

In any case, the phonological problems may have a direct bearing on other aspects of language production. Phonological complexity, or at least preferences, has been reported to influence the early productive lexicons of both the NLI (Ferguson & Farwell, 1975; Schwartz & Leonard, 1982) and the SLI child (Leonard, Schwartz, Chapman, Rowan, Prelock, Terrell, Weiss, & Messick, 1982). Phonological problems have also been related to syntactic productions. In the population studied by Paul and Shriberg (1982) about half of the children with "delayed speech" had syntactic problems that could be attributed to a phonological simplification of phonetically complex morphophonemes. For example, grammatical morphemes involving the addition of consonant segments to words which resulted in the formation of final consonant clusters (e.g., the past tense of *jump* forms a final cluster of /pt/) were more likely to be omitted by these children than changes involving vowel changes (e.g., past tense of *say* changes only the vowel /e/ to /ɛ/). Adding a consonant segment to a word (e.g., past tense of *play* adds /d/) makes it vulnerable to final consonant deletion (a phonological process frequently used by language-impaired children, as noted above), while adding a consonant to a word ending in a consonant makes it also vulnerable to cluster reduction.

The hypothesis that phonological complexity may be related to SLI children's problems with grammatical morphemes was tested in one of the first cross-linguistic studies of SLI children (Leonard, Sabbadini, Leonard, & Volterra, 1986; Leonard, Sabbadini, Volterra & Leonard, 1986). The productions of certain grammatical morphemes by both English- and Italian-speaking SLI children were examined in an effort to sort out the role of phonological complexity. While in English most morphological inflections involve the addition of consonant segments, in Italian many of the grammatical morphemes are coded by adding a vowel or a stressed syllable to a word. Inflections and articles with vowel endings were more likely to be produced correctly by both the English and the Italian SLI children, suggesting that phonological complexity creates particular difficulty for SLI children in the use of grammatical morphemes.

Moreover, phonological sophistication is related to learning to read. Ability to segment language into words, syllables, and phonemes is necessary for the decoding of written language. Such metalinguistic skills (i.e., the ability to treat language as an object apart from its meaning—see Van Kleeck, 1984) are not well developed in SLI children. SLI children have more difficulty segmenting words, syllables, and phonemes than age- or language-matched peers (Kamhi, Lee, & Nelson, 1985). Whether this deficit is related to poorly developed phonological and other linguistic representations or to the cognitive skills considered necessary for metalinguistic activities is not yet clear.

Content and Content/Form Interactions. Comparisons of the content of utterances of SLI and NLI children have suggested more similarities than differences when the children are matched in terms of mean length of utterance (MLU).

Studies of early lexical development suggest that the kinds of words learned during the single-word-utterance period by SLI children are not unlike those learned by NLI children (Bloom, 1980; Leonard, Schwartz, et al., 1982). In their multi-word utterances, the SLI children who were studied talk about the same notions that NLI children (with similar MLUs) talk about (Bloom, 1980; Freedman & Carpenter, 1976; Leonard, Bolders, & Miller, 1976; Mattingly, 1978). But there are subtle differences. For example, in a longitudinal study of one SLI boy, Bloom (1980) noted that, unlike the NLI children she had studied, this SLI child's early first two-word utterances coded primarily attributive relations. Clinical observation suggests that a number of SLI children appear to learn attributive relations more readily than MLU-matched NLI children. This may be because the SLI children studied are often in an environment where attributes are stressed (as in a nursery school program), or it may reflect differences in their experience with and concepts of their environment. Other differences have been reported at higher MLU levels. For example, nomination (or existence) and action are coded more frequently by SLI children than MLU-matched NLI children (Freedman & Carpenter, 1976; Leonard, Bolders, & Miller, 1976). Furthermore, SLI children encoded fewer ideas per utterance and talked more about ongoing events than language-matched peers (Johnston & Kamhi, 1980) or NLI and retarded children matched for mental age (Kamhi & Johnston, 1982). If we had information on more NLI children, such differences may well fall within normal variation. Alternatively, these differences may reflect a more advanced level of the SLI children's cognitive development while they are first learning the linguistic code (since they are older than the normal child when they are at this language level), or it may reflect a restriction in their use of linguistic forms to code concepts.

A part of the restriction in the use of linguistic forms to code concepts may be in accessing the lexicon. SLI children are slower in naming pictures than age-matched NLI children (though faster than NLI children matched on language level) (Leonard, Nippold, Kail, & Hale, 1983). For all children, naming times are shorter for frequent words than for infrequent words, and are shorter for words presented in context than those presented out of context (Kail & Leonard, 1986). From these data, Kail and Leonard concluded that the semantic memories of the SLI children contain "weaker links between entries as well as fewer connecting links" (p. 24)—that is, that the representation of words is less elaborate. While most authors have focused primarily on the *semantic* representation of words in interpreting such findings, it is possible that the problem may be related to the *phonetic* representation of the word for some children. Problems with phonetic representation in memory have been suggested for older children labeled as learning-disabled (see Mann, 1986). Furthermore, the language disordered children studied by Dollaghan (1987) were able to recognize new words presented only once as well as normal age-matched peers, but recalled fewer phonemes in attempts to produce these words.

Use.   Evaluation of the SLI child's ability to use language has been the subject of considerable interest in the past decade. Earlier studies on linguistic forms used by both SLI and MLU-matched NLI children suggested that questions might be less frequently asked by SLI children (Morehead & Ingram, 1973), but no analysis was made of function and so it was not clear that the SLI children were not requesting information, for example, by using other forms. In one of the first studies of SLI children's pragmatic abilities, Snyder (1975) reported that SLI children using only single-word utterances were less likely to use words to communicate imperatives and declaratives than NLI children using only single-word utterances; rather, the SLI children communicated these intents by nonlinguistic means. This finding was not, however, replicated by Rowan, Leonard, Chapman, and Weiss (1983) with somewhat older SLI children who were more advanced in the single-word-utterance period as determined by a larger vocabulary; these SLI children used words in a similar manner as language-matched NLI children.

More similarities than differences have been found in the variety and frequency of functions for which language is used when SLI children are compared with NLI children matched for language level (e.g., Leonard, Camarata, Rowan, & Chapman, 1982; Rom & Bliss, 1981). However, some differences in the frequency of use of certain functions have been reported. For example, in the single-word-utterance period NLI children are more likely to name objects than SLI children; while SLI children give proportionally more answers (Leonard, Camarata, Rowan, & Chapman, 1982). A greater use of replies and a greater variety of types of replies by the SLI have been interpreted as a greater degree of conversational sophistication for the SLI in comparison to MLU-matched NLI (Leonard, in press). However, these difference may be reflecting the more advanced comprehension skills of the SLI children in comparison with the MLU-matched NLI children included in this study. Finally, requests by SLI children from 3 to 9 years of age are more likely to be direct than indirect in form and to be requests for action rather than for information (Prinz & Ferrier, 1983). These investigators also found a direct relationship between measures of content/form development and the use of requests. Thus, in comparison to peers of the same chronological age, SLI children were not as sophisticated in asking, comprehending, or judging requests.

Dyads of SLI children are also more likely to ignore or respond inappropriately to requests than age-matched (5:6 to 6-year-old) NLI dyads and are less likely to request clarification (Brinton & Fujiki, 1982). Some of these differences may be related to their lower level of linguistic maturity (that is, they may not have understood the requests) and to their histories of not understanding others (and so why ask for more talk that is not understood). SLI children have been found to respond to questions less frequently than MLU-matched NLI children (Rosinski-McClendon & Newhoff, 1987), but this too may relate to differences in levels of comprehension. These same children were as assertive as MLU-matched NLI children in maintaining and continuing a topic that they themselves had initiated.

While SLI children have demonstrated sensitivity to listener needs, they do not always use the linguistic code to adapt to those needs in the same way as NLI children. When SLI children were asked by an adult for clarification (first with "huh?", then "what?" followed by "I didn't understand that") regarding their description of a picture, they responded as frequently as age-matched NLI children, but with more inappropriate responses and fewer responses that added information (Brinton, Fujiki, Winkler, & Loeb, 1986). Even when subjects were matched by MLU, responses to requests for repairs did not change with MLU for SLI children as it did for MLU-matched NLI children (Gallagher & Darnton, 1978). The children did respond to the investigator's "what?," but they made mostly primitive changes (e.g., phonological versus word substitutions) in their original utterance.

Other evidence suggests that use of alternative forms to adapt to listeners is similar between SLI and NLI children at the same level of language development. For example, SLI children change the content of their utterances as a function of the listener's age in a manner similar to MLU-matched NLI peers (Fey, Leonard, & Wilcox, 1981), and within a sentence they distinguish shared (or old) information from new information in a similar manner as NLI children. In fact, they are apparently linguistically superior to MLU-matched NLI peers in their ability to use pronouns as a means of coding old information (Skarakis & Greenfield, 1982).

Other aspects of discourse skill seem more related to language level than to age or cognitive level. SLI children are similar to language-matched NLI children in the use of cohesive devices of discourse such as repeating or substituting items from a prior utterance (Van Kleeck & Frankel, 1981). Another important skill for processing discourse (as well as for reading) is inferencing (or understanding information implied within and across utterances). Again SLI children fall short of age-matched peers even when the specifics of the linguistic input are understood, but behave much like NLI children matched for comprehension level (Crais & Chapman, 1987; Snyder, 1984; Weismer, 1985). For the most part then, pragmatic skills, or the use of language, in the SLI population seems similar to that of children with similar levels of content/form development. Differences that have been found may be related to difficulties in matching SLI children with NLI children.

One of the major problems in comparing NLI and SLI children has been in matching the two groups. In general MLU has been the measure used (except see Crais & Chapman, 1987; Rowan et al., 1983; Weismer, 1985). It is not, however, very useful at the single-word-utterance stage where considerable language learning is not reflected in longer utterances, nor does it take into account differences in level of comprehension which are so essential when studying discourse skills. In addition, MLU is but a superficial measure of change in form in the very early stages of syntactic learning; it is not even very useful after an MLU of 3.0 when it varies considerably, and even complexities in form are not always reflected in increased length (for a discussion of the problems of using MLU as a measure of language see Bloom, Lifter, & Broughton, 1985; Gerber, 1987; Lahey, Launer, & Schiff-Myers, 1983; Wollner, 1983).

Summary. In summary it appears that it is not easy to describe the language of a "typical" child with specific language impairment—variation is prevalent here as with the non-language-impaired child. The label of *SLI* does not predict what language behaviors we can expect. While more similarities than differences exist when SLI children are compared with NLI children at the same MLU, the language of the SLI child is not exactly like that of NLI children with similar MLUs. Some of these differences may well be found in NLI children when larger populations of NLI children have been studied; others may be related to problems in matching; and still others may be unique to this syndrome. By far the most outstanding characteristic of this group of children, and one that they all share, is late and slow development of form with better development of content and use inter-

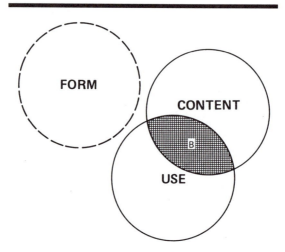

FIGURE 4-1 *Disruption in the Form of Language.*

actions, as illustrated in Figure 4-1. Certainly, the label of *SLI* (even when MLU is known) does not tell the clinician or teacher what it is that the child needs to learn nor what the child currently knows about language as a system for communication.

Hearing Impairment

Children with severely impaired hearing have a delay in onset and are slow in the rate at which they learn *auditory-vocal* language.* In this way they are like children labeled *specific-language-impaired.* Characteristics used to differentiate these two syndromes focus on the superior performance of the hearing-impaired children (compared with the SLI children) in terms of use of gestures and symbolic play; consistency on measures of auditory skills and intelligence; and motor coordination, social maturity, and social perception (Myklebust, 1954). Of course, the major criterion for the syndrome of hearing impairment is a hearing loss as determined by the results of standardized audiometric procedures.

Terminology

Terms used to describe the hearing-impaired individual vary with the purpose of the description. (See Chapter 1 for a discussion of this same point relative to definitions of language.) For example, hearing impairment can be defined according to the degree of loss, the time of onset, causal factors, site of dysfunction in

---

* It should be emphasized, however, that hearing-impaired children raised in an environment where sign language is their native language would not, necessarily, demonstrate a language disorder; they may have no difficulty at all learning their *native* language, which is not dependent on the auditory modality.

BOX 4-4   Classification of Hearing Loss

A classification developed for the American Academy of Ophthalmology and Otolaryngology (as presented by Silverman, 1971b) includes six classes of loss according to the degree of difficulty in understanding speech:

1. 25 decibels (ISO) or less, not significant
2. 25 to 40 decibels (ISO), a slight handicap—difficulty in understanding faint speech
3. 40 to 55 decibels (ISO), a mild handicap—frequent difficulty with normal speech
4. 55 to 70 decibels (ISO), a marked handicap—frequent difficulty with loud speech
5. 70 to 90 decibels (ISO), severe handicap—understands only shouted or amplified speech
6. 90 decibels (ISO) and up, extreme handicap—usually cannot understand even amplified speech

---

the auditory system, or social impairment (Myklebust, 1954; Silverman, 1971a, 1971b).

The degree of hearing impairment is usually described in terms of thresholds of sensitivity to pure tones in the so called speech frequencies (500 to 2000 hertz), as, for example, in Box 4-4. The term *deaf* refers to "those who do not have sufficient residual hearing to enable them to understand speech successfully even with a hearing aid, without special instruction" (Silverman, 1971a, p. 399). In this same sense the term *hard of hearing* refers to those whose hearing, although defective, is functional either with or without amplification.

The terms *deaf* and *hard of hearing* are also used, however, to refer to educational potential and to distinguish between those who have acquired language and those who have not (Myklebust, 1954). Such a distinction is often closely related to time of onset of the hearing impairment as well as to degree of impairment. However, acquisition of language is related to criteria other than degree of hearing impairment and time of onset.

Associated Factors and Explanations

A number of factors have been associated with severe hearing impairment and have served as a high-risk register in order to determine which newborn infants should participate in hearing screening programs. These factors, compiled by the Joint Committee on Newborn Hearing in 1981, are discussed by Gerkin (1984) and are briefly reviewed here. The first factor is asphyxia at birth. This condition is reflected by a low (i.e., 0–3) Apgar score (which includes measures of heart rate, color, muscle tone, respiration, and reflexes taken shortly after birth). Low Apgar scores are more common in premature infants and can result in high-frequency hearing loss. Bacterial meningitis is a second factor. In many cases it is not clear whether resulting hearing losses are related to the infection itself or to the antibiotics used to combat the infection. Resulting losses range from mild to profound and may be progressive. The third factor is congenital or perinatal infections including rubella, herpes, and cytomegalovirus (CMV). Incidence and type of loss vary with the infection. Fourth on the list are defects of the head and neck such as, but not limited to, cleft palate. Again, the incidence and type of loss vary with the type of defect. The fifth factor is jaundice, or an excess of bilirubin in the blood, which can result in losses ranging from mild to profound. Sixth is family history of hearing loss other than presbycusis. According to Gerkin, there are over 50 types of hereditary hearing loss. Some of these are present at birth; others develop later. Finally, low birth weight (less than 1500 grams) is associated with severe hearing impairment. Since these infants are more prone to many problems (e.g., many have jaundice and low Apgar scores), it is not clear what underlies the sensorineural high-frequency hearing problems often found in such infants.

Factors Related to Development of Communication Skills

A number of factors were found to correlate with degree of linguistic ability in a large-scale longitudinal study of hearing-impaired children (Levitt, McGarr, & Geffner, 1988). As expected, children who lost their hearing after they had learned language were superior in both speech and language skills to those who became deaf prelinguistically. There was some correlation between speech skills and hearing loss, but language skills did not correlate well with the degree of hearing loss. Although a marked reduction in language skills occurred when losses were greater than 115 decibels, only a slight reduction in language skills was found as loss increased from 40 to 80 decibels, with no change from 80 to 115 decibels. Lack of correlation between level of hearing loss and language skills has been reported by others (e.g., Curtiss, Prutting, & Lowell, 1979; Davis, Elfenbein, Schum, & Bentler, 1986). Better correlations were found between linguistic ability and the level of aided thresholds by Curtiss et al. (1979) and between linguistic ability and speech reception and/or recognition by Davis et al. (1986).

One of the best predictors of language skills in the Levitt et al. study was age at which intervention was begun. A positive effect of "early" (i.e., age 3 or sooner) intervention was found, and it was most marked for deaf children of hearing parents. On a less optimistic note, language scores do correlate with age with little change noted between children 6 and 10 years of age (Watson, Sullivan, Moeller, & Jensen, 1982); even in the less severely hearing-impaired children studied by Davis, Shepard, Stelmachowicz, and Gorga (1981), the gap between chronological age and language age increased from 5 to 12 years of age.

With a different population, teacher ratings of spoken-language ability at age 11 were highly correlated with scores on a spoken-language index obtained in *preschool* (Geers & Moog, 1987). This index assigned weighted scores to five factors —hearing capacity (including speech-reception capability and aided articulation index), language competence (including comparisons of oral and/or nonoral English skills with those of other hearing-impaired individuals), nonverbal intelligence, judgments of the amount of family support, and the child's speech communication attitude. Linguistic skills (as measured by verbal intelligence quotients and vocabulary comprehension) were related to academic achievement in the study by Davis et al. (1986). Nonverbal intelligence was correlated with measures of language performance in the study by Watson et al. (1982), but was not related to academic achievement or to verbal IQ or vocabulary comprehension in the Davis et al. data.

Although educational philosophy (i.e., oral, total, or manual approaches) is a source of great debate, no differential effect of approach could be sorted out by Levitt et al. (1988) despite the fact that their study involved almost 200 children from different educational settings. Likewise, a comparison of oral-aural (OA) and total communication (TC) approaches in profoundly deaf children from 5 to 9 years of age indicated no significant differences between combined signed and spoken productions of the TC children and the oral productions of the OA children (Geers, Moog, & Schick, 1984). However, children in the OA group were superior in spoken language. While, on the whole, children in the Levitt et al. study who were mainstreamed did better on measures of speech and language than those in schools for the deaf, their language skills were not uniformly better. Many mainstreamed children had language skills below those of children in the schools for the deaf.

As a general pattern, deaf children of hearing parents had better speech production skills than deaf children of deaf parents (Levitt et al., 1988). In contrast, deaf children of deaf parents had better language skills. As might be expected, children with other impairments (such as neurological impairments, emotional and behavioral problems, and visual deficits) in addition to the hearing loss had more difficulty with language than children without such additional handicaps. Multiple handicaps occurred in 33% of the deaf population studied by Levitt et al., but in only 13% of the less severely hearing-impaired children in public school studied by Shepard, Davis, Gorga, and Stelmachowicz (1981). Despite multiple handicaps, the longitudinal data of Levitt et al. indicated a steady, though slow, increase in their language skills with intensive special education. A major conclusion of Levitt et al. was that language training had an impact.

Description of Communication Skills

Hearing-impaired children appear to be more similar to hearing children in their development of content and use than in their development of form.

Content. Deaf individuals' ideas of the world, from which the content of language derives, develop in the same sequence as for the hearing child, and with only slight delay (Furth, 1966). Early (Bellugi & Klima, 1972) and more recent reports (Launer, 1982) suggest that the deaf child who is learning sign language codes the same semantic notions as the hearing child who is learning to speak; although the form of the communication differs, the *content* is the same. Indeed, even the sequence of acquisition of semantic relations is similar (Launer, 1982). Hearing-impaired children learning oral language also express similar semantic relations as language-matched hearing children. For example, action utterances accounted for the greater proportion of semantic relations expressed by both groups (Hess, 1972, as cited by Kretchmer & Kretchmer, 1978; see Kretchmer & Kretchmer for a review of such studies).

Some differences in the frequency with which certain content categories are expressed by hearing-impaired children were reported by Curtiss et al. (1979).

They examined the linguistic and nonlinguistic expression of semantic relations and communicative intentions in 12 preschool children who were severely to profoundly deaf (i.e., had losses greater than 90 decibels). In comparison with the literature on hearing children, the deaf children (in particular the 3- and 4-year-olds) more frequently pointed out and named objects (as reported for SLI in the prior section of this chapter) and used a greater number of performatives (i.e., gestures or vocalizations without specific semantic content) than expected for their ages. However, comparisons were not made with children of the same linguistic ability, and as pointed out by the authors, certain semantic relations are difficult to express nonlinguistically.

In fact, the form of coding semantic relations influences when a semantic relation will emerge. For example, few verb forms are found in the single-word utterances of hearing children, but action signs are frequent in the lexicons of deaf children learning sign language (Launer, 1982). Furthermore, Launer reported that the early verb forms used by the deaf children are more specific than the early verb forms used by the hearing child. As a possible explanation for this difference, Launer pointed out that the specific verb forms used by these children symbolized both the object of the action and the action itself within one sign. For example, in American Sign Language, there is one sign for "open door" and a different sign for "open jar." In order to code such actions on objects the child learning sign language does not need to learn syntax (i.e., the child does not need to learn to code meaning relations between words using word order). Thus, form may influence the sequence in which content is first expressed—or at least the frequency of the expression of certain content categories.

Use. The children studied by Curtiss et al. (1979, and described above) communicated a wide variety of functions using both verbal and nonverbal means. At the age of 2, the children appeared similar to hearing children in their ability to communicate various intentions, but these were expressed primarily by nonlinguistic means. Thus, the expression of functions exceeded the expression of content (by either conventional words or idiosyncratic gesture). Despite this apparent skill in communicating intentions, the quantity of communicative behavior was much less in these children than in hearing children. (A similar finding was reported by Goorell, 1971, as cited in Kretchmer & Kretchmer, 1978.) Most important, there was considerable variability among the children that was not predicted by level of hearing (as reported by Levitt et al. for measures of form) or by MLU. While MLU was a good predictor of linguistic ability, it was not predictive of overall communicative skill (see also under the previous section on specific language impairment). MLU did, however, account for the use of contrastive stress. No differences were found in the production of contrastive stress for coding new information when moderate-to-severely hearing-impaired children were matched to hearing children on mean length of utterance.

Implicit content (or meaning beyond that explicitly stated) in stories is understood as well by deaf adolescents as hearing adolescents, although the hearing students recall more of the explicit propositions (Sarachan-Deily, 1985). Likewise, deaf adolescents are able to comprehend metaphorical use of language although their tendency is toward a literal interpretation—a bias that may be exacerbated by some educational practices (Iran-Nejad, Ortony, & Rittenhouse, 1981). In the production of stories using sign language, deaf children produced as many figurative constructions as hearing peers (Marschark & West, 1985). In general, then, use of language (as has been studied to date) is not a major problem for deaf children. Most of their difficulties lie, as might be expected, with the learning of the auditory-vocal forms of language.

Form. Typically, the oral linguistic productions of the severely hearing-impaired are difficult to understand and have a distinctive voice quality. However, in the first half of the first year of life the vocalizations of the deaf infant appear similar to those of the hearing infant (Oller, Eilers, Bull, & Carney, 1985; Smith, 1982). But after that point important differences are apparent. Normal hearing and Down's syndrome children frequently produce forms that obey the timing constraints of syllables in the form of reduplicated babbling by at least 10 months of age (Smith & Oller, 1981). The deaf infant studied by Oller et al., (1985) however, did not produce repetitive syllables at all in the first year of life. Thus, by at least 10 months of age, the influence of auditory deprivation can be evidenced in vocal productions.

Since deaf individuals usually lack intelligible oral speech, their language has most often been studied in its written form. On the basis of a series of studies that compared syntactic knowledge of deaf children age 10 to 18 years with that of hearing children age 8 to 10 years, Quigley, Wilbur, Power, Montanelli, and Steinkamp (1976) concluded that "syntactic structures develop similarly for deaf children as for hearing children but at a greatly reduced rate" (p. 189). Both groups of children had the most difficulty with sentences that deviated from the usual subject-verb-object word order (such as passives or relative clauses) and with verbal auxiliaries, although the younger hearing children surpassed the deaf in most tasks. "Most of the oldest deaf students in the study (between 18 and 19 years of age) did not have syntactic development equal to the 8-year-old hearing children" (p. 193). Although there were some different syntactic structures used by the deaf children, "none of those structures was common to all subjects and most were used by fewer than 50%" (p. 193).

A somewhat different conclusion was reached by Levitt et al. (1988), who administered similar tests to children in schools for the deaf (age 10 to 13:9) for four consecutive years as well as to a group of 10-year-old hearing-impaired children mainstreamed into the regular school system. The pattern of findings was similar to that reported by Quigley Wilbur, Power, Montanelli & Steinkamp. But in a comparison of their findings with the literature on language development in hearing children, considerable differences were found on the more advanced structures. In contrast, few differences were found on the earlier learned structures. They concluded that extremely slow progress in language learning produces deviant patterns of development. Delay in the development of earlier forms creates deviant patterns on more advanced forms, since the advanced forms are being learned before the earlier forms are fully acquired.

Other comparisons with hearing children have found that fewer compound and complex sentences are used, and that stereotype carrier phrases and sentence frames are common (Heider & Heider, 1940; Simmons, 1962). The total number of words used by deaf children is similar to that of hearing peers in written composition (Heider & Heider, 1940) although the number of words is less than hearing peers in spoken language (Brannon, 1968). Even when amount of verbalization is taken into account, the diversity of vocabulary is not as great (Brannon, 1968; Simmons, 1962), and the frequency with which different classes of words are used differs from that of the hearing child (Brannon, 1968; Levitt et al., 1988; MacGinitie, 1964). When sentences are elicited, the deaf tend to use a greater proportion of nouns, verbs, and articles in their utterances and fewer adverbs, auxiliaries, pronouns, prepositions, and question forms than the hearing child (Brannon, 1968; MacGinitie, 1964). Brannon found that this difference was more pronounced with a severe hearing loss than with a moderate hearing loss. In less structured samples, articles and main verbs (particularly the verb *to be*) are also often omitted (Taylor, 1969; Tervoort, 1967; both as presented by Quigley, Wilbur, Power, Montanelli & Steinkamp, 1976). Reading scores are generally low, with little progress noted after the middle elementary grade levels.

As poor as the written skills of the hearing-impaired may be, they are apparently superior to those of some specific-language-impaired children (Cromer, 1978). While the deaf made more errors, they used more complex sentences and more different categories (e.g., noun phrases, verb phrases, adverbial phrases) per sentence even when the sentence lengths were comparable.

In a study of the oral language productions of deaf speakers, de Villiers and de Villiers (1986) also suggest that deaf children learn to code the basic grammatical relations. These researchers were able to elicit oral productions of structurally complete complex sentences and pragmatically appropriate *wh* questions from profoundly deaf children from 7 to 18 years of age. Comparing oral productions of the deaf adolescents with those of normal-hearing preschool children, differences were greatest in the use of grammatical morphemes. For example in *wh* questions the auxiliary was usually omitted by the deaf, but not the hearing, children. The deaf children also frequently omitted markings for past tense and rarely overgeneralized like the younger hearing children. Finally, differences were apparent in the use of the indefinite, but not the definite, article (the deaf children produced the definite article when the indefinite was appropriate). The de Villiers suggested that the learning of grammatical morphemes is more sensitive to environmental input than the learning of basic grammatical relations. Furthermore, they pointed out that grammatical morphemes are less important for the communication of information and that grammatical morphemes receive less stress in that input than content words.

Summary.   It appears that deaf children know sentence frames and can determine the form class that should be inserted in a frame, but they do not understand the use or meaning of specific functor words (Blanton, 1968). Thus, the deaf learn the *form* of language as it is written, but possibly do not learn language as a vehicle for coding *content* or for fulfilling a particular *use.* This may, however, tell us more about the training methods that have been used to teach language to deaf children than about the effect of the loss of the auditory channel on language learning. Instructional methodology has often focused more on structure and syntax than on communicative language.

Thus, it appears that the language disorder accompanying hearing loss can be described as a dysfunction in the interaction of form with content and use, as illustrated in Figure 4-1. Deaf children may know what they need to know about objects and events in the world and may know how to interact with others in order to communicate, but they have difficulty learning the auditory-vocal conventional forms used for communication by the community at large. This difficulty may, for some, influence the amount of communicative interactions, the frequency with which certain ideas are expressed, and the accuracy and sophistication of the auditory-vocal system of forms expressed and understood.

To know that a child is hearing-impaired does not tell the clinician what the child needs to know about language. Considerable variability is found among these children—variability that is not easily predicted given level of hearing loss, MLU, grade in school, nonverbal IQ, or age of onset. Unquestionably, the categorization of hearing impairment does lead to hypotheses about how the child might learn language; it certainly requires that techniques of teaching language modify the auditory signal and perhaps supplement the auditory channel. In all other respects, however, the category is too global to specify other techniques or the specific goals of a language intervention program.

Mild Fluctuating Hearing Loss

The information above has focused on children with moderate-to-profound hearing loss. A larger group of children suffer from intermittent ear infections that temporarily cause mild (15 to 40 decibels) hearing impairment. Some evidence suggests that children who have recurrent attacks of otitis media score lower on measures of language, academic achievement, and intelligence than children who do not have histories of such repeated infections (e.g., Burgener & Mouw, 1982; Downs, 1983; Holm & Kunze, 1969; J. Katz, 1978; Needleman, 1977). But not all studies agree—some find no evidence of differences (see Garrard & Clark, 1985, for a recent summary of relevant studies). Unfortunately, there have been problems with many of the studies, particularly in the choice of controls (see Ventry, 1980, 1983). Until the data indicate otherwise, however, these children should be considered at risk for language-learning problems and should be the concern of the speech-language pathologist. A child with a fluctuating mild loss can be a puzzle to parents who do not understand the child's problem and who may be annoyed by the many "what" questions that appear inconsistent. Interactional patterns may be upset, and incidental language learning may be decreased. Parent counseling and preventive programs can be established without undue hardship to the families and children. Extra language stimulation may be important for these children, and continual monitoring of speech and language skills as well as hearing is a necessity.

Mental Retardation

While the child with specific language impairment and the hearing-impaired child appear to be developmentally delayed primarily in language (although the hearing-impaired child could be delayed in many other areas), the mentally retarded child is characterized by delay in most, if not all, areas of development.

"Mental retardation refers to significantly subaverage general intellectual functioning existing concurrently with deficits in adaptive behavior, and manifested during the developmental period'' (Grossman, 1973, p. 1). ''Significantly subaverage general intellectual functioning'' means scores on standardized tests of intelligence that fall 2 or more standard deviations below the mean (e.g., an IQ of 70 on the *Wechsler Intelligence Scale for Children* where the mean is 100 and 1 standard deviation is 15). As with any test score, the dividing line is not that precise and the standard error of measurement for each test needs to be considered in interpreting the score (see Chapter 7 for further discussion of this point).

Perhaps more important than the IQ score is an estimate of the child's adaptive behavior or the effectiveness with which the child meets the levels of personal independence and social responsibility expected of peers in the same cultural group. The judgment is often made by observation of the child in different settings and by information provided by caregivers and teachers. In some instances the *Vineland Social Maturity Scale* (Doll, 1965) or the *Adaptive Behavior Scale* (Kennett, 1976) is used.

If a child had normal intelligence at one time, but develops this clinical pattern after the age of 18, the diagnosis is usually dementia rather than mental retardation; if the pattern develops before the age of 18 following normal intelligence, the diagnosis suggested by the American Psychiatric Association (1980) is both mental retardation and dementia.

Approximately 1% of the population meets the criteria of mental retardation. The prevalence of other behavioral problems, such as infantile autism, attentional deficits, and hyperactivity, is three to four times greater among individuals who are categorized as mentally retarded than among the general population; neurological abnormalities such as seizures are also common among the severely retarded (American Psychiatric Association, 1980).

Terminology

Within the category of mental retardation, children are sometimes categorized according to level of IQ. Mild retardation includes children with IQ scores from 55 to 69; moderate retardation, 40 to 54; severe, 25 to 39, and profound, below 25. The mildly retarded, or ''educable,'' constitute the largest segment of the retarded, approximately 89%. They are sometimes referred to as those who acquire the problem in school and are cured when they leave an academic setting. As preschoolers, they do achieve developmental milestones, albeit a bit later than their peers, and are often not identified as needing special assistance; as adults, they can generally be self-sufficient by holding simple jobs. However, in school they fall behind their peers and are usually identified as children in need of special educational programs.

Those described as moderately retarded, or trainable, account for about 6% of the retarded. While this group does learn to talk, they have difficulty with aspects of communication and are likely to be identified during the preschool years; as adults, they can work at routine tasks with supervision. The severely retarded make up 3.5% of the retarded population, and the profoundly retarded another 1.5%. Both groups evidence motor coordination problems and are very late (i.e., school age) in developing speech. They are rarely ever competent at conversation and require close supervision throughout their lives. Retarded individuals are also subcategorized according to the presumed cause (brain injury, familial, Down's syndrome, etc.). (See Menolascino & Egger, 1978, for further information on categorizations.)

Associated Factors and Explanations

Mental retardation may be the result of biological factors, environmental factors, or an interaction between both. The most common biological factors include chromosomal and metabolic disorders. Perhaps the best known and most frequent chromosomal disorder is Down's syndrome, or trisomy 21, which accounts for approximately 10% of retarded children (Coleman, 1980). In other instances of chromosomal disorders involving an extra chromosome, as trisomy 18 or 13, severe retardation results, but the children do not often live beyond 1 year. Chromosomal problems are more likely among infants born to older parents (i.e., females over 35 or males over 55). One of the most common metabolic disorders is phenylketonuria (PKU), which can now be screened for in infancy and which can be treated.

Other organic problems are congenital but not hereditary. For example, infection (e.g., rubella) or the use of certain drugs during pregnancy can result in retardation in the infant. Another problem that is drawing increasing attention is what is referred to as fetal alcohol syndrome—the result of either excessive amounts of or sensitivity to alcohol ingested during pregnancy. Other cases of retardation are the result of genetic defects plus some insult at birth (e.g., spina bifida, which is a neural tube defect). In addition, postnatal factors may also lead to retardation (e.g., meningitis or lead poisoning).

Although there is a disproportionate number of retarded children in lower socioeconomic families, the role of environment in retardation is not clear. The correlation of retardation with lower socioeconomic class may be related to the way intelligence is measured and the nature of the academic setting, or other environmental factors could be responsible. Children in lower socioeconomic areas are also at a higher risk for prematurity and low birth weight (Menolascino & Egger, 1978), and teenage parents are more common. Poor prenatal and postnatal nutrition and poor prenatal and child health care compounded over a number of generations may account for some of the higher incidence.

Language

Many quantitative analyses have been made of the speech of children described as mentally retarded (see, for example, Naremore & Dever, 1975). Descriptions have pointed to impoverished vocabulary, less complex sentence structure, and later development of the use of verbal mediation. In general, an overall relationship has been found between language and IQ, for example, between sentence length and mental age (Goda & Griffith, 1962; Mecham, 1955; Schlanger, 1954) and between mental age and size of vocabulary (Mein & O'Connor, 1960). Although quantitative studies pointed to differences between the language of the normal child and the retarded child, qualitative analyses have pointed to similarities between the two populations.

Form.   One of the first indices of the development of form in the infant is the emergence of reduplicated babbling and of consonant-type vocalizations. Although Down's syndrome infants are typically retarded in both motor and cognitive domains, their early speech development resembles that of nonretarded infants in terms of age of onset for reduplicated babbling and in terms of types of vocalizations (B. Smith & Oller, 1981).

A number of studies have described the morphological development of retarded children according to their performance on tests that ask the children to apply morphological inflections (such as plural or possessive -s) to either nonsense words or familiar lexical items and their performance with grammatical morphemes in free speech contexts. The results have suggested that such children's spontaneous speech (outside the test situation) yields more advanced levels of performance than test results do, and that test scores do not improve with length of time in school. While morphological inflections were learned in the same sequence by both retarded and normal populations, the performance of the retarded children was poorer than that of normal children matched for mental age (Dever, 1972; Lovell & Bradbury, 1967; Newfield & Schlanger, 1968), but better than that of SLI children matched for mental age (Kamhi & Johnston, 1982).

Similarities between retarded and nonretarded children have also been found in the sequence of development of grammatical rules. Lackner (1968) wrote rules of grammar for the spontaneous speech of retarded children and concluded that their rules were the same as those found in the adult model and that their grammars became more complex as mental age increased. To test similarities in development between retarded and nonretarded children, he presented, as imitation and comprehension tasks, the structures generated by the grammars to a number of nonretarded children (ages 2:8 to 5:9). The results indicated "an ordering . . . between the complexity of grammars and the mental ages of the retarded children, and the chronological ages of the normal children," suggesting "that the language behaviors of normal and retarded children are not qualitatively different, that both groups follow similar developmental trends . . ." (p. 309).

A similar conclusion was reached by Evans and Hampson (1968) on the basis of a review of research on the language of children with Down's syndrome. They quoted the findings of Lenneberg, Nichols, and Rosenberger (1964) as evidence that the language development in this population is similar to that of normal children at a younger age. Analysis of language samples using *Developmental Sentence Scoring (DSS)* (Lee, 1974) revealed no significant differences between total scores of the normal children and those of mental-age-matched retarded children although subcategory analysis indicated fewer questions and earlier-level conjunctions were used by the retarded (Kamhi & Johnston, 1982).

Furthermore, when children are matched according to average length of utterance, it appears that the retarded children's knowledge of syntax is similar to that of nonretarded children (Fowler, Gelman, & Gleitman, 1980). No differences were found in the proportion of complete sentences, incomplete sentences, cliches, or stereotype utterances or in the range of variety of verb transformations or types of errors (Ryan, 1977). Distribution of utterances with varying lengths was similar at MLU 3.0 (Fowler et al., 1980). Differences were found, however, in the mental ages of retarded and nonretarded children at similar MLU levels; the nonretarded children reached similar MLU levels at lower mental ages than the retarded (Fowler et al., 1980; Ryan, 1977). Since measures of mental age rely heavily on vocabulary, it appears that the retarded children learned vocabulary more easily than syntax. One further difference was in the continuation of language growth beyond an MLU of 3.0. In Fowler's (1986) longitudinal data on Down's syndrome children, a plateau in language learning occurred when MLU reached 3.0 and the children were in middle childhood. Some further growth took place when the children were about 12 years of age.

While Down's syndrome children appear to talk less than language-matched nonretarded children, their utterances are no less stereotyped, as evidenced by type-token ratios for single-word utterances and early syntactic utterances (Fowler, in press; Tamari, 1978). In fact, the children demonstrated some of the same variability in learning form as the nonretarded; some of the children followed longitudinally by Tamari used primarily pronouns in their early syntactic utterances, while others focused on nouns—a finding similar to that reported for nonretarded children by Bloom, Lightbown, and Hood (1975) and K. Nelson (1975). While the distribution of nouns and verbs used by the retarded does not differ from that of MLU-matched nonretarded (Fowler et al., 1980), and many of the same lexical items are used, the variety of different verbs may be somewhat less (Tamari, 1978). In general, few differences exist in syntactic skills between the two populations when MLU is 3.0, including the frequency of complex sentence production (Fowler et al., 1980).

Content.   Studies that have examined the content of retarded children's utterances also suggest that, at equivalent levels of language development, similarities in development exist between the retarded and the nonretarded child. The relational utterances produced by Down's syndrome children code similar semantic notions to those of the early utterances of nonretarded children (Coggins, 1979; Tamari, 1978). Furthermore, the sequence of emergence and the relative frequency of use of different semantic categories are like those reported for the nonretarded (Tamari, 1978). In terms of the coordination of content categories (i.e., the number and type of relations expressed beyond the main verb relation, such as attribution, recurrence, and place), the retarded children were similar to mental-age-matched normal language learners (Kamhi & Johnston, 1982).

Use.   There is evidence that communicative interactions are less well developed in some retarded individuals than in the nonretarded. Children with Down's syndrome vocalize less for social-communicative purposes than the nonretarded child (Gaines & Prutting, 1982; Greenwald & Leonard, 1979). In addition, Down's syndrome children evidence more object than social schemata and less complex coordination of object and social actions (Bricker & Carlson, 1980; Gaines & Prutting, 1982). Even as adults, retarded individuals are less likely to take a dominant role in conversation with other adults or children (Bedrosian & Prutting, 1978).

However, others have reported that the use of language by Down's syndrome children is superior to that of MLU-matched (and, thus, younger) normal children in terms of topic maintenance, turn taking, conversational relevance, and production of speech acts (Beeghly & Cicchetti, 1986). Similarly, mildly retarded 6-year-old children and nonretarded 5-year-old children were very similar on a number of measures of use when interacting with each other and with more retarded children (Guralnick & Paul-Brown, 1986). Each group adjusted the communicative patterns in similar ways to the varying developmental levels of those addressed.

Language and Cognition

As with nonretarded children, there is a high correlation between symbolic play and language development (Casby & Ruder, 1983; Wing, 1975). While for most retarded children there is a delay in all aspects of development, this is not so for all retarded children. For example, Wing (1975) describes children who speak well and comprehend language but have poor nonverbal skills. In addition, she describes children who have higher-functioning visual-manual skills than language skills. Likewise, Curtiss (1981) provides illustrations of the disassociation between cognition and language—in one case cognition exceeded language, and in another language exceeded cognition. Another example of such disassociation where language skills far surpassed cognitive skills has been presented by Cromer (1986). It has also been found that mental age does not always predict language skills (e.g., Fowler et al., 1980; and see Fowler, in press for a review of these studies).

Such patterns lead to three conclusions. First, intelligence is probably best thought of as individual functions that may operate at different levels of efficiency (Wing, 1975). Second, language is best thought of as the interactions among content, form, and use and cognition may differentially affect these components and their interactions. Third, language skills, or potential language skills, should perhaps not be judged by mental age or IQ.

Summary

It is clear that the syndrome of mental retardation does not define a language pathology that is particular to, or unique with, children who are considered to be mentally retarded. At least in terms of content and form, development seems similar to that of the nonretarded child (the evidence on use is still contradictory). But neither the diagnosis of "mental retardation" nor information about level or cause of retardation currently provides information that is directly useful for facilitating language learning—they do not tell us what it is that a particular child must learn about language nor what procedures to use in teaching language to that child. This is not to say that research with this population is not useful. It is. Continued research in terms of etiologies of retardation has already led to some means of prevention (e.g., genetic counseling) and may eventually lead to further avenues of prevention. Continued research into the effect of cognitive differences on language learning may eventually help us to understand language development in general and language disorders in particular. It is hoped that implications for intervention will ultimately emerge.

Emotional Disturbance—Autism

The last common clinical category associated with childhood language disorders is severe emotional disturbance, primarily autism. As the name implies, the major distinguishing feature of the children placed within this category is impaired

> ## BOX 4-5 Diagnostic Signs of Childhood Psychosis
>
> 1. Gross and sustained impairment of emotional relationships with people (including using people, or parts of people, in an impersonal way, or as though they were inanimate objects).
> 2. Apparent unawareness of personal identity as demonstrated by abnormal behavior toward self, repeated self-directed aggression, and/or, when language is used, a confusion in the person identity of personal pronouns (for example, substituting "you" for "me," etc.).
> 3. Pathological preoccupation with a few particular objects, to the exclusion of most other objects in general.
> 4. Continued resistance to change in surroundings, with extreme reaction to any change in daily routine or environment.
> 5. The occurrence of abnormal perceptual experience with either excessive, diminished, or unpredictable responses to sensory stimuli.
> 6. Illogical anxiety, possibly precipitated by change in the environment or by certain objects, and yet, a lack of fear when presented with real danger.
> 7. A specific and unaccounted for dysfunction in body movements (hypertension, immobility, bizarre postures, ritualistic mannerisms).
> 8. Severe and generalized retardation in intellectual functioning, often along with isolated areas of normal intellectual ability.
> 9. Loss of, lack of, or late development of speech, possibly accompanied by confusions in the use of personal pronouns, echolalia, or other mannerisms of use and diction—as when words and phrases are uttered but convey no sense of meaningful communication.
>
> *Note:* From Creak and Committee, 1961.

interactional patterns. How different are these children from the children given different categorical labels, such as specific-language-impaired, mentally retarded, or severely hearing-impaired? To answer this question we will first look at the defining characteristics of the syndrome and review the different terminology used in this area.

Terminology

Childhood psychosis is a term used to describe children whose relationships with their environments are disturbed. Nine diagnostic signs of childhood psychosis were agreed upon by Creak and Committee (1961) and are listed in Box 4-5.

Psychotic children have often been subcategorized by age of onset: psychosis that begins in adolescence and is similar to schizophrenia in adults; psychosis that becomes evident between 30 months and 5 years of age, referred to as *childhood schizophrenia;* and psychosis that becomes apparent before the age of 30 months, which is referred to as *infantile autism* (Eisenberg, 1967; Rutter, 1968). According to Rutter (1968), childhood schizophrenia differs from autism in terms of factors other than age of onset: the sex ratio of children affected (a greater incidence among males for autism); social class of parents (higher for autistic children); family history of psychosis (greater in families of schizophrenic children); intelligence (lower for autistic children and a tendency for uneven scores on subtests); delusions (in schizophrenic children only); and the course of the problem (symptoms of schizophrenia tend to become more severe with time, while autistic symptoms tend to lessen in severity).

During the 1960s, however, there was little consensus about the characteristics that distinguished the two terms used to describe childhood psychosis—childhood schizophrenia and infantile autism (De Myer, Hingtgen, & Jackson, 1981). Different studies tended to label apparently similar children with one or the other label. More recently, autism has been considered separate from schizophrenia and is included under the term *pervasive developmental disorder*, while schizophrenia in children is still grouped in the same category as adult schizophrenia (American Psychiatric Association, 1980). This change in attitude is also reflected in the change in the name of the *Journal of Autism and Childhood Schizophrenia* to the *Journal of Autism and Developmental Disorders.*

The syndrome of autism was first outlined in the American literature by Leo Kanner in 1943 when he described 11 psychotic children who were different from children with other psychiatric disorders. The features noted by Kanner included differences in speech (e.g., delay in acquisition, noncommunicative use of speech, delayed echolalia, pronominal reversals), normal physical appearance, poor relationships with people, an obsessive insistence on sameness, good rote memory, and poor imagination. Rutter (1978) found three broad groups of symptoms in most children diagnosed as autistic—"a profound and general failure to develop social relationships; language retardation with impaired comprehension, echolalia and pronominal reversal; and ritualistic or compulsive phenomena (i.e., an insistence on sameness)" (p. 4). In order to distinguish these children from those who develop degenerative diseases and schizophrenia in adolescence, Rutter pointed out that an important criterion for the diagnosis of autism is onset before the age of 30 months. These criteria are similar to those used by the DSM III classification system (American Psychiatric Association, 1980) outlined in Box 4-6. The criteria still allow for considerable variability among children so defined and make comparisons of research studies difficult. There is a need for more detailed description of symptoms so that core behaviors that distinguish the autistic child from other children can be more operationally defined (Denkla, 1986).

The prevalence of autism ranges from 2 to 5 per 10,000 children (American Psychiatric Association, 1980; Ritvo & Freeman, 1978; Wing, 1981). However, Wing, (1981) noted that 21 children in 10,000 have many of the symptoms characteristic of the autistic syndrome. The prevalence of autism among siblings of autistic children is 2 per 100 (Rutter, 1968), much greater than that noted above for the entire population, and the ratio of males to females with autistic symptoms is approximately 4 to 1.

Associated Factors and Explanations

In a large-scale epidemiological study carried out in a section of England, Wing and her associates identified all children 15 years of age and under who had any of the symptoms characteristic of autism. Each of the subjects had at least one (but not necessarily all) of the following symptoms: problems with communication, problems with social interaction, stereotyped and repetitive behavior, and severe

---

BOX 4-6   DSM III Diagnostic Criteria for Infantile Autism

Infantile Autism
1. Onset before 2½ years of age.
2. Pervasive lack of responsiveness to others.
3. Major deficits in language development.
4. If the child talks, peculiar speech patterns including immediate and delayed echolalia, metaphorical language, and pronominal reversals.

Residual State
1. The child once had all of the above, but currently does not meet all of the criteria.
2. There may be some odd communication patterns and social awkwardness.

Childhood Onset of Pervasive Developmental Disorder
1. If onset after 2½ years but before 12 years of age.
2. Severe and continued impairment in social relations (such as lack of appropriate affective response, inappropriate clinging, asocial behavior, and lack of empathy).
3. At least three of the following: excessive anxiety, inappropriate affect, resistance to change, odd motor movements, abnormal speech (including question-like melody and monotone), hyper- or hypo-sensitivity to sensory stimuli, and self-mutilation.
4. No delusions or hallucinations.

Note: Adapted from the American Psychiatric Association, 1980.

---

mental retardation (Wing, 1981). They found that one group of these children was sociable; that is, they appeared to enjoy social contact at a level appropriate to their communication skills. Another group, regardless of their communication skills, did not evidence appropriate social interactions. In a follow-up study of these children, there was little movement of the individuals from one group to another. Only a few of the socially impaired children became more sociable, but none became normally sociable.

The sociable children understood and used nonverbal communication at a level expected for their mental age, and when their language comprehension skills were comparable to a 20-month-old child, they all began to demonstrate some symbolic play. However, the socially impaired children were limited in symbolic play, regardless of their level of language comprehension, and had difficulty with nonverbal communication. Thus, social impairment, poor imaginary play, and communication problems generally co-occurred. In addition, this triad of problems was often associated with complex stereotyped movements.

The socially impaired group included all those children previously identified as having "early childhood psychosis." They differed, however, in their social behaviors. Some were aloof, others were passive, and others were "active but odd." Only rarely were children found who fit Kanner's original description of aloofness with some speech and complex repetitive routines (which require good motor skills). Most of the aloof children in Wing's study had no speech and had poor motor skills.

The triad of social impairment, communication problems, and poor imaginary play was related to low intelligence. Those children with histories of typical autistic children were most often found in the IQ range of 20 to 49. This finding is similar to that noted in prior studies of autistic children where 74% of preschool autistic children had IQ scores below 52 and only 2.6% had scores above 85 (De Myer et al., 1981). Performance scores are generally higher than verbal scores, and the discrepancy between performance and verbal scores is greater than for SLI children (Bartak, Rutter, & Cox, 1975). Generally the autistic children score best on perceptual-motor tasks [such as block design and object assembly (Rutter, 1968)]. Their IQ scores are relatively stable over time and do not change much even if social skills improve (M. Campbell, Hardesty, Breuer, & Polevoy, 1978; De Myer et al., 1981; Rutter, 1968). However, low intelligence does not explain the triad of impairments. Many retarded children are sociable—even those who are severely or profoundly retarded—and some autistic children have normal intelligence.

While at one time, explanations of autism focused on problems with parental interactions (e.g., Bettelheim, 1967), a number of studies have contradicted this view. For example, no differences have been found in comparisons of mothers of autistic children with mothers of SLI children (Cantwell, Baker, & Rutter, 1977; Cox, Rutter, Newman, & Bartak, 1975).

Most theorists now tend to organic explanations (e.g., Damasio & Mauer, 1978; De Myer et al., 1981; Rutter, 1978; Wing, 1981). A number of hypotheses have been suggested concerning specific areas of the brain that may be affected in autistic children either structurally or functionally (e.g., Damasio & Mauer, 1978; Rimland, 1962; Wetherby, Koegel, & Mendel, 1981), but as yet there is no clear direct evidence to support specific lesions or specific areas of dysfunction common to the syndrome. However, many mothers of autistic children have histories of troubled pregnancies and labor with these children, and autistic children show signs of neurological dysfunction and have minor physical abnormalities (suggesting problems in the first trimester of fetal life) (e.g., De Meyer et al., 1981; M. Campbell, Geller, Small, Petti, & Ferris, 1978). Computerized tomographic scans indicate abnormalities in the brains of a number of autistic individuals (e.g., Damasio, Mauer, Damasio, & Chui, 1980). Moreover, later epileptic fits occur in one-sixth of autistic children who have shown no earlier evidence of neurological defects, and the autistic syndrome is much like the clinical picture found in children after overt brain damage, such as encephalitis (Rutter, 1968).

Evidence for a genetic factor comes from studies of siblings of autistic children, in particular twins (see Silliman, Campbell, & Mitchell, in press, for a review). For example, if one twin is autistic, the likelihood of autism in the other twin is much higher among monozygotic twins (9 of 11) than among dizygotic twins (0 of 10) (Folstein & Rutter, 1977). Furthermore, in cases where autism was not found with the other monozygotic twin, early histories showed prenatal or perinatal injury to the autistic twin and not to the nonautistic twin, suggesting a possible multidetermined etiology. Even more striking was the high incidence (82%) of cognitive and linguistic impairment among the monozygotic twin siblings in contrast to that in the general population or among the dyzygotic twins (10%).

Prognosis

IQ is a good predictor of future functioning (M. Campbell, Geller, Small, Petti, and Ferris, et al., 1978; Rutter, 1968). While uneven IQ scores in early childhood often level off in adolescence, measured IQ levels remain stable, and those children who make the best social adjustment have IQs of at least 60 or 70. Both the course of language development and the time of onset are also important prognostic indicators. A history of regression in language development is a negative factor in terms of future prognosis (Swisher, Reichler, & Short, 1976). Likewise, unless there is a history of vocalizations during the first year of life, and the development of some useful speech before the age of 5 years, prognosis for eventual improvement in social conformity and adaptability is poor (Kanner & Eisenberg, 1956; Ruttenberg & Wolf, 1967). But not all children who talk early, who do not regress in language development, or who have IQs above 70 *do* make good adjustments. In general, withdrawal symptoms may decrease, but even as adults, the autistic individual remains lonely and aloof, unrelated to family except for the satisfaction of personal needs.

Language

A language disorder is an important part of the syndrome of autism. In fact, Wing (1972) stated that "unless there are marked problems with both spoken and non-spoken language the diagnosis cannot be made" (p. 2). In fact, it is the language and cognitive deficits that have been suggested as the primary deficits rather than the social problems (Rutter, 1968). Onset of speech is late in the autistic child. For those with IQs below 70, first words appear at a mean age of 4:7 and phrases at 6:5. Age of onset for autistic children with IQs above 70 is 2:6 for first word and 4:8 for phrases (Bartak & Rutter, 1976). However, the language disorder involves more than late onset. Differences in language development are seen in form, content, and use and in the interactions among these components.

Use.   Differences in the autistic child's use of language are among the more prominent features of the syndrome. Some of the differences in use may be related to knowledge of form. For example, deictic terms (i.e., terms that shift their meaning with the context, such as past tense markers, personal pronouns, and articles) are inappropriately used (Bartolucci & Albers, 1974, but see Geller, in preparation). Appropriate use of deictic terms involves both an awareness of listener needs and the effect of the context on the use of these forms.

Other differences in use are, however, less clearly tied to linguistic knowledge. As mentioned above, many of these children have difficulty with nonverbal communication as well as with vocal communication. Few of the children use gesture spontaneously at home, although they can produce and comprehend gesture to a limited extent on demand. Both their spontaneous use of gestures and their ability to perform on demand are at a lower level than that for SLI children of similar MLU and age (Bartak et al., 1975).

Communications in general are limited to immediate perceptions and satisfaction of immediate needs, such as requests for objects, food, or some change in the environment (Baltaxe & Simmons, 1975; Fay & Schuler, 1980; Layton, Strawson,

& Baker, 1981). The listener is rarely taken into account. For example, changes in topic are not signaled (Baltaxe, 1977). In addition, attention-getting devices are rarely used when these children begin talking, back-channel responses (i.e., responses that indicate the listener is following, such as a head nod or "um") are not given when another is talking, and many of the children talk incessantly without responding to a listener's questions or attempts to interrupt (Fay & Schuler, 1980). Few autistic children converse spontaneously or continue a conversation with linguistically contingent responses that are not imitations (Bartak et al., 1975) unless the prior utterance was a question (Hurtig, Enarud, & Tomblin, 1982). Questions asked by these children are rarely used to obtain information; they often seem to be used as a discourse device (e.g., a means of making contact) (Hurtig et al., 1982). Furthermore, autistic children make more inappropriate remarks than MLU-matched SLI children (Bartak et al., 1975) or MLU-matched mentally retarded children (M. Cunningham, 1968). Thus, many of the differences in use appear not to be attributable to level of language development, as measured by mean length of utterance.

However, autistic children were found to have more severe comprehension deficits than SLI children with similar MLUs (Bartak et al., 1975). Therefore, it is not clear how many of the differences in language use are attributable to knowledge of content/form interactions in contrast to social knowledge.

Form. The articulatory productions of autistic children are reportedly superior to those of MLU-matched SLI children (Bartak et al., 1975) and equivalent to those of mentally retarded children matched for mental age (Bartolucci, Pierce, Streiner, & Eppel, 1976). While there may be delays relative to chronological age, the development appears to follow a normal sequence, and the pattern of production is not noteworthy (Bartolucci et al., 1976). However, Needleman, Ritvo, and Freeman (1980) found "imprecise articulation" in a large proportion of autistic children.

In contrast, voice quality is apt to be unusual. It is frequently high-pitched with a monotone or singsong pattern. Loudness is not well monitored, and stress is often not pragmatically appropriate (Fay & Schuler, 1980). According to parent reports, babbling is limited and of odd quality in many autistic children (Bartak et al., 1975), and unlike normal or Down's syndrome children, autistic children imitate their own babbling but not that of other children (Ricks, 1975). Prelinguistic vocalizations also are different from the those of nonautistic children. While the vocalizations of nonautistic children (including Down's syndrome children) can be identified in terms of context (e.g., request, displeasure) by parents of other children, the vocalizations of autistic children can only be interpreted by their own parents (Ricks, 1975).

Form/Use Interactions. Repetition of the spoken utterances of others is frequent with autistic children and is referred to as *echolalia*. In some instances these repetitions immediately follow the prior utterance and are referred to as *immediate* echolalia; the children may copy the utterance of another exactly or make some change. In other instances, the repetition is separated in time from the original utterance and is referred to as *delayed* echolalia.

Immediate echolalia has been associated with lack of comprehension (Fay,

1969; Fay & Schuler, 1980) of the echoed utterance. At times it appears to be used for certain communicative functions such as affirmation or requests (Kanner, 1943; Prizant & Duchan, 1981). While the imitation of prior utterances is found among nonautistic children (e.g., Bloom, Lightbown, & Hood, 1975), the autistic child's imitations are more rigid (Shapiro, Roberts, & Fish, 1970). Just as for the nonautistic child, however, the frequency of these immediate imitations decreases as mean length of utterance increases beyond 1.9 (Shapiro, Chiarandini, & Fish, 1974) and as language becomes more complex (Howlin, 1982).

Delayed echolalia has also been associated with communicative functions (Fay & Schuler, 1980; Kanner, 1946; Prizant, 1983) such as requests, protests, or directives. However, there is no evidence to suggest that delayed echolalia is related to or derived from immediate echolalia. Rather, delayed echolalia appears to be an association of a unit of form, which is often a sentence, with an aspect of context (see Box 2-7 for examples). The aspect of context is not always one that is relevant to adults and makes many of the delayed echoes appear inappropriate; the utterances are often more related to some past experience that matches the child's current internal state or desire than to currently observable events. Thus, the classic example mentioned by Kanner, "Don't throw the dog off the balcony," was uttered by the child in many contexts where there was no dog or balcony, but when the child was about to do something wrong. The utterance was first spoken in an attempt to stop the child from throwing a toy dog off a balcony and was apparently used by him after that when he was tempted to throw something.

Content/Form Interactions. While the utterances of autistic children are generally syntactically correct, there are often errors in semantic constraints (Simmons & Baltaxe, 1975). The children's concept of reference, or their labeling of objects and events, seems more readily established and is developmentally more advanced than their coding of relationships. Their understanding of functional relations is weak and late in development (Baltaxe & Simmons, 1975), and the productive use of relational words, such as prepositions, is rigid. Sentences are often used as a label for a situation or event (Baltaxe & Simmons, 1975) rather than as a means to express relationships among objects and events. Further evidence of problems with content/form interactions is found in the private metaphors and neologisms the children often use (Kanner, 1946) and with some of the children's ability to read well aloud without comprehension of what they are reading (referred to as hyperlexia). In reading, as in speech, reference, or word identification, is developmentally superior to sentence comprehension (Bartak et al., 1975).

Variation. The above descriptions should not be taken to suggest that there is one syndrome of language behaviors among children diagnosed as autistic. Rather, variation is the rule here as with other children learning language. Two clusters of language patterns emerged in the language of the psychotic children studied by M. Cunningham (1968). The children were all verbal and included children diagnosed as autistic, as schizophrenic, or as psychotic but not autistic and in whom symptoms were evident in early childhood. In one cluster were children who used longer sentences, asked questions, and were not excessively echolalic. The second cluster consisted of children who had shorter sentences, poor pronunciation, peculiar intonation patterns, incorrect or inconsistent sentence structure, and a large

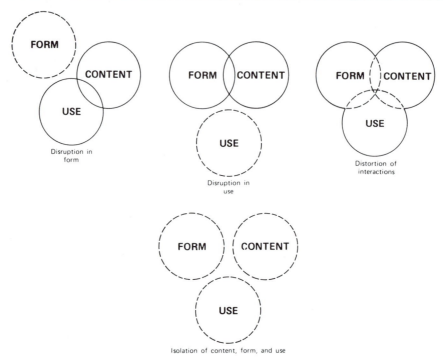

FIGURE 4-2   Disruptions in Content/Form/Use Interactions Found in Children Categorized as Emotionally Disturbed

amount of echolalia; these children rarely asked questions or used personal pronouns. This dichotomy did not correlate well with psychiatric diagnosis or age of onset.

Three groups of "severely disturbed" children were defined by Shapiro, Chiarandini, and Fish (1974) on the basis of categorizations of form and use of language. One group was made up of children who were severely retarded in the development of form. The remaining children were divided on the basis of their communicativeness. Group 2 demonstrated echoing and contextually inappropriate utterances so frequently that less than 75% of their utterances were communicative. The children in Group 3 differed from those in Group 2 in that greater than 75% of their utterances were communicative. Children's placement within a group was highly correlated across three points in time, and the authors concluded that the groups defined a spectrum of deviant language patterns.

Summary.   The patterns that emerge may be described in terms of the disruptions in content/form/use interactions discussed in Chapter 2 (see Figure 4-2): disruptions in form, disruptions in use, distorted interactions of content, form, and use, and isolation of the three components (the children who utter stereotypic forms for no apparent function). In general, language form appears better developed than the interaction of form with content and use. The wide diversity of behaviors that is manifested by children who are labeled emotionally disturbed or autistic negates the usefulness of these diagnoses as descriptions of specific language pathologies or as an explanation of the language disorders. Within the category of autism there appear to be qualitative differences in the type of language behaviors that are observed.

Other Syndromes

While the four syndromes discussed above are those more commonly associated with childhood language disorders, language disorders are also a symptom of other clinical categories (e.g., cerebral palsy, cleft palate, fetal alcohol syndrome). In most of these cases, language skills have not been considered a major differentiating factor; often, problems with language are a part of general retardation. One rather substantial group of children is at high risk for speech and language problems and must be of concern to the speech-language pathologist—children born prematurely and with low weight at birth. The chance of survival for infants born before full term is increasing; however, it is not clear what subtle language and learning problems may result. The results of the Collaborative Perinatal Project of NINCDS (Lassman, Fisch, Vetter, & LaBenz, 1980) found that premature and low-birth-weight children were at a higher risk than other children for problems with articulation, language comprehension, and language production. Premature infants with respiratory distress (a problem with almost of one-third of premature infants) were late in the acquisition of language, remained longer in the single-word-utterance period, were lower in volubility (i.e., number of utterances per unit of time), and had a lower receptive vocabulary than normal-term infants although they had "passed" the *Denver Developmental Screening Test* (Frankenburg & Dodd, 1969) and had IQ scores over 80 (Hubatch, Johnson, Kistler, Burns, & Moneka, 1985). It is possible that a stimulating home environment may help in reducing problems (Siegel, 1982), but further longitudinal research is needed. In the meantime, it is probably wise to follow such children and to initiate stimulation programs where such programs are practical and acceptable and can be carried out without creating alarm or expectations of failure.

In other cases (as acquired aphasia and learning disabilities) problems with language are major symptoms within the syndrome. These two categories are discussed below along with the language-learning problems that some blind children experience early in life.

Acquired Aphasia

In contrast to SLI (sometimes referred to as developmental aphasia), children with acquired aphasia have histories of normal language development. Loss of language is usually associated with cortical lesions or seizure activity.

As with adults, aphasia is more common in children when lesions occur in the left hemisphere. Right-handed children with left-sided lesions are, in fact, slightly more likely to have aphasia (73%) than right-handed adults with left-sided lesions (63%), and the frequency is even higher (85%) for children under 10 years of age. Right-sided lesions in right-handed children are not frequently reported in the literature, but when reported, the incidence of aphasia is less (14%) and the aphasia is very mild. Similarly, the prevalence of aphasia when right-sided lesions occur in left-handed children is less frequent (50%) than when left-sided lesions occur in left-handed children (83%). However, the information on left-handed children is based on a smaller number of children. These prevalence figures are taken from Hecaen (1983).

Hecaen also reports that the symptoms of acquired aphasia in children are somewhat different from adult symptoms and appear to be related to both lesion localization and the rapidity of the lesion onset. Anterior lesions are more likely to result in language difficulties of all sorts (including auditory and visual-verbal comprehension) than are temporal lesions; mutism (or complete suppression of speech) is most often associated with rapid onset. Disorders of auditory comprehension occur in about one-third of the cases reported, and tend to disappear rapidly and completely. Likewise, reading disorders are common in the early periods, and also disappear quickly and completely. In contrast, naming difficulties are frequent (44%) and tend to persist; writing disorders are even more common (63%) and persist the longest (see also Woods & Carey, 1978). Excessive talking and paraphasia are rare, but difficulties with mathematics are frequently reported.

Recovery appears to be related to the size or bilaterality of the lesions. While Lenneberg (1967) had suggested that both hemispheres could develop language until puberty, this notion has been questioned in terms of age (e.g., Krashen, 1975) and more recently as perhaps existing at all once language has developed (Hecaen, 1983; Satz & Bullard-Bates, 1981). In fact, according to Hecaen, the evidence suggests an early cerebral lateralization in the left hemisphere that may be of a more diffuse nature than found in the adult. If this is the case, "recovery of language capability after early brain damage might depend more on the tissue adjacent to the lesion in the left hemisphere than on cerebral tissue in a symmetrical region of the opposite hemisphere" (Hecaen, 1983, p. 586).

The spontaneous spoken language of children with unilaterally acquired left- and right-hemisphere lesions was described by Aram, Ekelman, and Whitaker (1986). In comparison with nonlesioned controls and children with right-hemisphere lesions, children with left-hemisphere lesions produced less complex and fewer *wh* questions, produced fewer complex sentences with more errors on those sentences, and had lower MLUs. No differences were found between right- and left-hemisphere-lesioned subjects in use of grammatical markers, conjunctions, or errors on simple sentences; in most cases, however, the subjects did less well than controls. These results were interpreted as support for the importance of the left hemisphere in syntactic processing—particularly, processing of complex syntax.

Acquired aphasia secondary to convulsive disorder results in different symptomology. The information presented here is taken from a review of the literature by J. Miller, Campbell, Chapman, and Weismer (1984). Difficulty comprehending oral speech is usually the first symptom and the one most commonly associated with this syndrome. Expression difficulties follow later, with jargon and abnormal prosodic patterns sometimes occurring. These symptoms are apt to co-occur and to precede or follow the onset of seizures, and for more than 80% of the children they persist for at least 6 months. Onset is usually abrupt, but in 25% of the cases reported it was gradual. Aphasia related to seizure activity is twice as likely to occur in males as females between the ages of 1 and 13, with most occurrences between 3 and 7 years of age. This syndrome appears to include a diverse pattern of language behaviors and a diverse, and not well understood, set of etiologies.

Learning Disabilities

The National Joint Committee for Learning Disabilities agreed that the term *learning disabilities* was a generic term referring to a heterogeneous population who exhibited difficulties with oral language, written language, mathematics, and/or reasoning abilities that are not a result of some other handicapping condition (Hammill, Leigh, McNutt, & Larsen, 1981). Children labeled as *learning-disabled* constitute the largest enrollment of any category of exceptional children in our schools°, and this number has increased in the past decade; prevalence estimates range from 2 to 20% of the school population (Kirk & Chalfant, 1984).

If the upper range of these estimates is accurate, then learning disabilities is a problem that is reaching epidemic proportions. However, Kirk and Chalfant report results of a survey of teachers of learning-disabled students that suggests that at least 30% of the children so classified do not belong in that category. The syndrome is basically defined by exclusion of known etiologies for learning problems (e.g., hearing loss, retardation, poor instruction)—thus classification depends on the success of identifying such other handicaps. Perhaps motivational factors and environmental factors are most difficult to assess given current assessment procedures. For example, in some cultures the language of the home is so different from the language of the school that without careful instruction in school these differences may interfere with learning to read (see, for example, Westby, 1985). Without rich knowledge of the child's home environment, such differences may not be discovered and the child may be assumed to have some intrinsic learning deficit. Furthermore, definition of a problem is often defined by discrepancy of reading scores from IQ scores. Not only is the amount of discrepancy necessary still open to question, but the use of discrepancy scores has been challenged (see Rudel, 1985; Silliman, in press). Thus, the method of assessing and defining the problem as well may make the syndrome appear more prevalent than it actually is. Finally, by all accounts the population is diverse (e.g., Lahey, 1981; Rudel, 1985; Silliman, in press; Wallach & Liebergott, 1984). Using neuropsychological tests, Mattis, French, and Rapin (1975) identified at least three subgroups. Denkla (1985) found differences in motor tasks on learning-disabled children with and without accompanying attentional deficits. Prevalence figures are, therefore, probably describing a wide variety of syndromes that manifest themselves in what was at one time referred to as underachievement.

As noted earlier, the syndrome of learning disabilities closely resembles that of specific language impairment. Definitions of both learning disabilities and SLI state that the language-learning problems are not the result of sensory impairment, motor problems, mental retardation, emotional problems, or environmental deprivation. In many definitions the two syndromes overlap. The federal definition in Public Law 94-142 (1976) states that "the term [learning disabilities] includes such conditions as perceptual handicaps, brain injury, minimal brain

---

° According to a recent article in *Asha* (July 1987, p. 9) they account for just over 42% of the handicapped children being served under Public Law 94-142.

dysfunction, dyslexia, and *developmental aphasia.*"° In this text, *SLI* will be used to refer to difficulties in learning auditory-vocal language skills that are normally achieved by exposure to caregiver interactions and without direct conscious instruction; the term *learning disabilities* will be used to refer to difficulties with academic language skills that are normally learned through schooling. In both instances, these terms refer to problems that exist despite what appears to be normal intelligence, normal peripheral hearing, no severe emotional problems or environmental deprivation, and adequate input or instruction. In this section we will focus on those children who have difficulties with the learning of written language. Such children constitute 60–70% of the children labeled as learning disabled (Kirk & Chalfant, 1984).

Factors associated with learning disabilities include motor problems, attentional deficits, and language disorders. Motor problems are evidenced by difficulty with rapid alternating finger movements, difficulties copying despite good perception of copying accuracy (Denkla, 1985; Rudel, 1985), and inaccurate productions of polysyllabic words (Kamhi & Catts, 1986). Attentional deficits, usually accompanied by hyperactivity, are frequently associated with learning disabilities; however, a substantial proportion of children are classified as learning-disabled without accompanying attentional problems (see Denkla, 1985; Simon, 1985). In addition, deficits in oral language performance are frequently reported in populations of learning-disabled children (Donahue, 1986; Vellutino, 1977; and see below). While motor and attentional deficits reportedly improve with age, increasing differences are found in language scores between learning-disabled children and age-matched peers (Rudel, 1985).

Clearly, children who have difficulty learning early language skills (e.g., SLI children) are at risk for academic learning problems. Retrospective follow-up studies of children with language problems in the preschool years report that these children often have difficulties with reading and other academic subjects in school (see Chapter 3 and Maxwell & Wallach, 1984, for a review of some of these studies). Furthermore, a greater percentage of poor readers have a history of delayed onset of speech than is found in the general population (Rutter, Tizard, & Whitmore, 1970, as cited by Mattis et al., 1975). The fact that children who have difficulty with written language continue to exhibit difficulties with auditory-vocal language skills in the school years has led many to suggest a verbal deficit may be responsible for the problems with learning written language (e.g., I. Liberman, 1985; Vellutino, 1977).

A number of studies have pointed to a word-finding or naming problem with these children (e.g., Denkla & Rudel, 1976a, 1976b; Denkla, Rudel, & Broman, 1981; Johnson & Myklebust, 1967; Mattis et al., 1975; Rubin & Liberman, 1983; Wiig, Semel, & Nystrom, 1982; Wolf, 1986). Naming problems refer to a child's difficulty naming pictures or objects that can be identified (thus suggesting that the difficulty in naming is not a result of a vocabulary deficit). Successful retrieval of words requires an accurate initial phonetic representation and an efficient

---

° Italics added for emphasis. Recall that *developmental aphasia* is a term used to refer to the syndrome of SLI; and SLI in preschool children is often considered to be an early manifestation of a learning disability (National Joint Committee on Learning Disabilities, 1987).

short-term storage of this representation (Rubin & Liberman, 1983), as well as efficient semantic organization of lexical items.

Difficulties in naming are evidenced by inaccurate productions of names of pictures as well as by a slower rate in the production of accurate names. Inappropriate names that are semantically related to the target word (e.g., *stairs* for *escalator*) or circumlocutions (i.e., talking about the object but not giving its name) account for the majority of errors; other errors are phonetic in nature, generally capturing some phonological aspect of the target word such as its initial consonant and/or number of syllables (Rubin & Liberman, 1983). A high correlation is generally found between accuracy of oral naming and skill with written language (e.g., reading and spelling skills). In fact, poor naming ability in kindergarten children has been considered a predictor of reading failure in later years (Jansky & de Hirsch, 1972, as cited in Denkla & Rudel, 1976a). In addition to providing the wrong label for pictures, children with learning disabilities and specific language disorders are often slower to name objects, numbers, colors, and letters than their age-matched peers although slightly faster than language-matched peers (e.g., Denkla & Rudel, 1976a, 1976b; Kail & Leonard, 1986). Again, this measure of naming skill correlates with reading ability. Rate of response on confrontation naming best discriminates boys with learning problems related to reading from boys with other types of learning problems (i.e., problems with writing, math, attention, etc.) (Denkla et al., 1981).

Evidence of problems with content/form interactions is not limited to lexical tasks. Learning-disabled children also have difficulty with comprehension and production of complex syntactic structures (e.g., Donahue, Pearl, & Bryan, 1982; Maxwell & Wallach, 1984; Wiig & Semel, 1976) as well as with use of morphological inflections (Donahue, 1986b). Some authors have related the children's problems with complex syntactic constructions to their problems with finding words (e.g., Kail & Leonard, 1986). In turn, problems with syntax and word finding apparently lead to difficulties with language use.

The spontaneously generated oral narratives of learning-disabled children are shorter and contain fewer complete episodes than those of age-matched non-learning-disabled children (Roth & Spekman, 1986). In addition, learning-disabled children are less likely to include complete orientations (minor settings, in the terms of Roth and Spekman) and information about the internal states of the characters (responses and plans) as well as attempts at reaching goals. Story recall and inferencing skills are more like those of younger children with similar vocabulary comprehension than of their age-matched peers (Crais & Chapman, 1987).

Some evidence suggests that learning-disabled children are less adept at using alternative forms for communicating messages that take into account listener perspective, status, and feelings and less likely to request clarification from other speakers (Donahue, 1986b). Because many of these adaptations do not involve more complex syntax or vocabulary, Donahue has suggested that learning-disabled children exhibit social deficits as well as language deficits. It is, of course, difficult to sort out whether a history of difficulties in using content/form interactions may result in such problems with use and in social deficits or whether such problems with use (and perhaps content/form interactions) are the result of social deficits. Finally, learning-disabled children evidence problems with metalinguistic skills.

They are less able to segment language into words, syllables, and phonemes (e.g., Kamhi & Catts, 1986) and to identify errors in syntax (Kamhi & Koenig, 1985) than age-matched children who are not having difficulty learning to read.

Certainly the learning-disabled population is no more homogeneous than any of the other populations that have been described in this chapter. There have been many attempts to define subgroups. Some have been based on neuropsychological tests (e.g., Mattis et al., 1975), while others are more related to differences in processing skills (see, e.g., Fletcher & Morris, 1986). In terms of language, Donahue (1986b) has suggested that at least three groups may exist: those who have obvious language-learning problems in preschool; those who have not been identified in preschool and whose casual conversational skills are adequate, but who have subtle language problems as measured by structured tests and rapid word retrieval; and those whose oral language problems may well be the result of less exposure to written language because of difficulties with reading. But even subgroups do not describe the specific language problems of these children. Again we find that information necessary for improving language skills must come from careful description of each child. What the research does emphasize is that casual conversation is not an effective way of determining whether the learning-disabled child has the auditory-vocal language skills necessary for proficiency with written language.

Blindness

While blind individuals do not necessarily have a language disorder, there are some interesting patterns that emerge in their early language learning. At first thought, it may seem that vision would play a small part in language learning. Yet many blind children are late in the development of vocabulary, syntax, and the use of words to communicate wants. Indeed, they are also late in walking, in the development of object concepts and symbolic play, and in the use of their hands to explore their environment (Fraiberg, 1977). Fraiberg also observed that their spontaneous vocalizations were limited and that there tended to be little child-initiated dialogue between caregiver and child.

When speech does develop, many similarities are found in the early development of language. The meanings coded by single-word utterances and early syntactic constructions appear to be the same as for normal children (Landau & Gleitman, 1985). While the onset of syntactic constructions is late, rapid advances are made so that MLU is similar by the age of 3 (Landau & Gleitman, 1985). In fact, other than some difficulty learning the auxiliary forms of English and the delay of onset, Landau and Gleitman report remarkable similarities between the blind children they studied and the literature on sighted children, including the use of "sighted" verbs such as *look*.

Others have reported more differences, particularly in the use of language, but some also in form. In the early stages of language learning, some young blind children are apt to display many routine phrases, considerable echolalia, pronominal reversals, flat intonation, articulation difficulties, and a limited range of prepositions and questions—in general, their language lacks creativity (Fraiberg, 1977; Urwin, 1976, 1984). According to Urwin, language is first used in self-play and only later in communicative fashion. Phrases are associated with some aspect of context, and so expressions like "cuppa tea yeah" will be uttered to ask for a drink and "bathtime" will be uttered whenever water is heard. In some ways this pattern of early language learning resembles that discussed under autism; yet these children usually develop into loving social individuals, and language skills eventually seem indistinguishable from those of sighted individuals.

Early infancy is not an easy time for socialization between caregiver and child. The early social signals most mothers expect to receive are absent—blind infants do not gesture to objects in the environment, do not lift up their arms to be picked up, do not smile as mother looks or enters the room, and do not gaze at objects with mother in joint attention (Fraiberg, 1977; Urwin, 1976). Fraiberg worked with mothers to help them understand their children's apparent lack of affective input and to teach them how to read communicative cues that the child may be giving, such as finger movements. While most blind children eventually learn language, many blind infants and their parents might benefit from support and intervention in the early years (Fraiberg, 1977; Urwin, 1984).

The Uniqueness of Clinical Categories

Having spent some time discussing the syndromes that define the categories associated with childhood language disorders, it is important to ask whether these categories are reliable groupings and how they contribute to our understanding and education of these children. First let us explore the uniqueness of the categories.

Unquestionably, some children fit the classical descriptions of behavior patterns associated with each category. However, it is rare to find many children who clearly fit into only one category. "The same child may receive four or five different diagnoses, as successive clinics diagnose the case in terms of their special area of interest and experience" (Kessler, 1966, p. 260). For example, as many as 80% of the SLI and autistic children studied by Bartak et al. (1975) were diagnosed as deaf at some time. Considerable overlap among categories was found by Needleman et al. (1980) when comparing language behaviors, such as echolalia, and communicative use.

Why should this be so? For one reason, precipitating factors themselves are not mutually exclusive; they can and do easily coexist with one another. Just as a child may be both blind and deaf, a child may also have both a peripheral hearing loss and a central nervous system dysfunction. Multiple handicaps certainly account for some of those children who are not easy to place within an etiological category.

Another reason why the same children may be categorized with more than one label is that the manifestation of a dysfunction can be influenced by the way in which the environment interacts with a developing organism. A child who is nonverbal, for whatever reason, may well show signs of emotional disturbance and mental retardation by virtue of the reactions that are, or are not, received from other individuals. It is usually not possible to separate cause-and-effect relations when a child is seen for diagnosis. Such children, then, fit the syndromes associated with more than one category and are prone to different diagnoses by different persons.

A final reason why the same child can be diagnosed differently is that it is difficult to associate certain behaviors with only one kind of dysfunction. A child who is neurologically limited in the amount of information that can be processed from the environment may well attempt to control the amount of surrounding stimulation by "turning off" or "tuning out." Thus, what can be described as *autistic* behavior (reducing contact with the environment) may, for one child, be a useful coping mechanism that was motivated by difficulties in dealing with information from the environment. For another child, however, and for other reasons, the same behavior may be motivated by a desire to withdraw from and avoid interaction with other persons. "The more one investigates child behavior, the more one realizes that identical behavior can be the result of radically different causes" (Kessler, 1966, p. 287). For various reasons, then, it is difficult, if not impossible, to agree on a diagnosis for many children.

Are the clinical categories in fact unique or independent of each other? In an attempt to empirically verify the independence of diagnostic categories used with language-disordered children, Rosenthal, Eisenson, and Luckau (1972) examined the medical, psychological, and language evaluations of 82 children who had been assigned with "high reliability" to diagnostic categories [such as mentally retarded, severe hearing impairment, neurologically handicapped/aphasic, maturational lag (organic), and autistic]. A cluster analysis of the 32 variables derived from the records yielded only two clusters—one cluster included the mentally retarded and autistic children and the other included the children in the hearing-impaired, aphasic, and maturational-lag categories. The factors that separated the two clusters were primarily measures of nonverbal intelligence rather than medical, language, or other psychological measures. The authors concluded that the categories were "neither unique nor homogeneous with respect to measurements routinely collected in the course of clinical evaluation" (p. 135). Not only, therefore, is there a problem in placing a child within only one category, but analyses of the data used to make diagnoses do not support the uniqueness of the categories. But even when a fit is readily agreed on and the categorical placement does describe a child in comparison with other children, it is necessary to consider whether the category *explains* the child's language disorder.

The Explanatory Value of Clinical Categories

The category in which a child is placed (i.e., the diagnosis) is determined by descriptions of behaviors felt to be associated with dysfunctions of sensory systems, nervous systems, mental abilities, or emotional interactions. The implication is often that each category represents a precipitating factor. The representation of the precipitating factor is, however, generally inferred from behavior; the factor itself is not tangible or directly observable. For example, it is not possible to observe the inner ear or the central nervous system directly in a diagnostic session, and so their dysfunction is generally inferred from the individual's behavioral responses to certain tasks. Verification of an etiology, by other than the behavioral manifestations that were used to define the category in the first place, is rarely possible—with some exceptions such as the use of impedance audiometry as an objective measure of certain types of hearing loss (Jerger, Burney, Mauldin, &

Crump, 1974) or postmortem examination of brain tissue (W. M. Landau, Gold-stein, & Kleffner, 1960).

In the future, more sophisticated procedures and methods of analyses may assist in validation of all categories that are attributed to organic dysfunctions. At present, however, most statements about organic dysfunction, particularly state-ments about central nervous system dysfunction as a cause of a language disorder, are highly inferential. For example, EEG tracings have not clearly differentiated among categories where the precipitating factor was felt to be some central ner-vous system dysfunction (Goldstein, Landau, & Kleffner, 1958; Kessler, 1966). Thus, a diagnostic label that infers central nervous system dysfunction, such as developmental aphasia or specific language impairment, represents and is a short-hand description of behavioral patterns—patterns that include a language disorder.

The assignment of different labels to different children does not mean that the cause or precipitating factor of any of the observed behaviors, including the lan-guage behaviors, has been isolated and identified. Inadequate language skills are an important part, if not the major part, of the syndromes that define autism, mental retardation, and SLI. It is intuitively unreasonable and unsatisfactory to say that a child is autistic because of certain behaviors and then to state that the reason the child behaves in those ways is because he or she is autistic. This circularity of reasoning results when certain behaviors lead to a diagnostic label, and then the diagnosis is used to explain the behaviors.

We are left then with global categories that give us a broad indication of certain patterns of behavior. Even when a fit is readily agreed on, the categorical place-ment does not explain the language disorder—one does not know the reason for a language disorder when one knows the categorical label assigned to a child. Why are they used? Are they perhaps useful in the educational management of the child?

The Usefulness of Categories for Educational Management

Because many schools and private facilities have programs designed for neurologi-cally impaired, learning-disabled, SLI, deaf, or mentally retarded children, and because much funding of special services is tied to categorical labels, placement within a treatment program is often dependent on such categorical classification. In such cases, a categorical label must be assigned to each child before admitting the child to any program—and the label determines the program to which the child is admitted. Are the programs unique and actually different from one another in terms of what they provide for the supposedly different children who are assigned to them? Usually the distinctions among such programs exist more in title than in content, which is not surprising, considering that what a child with a language problem needs to learn about language is precisely what the non-lan-guage-impaired child needs to learn about language at some point in development. The model language is the same for all. At present there is little reason to suspect that the sequence in which that model is achieved does, or should, differ for different groups of children.

Although the clinical categories do not specify what language behaviors should be emphasized in intervention, the orientation does stress observing behaviors that may provide information about how language intervention should be presented. Information about a child's hearing, social interactions, play behavior, and conceptual development is important in planning procedures to be used in facilitating language learning. Unfortunately, the categorical label itself abstracts this information and too often decreases the understanding of the child by making the child fit a preconceived notion of the classic syndrome.

An additional danger in the use of categorical labels to define children and their problems for educational management is the function it may serve as a self-fulfilling prophecy. Children are often treated in certain ways because of the label applied to them. Some educational and clinical programs are closed to children because of one or another diagnostic label, not because of the child's success or failure within the program. Parents and teachers expect certain behaviors of children who are retarded, emotionally disturbed, or neurologically impaired. Expectancy is an important element in learning. Thus, while many children do manifest common behavior patterns, seeking to categorize children according to etiological syndromes is rarely useful to educators or clinicians interested in developing language skills. Careful description of the child's behaviors is more important in determining what and how the child will learn.

To say that the categorical orientation is not currently useful for educational management is not to say it has no value at all. Nor is it to say that we should not be concerned with discovering etiological factors. Rather, the attempt to define groups of children with similar patterns of behavior is an important research topic that may lead to better understanding of language learning in general and language disorders in particular. The current groupings may, or may not, be the most appropriate, and certainly better descriptions of language behaviors are in order. Such research has theoretical implications and may have clinical and educational implications in the future. Eventual understanding of etiology is important for the development of prevention programs.

Summary

The categorical orientation focuses on the primary cause of the language disorder, with the resulting clinical categories of deafness, mental retardation, specific language impairment, and autism. The categories that have been formed represent dysfunction of one or another of the factors thought to be necessary for the development of language (i.e., an intact sensory system, adequate cognitive function, an intact central nervous system, and appropriate psychosocial development). This orientation to precipitating factors has had a major influence on diagnosis, on placement within educational programs, on funding for educational programs, and on research having to do with the nature of language disorders.

The children placed in the clinical categories are not homogeneous. Furthermore, the supposed etiologies of a language disorder are rarely reversible without programs directed to the symptoms (i.e., the language itself). The behaviors of each child, viewed in terms of some ultimate goal (as effective communication or the learning of specific communicative interactions), determine the content of an intervention program. Certain other factors (e.g., emotional and physical factors) must be considered in all learning whether they were the factors precipitating difficulty in learning or not. Thus, the categorical orientation has not been particularly useful for educational or clinical management, and in the past two decades, less time has been spent on determining such categorical placement than was done earlier.

However, it is through such subgrouping of children that we may eventually come to learn more about factors that effect language learning in all children. Eventually, this may lead to a better understanding, and perhaps prevention, of language-learning difficulties. The categorical orientation has considerable heuristic value, particularly if the defining syndromes are gradually changed (and subdivided) to incorporate more sophisticated descriptions of both linguistic and nonlinguistic behaviors.

Suggested Readings

Ceci, S. (Ed.). (1986). *Handbook of cognitive, social, and neuropsychological aspects of learning disabilities.* Hillsdale, NJ: Erlbaum.

Fay, W. H., & Schuler, A. L. (Eds.). (1980). *Emerging language in autistic children.* Baltimore: University Park Press.

Fowler, A. (in press). The development of language structure in children with Down syndrome. In D. Cicchetti and M. Beeghly (Eds.), *Down syndrome: The developmental perspective.* N.Y.: Cambridge University Press.

Fraiberg, S. (1977). *Insights from the blind.* London: Souvenir Press.

Hecean, H. (1983). Acquired aphasia in children: Revisited. *Neuropsychologia, 21,* 581–587.

Holland, A. (1984). *Language disorders in children.* San Diego: College-Hill Press.

Kretschmer, R. R., & Kretschmer, L. W. (1978). *Language development and intervention with the hearing impaired.* Baltimore: University Park Press.

Landau, B., & Gleitman, L. (1985). *Language and experience: Evidence from the blind child.* Cambridge, MA: Harvard University Press.

Rosenberg, S. (Ed.). (in press). *Advances in applied psycholinguistics, Vol. 1: Disorders of first-language development.* New York: Cambridge University Press.

Rutter, M., & Schopler, E. (1978). *Autism: A reappraisal of concepts and treatment.* New York: Plenum.

Swisher, L. (1985). Language disorders in children. In J. Darby (Ed.), *Speech and language evaluation in neurology: Childhood disorders.* New York: Grune & Stratton, pp. 33–96.

Torgesen, J. K., & Wong, B. Y. (Eds.). (1986). *Psychological and educational perspectives on learning disabilities.* New York: Academic Press, 1986.

Wallach, G., & Butler, K. (1984). *Language learning disabilities in school-age children.* Baltimore: Williams & Wilkins.

5

The Language-Disordered Child Viewed From a Specific-Abilities Orientation

Another major approach to language-disordered children has focused on specific abilities and processes that are felt necessary for the development and use of
language. For some, a specific-abilities orientation has had heuristic value for

looking at children who are considered specific language-impaired, learning-disabled, or autistic. Research efforts have tried to explain their language-learning problems by looking for breakdowns at various levels of processing—most such attempts have centered on perceptual processing.

For others, the specific-abilities orientation has served as a model for clinical assessment and educational management. Assessment has been geared to describing the specific abilities hypothesized as being necessary for language learning and use; results of assessment have been used not only as a means of explaining the problem, but also as a means of determining the goals of intervention. Intervention goals derived from such assessment have generally related to strengthening weaknesses that were found. This orientation, which became popular in the 1960s, was a shift from interest in factors that may have precipitated the language-learning problem to descriptions of the child's present skills. It also represented a shift from a main focus on which category best fit the child (i.e., the categorical orientation that was concerned with interchild comparisons) to a focus on how various abilities of a particular child were like the same child's other abilities (i.e., an intrachild comparison).

In this chapter, certain applications of this orientation are described. First, certain abilities commonly associated with language disorders in children are discussed. Following this, some more direct applications of the orientation to assessment and educational management are presented and evaluated in terms of their value for facilitating language learning. Two major challenges connect the discussion throughout the chapter. First, questions are raised about the assumption that poor performance on any of the measures used to infer these abilities can be considered as an explanation of language-learning difficulties. It is argued that the model of serial processing abilities is probably not valid and that other factors, such as knowledge of what is being processed, could account for performance on measures of the specific abilities. In some cases, an alternative model based on utilization of attentional capacity (e.g., Case, 1985) will be proposed. Second, and following from this, questions are raised concerning the assumption that information about specific abilities, as now assessed, aids us in planning educational programs for language-disordered and/or learning-disabled children.

Specific Abilities Related to Language Learning

Various models have been proposed to represent the cognitive processes involved in language learning and use; each attempts to get inside the human mind and explain *how* an observable stimulus elicits an observable response.

Most of the models of language processes that have been proposed include at least three major components: a perceptual component that involves the initial processing of the input signal, a conceptual or representational component that involves meaning and symbolic thinking, and an output component that has to do with planning and command of motor responses. In addition, some models include a feedback component. The perceptual component generally includes signal recognition, discrimination, retention, and intersensory integration. Some of the research related to the perceptual component has been concerned with the perception of linguistic stimuli; other research has dealt with nonlinguistic stimuli. The conceptual component includes the association of meaning with the input or output signal, and the use, or manipulation, of symbols to carry out various tasks. Problem-solving tasks such as analogies and similarities have often been used to evaluate or measure the function of this component. The output component includes a plan for the production of the motor response, for example, the speech signal. Most models also stress the independence of modalities (e.g., visual and auditory). The arrangement and ordering of the different components or elements vary from one model to another, but many schemes suggest some degree of linear processing (e.g., Osgood's 1957 model of language). (See Figures 5-1 and 5-2 for examples of two models.)

The levels and components of language processing are often discussed and schematized as though they were discrete and separate from each other, but it would seem that they are actually and necessarily interdependent. Such interdependence among the components is a large factor in the interpretation of much of the research having to do with specific abilities and with the attempts that have been made to apply such information to clinical situations.

Specific Abilities Related to Language Disorders

In an article emphasizing the importance of considering specific abilities in relation to language disorders, Hardy (1965) pointed out the importance of knowing the modalities of input that are intact when planning remediation for children with language disorders. Considerable research within the specific-abilities orientation has focused on the perceptual processing of auditory stimuli. The interest in the processing of auditory signals spurred the development of a number of tests of auditory perception and the viewing of etiology of language problems in terms of a child's inability to process information in the environment—particularly the inability to process verbal stimuli. Much of the research has considered specific abilities in relation to various clinical syndromes. That is, deficits in auditory processing, or the search for other specific-ability dysfunctions, have been related to the clinical categories that were discussed in the preceding chapter.

Categories of particular interest are the populations of children who may be labeled *specific language-impaired* (SLI), *learning-disabled* (LD), or autistic (in earlier research these categories may have been referred to by different names; e.g., SLI and LD may have been called *brain-damaged* or *minimal brain dysfunction,* while autism may have been included with childhood schizophrenia or with emotional disturbance). To be discussed in this section are auditory memory, the use of temporal cues, and the processing of multisensory input.

In examining this research it is important to keep in mind how the child's knowledge of language may have influenced the findings. Unfortunately, this factor is not always considered in the design of studies. Input does not impinge on a blank or static mechanism. Processing is done to some knowledge structure. It is difficult to separate any aspect of processing from knowledge of what is being processed (see, for example, Chi, 1983; Keil, 1984; Rees, 1973b, 1981). It is most likely that when tasks that measure perceptual function use language as stimuli (whether it be digits, single words, or sentences), the tasks are actually a test of the children's knowledge of language rather than a measure of some independent

FIGURE 5-1 A Clinical Model of Communication Processes

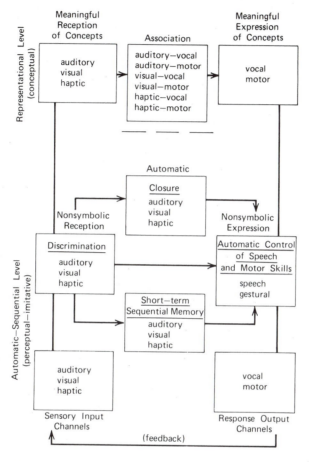

This adaptation of Osgood's model (Kirk and Kirk, 1971) illustrates linear processing from perceptual to conceptual and an independence of the perceptual level from the conceptual level. As do many models, this model suggests that the conceptual level can be bypassed—note the automatic loop (the perceptual-imitative level).

auditory-perceptual skills. Whenever units of language are used as the stimuli to be processed, the question arises about whether perceptual dysfunction, identified by response to such stimuli, is a cause or a reflection of a language disorder. (Recall the earlier discussion about the interdependence of levels of processing.)

Auditory Sequential Memory

Auditory memory span has been one of the most studied specific abilities. It is logical that to learn and use language, one must be able to hold in mind units of stimuli long enough to process their relation to other units and to the context.

FIGURE 5-2 *An Operational Diagram of the Levels of Function in the Central Nervous System*

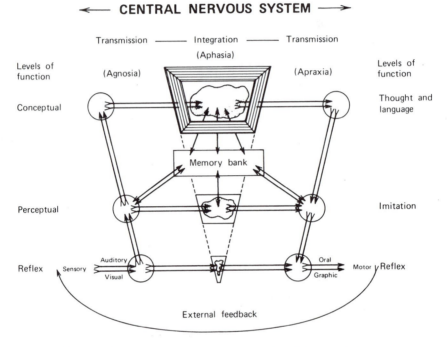

In contrast to the model by Kirk and Kirk (1971, in Figure 5-1) the model by Wepman, Jones, Bock, and Van Pelt (1960) presented here suggests some degree of interdependence between conceptual and perceptual levels through a memory bank. Although the discussion of the model by Wepman et al. focused mainly on the traces imitation can leave in the memory bank, the arrows suggest recognition of the fact that the memory bank, which is also influenced by the conceptual level, can also influence processing on the perceptual level.

The correlation between age and short-term memory span is well established —for example, older children and adults can repeat more words and digits than younger children (e.g., Case, 1985; Chi, 1978; Dempster, 1981; Huttenlocher & Burke, 1976). Moreover, children with language disorders and learning disabilities generally recall fewer digits and words in sequential order than do their age peers (e.g., R. Katz, Healy, & Shankweiler, 1983; Mahecha, 1981; Masland & Case, 1968; J. Stark, Poppen, & May, 1967; Torgesen, 1985). In a study of the relationship between auditory memory span and language skill in a retarded population, Graham (1968) reported that the ability to imitate and comprehend sentences varied directly with the length of digit-span recall. Why should memory span increase with age, and why should it be related to language level and language disorders?

Some have suggested that the capacity for storage increases with age (as if a loop of tape records the incoming stimuli for playback and the tape increases in length as the child grows older, or as if a basket that collects the incoming information grows larger as the child grows bigger). In line with this hypothesis, it has been suggested that children with language and learning problems have reduced capacity and that this reduced capacity may be a causal factor in their learning problems (e.g., Eisenson, 1968; Masland & Case, 1968; McGinnis, 1963; Wepman & Morency, 1973).

It is easy to assume that a deficiency in the reproduction of sequences of auditory stimuli reflects the cause of a language disorder—or that such a deficiency interferes with learning language. Certainly learning and using language involve the processing of sequences of auditory information. The sequence of words within a sentence is a major cue for speech processing by children (e.g., Bever, 1970; Hsu, Cairns, & Fiengo, 1985; Lahey, 1974; Sinclair & Bronckart, 1972; Stanton, 1986), but the sequence of words within a sentence is motivated by the semantic relationships among the words. Three-year-old children who can only repeat a list of two or three unrelated words are able to produce and comprehend some rather long sentences because of the semantic relations that are cued by the words in sequence with one another. Such children also know how to use information about word order to express semantic relations in their own speech. It is not clear how many unrelated words one must be able to repeat in order to learn language—perhaps only one or two, or perhaps none. The correlation between memory span for sequential auditory information and language development in children may be related to some third factor influencing both. Alternatively, it may be that poor language skills are the cause of the depressed memory span in younger children and in language-impaired children.

To assume that poor memory span causes a language disorder is to assume a linear, unidirectional model of language processing as discussed previously and schematized by Kirk and Kirk's model of communication (1971, Figure 5-1). On the other hand, if one assumes that language processing involves *inter*dependence of processing levels, as schematized by Wepman, Jones, Bock, & Van Pelt (1960, Figure 5-2), the finding of poor auditory memory span in language-disordered children may itself be *explained* by the language disorder; the shorter memory spans of younger children in comparison with older children may be related to their less well-developed knowledge of language. If this is the case, then the recall of auditory sequential information (as measured by repetition of lists of words) is a sensitive index of an individual's familiarity with a linguistic code and not a processing ability on which language learning depends.

The notion that auditory memory span may reflect a child's ability to handle verbal information and may not itself be a measure of processing capacity was suggested by Olson in 1973. Evidence to support this notion was presented by Brenner as early as 1940. Brenner reported that meaningful words are recalled better than nonsense words, and concrete words are recalled better than abstract words. Thus, familiarity with words influences the ability to recall lists of such words. Further evidence supporting the influence of stimulus familiarity on the ability to recall has been obtained using nonnative languages. College students recall digits, words, and sentences better in their native language than in a language they were studying in college (French); and the difference between the two decreased with increased ability and experience in the second language (Connelly,

1974). Likewise, American elementary school children learning Hebrew had longer spans in their native English language than in Hebrew (Diamond, 1979). Similar findings have been reported for visual stimuli by Vellutino (1977, 1979) and Vellutino, Pruzek, Steger, and Meshoulam (1973).

Using nonlinguistic stimuli, Chi (1978, 1983) also demonstrated the importance of subjects' knowledge of stimuli in recall. When children are more knowledgeable about stimuli than adults, they are able to recall more about those stimuli than adults (i.e., their memory spans for topic-related items are greater). In Chi's study, children recalled positions on a chessboard better than adults. On an independent measure, these children were more skilled at chess than the adults in the study. If the children's capacity to recall was smaller than that of adults, as the results of digit spans might suggest, then such a finding would not seem likely.

A number of studies have attempted to control linguistic familiarity at both the semantic and the phonological level and to observe the effect on memory span. Adults with expertise in soccer were able to recall more soccer-related words than adults without such expertise although they were similar on other measures of memory (Naus & Ornstein, 1983). Likewise, adults' memory spans were shortened when nonsense syllables (which eliminate semantic familiarity) were the stimuli as demonstrated by Brenner (1940) and considerably shortened when nonsense syllables containing non-English consonants (which reduce phonological familiarity) were used as stimuli (Case, 1985).

The second such study was a direct test of the capacity hypothesis in SLI children. Children diagnosed as SLI were compared with a group of non-language-impaired (NLI) children (Mahecha, 1981; Mahecha & Lahey, in preparation). The groups were comparable on measures of age, sex, and nonverbal intelligence, but differed in terms of language skills as reported in school records, their placement in special classes for the communicatively handicapped, and their scores on the grammatic closure subtest of the Illinois Test of Psycholinguistic Abilities (Kirk, McCarthy, & Kirk, 1968). As would be predicted from previous research, the two groups differed on sequential and item recall of meaningful linguistic stimuli including digits and words. The differences were less striking when the groups were compared on nonsense syllables—stimuli that were familiar in terms of English phonology but had no semantic referent. The span of the NLI children dropped considerably, while that of the SLI children dropped only slightly. On the last set of stimuli, familiarity was reduced even further—nonsense syllables were again presented, but this time the initial consonant of each was non-English. In this condition there was no significant difference between the two groups on item or sequential recall.

Thus, it seems unlikely that there were capacity differences between the language-impaired and non-language-impaired children; rather, it appears that the children's familiarity with the stimuli had a major effect on how many items they could recall. This effect on sequential recall was primarily a function of the decrease in memory span for the NLI children as familiarity of the stimuli decreased —the scores of the SLI children changed little with the change in the stimuli. The results of this study suggest that memory deficits in language-impaired children are a reflection of their lower levels of language knowledge and not a cause of that problem. When matched on equally unfamiliar stimuli, SLI children did as well as their age peers. Similar findings have been reported for LD children—memory span for nonsense syllables is similar to academically achieving children although memory span for words is considerably less (Torgesen, 1985). How might knowledge of language influence memory span?

According to some, speed of processing influences memory span (Dempster, 1981; Huttenlocher & Burke, 1976). It appears that children take longer to encode information than adults or older children. For example, children take almost twice as long to name a familiar person from a picture of that person than do adults (Chi, 1978), and children increase their speed of counting dots from kindergarten to sixth grade (Case, 1985). LD children take longer to encode the names of digits, pictures, and colors than normal children (e.g., Denkla & Rudel, 1976a, 1976b; Spring, 1976; Wiig, Semel, & Nystrom, 1982), and SLI children take longer to name pictures (e.g., Kail & Leonard, 1986). Furthermore, reaction time for identification of words as real words is faster for frequent words than for infrequent words or nonwords—suggesting that familiarity with the word influences processing time (Forster, 1976).

Speed of articulation has also been related to memory span and to age. A high correlation was found between subjects' (aged 3–22 years) rate of repeating word pairs 10 times and their memory spans (Hulme, Thomson, Muir, & Lawrence, 1984). Moreover, the time it takes 3-year-old children to imitate individual words is longer than that for 4-year-old children, and 4-year-old children take longer than 5- and 6-year-old children (Case, Kurland, & Goldberg, 1982). Memory span was directly related to the speed with which the children studied by Case et al. could imitate the individual words that they were subsequently asked to recall, and the correlation between speed of imitation and span of recall was significant even with age partialed out.

Adults behaved much like the 4-year-old children in terms of speed of imitation and span of recall when the stimuli used were foreign nonsense syllables—rate was slower and span was shorter (Case, 1985). Thus, again, a strong tie exists between speed of imitation and span of recall and the influence of familiarity on both span of recall and speed of imitation.

While rate of articulation of word pairs or speed of imitation of individual words has not, to my knowledge, been directly related to memory span in language-impaired children, it is obvious that such a relationship might well exist. [This possibility is currently under study (Lahey & Edwards, in preparation).] Language-impaired children are slower in naming pictures than age-matched peers (e.g., Kail & Leonard, 1986) and slower in articulating multisyllabic words (Tallal, Stark, & Mellits, 1985b). The language-impaired children that do *not* generally evidence deficits in short-term sequential memory for unrelated words are autistic children (Hermelin & Frith, 1971). Verbal autistic children reportedly produce fluent articulate utterances; their difficulties in language are related to the integration of form with content or with use. (See Chapter 4.) It is likely that their rate of articulation is more rapid than that of SLI children with similar levels of productive content/form/use interactions.

The relationship between speed of processing and memory span has been interpreted by Case as support for the hypothesis that increases in memory span with age are related, not to increased capacity, but to increased operating efficiency. According to this view, there is a limited amount of total processing space, or attentional capacity, available to any of us and the amount of this space does not increase with age. What does increase is the amount of space needed for executing operations. "The gradual increase in working memory does not stem from a structural increase in the attentional capacity of the organism but rather from an increase in the automaticity of the basic operations it is capable of executing. As these operations become more automatic, their execution requires a smaller proportion of total attentional capacity" (Case, 1978, p. 64). It would appear that accessing the phonetic representation and the motor commands and executing the actual articulation of syllables are operations that take up some of the attentional capacity available to children and adults; it would further appear that such operations become more efficient and automatic as we gain experience utilizing them. This view provides a framework that could explain the data on variation in memory span including the low memory spans found in SLI and LD children.

Another factor related to memory-span differences (as well as other differences in performance on language tasks including the speed of encoding and producing words) is differences in the children's use of phonetic representations of words (see, for example, Mann, 1986; Shankweiler, Liberman, Mark, Fowler, & Fisher, 1979; Torgesen, 1985). Some evidence suggests that phonetic representation of stimuli is better utilized by children with more developed language skills. For example, the recall of younger children and poor readers is less affected by acoustic similarity of words than that of older children and good readers (Hulme, 1984; Mann, 1986). It is possible that some SLI children (particularly those with good comprehension but poor production skills) may even have less well-developed phonetic representations of words stored in their lexicon.

Alternative explanations of the data are also possible. For example, memory span may be influenced by the amount of time available for rehearsal. The longer it takes to articulate the words in rehearsal, the fewer the number of words that can be recalled (Hulme, 1984; Hulme et al., 1984; Salame & Baddeley, 1982).

In any case, the data support the notion that poor short-term memory, as currently measured, is most likely not the cause of a language disorder. While it may be that some children do have memory deficiencies, it seems that we are not assessing memory apart from what is being remembered—perhaps we never can. Certainly our current knowledge and theory suggest that it is not memory that needs remediation, but the operations on language encoding and production— that is, we should not be remediating the tested deficit of memory in order to help a child learn language. Rather, we should be teaching language that, in turn, may increase short-term recall.

Temporal Cues

Familiarization with both the form and the content of a language influences the rate at which we can process that language. When you are first learning a language, it is easier to understand if the speaker speaks slowly, but once you have mastered the language, you can understand the input at rather rapid rates of presentation if you are familiar with the content. This observation has been made by many of us: when we attempt to learn a second language; when we are less familiar with the content/form/use interactions (i.e., the natives talk so fast!); and when we attempt to understand a lecture in our native language where the topic is over our heads (i.e., we wish the lecturer would slow down). Yet the same rate is easily understood when someone is talking to us about everyday activities. Parents apparently sense that a slower rate enables their young children to process the signal more easily; they speak more slowly to young children learning language than they do to older children (e.g., Broen, 1972; Snow, 1974). Research on the influence of rate on processing has supported these observations.

When speech is compressed electronically, thereby increasing the rate of speech, younger children have more difficulty than older children (Beasley, Maki, & Orchik, 1976; Bonvillian, Raeburn, & Horan, 1979), and children with language problems have more difficulty than age peers (e.g., Manning, Johnston, & Beasley, 1977, N. Nelson, 1976). For both younger children and language-impaired children, rapid rate has also been reported to influence discrimination and sequencing of nonlinguistic stimuli, as tones, and of speech sounds and nonsense syllables.

In a replication of Efron's (1963) findings with adult aphasics, Lowe and Campbell (1965) and Schnur (1971) found that SLI children needed considerably more time between the presentation of two successive pure tones than normal listeners in order to identify which tone came first. In contrast to NLI children, SLI children had more difficulty discriminating speech sounds that are different because of temporal cues, such as /ʃ/ and /tʃ/, than between those that are different because of frequency cues, such as /s/ and /ʃ/ (Rosenthal, 1972).

In a series of studies, Tallal and her associates (Tallal, 1976, 1980; Tallal & Piercy, 1973a, 1973b, 1974, 1975) have reported gross deficits in rapid auditory processing by SLI children. There was no difference between the SLI children and their age-matched peers in their ability to discriminate and sequence visual stimuli as well as two pure tones or vowels when the stimuli were presented at a slow rate. However, when the auditory stimuli were presented at a rapid rate or when a longer series of auditory stimuli were presented, the SLI children had difficulty discriminating and sequencing. Furthermore, over half of these children had problems with the discrimination of synthetic speech stimuli that included consonant-vowel combinations with rapid formant transitions such as /ba/ versus /da/. However, when Tallal artificially extended the formant transitions to twice their duration (thus making the transition less rapid), all the SLI children could discriminate the syllables. The conclusion reached by Tallal and her associates was that a constraint on the speed of auditory perception affects the processing of certain speech sounds and underlies the difficulty with language learning.

An important question is how does this apparent difficulty with processing of rapid formant transitions by SLI children relate to the children's production of speech sounds and to their understanding of language. If there is any relationship between these findings and the children's learning of language, it should be reflected in these two measures.

In fact, a relationship was found between the kinds of errors on the perception of the synthetic speech stimuli and the kinds of errors in speech production (R. Stark & Tallal, 1975, 1979). Moreover, voice onset time (VOT) for voiceless stops was less well defined (i.e., more variable) for the SLI children than for NLI age peers (R. Stark & Tallal, 1979). (According to Stark and Tallal, such variability has also been reported in younger children.) The authors concluded that the production difficulties could be related to difficulties with precise timing and that perceptual problems may be causing the production problems. They conceded, however, that the production problems may be interfering with perception. In any case, a relationship was established between performance on the perception of synthetic productions of stop stimuli and the production of these same speech sounds. Furthermore, responses to the auditory-speech-perception tasks (using the synthesized stop consonant-vowel stimuli) correlated highly with the level of receptive language functioning (as measured by a number of standardized tests) for both SLI and normal children (Tallal, Stark, & Mellits, 1985a).

These were rather elegant studies in which the auditory signal and the tasks were systematically manipulated to try to determine which variables influenced perception. In this sense they serve as a model of how we might proceed to further understand auditory perception. But there is still some question about findings and interpretation. First, as with any finding, there is a need for replication by other investigators. One replication of procedures reported that training influenced performance, suggesting that, to some extent, results of these studies reflect "perceptual learning" rather than some basic process (Tomblin & Quinn, 1983). In this sense the results of Tallal and her associates may simply be another reflection of some children's difficulty in learning. Finally, it is hard to understand how results with normals can be reconciled with the interpretation that deficits found in processing rapid auditory information underlie language-learning problems.

As pointed out by Tallal (1976, 1980), the ability to respond correctly to rapidly presented auditory signals develops with age. Non-language-impaired children below 4:6 would not perform the tasks; those from 4:6 through 7:6 had difficulty sequencing two tones presented rapidly; and those 4:6 and 5:6 even had difficulty when they were presented slowly (Tallal, 1976). In addition, 5-year-old normal children had considerable difficulty with detection and association of the synthetic consonants, but their performance improved with age (Tallal, Stark, Kallman, & Mellits, 1980). Despite these apparent problems with processing rapid auditory stimuli, children by the age of 4 and 5 have considerable language ability. Is it possible that problems with rapidly presented material are influenced by knowledge of the phonology of the language, the ability to manipulate phonetic representations, some general mediational or metalinguistic skill, or experience with listening tasks? In any case, the developmental data again suggest that difficulty with these tasks may reflect, rather than underlie, problems with language learning.

More recently, a general timing mechanism (which involves both production and perception) has been implicated as a source of pathology in language-disordered children (Tallal, Stark, & Mellits, 1985b). In a study of 25 SLI and 33 NLI children (matched on age, 5:6 to 8:6, and performance IQ), Tallal, Stark, and Mellits administered a battery of perceptual, motor, and neurodevelopmental tests. While the SLI children were significantly inferior to the normals on a number of measures (including almost all of the auditory-perceptual tests, some of the visual tests, sequenced oral nonspeech movements, and tactile perception), six measures correctly discriminated between the two groups in the predicted direction with 98% accuracy. These measures included rapid speech production of three-syllable words, ability to identify two fingers touched simultaneously, discrimination of computer-synthesized syllables /ba/ versus /da/ with 40-millisecond formant transitions, sequencing of cross-modal nonverbal stimuli (light flashes and tones) presented rapidly, sequencing of the letters *e* and *k* presented rapidly, and the location of two touches presented simultaneously to the cheeks and/or hands on either side of the body. The authors claim that each of these variables involved temporal processing (either simultaneous or successive) and, since similar tests that involved slower presentation rate did not discriminate between the groups, that the SLI children may have difficulty with temporal information in production and perception. Quoting work by Ojemann (1983) and Ojemann and Mateer (1979), they hypothesized that the anatomical site for such a temporal mechanism may be the perisylvian cortex in the dominant hemisphere.

It is certainly not clear that these measures are free of the child's knowledge of language. First, the rate of producing multisyllabic words is no doubt related to the child's familiarity with these words, as discussed in the prior section, and may be more a measure of the child's knowledge of language than of some timing mechanism. Likewise, the rate at which one can sequence letters is no doubt dependent on familiarity with those letters, as discussed in the prior section. Finally, verbal mediation may have been a factor in the sequencing of tones and lights, and the child's knowledge of the phonology of language may influence the rate of perception of nonsense syllables. Thus, it is possible that many of these variables could again be a reflection of the child's knowledge of the language system. In addition, unlike the interpretation in this study, processing of simultaneous stimuli and processing of successive stimuli have usually been considered distinct types of processing (Das, Dirby, & Jarman, 1975); it would be interesting if both were associated with the same cortical mechanism. Regardless of these potential problems with interpretation, the linking of perception and production and the hypothesis that a timing mechanism may serve as the biological basis for language development is provocative and will, no doubt, generate more research in this area.

Do these data mean that children with SLI have qualitatively different processing skills and that these differences interfere with language learning? Not necessarily. It is possible that perceptual and/or motor learning in children with language disorders may be late in development rather than qualitatively different. In a follow-up study done 3½ to 4 years later on some of the same children, improvement had occurred on both the measures of perception and the measures of language (although most of the SLI children still had language problems) (Bernstein & Stark, 1985). This finding, plus the finding that normal children improve on these tasks with age (Tallal, 1976), suggests that both the processing of rapid speech stimuli and language reception skills change together—it does not, unfortunately, sort out any causal relations.

While it seems logical to assume that the processing of the nonsense syllables is the basic task and that language learning must depend on such a skill, it is quite likely that success at these tasks may reflect other skills—possibly language itself. Further research is needed before we will know whether such tasks are measuring some prerequisite to language learning, familiarity with language, or some "higher-level" cognitive processing that is related both to the task and to language learning. At this time the work on temporal cues and language disorders is of heuristic interest. It does not, however, appear to be directly applicable to intervention strategies other than to reinforce what has been known for a long time— that a slow rate of speech is usually a good idea when teaching or communicating with any person who is at the early stages of learning a first or second language.

Processing Multisensory Input

One aspect of perception that is logically related to language learning is attention to and integration of separate sensory stimuli from different modalities. It would seem that visual and tactile features of input from the context must be attended to and integrated with auditory impressions, if the interactions between content, form, and use are to develop. That is, children need to experience the objects and events referred to by the speech that they hear in order to learn the coding relation between meaning and sound.

In a comparison of the auditory-visual integration skills of schizophrenic children with those of normal children, Walker and Birch (1970) found that the schizophrenic children's responses to the integrative task were significantly inferior to the responses by the normal population. Walker and Birch concluded "that the schizophrenic children manifest a clear inability to organize and integrate information coming to them from the environment through the separate organs of sense and that this inability probably reflects a primary peculiarity in the organization of their central nervous systems" (p. 111), which contributes to childhood psychosis. The schizophrenic group was not homogeneous; some of the schizophrenic children performed as well on the integration task as the normal population. No description of the children's language was presented, so it is impossible to relate such integrative skill to language behaviors.

If these experimental tasks are representative of the integration of auditory and visual stimuli in real-life situations, then the difficulties exhibited by the child who does not integrate multisensory stimuli might account for difficulties in the interaction between content and form in language development. The child might conceivably learn a lot about the system of linguistic signals through the auditory channel and be able to utter long, complex sentences. But the child might be unable to learn the semantic-syntactic relations in sentences and also their relation to social situations—the connection of form with content and use—because of an inability to integrate knowledge of the world obtained through vision and tactile senses with the vocal linguistic signals. The language of many psychotic children presents such a pattern—referred to as distorted interactions or separation of content, form, and use in Chapters 2 and 4. Since the integrative task presented in the Walker and Birch experiment was nonverbal, and since no description was given of the language of the nonintegrating children, such conjecture is only of heuristic value at the present time. Furthermore, the evidence that speech perception may be bimodal (e.g., Kuhl & Meltzoff, 1982) suggests that the children could not have developed form without some degree of bisensory integration.

Rather than a problem with the integration of multiple sensory input, it may be that the problem is one of selective stimulus control or selective attention. Some children may attend to only one type of stimulus during multisensory stimulation. Such a possibility was demonstrated by Lovaas, Schreibman, Koegel, and Rehm (1971). Three groups of children (normal, retarded, and autistic children of similar age) were reinforced for responding to multisensory stimuli and then tested to see which of the stimuli were responded to when presented separately. They found that the autistic children responded primarily to only one cue, the retardates responded primarily to two cues, and the normal children uniformly responded to all three cues. No one modality was preferred for any group, and the first modality preference of a particular child could be changed, suggesting, according to the authors, a problem of "stimulus overselectivity." The results cannot, however, be used to account for differences in verbal behavior, since the language behaviors were not specified; the autistic children were described as severely impaired, with all but one "mute," but the language of the retarded children was not described.

Certainly, a problem with selective stimulus control could also inhibit language learning, since language learning involves processing the simultaneous or near contiguous presentation of both linguistic and nonlinguistic stimuli. Selective attention may account for lack of auditory-vocal language (if the auditory modality is continually ignored) or for auditory-vocal behaviors that may be described as a distorted interaction or separation of content, form, and use. On the other hand, selective attention to only one modality may reflect the inability to learn language for some other reason. The inability to attach meaning to sound may cause a child to "tune out"—either to complex input or to a particular type of input. It is not clear, therefore, that attentional deficits are, in fact, distinct from integrational deficits, nor is it clear whether either is a cause or a reflection of a language disorder.

To determine the cause-effect relationship between poor performance on tasks designed to measure perceptual skills and a language disorder, more information about the language behaviors that differentiate between children who do well and children who do not do well on such tasks is needed (thus, an integration of a specific-abilities orientation with a communication-language orientation), as well as developmental information on these skills in both normal and language-disordered children.

Does the specific-abilities orientation have other than heuristic interest—can it be useful for the educational management of children with language disorders? Are the molecular categories—the elements of processing evolved from models of cognitive functioning—useful to the educator or clinician responsible for developing language skills? Can we measure such functions, and if so, what do they tell us about goals or techniques of intervention related to language learning?

The Usefulness of the Specific-Abilities Orientation for Educational Management

Much of the impetus behind the specific-abilities orientation to language disorders came originally from educators. These educators were interested in schoolchildren who had problems learning academic skills despite normal overall intelligence and no evidence of severe emotional problems. The concept of weakness in certain specific abilities underlying language and learning in general was appealing, both as an explanation of language and learning problems and as a model for intervention. Much of the research within this orientation has been done with children labeled *learning-disabled*. While this book is about language disorders, learning-disabled children are included in the discussion of this orientation because so many of these children have difficulty with auditory-vocal language functioning as well as with written language and other academic skills. In fact the terms *language-disordered* and *learning-disabled* are often used interchangeably (see, for example, Kirk & Kirk, 1978, p. 71, and Chapter 4). Unfortunately, the language behaviors of the children under investigation are not always independently described.

Three different approaches to children with language-learning problems can be considered related to the specific-abilities orientation. One, the most popular, has focused on delineating weaknesses in cognitive abilities and directly teaching to these weaknesses with the goal of improving such skills and indirectly language skills—a specific-disabilities approach. Another has assessed various abilities in order to infer central nervous system dysfunction. The results are used to classify children and/or make general recommendations and to gauge prognosis (but not to directly remediate particular abilities)—a neuropsychological approach. The third approach also infers central nervous system dysfunction from behaviors, but here the focus is on attempting to change brain functioning more generally (and thus remediate deficits in cognitive skills) through indirect means such as sensorimotor training—a motor approach.

Each is more concerned with components of language processing or the nonlanguage skills of the children than it is with description of the language behaviors themselves. Most are more concerned with remediating the weaknesses that have been tested than they are with facilitating language learning directly (and, thus, they differ from the communication-language orientation) or than they are with classifying the child relative to other children (and thus they differ from the categorical orientation).[*] The impact of each approach has varied with time, with section of the country, with the extent to which other professionals are involved in the assessment of a particular language-impaired child, with state and federal regulations for funding educational programs, and with each of the different children with whom we work. Each approach is discussed in the following sections from the viewpoint of its usefulness for facilitating early language development.

A Specific-Disabilities Approach

The assessment of various abilities felt necessary for language learning and use has been rather common. For example, it is not unusual to read a file on a child with a language disorder and see reference to the child's auditory memory, auditory discrimination, or other abilities. A number of assessment instruments have focused on this type of description. However, the most influential and the most elaborate attempt to diagnose specific disabilities has been the *Illinois Test of Psycholinguistic Abilities (ITPA)*, published first in an experimental form (Kirk & McCarthy, 1961) and later revised (Kirk, McCarthy, & Kirk, 1968). The objective of the ITPA is to "delineate specific abilities and disabilities in children in order that remediation may be undertaken when needed" (Kirk et al., 1968, p. 5). The purpose of diagnosis is to identify specific areas of defective functioning, and the purpose of intervention is to provide appropriate remediation in the areas so identified.

The ITPA was based on a three-stage mediational model of language (Osgood, 1957) that included the processes of reception, association, and expression; the modalities of input and output; and levels of processing. (See Figure 5-1 for an adaptation of this model.) The authors of the ITPA modified Osgood's model

---

[*] While the neuropsychological approach also classifies children, it seems more closely aligned with the specific-abilities orientation.

somewhat to apply it to a clinical population and to the practicality of a testing situation. The test purports to tap both auditory and visual channels of sensory input and motor and vocal channels of output. Each of these channels is considered for the processes of reception, association, and expression at two levels of processing. One level of processing is called the automatic level where information is integrated and organized but does not involve any mediation of meaning. It includes rote learning, automatic production of a sequence of items, and utilization of the redundant codings in heard speech, such as *two* shoes. The second level is called the representational level and involves the processing of meaning and the use of symbols. Twelve subtests are included in the test to observe specific processes through each channel at each level. Each subtest was designed to represent a specific ability, and normative data were presented so that each ability could be compared with a general population of normal children and with the other abilities of the same child. Remedial programs, based on this approach to specific abilities, are designed with the goal of strengthening each ability. The following section discusses the relevance of this approach to language learning and its application to children who are having difficulty learning a first language (i.e., to language-disordered children).

Several assumptions are implied in any orientation to language disorders that attempts to delineate and remediate specific abilities: (1) that the abilities for language are distinct from each other in the learning and use of language; (2) that each ability is a necessary prerequisite for the development and use of language, and weak abilities therefore interfere with the learning or use of language; and (3) that weak abilities can be strengthened by training, and that strengthening specific abilities through remediation training will transfer somehow to general improvement in the knowledge and use of language. These three assumptions are examined below, using the ITPA as a model of such an approach.° (See Mann, 1971, and Hammill & Larsen, 1974, for further discussion of many of these same points.)

Can Abilities Be Isolated from One Another?   First, are the abilities that have been defined in the model of language on which the ITPA was based actually distinct from each other in language learning and use?

One way of inferring this is through factor analysis of test results. This type of analysis has been carried out by a number of investigators, with conflicting results. For example, the concept of distinct abilities as tested by the ITPA was substantiated for fourth-grade children by Newcomer, Hare, Hammill, and McGettigan (1973). They concluded that "all subtests except Visual Reception, Auditory Reception, and Visual Sequential Memory can be regarded as measuring separate psycholinguistic abilities . . ." (p. 17). With the use of a different statistical technique, the process and channel distinctions were supported in other studies, but the Grammatic Closure Test factored out as a part of the representational level instead of the automatic level (Cohen, 1973, and Elkins, 1972, as cited by Kirk & Kirk, 1978).

Other factor-analytic studies have not supported the distinct 12 abilities tested

---

° The ITPA has been selected for discussion because it represents the best organized and most researched attempt to apply this approach. It should be noted that the critique applies only to first oral language learning and not to the application of this approach or this instrument to later academic learning, such as learning to read.

on the ITPA, but have found differences with age. The subtests of the ITPA were more highly intercorrelated for younger children than for older children. In contrast to the findings by Newcomer et al., the modality distinction was the one factor that did receive support (Rykman & Wiegerink, 1969). These discrepancies may be related to differences in the studies (e.g., some, as Newcomer et al., used additional criterion tests in their data, while others did not), or to changes in the interrelationship of such abilities with increases in age or level of language knowledge. The question (Can the abilities be isolated from each other?) remains unanswered. On the basis of the above data and the data presented in the first part of this chapter, however, it appears the answer is quite likely negative—at least for the child in the early stages of language learning.

Are the Specific Abilities Necessary for Language Development?   Even if the abilities were isolated, is each ability essential for the development and use of language, and do weaknesses within each ability interfere with the learning and use of language? These are difficult questions to answer because of the manner in which most of them are tested—and, probably, because it is not possible to test them in a manner that is free of the influence of language knowledge (as discussed in the earlier section on auditory sequential memory).

While, theoretically, some of the abilities may be necessary for language learning (e.g., the ability to associate sound and meaning), most published tests that assess association skills are tests of language knowledge. Failure on subtests such as auditory reception, auditory association, grammatic closure, verbal expression, and auditory memory indicates a low level of language knowledge, but does not indicate whether that particular ability is responsible for the low level. For example, the grammatical closure subtest measures the child's knowledge of morphological inflections. While the test is placed on the automatic level of processing, it is quite clear that such learning is not automatic, but has to do with important inductions about correspondences between sound and meaning. Attempting to remediate this as a deficit in automatic processing usually results in exercises for sentence completion, repetition, and memorization of grammatical sentences out of context. Such training is not likely to help a child learn the necessary inductions of content/form/use interactions.

Other subtests are less clearly related to the development of auditory-vocal language, although they may well be related to the learning of written language.

One such subtest, sound blending, taps the ability to synthesize separate phoneme-sized segment. However, research in speech perception (A. Liberman, Cooper, Shankweiler, & Studdert-Kennedy, 1967) and coarticulation studies of speech production (Amerman, Daniloff & Moll, 1970) have indicated that individuals neither perceive nor produce words by connecting one separate phoneme-sized segment with another. The acoustic signal of speech cannot be segmented to individual phoneme-sized units. For example, the acoustic signals that are perceived as plosives (/p/, /b/, /d/, /g/, /t/, /k/) vary in frequency, and the direction of frequency changes depending on the vowels that precede or follow them. If a perceived plosive such as /p/ is separated, by tape cutting, from the word in which it is embedded and placed in front of a different vowel, the resulting segment may sound different—for example, the /p/ burst of the syllable /pi/ will sound like a /k/ if the /p/ burst is followed by /a/ (A. Liberman, Delattre, & Cooper, 1952; Schatz,

FIGURE 5-3   The Influence of the Vowel Context on a Plosive Consonant (from A. Liberman, Cooper, Shankweiler, and Studdert-Kennedy, "Perception of the Speech Code," Psychological Review, 74, 1967, 431–461. Copyright © by the American Psychological Association. Reprinted/adapted by permission of the author.)

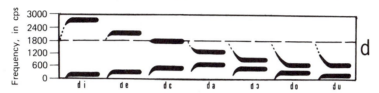

Note that the initial part of the acoustic signal in the figure above is different in each syllable although both syllables are perceived as beginning with /d/.

1954). Thus, it has not been possible to describe invariant acoustic characteristics that correspond to phoneme-sized segments: see, for example, Figures 5-3 and 5-4. It is not clear what unit of speech is the unit of perception nor where in the process of speech production this unit is represented.

FIGURE 5-4   The Interdependence of Phonemes (from COGNITIVE PSYCHOLOGY by A. Liberman, copyright © 1970 by Harcourt Brace Jovanovich, Inc. Reprinted by permission of the publisher.)

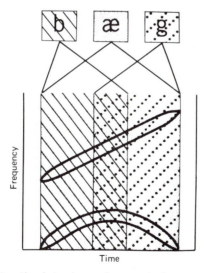

This figure illustrates the interdependence of phonemes; both consonants are influenced by the vowel and the vowel is, in turn, influenced by both consonants.

A skill in phoneme synthesizing, thus, is certainly not a prerequisite for learning to talk or understand language. It is, in fact, even difficult to teach such skills to normal preschool children (I. Liberman, Shankweiler, Fischer, & Carter, 1974).° The development of the ability to synthesize speech sounds appears to be more necessary to the use of written language than oral language, and perhaps is best reserved for such academic or remedial training in reading and writing where sounds are necessarily represented by separate letters of the alphabet. Certainly the speech-language pathologist should question teaching sound synthesizing or blending to a child with a language disorder whose language skills are comparable to those of a 2- or 3-year-old child, who, research has shown, is not capable of performance with sound blending tasks. Nevertheless, in many clinics and schools, children who are speaking with syntactic constructions of two and three words that are typical of early language development have been given training on such skills. The ability to separate and integrate the separate sounds of a word or phrase is a metalinguistic task that has to be taught, and it is not usually taught to children until they demonstrate their readiness at about age 6 or 7 years.

Thus, the question regarding whether the abilities are necessary for the development and use of language and whether weaknesses within each ability can interfere with the learning and use of language cannot be answered as long as the abilities are measured with language or with tasks that are sensitive to level of language knowledge.

Can the Specific Abilities Be Remediated, and Do Remedial Programs Lead to Improvement in Language Skills? Again, conflicting evidence is reported on the success with which deficits on the subtests of the ITPA can be remediated. In a review of 38 studies that measured the effectiveness of training specific abilities, Hammill and Larsen (1974) concluded, "It is apparent that for the most part, researchers have been unsuccessful in developing those skills which would enable their subjects to do well on the ITPA" (p. 10). They suggested that either the test may not be an appropriate measure of the abilities, the abilities may not be trainable, or the intervention programs reported in the literature may be inadequate.

In contrast, Kirk and Kirk (1971) have presented treatment case histories as evidence that subtests of the ITPA can be improved with remedial training. Furthermore, K. A. Lund, Foster, and McCall-Perez (1978) reanalyzed 24 of the studies reviewed by Hammill and Larsen and concluded that some studies did show positive results and others were inconclusive.

The exact nature of the intervention in the reviewed studies is not always clear from published reports, but certainly many intervention programs designed around the ITPA appear to be training tasks similar to the testing tasks (e.g., memory is trained by having the child repeat lists of words). It would not be surprising if test scores did improve when intervention programs were designed

---

° Although the norms on the sound blending subtest of the ITPA go as low as 2½ years of age, thus indicating early acquisition of such a skill, sound blending ability is not really tapped in the early items of the test. On the first eight items of the test, children are asked to choose a picture in response to a phoneme-by-phoneme presentation of the name of an object (e.g., b-a-t). A correct response can very conceivably be made on the basis of the recognition of a part of the word, and actually blending the sounds is really not essential to such recognition. In fact, a psycholinguistic age of 5 years can be reached on the test items without the necessity of phoneme synthesis, and 5-year-old children already have considerable facility with their native language.

around the test—that is, if the programs were, in effect, teaching the test. Familiarity with a task and with test-taking procedures may well result in improved scores. A more basic question is: Does the improved score represent improved skills within the entire domain of the ability supposedly measured by the test or only in the specific type of skill used to measure the domain of that ability?

Even more important is the question: Is there evidence that remediation of specific abilities transfers to a general improvement in the knowledge or use of language? According to Bortner (1971), no body of evidence exists to support the practice of remediation of specific abilities. We are not aware of any studies that have found improvement in general language development after the remediation of specific abilities—perhaps because few studies have looked for such transfer of improvement in language use. Without such evidence, however, and without evidence that such abilities are necessary for the development and use of oral language, it is questionable that the remediation of specific abilities should dominate a remedial program for children who are learning language slowly and with difficulty.

One problem with focusing intervention on these abilities, instead of focusing on language itself, is the resulting tendency to teach these abilities alone. Such teaching often isolates these abilities from the other language skills that the child exhibits and from the sequence in which these abilities are manifested by children who are learning language without difficulty. For example, the problems with remediating sound blending with children who do not have language skills comparable to that of a 4-year-old have already been discussed. At a different level, training on analogies and categorization is a part of the procedures generally suggested for remediating deficits in auditory association (note that forming analogies is the task used to test auditory association). A potential problem with teaching analogies to children who do poorly on this subtest also lies in the selection of priorities for sequencing goals of intervention. Younger children of 2 to 4 years of age who are developing language normally do not readily use or understand analogies.° A developmental approach would question an intervention program that stressed analogies with any age child who did not have the language skills of a 3- or 4-year-old. Thus, teaching to specific abilities for the purpose of improving language and other communication skills has not been supported. Moreover, there is the possibility that an intervention program centered on specific abilities that are beyond the child's current language level could even impede language learning.

Conclusions. The specific-disabilities approach represented a shift away from the search for precipitating factors, to a concentration on present abilities. It also represented a shift from global to molecular categorization. Each child was viewed in terms of strengths and weaknesses; remediation was based on assessment. This orientation represented a major thrust forward in diagnostics in that it stressed assessment of present functioning with the purpose of determining the goals and procedures of a remedial program. However, when the specific-disabilities ap-

---

° Even though the auditory association subtest tests analogies and provides norms that extend as low as 2½ years of age, it is nevertheless possible to reach a psycholinguistic age of 4½ on the test without dealing with analogies. Most of the first 14 items on the test can be responded to correctly by understanding only the second of the first and second ideas in the analogy.

proach is used as a search for weak cognitive skills that need remediation before language can be learned, this orientation is also etiological, as was the categorical orientation, but simply on another level.

The information on perceptual processing would appear to be most applicable to determining the procedures or context of intervention, not the goals of intervention; for example, children high on visual skills and low on auditory skills might learn better through the visual than the auditory channel. [As yet, however, even this hypothesis has not been substantiated (I. Liberman, 1985, Newcomer & Goodman, undated; C. M. Smith, 1971) with schoolchildren, although it may be relevant at preschool ages.] Information from the specific-disabilities approach may lead to hypotheses about the procedures of teaching, which can be tested through diagnostic teaching. Certainly research within this approach will increase our understanding of children with a language disorder and, as more information is gained, may lead to important information on procedures of language intervention.

It would seem that the dominant theme and goals of a remedial program for children with a language disorder should be the meaningful use of language. Any instrument geared to measuring specific abilities does not give the clinician or teacher information on what the child knows about language or what it is the child needs to know, nor by itself does it tell what uses the child can make of language for problem solving or communication. Such instruments cannot be considered an evaluation or assessment of *language*—they were not so designed and should not be used as such. Language programs should be based on what a child knows about language and what the child is best ready to learn next.

Neuropsychological Approach

A neuropsychological approach examines certain motor and cognitive abilities in an attempt to infer functioning of the central nervous system rather than to plan which abilities need to be remediated. Most of the tests and hypotheses regarding brain-language relationships have been derived from information obtained from adults or animals—from studies of induced brain lesions (in the case of animals), accidental insults (as in adults with tumors or strokes), electrical stimulation of the brain (done during brain surgery), or, more recently, passive measures of brain function through electroencephalographic (EEG) data or PET and CAT scans. Usually, the tests administered to children and the inferences drawn from children's responses have been adapted from the research with adults.

Traditionally, specific language impairment and learning disabilities are considered to be the result of neurological dysfunction. Terminology was taken from the terms used to describe adult aphasics where language use was impaired as a result of neurological insult. In the case of developmental language disorders and learning disabilities, however, there is rarely clear evidence of any neurological dysfunction, and the assumption of such dysfunction has come by default. After all, if the child can hear, appears intelligent enough to learn language, and interacts appropriately with people, what other explanation could there be? Besides, all behavior, including language, is mediated by the central nervous system—thus, problems in learning a behavior seem logically related to some problem with the central nervous system. While traditionally autism was not considered a result of neurological dysfunction, most researchers are now suggesting a neurological basis for the problem (see Chapter 4). A neuropsychological approach has been used in the study of these three syndromes to test such hypotheses and, in some cases, to attempt to locate the site of dysfunction. Most of this work has been experimental, but some has been used for the clinical management of these children. Two exemplars of this approach, which are currently used *clinically*, are the central auditory testing performed by some audiologists and the neuropsychological testing performed by some psychologists. Each is briefly discussed below.

Central Auditory Testing.   Auditory-perceptual problems have, for many years, been implicated' as a correlate, if not a cause, of language-learning problems (Eisenson, 1968, 1972; Hardy, 1965; Monsees, 1968; Myklebust, 1954; and see earlier sections of this chapter). However, beyond traditional testing of peripheral sensitivity, the audiologist was rarely involved in the assessment of language-impaired children until the 1970s.

With adults, audiologists have been able to confirm lesions in the central auditory pathway and to identify site of lesion (i.e., brain stem versus cortical) through the use of a battery of tests designed to test central auditory function in contrast to peripheral function. These tests generally tax the processing skills of adults by degrading the auditory stimuli or in some way reducing the redundancy of linguistic input (by filtering certain frequencies from the speech signal, presenting competing messages, etc.). Validation of these tests has been obtained by subsequent surgery or autopsy, by research with split-brain patients, and in some cases by correlations with electrophysiological measures. In the 1970s, audiologists began using similar batteries of central auditory tests with children (over the age of 5) diagnosed as having language impairment, auditory-perceptual problems, and/or learning disabilities.

Some of these tests are discussed below with information on how non-language-impaired and language- and/or learning-disabled children responded to the tasks. The tests most commonly administered are derived from the battery presented by Willeford (1977) and Willeford and Billger (1978) and the experimental tapes circulated by Willeford. Most have speech as stimuli. Some of the tests designed for adults have not been found helpful with children. One of these, the rapid alternating speech test, requires the listener to repeat sentences that alternate between the ears every 300 milliseconds. This task is easily performed by 5- to 10-year-old children and was not a problem for children diagnosed as having auditory-perceptual problems (Musiek, Geurkink, & Kietel, 1982).

In contrast, other tests show a pattern of improving scores with age, and these tests often are difficult for children with language disorders and/or learning disabilities. One example is the test of binaural fusion. In this test the child is asked to repeat spondee words (i.e., bisyllabic words with equal stress on both syllables, such as *baseball*) which have been passed through a low-frequency and a high-frequency band-pass filter. The low-band-pass version is given to one ear and the high-band-pass version to the other ear. High variability in performance is found in normal children until the age of 10, and the task is considered by some to be a closure task and language-related (Keith, 1981, 1984). Conflicting data exist on the performance of children referred for clinical testing. Matkin and Hook (1983) reported that it was one of the most discriminating central auditory tests administered to a rather heterogeneous group of 7- to 11-year-old children diagnosed as learning-disabled; over two-thirds of the children failed the test. However, with a group of 5- to 8-year-old children diagnosed as having auditory-perceptual deficits, Musiek et al. (1982) reported that the test had little discriminating value; only about 20% of the children failed the test. This discrepancy between the studies may have been related to differences in the pass/fail criterion applied in each study, differences in the acoustic characteristics of the tapes (see discussion of this latter point below), or differences in the groups of children used as subjects in each. The data were not presented in a manner that allowed these factors to be sorted out. In an earlier study (D. B. Harris, 1963), a similar-type task did not discriminate brain-damaged from non-brain-damaged children nor normal from learning-disabled children when statistical analyses were applied to the raw scores (note that most studies use only a pass/fail criterion).

Tests that involve the simultaneous presentation of speech to opposite ears (i.e., dichotic presentation) and require the child to repeat the stimuli heard at one or both ears tend to show variable scores among younger children for responses to the left-ear stimuli. Improvement in left-ear performance on this task is found as children reach 8 or 9 years of age. One such test is the competing-sentences test—a test that is sensitive to temporal-lobe pathology in adults. In this test two different sentences are presented—one to each ear—with one sentence, considered the primary message, delivered at an intensity that is 15 decibels less than the other. The task is to repeat the primary (or quieter) message while ignoring the sentence in the opposite ear. Children do well with this task when the primary message is presented in the right ear. When the primary message is presented in the left ear, however, considerable variability exists among children 5 through 8 years of age and among children with learning disabilities. This test was failed by almost 90% of the subjects in the study by Musiek et al. (1982), but by less than 33% of the subjects studied by Matkin and Hook (1983). Again, it is difficult to account for the differences except for the possibilities raised in the previous paragraph.

Tests involving repetition of dichotically presented words (in contrast to sentences) provide more consistent results across studies. Such a task (using words) was failed by over 60% of the subjects studied by Matkin and Hook, and a similar task (with digits as stimuli) was failed by over 60% of the children in the Musiek et al. study. This type of task has also been reported by others to differentiate learning-disabled and language-impaired children from children with no reported problems with language (Hynd & Obrzut, 1981; Pettit & Helms, 1979). By the age of 5, normal children typically do well repeating the stimuli presented to the right ear (this has been referred to as a right-ear advantage). Considerable variability exists, however, in young children's responses to stimuli presented to the left ear. The learning-disabled children tested by Hynd and Obrzut and the children with auditory-perceptual impairment tested by Musiek et al. also showed a right-ear advantage. However, Musiek et al. reported that the children's performance in the left ear was consistently much lower than those of normal children. Both studies concluded that this may be the result of problems with transferring information from the right to the left hemisphere (involving the corpus callosum).

A final example of a central auditory test using speech presented simultaneously to opposite ears (i.e., a dichotic task) is the *Staggered Spondaic Word Test* (SSW) developed by J. Katz (1977). In this test the first syllable of one word (such as *up* from *upstairs*) is presented in noncompeting condition to one ear (e.g., the right ear). The second syllable (in our example *stairs*) follows to the same ear while the first syllable of another word (e.g., *down* from *downtown*) is simultaneously presented to the opposite ear (e.g., the left ear). Thus, these syllables are delivered in competing condition (e.g., *stairs* is presented to the right ear at the same time as *down* is presented to the left ear). Finally, the second syllable of the second word (e.g., *town*) is presented in a noncompeting condition (in our example to the left ear). Measures of correct responses in the competing condition for the right ear are better than for the left ear, but the variability among children is very high (Keith, 1981). This test is significantly correlated with a number of measures of language performance in children 6 and 7 years old (Keith, 1984) and was failed by about half of the subjects studied by Musiek et al. (1982). (It was not administered by Matkin & Hook, 1983). Thus, tests where stimuli are presented simultaneously to opposite ears show a pattern of improved performance in the left ear with age and a more consistent pattern of low scores in the left ear for clinical populations.

The assumptions and purposes of the testing have been discussed by Keith (1984). According to Keith, it is assumed that tests as these reflect fundamental auditory abilities if they are not loaded with language comprehension, do not require linguistic manipulation, and limit cross-sensory processing. Furthermore, it is assumed that the tests yield information about why an auditory learning problem exists. The rationale is that if the nervous system is not sufficiently mature, it will have problems with degraded stimuli. Therefore, the tests that we have described (which all reduce the redundancy of the stimuli) can be used to determine neuromaturational age by comparing a child's score with normative data. Following from these assumptions, low scores represent difficulties with fundamental auditory abilities which underlie the auditory learning problem and are the result of delay in neuromaturation.

These assumptions, and the subsequent interpretation of findings, are open to question. For one, the tapes of the most widely used tests for children (the Willeford battery) have been criticized in terms of their acoustic characteristics (e.g., Shea & Raffin, 1983). The binaural fusion test discussed earlier was reported to have the least reliable intertape recording levels. According to Shea and Raffin, distortion on these tapes could make the task a test of language (where the subject must fill in the missing segments) rather than a test of binaural fusion—a conclusion also reached by Keith (1984).

A second problem with interpretation relates to the question raised throughout this chapter—can these perceptual abilities be examined independent of the stimuli that are being perceived? A number of audiologists (cited above) are recognizing this problem and have described *some* of the tests as more a test of language than of independent auditory ability. But are the other measures independent of the language knowledge base because they don't directly ask for language comprehension responses or ask for direct manipulation of the linguistic signal? This issue has been addressed in a number of studies by Keith (1984) and his colleagues. They report that familiarity with the stimuli (i.e., the words) has been found to influence performance on the SSW. As noted above, the SSW was significantly correlated with measures of language in children. In addition, adults whose native language was not English made more errors than native English-speaking adults in the competing but not the noncompeting condition (Keith, 1984). Similar findings are reported for other examples of degraded speech such as speech discrimination in the presence of noise (Gat & Keith, 1978, as reported in Keith, 1984) and for discrimination of nonsense syllables (Seller, 1981).

In contrast, other evidence suggests that language was not a factor. The nonnative English-speaking adults did not have trouble with dichotic presentation of CV nonsense syllables. This may mean that familiarity with language is only relevant at the semantic level for this task—unlike the memory tasks discussed earlier—or it may be that the adult's exposure to English (6 years) enabled them to process phonetically the CV syllables that were presented. Further study with different CV combinations and with more phoneically complex nonsense syllables may help sort out the answer to this problem.

One further type of evidence gives mixed results. Correlations of scores on central auditory tests with certain measures of language yielded significant correlations for only one of the tests, dichotic presentation of words (Matkin & Hook, 1983). Unfortunately, not enough information is presented (e.g., range of scores) to try to explain why, for example, dichotic words might be correlated while competing sentences might not. Clearly, further research is needed concerning the influence of familiarity and level of language knowledge on central auditory tests. More studies such as those done by Keith and his associates or studies using tasks such as those described under Auditory Sequential Memory might help us to understand better what is being measured by central auditory tests.

The current data do suggest that the child's ability to imitate a message under noncompeting conditions is not sufficient evidence to determine whether listening performance is based on auditory-perceptual or linguistic deficits as suggested by Keith (1984). Recall that speed of imitation was highly correlated with span of recall—not just the ability to imitate (Case, 1985). It no doubt takes attentional capacity to inhibit a competing signal (as on competing sentences). If the child is using a great deal of capacity to process the speech signal (at phonemic, semantic, or syntactic levels), capacity may be limited for inhibiting a competing signal (see also T. F. Campbell & McNeil, 1985). In other words, if processing language is not fairly automatic, any degradation may influence the results. Differences between left- and right-ear performance may well be due to neuromaturation in all children, but the delay observed with language-disordered and learning-disabled children may be more the result of language facility than differences in maturation of the corpus callosum.

A third problem with the interpretation of low scores as evidence of auditory processing problems is understanding how improvement in such auditory skills logically relates to the language learning that occurs between the ages of 5 and 8 or 9. The advances in language made in this age range seem less easily explained by improved auditory perception than do the advances made in the first 5 years of life. In fact, the development in language skills that does occur in this later age period seems more likely to influence how the child can respond to these tasks. For example, the child becomes more adept at metalinguistic skills, or the manipulation of language as an entity apart from its meaning—an advantage in any task that involves processing language apart from extracting the meaning. The young school-age child also learns to use language to mediate activities (which may account for results found on certain nonlinguistic measures such as pitch patterns). Furthermore, the child learns, with experience, to process language more rapidly and automatically. Thus, increased skill with language in terms of mediational skills and metalinguistic skills as well as automaticity with certain linguistic operations may influence performance on the tests.

Finally, the conclusion that low scores indicate a maturational delay that underlies the child's language and learning problems is difficult to accept given the wide variability in scores reported among the normal children tested. In some of the tests discussed above, the norms published by Keith (1977) indicate a range of 20 to 100% correct for children below the ages of 8 or 9. If the tests measure only maturation of the central nervous system, it appears that the age of such maturation is highly variable in the normal population. If this is so, and if low scores suggest auditory-perceptual problems that underlie the learning of language and certain academic skills, an interesting question arises. How do normal children who obtain low scores manage to be free of such learning problems—why do they not stand out in class and home as having auditory-perceptual problems? The answer to this question could have important remedial implications. Perhaps we should be studying, in more detail, other aspects of processing and learning in the normal children who obtain low scores on tests of central auditory functioning. This may be more profitable than searching for further evidence of dysfunctioning in children with language and learning problems—particularly, given the minimal influence that the present clinical use of this battery has had on remediation.

In some cases, low scores on the tests yield recommendations for auditory training as a means of remediating the deficits found during testing (Musiek & Guerkink, 1980). The assumption is that such training will help with auditory processing and the associated problems that instigated the referral in the first place. This is similar to the specific-disabilities approach discussed earlier, and the same criticisms apply. More typically, recommendations given to those working with children who fail one or another of these tests are rather general and refer to ways adults can deal with the dysfunction. Suggestions include using clear speech when talking to the child, ensuring minimal distraction, presenting feedback, using an experiential approach to learning, presenting material at the level of the child, giving praise, using other modalities, and taping instructions for the child to relisten to at home (Willeford & Billger, 1978). As noted by Matkin (1983), these are recommendations that are a part of any good teacher's or clinician's repertoire; they could be arrived at without the time and expense of such an extensive battery of tests. More extreme measures have been recommended, such as changing the speech signal (Lubert, 1981; Tedeschi, 1983) or blocking one ear with a muff. Unfortunately, the effectiveness of these recommendations has not been documented. Much time and money could be spent on sophisticated acoustic equipment (for changing the speech signal) that might better be spent on education and language facilitation programs. Furthermore, subjecting a child to earmuffs or to distorted speech signals could conceivably interfere with the child's adjustment and learning. Before a child is subjected to this type of treatment, ethologically valid evidence should be obtained that such measures are more effective than the more usual recommendations.

Audiologists have brought to the area of language disorders and learning disabilities sophisticated instrumentation and measures of processing. While the approach may eventually be informative and aid in our understanding of auditory processing, its clinical value for an individual language-disordered or learning-disabled child appears limited at this time. It is hoped that research will continue in this area. Until we have better normative data and more information on what test results actually mean, the tests of central auditory dysfunction are more useful as research tools than as clinical procedures. We have known for a long time that children with language disorders have difficulty, by definition, processing language. To date, applying the term *central auditory processing dysfunction* to these children seems to offer little that is new in terms of explaining or remediating language or learning problems in children.

Neuropsychological Test Batteries. Perhaps the most common clinically used neuropsychological tests are adaptations of the Halstead-Reitan Battery originally developed for adults. There are now three batteries—one for children 5–8 (the Reitan-Indiana Battery), one for children 9–14 (the Halstead Battery), and one for children 15 and older (the Halstead-Reitan Battery). No battery is available for children below the age of 5. A complete description of the tests can be found in the *Ninth Mental Measurement Yearbook, Vol. 1* (Mitchell, 1985) and in many texts on neuropsychological testing (e.g., Hynd & Obrzut, 1981). In conjunction with one of the children's batteries, the *Weschler Intelligence Scale for Children* (Weschler, 1974) is usually administered and the results are examined for differences in verbal and performance scores as well as for scatter among subtest scores within the performance and verbal areas.

The neuropsychological battery for younger children includes 12 tests (e.g., category test, tactual-performance test, finger-tapping test, sensory-perception test, aphasia screening test, target test, and matching-pictures test). The category test is a concept-formation task designed to tap ability to abstract and integrate. In the tactual-performance test the child completes a modified Sequin-Goddard Form Board without the aid of vision, first using each hand independently and then both hands. It is included in order to measure tactile discrimination, kinesthesics, spatial memory, incidental memory, and manual dexterity. The finger-tapping test measures the number of taps per 10 seconds for the index finger of each hand and is used to determine motor speed and dexterity. The sensory-perception test includes tactile, visual, and auditory stimuli on tasks such as identification of fingers touched both unilaterally and bilaterally. The aphasia screening test includes reading, spelling, articulation, naming, math, and right-left orientation. In the target test the child reproduces patterns of dots as a measure of the ability to attend to and copy a visual pattern. The matching-pictures test taps generalization and categorization ability by asking the child to match pictures of similar but not identical pictures (e.g., different-aged men with similar-aged women). Standardization or normative data are not available in the manual; and standard score transformations are not presented, making intertest comparisons difficult (Mitchell, 1985). In most cases measures of performance are cutoff scores below which functioning is considered impaired.

Studies have indicated that children with known brain damage consistently score lower on this battery than children without brain damage (e.g., Reitan & Boll, 1973; Selz & Reitan, 1979). In the same studies, the scores of children with learning disabilities usually fell somewhere between those of the normal and brain-damaged children; the scores of the LD children were often not statistically different from either the normal or the brain-damaged children. By examining only the profiles of test results, however, Reitan was able to accurately place the children in the independently arrived at diagnostic categories (i.e., normal, brain-damaged, learning-disabled) with good accuracy. It appears that interpretations depend more on the knowledge and experience of the psychologist than on the psychometrics of the battery (Mitchell, 1985). But even if experienced clinicians can distinguish children according to profiles on such test batteries, there is no independent evidence that children scoring between normal and brain-damaged children do in fact have brain dysfunction.

Furthermore, neuropsychological test batteries for distinguishing normal from learning-disabled are more reliable for children after 9 years of age than for younger children (Rourke & Gates, 1981). The relevance of testing "for the educational process must be viewed within a developmental context" (Rourke & Gates, 1981, p. 14).

At this time there is little link between educational procedures and test findings. The usefulness of such testing to those currently involved in facilitating the learning of language or other skills with language-impaired and learning-disabled children is not apparent. However, research with such neuropsychological batteries or other neuropsychological tasks may eventually lead to further understandings.

For example, some interesting research with autistic children has implicated dysfunction of the amyglia in the temporal lobe (Nadel, 1986). A nonverbal concept-formation task was found to discriminate between primates with and without ablation of the amyglia. This same task, as well as one sensitive to hypothalmic lesion, was presented to autistic children and to retarded children. The autistic children had difficulty with the task sensitive to lesions of the amyglia but did not have difficulty with the task that was sensitive to disturbances within the hypothalmus; the retarded children had difficulty with neither. This type of research may some day have clinical and educational implications.

The neuropsychological approach is fascinating and intrigues those of us who would like to know the whys of language disorders. Research within the area should continue—but continued research and correlational findings do not mean that immediate clinical implications are obvious. When you need to know what to do and how to help an individual child, neuropsychological test results are not yet very helpful unless funding in your location is dependent on certain test results.

A Motor Approach

Like the specific-disabilities approach, the motor approach has to do with improving cognitive skills; unlike the specific-disabilities approach (which stresses direct remediation of weak cognitive abilities), the motor approach stresses motor development as a means of improving cognitive abilities (e.g., Ayres, 1975; Barsch, 1967; Delacato, 1963; Freidus, 1964; Kephart, 1960). The motor approach directly remediates motor and perceptual-motor skills. There is considerable variation in the rationale given and the techniques used by proponents of this approach, but the assumptions are the same. When these assumptions are applied to the child with a language disorder, they include: (1) that motor development is a necessary prerequisite to language development and (2) that training in motor skills will lead to improvement in language. There is certainly a strong correlation between motor development and language development (see Lenneberg, 1967), but there is also evidence that degree of motor disability is not directly correlated with language skills. According to Myers and Hammill (1969), "Irwin and Hammill (1964, 1965) have consistently failed to find differences in perception, language, or intelligence between mild, moderate, and severe cerebral palsied youngsters" (p. 130). There is no evidence that supports the assumption that motor training alone improves language expression or comprehension. Thus, if improved language skills are the ultimate goal, this cannot be the primary approach.

Certainly no one would deny the importance of improving the motor skills of any child. Not only is it possible that such improvement will enhance a child's ability to orient in relation to the environment, but it will probably enhance social relationships as well, and, thus, improve self-concept (as the child is better able to participate in play). However, the assumption that training motor skills should precede or supersede direct help in language learning with a language-disordered child would appear to be misguided. In fact, there is no need for such priority; motor activities make excellent contexts for language stimulation. If a language-disordered child is under any remedial program, it is the task of the speech and language pathologist to ensure that language is also an important part of the program and to incorporate language, whenever possible, with other activities.

Most of the motor approaches have had more impact on intervention for the learning-disabled child than for the language-disordered child. However, it becomes more and more obvious that learning disabilities and language disorders are integrally related—that the learning-disabled child often has a language disorder, and vice versa; that the preschool language-disordered child may well be called learning-disabled when entering school; and that the move for early identification of learning disabilities will bring the preschool language-disordered child in contact with special educators interested in learning disabilities. Thus, the speech-language pathologist and the special educator must be aware of various approaches that exist so they can integrate their approaches for the benefit of the child.

Information and techniques from approaches within the specific-abilities orientation should not provide the goals of language intervention but may well be incorporated into planning the techniques or context for facilitating language learning.

Summary

In this chapter some cognitive processes felt necessary for language learning were discussed. Poor performance on tasks designed to measure these abilities are correlated with language disorders and learning disabilities. Most often noted are problems with auditory sequential memory, processing of rapid auditory information, processing of multisensory input, and processing of degraded language stimuli. These correlates are usually viewed as causative factors, but each of these correlates may, in fact, be a reflection, instead of a cause, of a language disorder. It was suggested that processes cannot be examined without consideration of the knowledge base underlying the stimuli to be processed.

Within this orientation three approaches have impacted the clinical and educational management of language-disordered children. One, referred to here as the specific-disabilities approach, focuses on delineating and remediating weaknesses in cognitive skills. The assumptions implied in using this approach as the focus of an educational or clinical program for a language-disordered child are discussed using the ITPA as a model of the approach. The conclusions reached are that specific abilities, as currently measured, may not be distinct from one another in language learning, do not appear to be prerequisites for language learning, and may not be improved in many children by current remedial programs. Most important, however, is that no evidence exists that remedial programs designed to remediate these abilities improve general language functioning.

The second approach discussed is the neuropsychological approach, which includes the central auditory testing done by audiologists and the neuropsychological test batteries administered by psychologists. Each infers central nervous dysfunction from behavioral observations. Problems with each were discussed, and it was concluded that each represented an important research approach but neither was currently useful for explaining or remediating language-learning difficulties. A similar conclusion was reached concerning the third approach, a motor approach, which stresses motor development as a means of improving cognitive abilities.

The conclusions reached apply only to the clinical application of the specific-abilities orientation and not to its heuristic value. The specific-abilities approach is of particular interest to those carrying out research with the language-disordered child. It is probably through a combination of this orientation with the categorical and the communication-language orientations that we will eventually arrive at a better understanding of language-learning difficulties. At present, an orientation that is concerned with describing and facilitating the communication skills of language-disordered children is most appropriate for clinical and educational management. The application of a communication-language orientation is the focus of the rest of this text.

Suggested Readings

Case, R. (1985). *Intellectual development: Birth to adulthood.* New York: Academic Press.

Chi, M. T. H. (Ed.). (1983). *Trends in memory development research,* New York: Karger.

Hynd, G. W., & Obrzut, J. (Eds.). (1981). *Neuropsychological assessment and the school-age child.* New York: Grune & Stratton.

Keith, R. (Ed.). (1981). *Central auditory and language disorders in children.* San Diego: College-Hill Press.

Kirk, S., & Kirk, W. (1978). Uses and abuses of the ITPA. *Journal of Speech and Hearing Disorders, 43,* 58–75.

Tallal, P., Stark, R., & Mellits, D. (1985). Identification of language-impaired children on the basis of rapid perception and production skills. *Brain and Language, 25,* 314–322.

Tomblin, J. B. (1984). Specific abilities approach: An evaluation and an alternative method. In W. Perkins (Ed.), *Language handicaps in children.* New York: Thieme-Stratton, 27–42.

6

Describing Deviant Language

The goal of studying both normal and deviant language development has been to describe what children know about language, and to compare that knowledge with some standard or model. In most cases the ultimate objective of describing deviant language is to identify children with a language disorder, to plan educational intervention, or to estimate prognosis. A related fourth objective is to determine whether differences between deviant and normal language development are mainly *quantitative* (i.e., later onset and slower rate of development) or *qualitative* (i.e., different content/form/use interactions or different sequences in their development). This latter objective is usually met by comparing the language of a group of children who are in some way similar (often having been assigned a similar categorical label such as mentally retarded, deaf, or autistic) to a normal population. The results of this comparison are used to define clinical syndromes and to support or reject hypotheses about the interrelationship of language learning and other factors (e.g., intelligence, perceptual processing). In contrast, the first three objectives are most common when describing the language of a particular child, and the results are applied to decisions concerning language intervention.

Describing a child's language behavior for the purpose of identifying a problem, planning intervention, or estimating prognosis is referred to as *assessment*. Assessment is carried out before intervention not only to determine if a particular child needs intervention but to describe what a child needs to know about language and how the child can best learn language. Such prior description of the child's language and learning patterns ensures that the educational program begins immediately with the most appropriate and reasonable goals and procedures for facilitating language learning. Assessment continues during intervention in order to chart progress, establish new goals, and make necessary changes in procedures.

A Plan for Assessment

To be most efficient, persons involved in assessment must operate with a *plan*. An overall plan for assessment differs from a specific program, set of procedures, or list of test instruments. Although a program specifies certain techniques, and perhaps their order of application, a plan stresses the objectives of assessment and categorizes procedural techniques that might be useful for reaching each objective. An overall plan is needed if the assessor is to evaluate the usefulness of new testing instruments that appear on the market and the new observational methods that are mentioned in the literature. Because children are different in the ways that they can respond to procedural techniques, one cannot become bound to a limited set of testing instruments or procedures. In addition, a *plan* of assessment that focuses on the goals and purposes of techniques may help to avoid the tendency to collect large quantities of information with one or another instrument, without need or use for that information.

While all information about a child may be interesting, the information obtained from assessment should bear directly on identifying whether there is a problem, on determining the goals and procedures for intervention, or on determining prognosis. In the process of assessment, the clinician must be continually aware of the purpose of each technique that is used. That awareness extends to the information that can be expected and also to the reason why that information is needed. When perplexed by a particular child's problem with language learning, we often tend to search for a new instrument in the hope it will resolve our perplexity. The answer might better be found by determining *why* more information is needed and specifying *what* that information is, and only then to be concerned with the procedures for obtaining that information.

A plan for clinical assessment entails certain objectives:

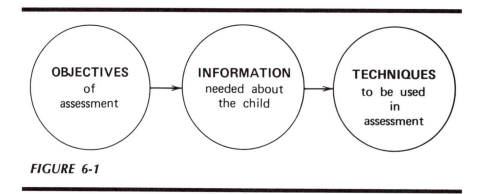

FIGURE 6-1

1. To determine whether there is a problem that needs further assessment and intervention
2. To determine the content/form/use goals of intervention, that is, to indicate what the child needs to learn, and what the child should be able to learn about language
3. To suggest procedures of intervention, that is, to indicate the factors that need to be taken into account for the child to be able to learn language skills most effectively
4. To determine, if possible, what kind of progress can be expected in an intervention program in contrast to progress made without such a program

Each objective of assessment determines the information that is needed to reach that objective; the information that is needed, in turn, determines the techniques to be used to obtain the information. Thus, the objectives of assessment lead to the information needed, and the information needed leads to the techniques as schematized in Figure 6-1. The objectives are outlined in Table 6-1 with examples of the information needed to reach the objectives.

In order to determine the existence of a problem and to determine the goals of intervention, information is needed about the child's language itself: what the child's purposes are for using the linguistic system and how the child chooses among alternative means in different contexts (use); what ideas of the world the child communicates (content); and how the child uses the conventional system of signals to represent what the child knows about the world and what aspects of the system the child uses (form). To determine the existence of a problem, given the definition in Chapter 2, a child's language will be compared with norms for other children of the same age. To determine the goals of intervention, a child's language performance will be compared with a sequence of language behaviors—a sequence presumed to represent a hierarchy of behaviors for language learning or at least a sequence presumed to be ordered from easiest to hardest to learn. Given a developmental approach, this sequence will be drawn from the developmental sequence of content/form/use interactions found among children learning language without difficulty.

To determine procedures for intervention and prognosis, it is necessary to obtain information about more than a child's language behavior. Are there factors

TABLE 6-1   Objectives of and Information from Assessment

Objectives: (Why use a procedure)	Information needed: (What the relevant procedure will produce)
1. To determine the existence of a problem.	A comparison of content/form/use interactions with those of children of comparable age.
2. To determine the goals of intervention	A description of the content/form/use of the child's language behaviors
3. To plan procedures of intervention: a. To reduce the effect of maintaining factors	Amount and type of language exposure in the environment; social and cognitive development; sensory acuity; general health
b. To determine the role others can play	Description of home and school environment; attitudes of others in the child's environment
c. To provide motivators and reinforcers	Child's interests, likes and dislikes
d. To plan structure of intervention sessions	Child's attention span and degree of distractibility in different contexts
e. To plan methods of presenting input	Sensory acuity and ability to associate meaning with a signal
f. To determine the form of the output	Oral motor capabilities; ability to make auditory-vocal associations
4. To determine prognosis	Results of previous attempts to facilitate language; all maintaining factors

interfering with language learning that can be changed? What aspects of the child's environment can be used to assist language learning? What conditions favor the child's language performance? Under what conditions does the child learn best? What conditions tend to disrupt the child? What interests the child? What seems to motivate and what appears to reinforce the child? What attempts have already been made to facilitate language learning and how have they succeeded? This information leads to suggestions about the *procedures* for intervention and to hypotheses about the progress that can be expected from future intervention. Thus, the information needed from assessment includes both a description of the child's current language performance and a description of factors that may influence the child's learning new language behaviors.

In order to plan the most effective procedures for intervention, it is necessary to know the role that the family and school might play in the intervention program; the most advantageous structure for an intervention program (e.g., a highly structured one-to-one relationship or a low-structured group experiential program); the necessity for manipulating the input signal (e.g., amplifying the signal, supplementing the signal with another sensory modality); the maintaining factors that might be eliminated; and both the topics and reinforcers that might best motivate the child to change language behaviors. Certainly no one set of intervention procedures is applicable to all children, just as no one set of intervention goals is appropriate to all children.

Given the objectives of assessment and the information needed to reach these

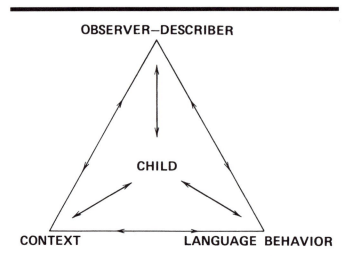

FIGURE 6-2 *A Schematic Representation of the Interactions That Influence the Evidence Obtained in Assessment (adapted from Henderson, 1961)*

objectives, we are left with the problem of how to obtain this information—how to collect evidence about the child and about the child's language and how to interpret the evidence that is obtained. Evidence of a child's knowledge of language is influenced by complex interactions among the child, the observer-describer, the contexts of observation, and the lnguage behavior to be described (see Figure 6-2). For example, the observer-describer brings to the observation certain preconceived ideas that influence what is observed and how it is described. In addition, when the observer is a part of the situation, the observer's personality and interactional patterns will influence the behavior of the child. Labov (1970) reported that both the familiarity of observers and the interactional patterns influenced the language sample obtained—only small restricted samples were obtained from many children when in the context of strange adults, while richer and longer samples were obtained in peer-peer interaction. The context of observation also influences what language behaviors are observed (Cazden, 1970). Low-structured settings have elicited samples that were more complex and longer than samples obtained in highly structured settings (Longhurst and Grubb 1974). Further discussion of these and other interactions is included in this chapter and in Chapters 12 and 13.

Obtaining the Evidence

Two major considerations involved in obtaining evidence about deviant language development are the observer, who chooses the behaviors to describe, and the context in which the language behavior is observed. Both considerations were discussed earlier in this chapter and are discussed further in the following sections.

Observer

Basically, all assessment techniques are observations under various conditions. Information from assessment is influenced by the acuteness and accuracy of the observer. To be an acute and accurate observer involves a number of factors; the most important factor is an understanding of the behavior being observed and of what aspects of that behavior are relevant to the purpose of the observation. For example, many individuals hear and enjoy operatic singers and can describe their voices. However, most descriptions probably would not help the singer who wished to improve singing skills. Likewise, we can all describe a book we have read and enjoyed, but few of us can describe the style of writing in a manner that would aid authors in improving their writing skills. It is possible to observe a child talking and interacting with someone else, and describe many important and interesting aspects of the situation. However, such descriptions may not provide the information that is necessary for understanding what the child knows about language or for determining what the child is ready to learn.

Thus, the first requirement for observation in assessment is knowledge of the behavior that is to be observed, including a framework for describing that behavior. The framework for describing deviant language behavior advocated in this text is a developmental framework that includes aspects of the content, form, and use of language and interactions among these dimensions.

Use of Other Observers.   If the observer must know the behavior being observed, can one use other nontrained observers (as parents or teachers) to obtain information about a child's language? It is possible to solicit from unsophisticated observers information about the child's use of language if one asks specific questions of the parent or teacher. In many instances teachers and parents can be quickly trained to keep a record of particular behaviors in school and home settings. In this way the speech-language pathologist obtains relevant information by imposing a framework for observation on others who interact with the child.

In addition to observations about language, other specialists can provide information that is important to planning the procedures of intervention—information that is beyond the expertise of the language specialists and requires different points of view as well as knowledge of different behaviors. For example, the medical person might provide information on the possibility of seizures; the educational specialist could contribute information on learning styles and academic areas in which language training could be embedded; the psychologist might describe social interactional patterns or cognitive skills; and the audiologist might suggest the need for a specific type of amplification. The usefulness of such reported observations is dependent on the evaluator's skill in (1) soliciting the information that is most applicable to the purposes of assessment and (2) interpreting the accuracy and relevance of the reports of others. Too often, reports are requested from other professionals without specification of the kind of information that is wanted. Such reports are often filed, and never referred to again. If the goals of assessment and the information that is needed to reach these goals are kept in mind, then one will not be asking for a "psychologist's report" or a "neurologist's report" but, instead, will be asking for particular information from the psychologist or neurologist. (For example, one might ask the psychologist for an estimate of nonverbal intelligence or of the social maturation of a child.) In this way one can tap the thinking of other professionals to assist in planning intervention.

In addition to other professionals, a child's family is a rich source of many kinds of information relevant to the goals and procedures of intervention. But much of this information is also lost if it is not solicited with its relationship to intervention kept in mind. Thus, two sources of information about the child are available in assessment—the observations made directly by the evaluator and the observations reported by other professionals or those in close contact with the child.

Context

Another consideration in obtaining evidence about deviant language development is the setting or context in which the observation occurs. As noted before, a variety of contexts are desirable for generating useful hypotheses about intervention (see also Gallagher, 1983; Muma, 1978).

How might contexts vary? They can take a number of forms. For example, contexts can vary in terms of the physical setting. The observation could take place in a familiar location (as home or school) or a strange location (as clinic or hospital). Different settings appear to influence the amount of data that is obtained, but not the type of grammatical structures observed (Olswang & Carpenter, 1978).

Contexts can also vary in terms of the persons who interact with the child. Children typically interact in everyday situations with persons they know, and so every opportunity should be taken to observe the child with familiar adults and peers. When possible, one should attempt to observe the child with family, friend, or teacher, not only as part of the observation session itself, but also in the waiting room, hallway, or cafeteria. Observation of interactions with different individuals allows the evaluator to determine whether the child adapts to listener needs by choosing alternative forms according to listener needs and status.

The observation could include a wide variety of settings within a particular location such as varying the types of objects available or the activities (e.g., playing with toys, eating, bathing, dressing, reading a book). Certain objects, such as blocks or objects that are difficult to manipulate and take a lot of concentration, tend to inhibit talking. The children are apparently so involved in the construction process that they talk little. Play with objects encourages talk about the "here and now" and may underrepresent the child's ability to talk of past events (French & Nelson, 1982). On the other hand, talking about events in the here and now may be easier than talking about events that are removed in space and time from the utterances since the child has the advantage of perceptual support in forming mental representations of the content. When moving away from the here and now, it appears to be easier to talk about familiar events (or scripted events, as discussed by French & Nelson). Actually, the influence of different settings (such as objects versus books or general conversation) and of "here and now" may vary with the age, cognitive level, and linguistic level of the child. In the observations of Lee and her associates (1974), older normal language learners gave more complex utterances when looking at pictures or retelling a story than when playing with toys. The reverse was true for the younger normal language learners. Similar comparisons have not been made with language-disordered children of different ages, cognitive levels, or language levels.

Finally, context can be varied in terms of the structure imposed by the observer or interactor. In certain situations the child is free to ask questions, respond to comments, and choose and direct his or her own activities as well as the activities of others; in other contexts the child is fairly passive and is expected to speak only when given permission, to follow commands of others, and to maintain rituals or schedules set by another.

Variations in context not only may affect the amount of data obtained (i.e., the number of words or utterances), but may affect the type of language behavior observed (e.g., the production of particular functions, alternative linguistic devices, or semantic-syntactic structures). For example, if a child is seen in a highly structured or ritualistic setting, there may be few examples of questions, requests, directives, or spontaneous comments; if the context of conversation is only about the here and now, the anaphoric reference or past tense may never be necessary and, thus, never be observed.

Many assessment contexts involve the child talking about activities that may not be easily retrievable from memory. For example, children are often asked to tell about an object; to describe what might be done given some hypothetical situation; to listen and answer questions about a story; to act out, recall, or imitate verbal comments or directions; or to tell a story about a static picture that does not necessarily represent a familiar scene or event. Such contexts tend to be highly structured; the child is moved from task to task, and little consideration is given to the ways in which tasks may influence the child's performance. In assessment contexts that are highly structured, the child is rarely able to use ongoing events (or even events well established in memory) to support the representations about the messages to be encoded or decoded. In contrast, less structured situations tend to allow support of context either from mental representations in consciousness or from ongoing events.

The techniques used in obtaining evidence about normal or deviant language development include observation in naturalistic interactions and observation of responses to the experimental manipulation of one or another of the components of content, form, and use. The difference between these two types of techniques can be thought of in terms of the degree of structure imposed by the observer. In the naturalistic observation the imposition of structure is minimal; this type of observation, when applied clinically, is referred to as obtaining a naturalistic *language sample*. In the observation of responses to experimental manipulation the imposition of structure by the observer is high; this type of observation, when applied clinically, is referred to as *standardized testing*. In addition, there are observations that fall somewhere on the continuum between high and low imposition of structure that are referred to here as *nonstandardized elicitations*. Each type of context has a role in assessment.

Standardized Testing

The highest degree of structure is imposed on a situation when a standardized test is administered. Observations of a child in highly structured situations are best used when one has need to compare a child's behavior with the behavior of his or her peers (as when attempting to identify children with a problem). In this case it is helpful to try to control for situational variables that may differentially influence comparisons among children.

In order to compare children's responses to particular tasks, it is necessary for the observer to keep constant as many of the situational variables as possible. To reduce the number of variables and keep the situation constant, many things need to be determined in advance, such as directions, the methods of presenting materials, the time devoted to certain tasks, and responses to the child's questions. By controlling the situation in these ways, the differences between children's responses to the task are more likely to be attributable to differences between children themselves than to differences in the situation. The structured situation generally provides information that is relevant for comparing children with respect to language behaviors—information that is important for identifying children with a language disorder. For this purpose, highly structured observations are useful (see Chapter 7). However, such highly structured observations are strictly etic—that is, they use preset categories for description and do not allow for other interpretations. In addition, they are less flexible in the contexts observed, and restrict the language behaviors that can be observed. Standardized testing is *not*, therefore, designed to provide information relevant for a *description* of a particular child's language system or his use of that system. Because of this, it is *not* helpful in providing information that would lead to hypotheses about what a child is ready to learn, that is, for planning the goals of intervention.

Standardized testing was a common means of obtaining evidence about deviant language (see language assessment procedures, for example, in Berry, 1969; Carrow, 1972; J. Irwin & Marge, 1972; and Myers & Hammill, 1969). Currently, there has been a trend away from the use of such highly structured observations (e.g., Bloom & Lahey, 1978; Leonard, Prutting, Perozzi, & Berkley, 1978; N. J. Lund & Duchan, 1983; Muma, 1978). This trend has been motivated by the desire to describe what a child knows about language as a system to be *used* for communication. Such information is needed to plan an intervention program or to specify qualitative differences between deviant and normal language. For these objectives a less structured situation is more helpful.

Naturalistic Observation (Language Sample)

Low-structured observations allow for both etic (i.e., use of preset categories) and emic (i.e., categories derived from the data themselves) interpretations.° To understand how the language of the child with a language disorder is both similar to and different from the language of the child with normal language development, and to best describe what the child knows about language, low-structured observations offer the most flexibility.

Settings should be used that permit the child to interact verbally both as an initiator and as a responder and that allow the child to talk about topics that are of interest and that are easily retrievable from the child's memory. Such settings are often termed *naturalistic* in that they are more like a child's "real life." While

---

° That is, if the process of observation does not involve severe data restriction before the observations are recorded.

structured settings are also a natural part of at least the schoolchild's daily life, and perhaps the home life of some children, they do not afford enough opportunity for the child to direct interactions and activities to make them useful for describing a wide variety of content/form/use interactions. Language is a form of communication and essentially a social interaction; its *use* can only be described in a social context—ideally one that is representative of the child's usual interactions. Some homes, school playgrounds, lunchrooms, or classrooms (during a free activity period) may be used as settings for naturalistic observations. In lieu of an actual visit to the child's natural environment (at home or at school), one might attempt to recreate a relaxed naturalistic-type setting within the clinical or educational facilities that are available to the observer.

Low-structured observations in the form of "language samples" have been frequently recommended as an assessment procedure (e.g., Blau, Lahey, & Oleksiuk-Velez, 1984; Crystal, Fletcher, & Garman, 1976; Hubbell, 1981; Lahey, Launer, & Schiff-Myers, 1983; Lee, 1974; N. J. Lund & Duchan, 1983; J. E. McLean & Snyder-McLean, 1978; Muma, 1978; Tyack & Gottsleben, 1974). (For more detail on language sampling see Chapter 12.) Information from such a language sample should be supplemented with information obtained through nonstandardized elicitation. Certain language behaviors may not occur (or may occur only rarely) in a low-structured context, but may be readily elicited (see, for example, Coggins, Olswang, & Guthrie, 1987).

Nonstandardized Elicitation

Sampling low-structured, or naturalistic, situations allows one to observe the child's spontaneous behaviors, and is the best situation for forming hypotheses that may be tested subsequently with more structured nonstandardized elicitations. Analyses of data obtained from a language sample and from elicitation tasks are used to plan goals of intervention.

Nonstandardized elicitations are midway between high and low degrees of observer-imposed structure. The situation is similar to the low-structured observation except that the evaluator takes a more active role in manipulating the context in order to elicit particular responses. The situation can be a naturalistic one in which the observer suggests certain tasks and probes in order to obtain responses. However, the child's responses and interests determine the exact procedures that are used. Children might be asked to describe what they are doing, to give directions to puppets, or to respond with actions to certain linguistic input. All these are carried out in a play context and, unlike standardized elicitations, use topics and objects that the child has chosen or event sequences with which the child is very familiar. Unlike the low-structured observation, the evaluator intervenes in the play and attempts to elicit particular content/form/use interactions; the interactions have been determined in advance, but the procedures for eliciting interactions evolve in the situations as they happen. The use of such techniques is discussed in detail in Chapter 13 and by Leonard, Prutting, Perozzi, and Berkley, 1978.

The function of nonstandardized elicitations is to observe some particular aspect of the child's language performance. The nonstandardized elicitation of responses is most useful for testing hypotheses about a child's language in order to plan the goals of intervention; such elicitation is also helpful for determining procedures of intervention, especially in regard to how particular responses might be obtained from a particular child. Nonstandardized elicitations are less useful for comparing children with one another and, thus, for identifying a problem with language learning.

In summary, the evidence obtained about deviant language is influenced by the observer's knowledge of the behavior to be observed, the variety of contexts observed, and the degree of structure imposed on the contexts by the observer. The objectives of observation influence decisions about how to obtain data and also influence how the data are interpreted. For further information on obtaining information see Chapters 12 and 13 as well as Dollaghan and Miller (1986) and the references cited above.

Interpreting the Evidence

To place the obtained evidence in some meaningful perspective, it must be categorized in relation to a model or standard of comparison, and it must be presented in a frame of reference that is relevant to the objective of comparison. Such activities have to do with forming taxonomies and presenting taxonomies once they have been formed.

Forming Taxonomies

A taxonomy is a categorization of the behaviors that are observed. Behaviors that are similar in some way (e.g., in terms of their content, form, or use or in the interactions among content, form, and use) are grouped together and labeled. In the study of deviant language development the taxonomies of form are usually etic (predetermined) and are based on the adult model of language or on descriptions in the literature of normal language development (i.e., a child model).

Taxonomies of Form. The formal characteristics of language structure, as outlined for the adult speaker by the science of linguistics, have most often provided the taxonomies used to describe the form of deviant language. There is not, however, a set of accepted or standardized categories. Both the theory of generative transformational grammar and procedures of structural linguistics have been drawn upon. The emphasis in each has varied with the preferences of individual researchers and clinicians, and the resulting categories of description have been different. For example, Menyuk (1964) described differences in the sentences produced by children with and without a language disorder according to grammatical transformations (being influenced by the theory of generative transformational grammar), while others (Dever & Bauman, 1974; Engler, Hannah, & Longhurst, 1973; Hubbell, 1981) recommended use of tagmemic or structural categories (being influenced by procedures from structural linguistics). Although the names of the categories may vary, most categories of form have represented one or another application of linguistic theory to the description of the structural characteristics of language form.

When the linguistic system of the adult language has served as the model for comparison, the children's behaviors have been described in terms of their ap-

TABLE 6-2 Frequency of Sentence Types in the 1000 Sentence Samples for Each Retarded Child

Mental Age of Retarded Children (Years and Months)	Chrono-logical Age of Retarded Children (Years and Months)	Sentence Type						
		Declarative	Negative	Question	Negative Question	Passive	Negative Passive	Negative Passive Question
2, 3	6, 5	563	275	162				
2, 11	13, 1	517	293	171	19			
3, 3	7, 10	516	337	99	37	11		
4, 9	16, 2	430	393	127	41	9		
8, 10	14, 4	438	351	119	45	24	18	5

Note: Adapted from Lackner, 1968.
These data illustrate the increasing use of adult sentence types as mental age increases.

proximations to the adult model (e.g., the sentence types, transformations or grammatical parts of speech, and features that are included, omitted, substituted, or incorrectly placed in their speech). Table 6-2 is an illustration of the use of sentence types from the adult model as a means of describing deviant language development. Table 6-3 illustrates an analysis based on adult parts of speech. And Table 6-4 demonstrates comparisons between normal language learners and language-disordered children on various adult structures (see also Menyuk, 1964). (Note that the data in each table are based on language sampling procedures, but that each of the studies reported the data in a different manner, such as frequency, proportion, or number of children. As noted on Table 6-4, different conclusions can be drawn depending upon the way the data are reported.)

Often the language of such children is described in terms of what is lacking—what the child must learn in order to become a fluent speaker. Parents and teachers, as well as the clinicians and educators, who are unsophisticated in linguistic analysis commonly use descriptions such as "the child confuses pronouns," "the child does not speak in complete sentences," and so on. These descriptions do not describe what the child *does* do or the system that the child has. Rather, they compare the child's performance with the adult model that the child is expected eventually to learn. Before the late 1960s, speech-language pathologists and educators concentrated on quantifying such adult-based descriptions. They employed measure such as the length-complexity index, which assigned points to sentence structures according to their complexity and completeness in relation to the adult model (see W. Johnson, Darley, & Spriestersbach, 1963, for procedures).

Although the above examples were drawn from low-structured observations, highly structured observations designed for clinical application (i.e., standardized tests) were, and are still, most often based on adult models of form. Responses are sometimes categorized according to parts of speech as adjectives, articles, and pronouns (see Carrow, 1974), but usually are categorized more globally into

**TABLE 6-3 Grammatical Structure of Responses by Matched Pairs
of Mongol/Non-Mongol Patients to Two Forms of Interview (N = 11 Pairs)**

Part of Speech	Conversation Mean Percent		Picture Description Mean Percent	
	Mongol	Non-Mongol	Mongol	Non-Mongol
Verbs	19.36	20.27	5.55	7.64
Nouns	31.91	26.91	66.73	50.55
Adjectives	10.00	10.36	8.09	10.36
Adverbs	6.09	6.55	1.27	3.36
Prepositions	7.36	7.82	2.00	3.64
Pronouns	9.64	11.00	2.18	3.09
Articles	7.00	6.18	7.73	12.91
Conjunctions	2.73	3.64	5.91	8.18
Miscellaneous	5.91	7.27	0.55	0.27

Note: From Mein, 1961, p. 57.

These data were based on an analysis of language samples collected in two contexts—a conversational interview and description of pictures. The two populations were matched on the basis of sex, chronological age (mean was 20 years, 9 months, for mongols and 20 years, 5 months, for nonmongols), and mental age (mean was 4 years, 6 months, for mongols and 4 years, 7 months, for nonmongols).

As might be expected, the percentage of nouns was higher for both populations when the subjects were describing pictures and a greater variety of word types was used in the conversational context. This analysis showed few differences between the groups except for the relatively higher percentage of nouns for the mongols in both contexts and a lower percentage of articles in the picture description context.

syntax (e.g., Lee, 1971) or vocabulary (e.g., Dunn & Dunn, 1981). (See Chapter 7 for categorization of tests to elicit language form.) In all cases tabulations are made of the number of correct and incorrect responses—correctness determined by conformity to the adult model.

Even when comparisons are not made directly with adult performance, most taxonomies of form ultimately rely on terminology and categories derived from the adult model. However, when child language has motivated the taxonomies of form, the comparisons focus on what the child *can do*, rather than on what the child cannot do. For example, the strings of lexical categories that the children produced were described by Morehead and Ingram (1973). The lexical types (e.g., noun, verb, modal) came from adult descriptions, but the strings were derived from the children's performance and comparisons were made with normal language learners at the same level of linguistic development; the children were not compared with the adult model. Thus, though some aspects of adult taxonomies were used, the categories of strings were adapted for child language.

Comparisons of the forms produced by language-disordered children with those produced by normal language learners at similar levels of development suggest that differences that do occur are more in terms of the frequency of occurrence of various structures than in terms of the type of structures (e.g., Leonard, 1972; Morehead & Ingram, 1973).

Taxonomies of Content. In a first report on the taxonomies of the content of deviant language, Leonard, Bolders, and Miller (1976) described and compared semantic relations expressed in the two-word utterances of normal and language-disordered children. Their descriptions were influenced by Fillmore's case grammar (1968), which was based on the adult speaker, with adaptations based on studies of normal child language. (See Table 6-5). Similarly, Freedman and Carpenter (1976) described and compared the number of differet semantic relations expressed in the two-word utterances of four normal and four language-impaired children. Their descriptions were based on the taxonomies of content that evolved in the studies of normal child language by, in particular, Bloom (1970) and Schlesinger (1971, 1974) and as summarized by Brown (1973). The categories derived by Bloom, Lightbown, and Hood (1975) in the study of normal children were applied by Tamari (1978) in a longitudinal study of Down's syndrome children and by Mattingly (1978) in a study of a heterogeneous group of language-disordered children. In each of these studies, comparisons showed few differences between language-disordered children and normal language learners when children were matched by mean length of utterance.

Taxonomies of content have less often been utilized in highly structured observations of language-disordered children. In a study of the comprehension of various semantic relations (agent-action, action-object, possession, and locative) presented with varying forms, Duchan and Erickson (1976) found no differences between normal and retarded children matched by MLU.

Since the late 1970s, taxonomies of content have also been suggested for clinical assessment where the objective of assessment is to determine goals of intervention (e.g., Bloom & Lahey, 1978; N. J. Lund & Duchan, 1983; J. Miller, 1981; Muma, 1978; J. E. McLean & Snyder-McLean, 1978). The taxonomies used have been based on child language as a model; that is, they evolved from the study of normal development. An extended taxonomy of content/form interactions based on the study of normal child language is presented in Chapters 8–11 as a part of the C/F/U Goal Plan for Language Learning.

Taxonomies of Use.   Taxonomies of use applied to low-structured observations before the late 1970s most frequently related to communicativeness and the relevance of utterances to context. For example, Shapiro, Chiarandini, and Fish (1974) divided utterances into communicative and noncommunicative. M. Cunningham (1968) classified utterances as egocentric utterances (e.g., echoes and inappropriate remarks) and socialized utterances (e.g., giving information and answering questions). Although Cunningham's first level of categorization was influenced by Piaget's (1955) study of child language (i.e., the distinction between egocentric and social speech), the basis of the subcategories is not clear. Descriptions of use by Kanner (1946) were combined with aspects of content/form interactions.

More recently, a wider variety of use categories have been applied to the study of developmental language disorders. Categories of various communicative functions (e.g., requests for object, requests for information, comments, answers) have been used (e.g., Curtiss, Prutting, & Lowell, 1979; Leonard, Camarata, Rowan, & Chapman, 1982; Rom & Bliss, 1981) to describe particular populations and to compare populations of language-disordered children. The use of language in the context of other language (e.g., use of anaphoric reference, request for clarification, use of cohesive devices) has been categorized by some to describe the com-

TABLE 6-4 Comparison Between the Normal and Deviant Language Users in Terms of the Number of Children Using Each Structure and the Frequency with which Each Structure Was Used. N = Normal Speakers; D = Deviant Speakers

Structure	Number of Children Using Structures		p^a	Mean Frequency		Standard Deviation		p
	N	D		N	D	N	D	
Negation (He is *not* smiling.)	7	2	ns^b	2.44	0.67	1.59	1.66	0.05
Contraction (She's happy.)	9	8	ns	17.67	8.78	6.33	6.34	0.01
Auxiliary *be* (The lion *is* jumping up.)	9	8	ns	22.00	7.78	6.48	5.83	0.001
Adjective (The *big* bear likes her.)	9	5	ns	6.78	1.44	4.21	1.59	0.01
Infinitival complement (I want to *sing*.)	9	9	ns	14.56	5.89	6.88	6.47	0.05
Indefinite pronoun (*It* was gone.)	9	8	ns	15.11	7.00	8.30	5.79	0.05
Personal pronoun	9	9	ns	30.56	16.00	12.70	10.09	0.05

(The ghost saw them.)

Main verb	9	9	ns	51.00	22.89	7.25	11.01	0.001
(The plane *flies* funny.)								
Secondary verb	9	8	ns	18.00	5.44	6.78	6.62	0.01
(He wants the boy to *sing*.)								
Conjunction^c	9	6	ns	7.00	2.44	5.17	2.46	0.05
(I want it *but* I won't get it.)								
Verb-phrase omission	5	9	ns	1.00	11.78	1.32	8.60	0.01
(That funny.)								
Noun-phrase omission	3	9	ns	0.44	5.22	0.73	4.55	0.01
(Wanna go.)								
Article omission	4	9	ns	0.78	3.22	0.97	2.39	0.05
(Ghost is gonna scare us.)								
Inversion verb number	8	5	ns	2.22	0.56	1.09	0.53	0.01
(There's the bears!)								

Note: From Leonard, 1972, p. 433. Reprinted by permission of the American-Speech-Language-Hearing Association.

[a] p = probability of this result occurring by chance alone; in other words, significance level.

[b] ns = not significant.

[c] Lee and Canter (1971) conjunction classification.

Language samples were based on children's responses to pictures following a predetermined set of prompts by the interviewer. Data were analyzed according to structures defined by Menyuk (1964) and by Lee and Canter (1971). Normal and deviant children were compared in terms of the number of children who used a structure and in terms of the frequency with which each structure was used. The table reports differences found between the groups on structures used by at least 50% of one of the groups. Results indicate there are differences between the populations in the frequency with which certain structures were used and not in terms of the number of children who used a structure.

TABLE 6-5 An Example of a Taxonomy of Language Content, with the Mean Frequency of Utterances Used to Express Each Semantic Relation Presented Here by Age and Mean Length of Utterance[a]

	Means					
Semantic Relation	3-Year-Old N[b]	3-Year-Old LD[c]	5-Year-Old N	5-Year-Old LD	MLU 5.03 N	MLU 4.97 LD
Essive + locative	3.90[d]	10.00[d]	2.20[d]	11.20[d]	4.43	5.14
Verb + agentive	3.70[d]	10.40[d]	7.70	10.40[d]	5.00	9.86
Locative + designated	3.00	3.70	1.80	2.10	3.86	3.57
Attributive + designated	3.00	1.50	2.30	1.50	4.29	3.14
Verb + agentive + locative	6.50	7.20	9.60	6.30	6.86	7.43
Verb + agentive + objective	3.60	4.10	6.40	3.60	3.00	5.43
Verb + agentive + dative	1.70	2.60	3.00	2.00	—	—
Utterances that reflected more complex semantic rules but were not used twice by half of the subjects	10.40[e]	2.10[e]	9.30[e]	1.50[e]		

Note: Adapted from Leonard, Bolders, and Miller, 1976.

[a] Data were based on a sample of 50 utterances. Only semantic relations that occurred at least two times by at least half of the children in each group were included.

[b] N = normal.

[c] LD = language disordered.

[d] Least significant difference < .05.

[e] Least significant difference < .001.

municative behaviors of language-disordered children (e.g., Brinton, Fujiki, Winkler, & Loeb, 1986; Geller, in preparation; Gallagher & Darnton, 1978; Van Kleeck & Frankel, 1981). Finally, some researchers have categorized various aspects of the children's use of language to adapt to their listeners (e.g., Fey, Leonard, & Wilcox, 1981). See Figure 6-3.

Presenting Taxonomies

It is rare that a mere listing of the taxonomies with exemplars is sufficient. Usually the data are quantified and compared with other data or with some frame of reference.

Quantification may take the form of frequency counts of the number of utterances or words that fit each category. In the example in Table 6-2 frequency counts were given, but also included was the total number of utterances produced so that proportions could be computed. The proportional use of particular categories is frequently reported and is illustrated in Table 6-3 and Figure 6-3. To know, however, that a child produced six utterances that were classified as negatives, and this was equal to 10% of the total utterances, or to know that a child responded correctly to 22 out of 60 utterances is still not meaningful until the information is

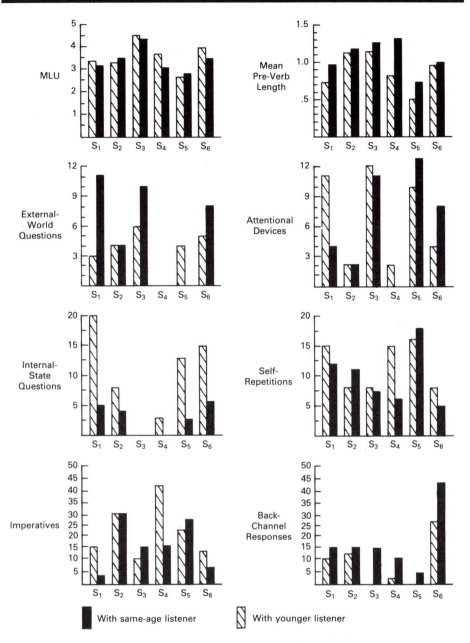

FIGURE 6-3 *Performance of Language-Impaired Subjects in Younger versus Same-Age Listener Conditions on Eight Linguistic Measures. Mean Length of Utterance (MLU) and Mean Pre-Verb Length are reported in morphemes. The remaining six measures reflect the percentage of total utterances falling into each category. These language-impaired children varied a number of factors when talking with younger children (e.g., the number of internal state questions, amount of feedback, and complexity), but they did not vary other factors. (From Fey, Leonard, & Wilcox 1981, p. 95.)*

placed in a context or perspective that relates to the original purpose of the observation.

Taxonomies derived from observations of a particular child during clinical assessment may be placed in meaningful context by three approaches; (1) norm referencing—comparison with a group; (2) criterion referencing—comparison with a predetermined standard of performance; and (3) communication referencing—comparison with some concept of communicative behavior that is without defined norms or standards of performance. Each provides important but different information. The approach used in reporting observations varies with the objective or purpose of observing. The value of each type of reference should be kept in mind when describing observations and when reading descriptions of observations.

Norm-Referenced Descriptions. Norm-referenced descriptions compare the behaviors of one child with the behaviors of other children. Norm-referenced descriptions may be reported as scores that reflect a child's standing relative to peers. For example, the number of correct responses on a test may be presented as a percentile rank. Percentile ranks represent the percentage of children whose scores were lower than the score being reported—a rank of 10th percentile indicates that 10% of the children in the normative population scored at or below this level and 90% scored above this level. Other means of comparing a child's score with that of peers include standard scores and stanine scores (see Chapter 7). Each of these comparisons is based on results of the same task administered to a number of children of the same age or grade level.

Another type of norm-referenced description is referred to as an equivalent (or status-level) score. Age-equivalent scores reflect the average age of children with similar language behaviors or with a similar score on a test—they do not necessarily compare a child with same-age peers. Sometimes informal observations are reported in terms of age-equivalent descriptions. For example, a teacher or parent may report that a child behaves like a 3-year-old, or that a child's language behaviors are most like those of a 1-year-old.

Since norm-referenced reports of observations are comparisons of a child with other children, they best serve the function of determining the existence of a problem. However, see Chapter 7 for a discussion of the problems with the use of age-equivalent scores for this purpose. Norm-referenced reports are helpful for determining *who* might be considered for intervention, but they are not helpful for determining the goals and procedures for intervention.

Criterion-Referenced Descriptions. In lieu of, or in addition to, a normative reference, observations can be reported in terms of an operational criterion of performance. Criteria of performance have become important in educational technology, where interest has focused on students' mastery of operationally defined instructional objectives. Tests designed to measure achievement in these terms have been called criterion-referenced tests; they compare the performance of a child or group of children to a preset standard or criterion. The difference between criterion-referenced and norm-referenced tests and the application of criterion-referenced instruments have been reported by B. Bloom, Hastings, and Madaus (1971); Glaser and Nitko (1971); Gorth and Hambleton (1972); and Popham and

Husek (1969). The purpose of criterion-referenced measures is to provide information about the performance of individuals or groups of individuals relative to certain tasks or goals. It is particularly relevant as a means of reassessing behaviors during intervention to determine the effectiveness of a program and the need to establish new goals. Normative scores cannot be used for this same purpose. Normative reference points are not defined with respect to the behaviors that are being observed, but, instead, with respect to how many other children behaved in the same way. The norm-referenced score gives certain comparative information but gives no information about the nature of the child's own behavior or its relevance to some specified skill. As such, normative scores do not directly relate to the kind of information that is needed for planning the specific goals of intervention.

In order to use criterion reference as a means of reporting taxonomies formed in assessment, a standard of performance must be established beforehand—one that indicates competence or productivity of that behavior in the child's repertoire of behaviors. Examples of such operational criteria have been used in the study of normal language development. One instance of a particular behavior is not enough. One instance cannot be considered adequate evidence that a child has mastered the rule that underlies the content/form/use interaction. The clinician feels more confident inferring such knowledge after observing many instances in different contexts. For example, if a child said "no juice," "no bath," "no get dressed," "no ball," in situations where the child was rejecting these objects or activities, we could reasonably conclude that the child knew a rule for negation. The rule specifies that *no*, a negative marker, can be juxtaposed with other words and used in different situations to express the same meaning in each situation—the meaning of rejection. Suppose that, at the same time, the child also said "don't do that" only once. Although one could conclude that the child knew something about the content of negation and the form of negative utterances (*no* plus a word), there is less evidence that the child also *knew* the contracted negative particle *don't*. Further exemplars of *don't* juxtaposed with other words (e.g., "don't eat it," "don't touch") spoken in different situations would be needed before such knowledge could be inferred.

If one instance is not enough, how many instances are needed? The answer is not clear, but there are a few precedents in the study of normal language development. The production of five or more different multiword utterances that represented a particular structure or semantic-syntactic relation was used by Bloom (1970) as a criterion. This criterion of five different utterances in 5 to 8 hours of observation was initially an arbitrary decision. However, it was later supported as an indication of rule-governed behavior when the sequence of development that resulted from the absolute frequency criterion was compared with the sequence obtained using proportional measures (a relative instead of an absolute measure) (Bloom, Lightbown, & Hood, 1975).

Brown (1973) set the criterion for the *acquisition* (i.e., full knowledge) of various grammatical morphemes at 90% occurrence in obligatory contexts in two consecutive samples. That is, the child must have used the morpheme at least 9 out of every 10 times the linguistic or nonlinguistic context required its use in the adult model. Brown counted the number of times that a morpheme (e.g., plural -*s*) was obligatory (i.e., the number of required contexts) in a sample of language, and then counted the number of times the child produced the morpheme in order to compute a proportion of morpheme use. (See also Johnston & Schery, 1976, in Table 6-6 for an application of this criterion to language-disordered children.) Such a criterion that compares the child's behavior with expected adult behavior represents a standard of performance based on an extrinsic measure—the adult model.

With either the frequency measure or the proportional measure, the behavior was specified and a quantitative criterion was set in advance. These are examples of criterion-referenced descriptions—a description in relation to a preset standard of performance.

Further examples of distinctions between norm-referenced and criterion-referenced descriptions can be found in your everyday life. As a student you have experienced both types of reference in the assignment of grades by your instructors. On certain types of tests some instructors may have set a percentage of correct responses as a criterion by which you were graded. In this case you might have received an A if you correctly answered 90% of the questions or a B if you correctly answered 85%. In this type of criterion-referenced grading every member of the class could obtain an A, or even a C or D. The criterion of description is not related to how the other students performed. Rather, your performance was compared with a preset standard of performance and is a good example of criterion-referenced description.

More than likely, you have also experienced grading that was based on norm referencing—that is, on comparisons of your performance with that of the other members of your class. This type of grading is common in large introductory classes and is usually referred to as "curving" the grades (implying a grade distribution that approaches the normal curve). To curve the grades simply means to take a certain percentage at the top and assign an A, assign a B to a certain percentage below that, etc. In this case it is virtually impossible for all students to obtain an A or for all students to fail. Students are graded according to comparisons with other students in the class—a norm-referenced description.

In language assessment, criterion-referenced descriptions are used when the purpose of the observation is to determine how well a certain behavior is established in a child's repertoire. Criterion-referenced descriptions are most helpful in initial assessment to determine the goals of an intervention program. Criterion-referenced descriptions are most useful in reassessment to determine when those goals have been reached and when new goals should be established.

Communication-Referenced Descriptions.   Communication-referenced descriptions° are those descriptions of observations made during assessment which make reference to the general communication behavior of a child without considering either norms or preset standards of performance. While it is usually the case that a standard of performance or norm has not been well defined for the behaviors described, some expectation is unquestionably implied or the behavior would not have been mentioned. For example, a techer describes a child to the speech-language pathologist as one who smiles a lot and who frequently touches other children's hair. The teacher may not have had a list of behaviors that included

---

° What is here called *communication-referenced* seems close to what Hively (1974) referred to as *domain-referenced.*

TABLE 6-6   Language Levels and a Taxonomy of Form

Mean Values for Summary Language Measures by Level

Level	N	Mean-Words-Per-Utterance	Mean-Morphemes-Per-Utterance	Mean-Words/Mean-Morphemes
1	10	2.29	2.58	0.890
2	17	2.78	2.95	0.944
3	51	3.67	4.05	0.907
4	76	4.59	5.12	0.895
5	133	6.19	6.97	0.894

Note: From Johnston and Schery, 1976.

Language Level (Johnston and Schery Criteria) at Which Each Morpheme was Used at All and Acquired (90%) by 50% of the Subjects at that Level in Three Research Studies

	Use At All J&S	90% Use in Obligatory Contexts		
		J&S	DeVilliers	Brown
Plural -s	1	2	1	1
In	1	2	2	1
On	2	3	2	1
-ing	1	3	2	2
Irreg. past	1	1.4	—[a]	2
Article	1	4	4	3
Copula uncontracted	3	5	4	2
Possessive -s	5	+[b]	—	3
Aux. "be" uncontracted	4	5	—	3
Past -ed	4	5	4	3
3rd person -s	4	5	4	3
Aux. "be" contracted	3	5	—	(4)[c]
Copula contracted	1	+[b]	3	(4)
Irreg. 3rd person	5	5	—	(4)

Note: From Johnston and Schery, 1976.

[a] Dashes indicate insufficient data.

[b] Did not reach criteria at any level.

[c] Numbers in parentheses are probable.

Johnston and Schery (1976) reported on the use of grammatical morphemes by 287 language-disordered children, aged 3 years, 10 months, to 16 years, 2 months. The data were based on 100-utterance language samples obtained and analyzed by teachers under the guidance of the authors. Children were grouped by language level—based on utterance length, as outlined in the Table above. Results were then compared with two previously reported studies in normal language development. The language-disordered children acquired (i.e., they used the morphemes in obligatory contexts 90% of the time) the morphemes in much the same order as the normal children, but this acquisition was at a later level of development, that is, when their MLU was higher than that reported for normal children.

smiling and touching hair, and yet when asked about the child's mode of communicating with others, these behaviors became relevant to the description. The criterion related to contact or communication, but it could not be quantified in terms of other children or in terms of how much is expected. Many descriptions of the language-disordered child fit into precisely this type of reference.

In initial assessment, communication-referenced descriptions are rarely quantified and are often anecdotal. They include behaviors that the observer feels are relevant to describing a child's communication skills. (See Box 6-1 for an example.) In later assessment sessions, one may look for regularities between the occurrence of the behavior and contextual factors. For example, the clinician may observe Nancy, who is described in Box 6-1, further to see if there is any context associated with the sounds produced. In this case the communication-referenced description may then switch to a criterion-referenced description as a certain frequency of sound-context co-occurrences will be needed to determine if this is a rule-governed behavior.

Remember, however, that taxonomies should record the regularities and consistencies that are to be found among the different behaviors a child may present. Isolated instances of behavior, although no doubt interesting and possibly important, are less important than a larger number of behaviors that share common elements or features. Regularities should emerge in almost any sample of behavior, and they may well be dissimilar across children or even for the same child at different times in the course of development.

Assessment Objectives in Relation to Context and Description. Observations for the purpose of identifying a child with a language disorder and for planning intervention are generally reported in all three frames of reference: norm reference, criterion reference, and communication reference. Each has a particular function. Norm-referenced descriptions help to determine the existence of a problem; criterion-referenced descriptions help to determine what will be taught in planning the goals of intervention; communication-referenced descriptions may lead to goals of therapy or to procedures. The structure of different contexts and the types of reference most often employed to reach each objective of assessment are summarized in Table 6-7.

Analyses of standardized observations are usually reported in reference to normative data (as a language age, standard score, percentile rank, etc.), but other forms of reference are occasionally utilized. For example, many reports of standardized observations comment on the child's behavior within the domain of a

---

BOX 6-1

Nancy was taken from her wheelchair and seated on the floor facing the interviewer. She immediately swiveled so she faced the opposite direction. When turned to face the interviewer, she repeatedly swiveled herself until a box of toys was placed in front of her. Facing the box, she remained in position and picked out toys from the box. She handled each without looking at it, and then dropped it to pick up another. Occasionally, she emitted the sounds /f/ or a nasalized /a/.

TABLE 6-7   Reference Used to Report Observations According to the Structure Imposed by the Observor and the Objective of Assessment

| Objective of Assessment | Degree of Structure Imposed by the Observer and Most Useful Reference for Descriptions | | |
| | High | | Low |
	Standardized Elicited Response	Nonstandardized Elicited Response	Relaxed Structure Nonelicited Response
Determine existence of a problem	Norm-referenced		Norm-referenced
Plan goals of intervention		Criterion-referenced	Criterion-referenced Communication-referenced
Plan procedure of intervention		Criterion-referenced	Criterion-referenced Communication-referenced

structured task (the child's attention span, frustration level, dependence on the examiner, etc.) and thus provide a communication-referenced description that may assist in planning the procedures of intervention. In addition, some clinicians try to use responses to particular items on tests to determine goals of intervention, that is, as a hypothesis about the child's knowledge of that structure. This procedure is not recommended.

Considerable research has indicated that responses to highly structured elicitations are not predictive of productions in free speech (e.g., Blau, Lahey, & Oleksiuk-Velez, 1984; Dever, 1972; Lahey, Launer, & Schiff-Myers, 1983; Prutting, Gallagher, & Mulac, 1975). Moreover, most standardized tests only *tap* a domain of language; they do not, and could not, sample all behaviors within a domain. A test that examines production of conjunctions may only include two or three different conjunctions with but one or two trials on each. While this may be sufficient to predict which children are not producing conjunctions as are their age peers, it is not sufficient to determine which conjunctions should be goals of intervention. Determining goals of intervention from item analyses of standardized tests is, therefore, of questionable value and is usually not necessary when information from low-structured and nonstandardized elicitation can be obtained. Thus, in Table 6-7, standardized elicited responses are listed as being most often norm-referenced and used to determine the existence of a problem. The results might be reported as "Mary scored below the third percentile in both the tests of vocabulary and the tests of syntax that were administered. These scores suggest a language disorder and she has been scheduled for further assessment in order to plan intervention."

Observations of situations that fall at the low end of the continuum of observer-imposed structure (i.e., naturalistic situations) are generally reported in communication-referenced terms and criterion-referenced terms and are used to plan goals and procedures of intervention. Communication-referenced reports of these naturalistic situations attempt to give a total picture of the communication behaviors that are observed. The communication forms may or may not be linguistic (e.g., they may include gestures, facial expressions, etc.), and they may or may not relate to the adult or child model of language discussed previously. The purpose of the description is to describe what it is the child does and to hypothesize what the child knows about communication in general. Norm-referenced descriptions of naturalistic observations generally refer to the developmental milestones (first words, single words, two-word phrases, simple sentences, etc.), and not to scores, or quotients. Such descriptions can be used to help determine the existence of a problem.

The criterion-referenced descriptions of low-structured observations can vary and can be similar to the criteria used for describing elicitation responses. One might, for example, go over a transcript of a recorded naturalistic observation and compute the productivity of different taxonomies of content, form, or use interactions (e.g., reporting that the -*ing* was produced 60% of the time it was obligatory, but that these utterances generally followed an utterance that included a similar verb inflected with -*ing*; that agents were mentioned in 20% of the agent-action-object relations, and that most of these were utterances that followed the child's production of two constituent action-object utterances; or that 80% of the child's single-word utterances were requests for objects). Otherwise one might describe an observation in a naturalistic setting with a particular criterion in mind to begin with, looking for, for example, X number of instances of contingent responses to prior adult statements or X number of rejection utterances. A low-structured setting lends itself equally well to communication- or criterion-referenced descriptions and provides information relevant to the goals and procedures of therapy. It can also aid in determining if there is a problem by reference to developmental milestones. Thus, in Table 6-7, all forms of reference are listed in the Relaxed Structure column. Most often, the communication-referenced descriptions that are obtained through naturalistic observation lead to hypotheses about the child's communication behavior. These hypotheses may be then tested by criterion-referenced descriptions of the behavior, elicitation of responses from the child, and solicitation of reported observations.

Nonstandardized elicited responses are most often obtained in order to plan goals and procedures of intervention and are most often criterion-referenced. An evaluator may design situations to elicit a particular content/form/use interaction. Although such situations can be communication-referenced, in a manner similar to that discussed for low structure, they rarely are. Thus, only criterion reference is listed in the column of Table 6-7 headed Nonstandardized Elicited Response.

Ongoing versus Initial Assessment

Throughout intervention, goals are constantly changing; as the child reaches one goal, another is established. In order to determine whether the child has achieved a particular goal, ongoing assessment is necessary. In this context, one is most concerned with comparing a child's behavior to a standard of performance relative to the mastery of the immediate goals that have been set for intervention. An additional aspect of ongoing assessment is the constant evaluation of the effectiveness of procedures used for facilitating language development. Procedures are changed based on this assessment.

Comparisons of the child with other children, or norm-referenced descriptions, are generally not relevant unless one suspects the child is now operating within normal limits and is ready to be dismissed from an intervention program. (Unfortunately, there are still some institutions that require annual or semiannual read-ministration of certain norm-referenced tests. The rationale for this is not always clear, but often it is simply to convince those responsible for funding that the need still exists.) Using norm-referenced descriptions as a means of measuring progress in intervention is almost always a less accurate gauge of change than criterion-referenced descriptions that are related to individual goals (such as particular content/form/use interactions). Now that most professionals are being pressured to be accountable for their efforts, accurate measures of the effects of intervention are important. Moreover, they focus parents and other concerned individuals on what is being learned rather than on comparisons with other children.

A great deal of ongoing assessment takes place within the intervention setting, but other settings must also be observed if goals include, as they should, the use of language outside of the intervention structure. The variety of settings for ongoing assessment includes both low and intermediate structure, rarely high structure; and the descriptions used to report observations include both criterion- and communication-referenced descriptions, rarely norm-referenced descriptions. As with initial assessment, both direct and reported observations are important.

Summary

In this chapter it is pointed out that the objectives of description determine both the methods of obtaining evidence about deviant language and the way that evidence is described and interpreted. Furthermore, the method of obtaining evidence can limit the way it can be categorized and interpreted; and the way evidence is categorized further limits conclusions that can be drawn.

The objectives of assessment include determining the existence of a problem, determining the goals of intervention, planning procedures of intervention, and determining prognosis. These different objectives demand different information that can be obtained from different contexts. The contexts for obtaining evidence range from high structure (e.g., standardized testing) to low structure (e.g., observations of the child during play). Information obtained from any context must be categorized and presented in comparison to some standard or model. Categories discussed include the content, form, and use of language and their interactions, while the standard of comparison is either the adult model or a child model of language. Both the categories used and the model of comparison may influence goals of intervention.

Differences in type of comparison (frame of reference) are related to the objectives of clinical assessment: norm reference for identification of a language disorder, and criterion or communication reference for planning intervention. Thus, methodological issues relate directly to the purpose of description and include the method of obtaining evidence, the aspect of language described, and the model used and means of comparison in interpreting evidence.

More specific information on assessment is covered in the following chapters. The next chapter is concerned with obtaining information that will help the clinician identify children with a language disorder—generally the first goal of assessment.

Suggested Readings

Cazden, C. (1970). The neglected situation in child language research and education. In F. Williams (Ed.), *Language and poverty, perspectives on a theme.* Chicago: Markham.

Fey, M., Leonard, L., & Wilcox, K. (1981). Speech style modifications of language impaired children. *Journal of Speech and Hearing Disorders, 46,* 91–96.

Gorth, W. & Hambleton, R. (1972). Measurement considerations for criterion-referenced testing and special education. *Journal of Special Education, 6,* 303–314.

Lackner, J. R. (1968). A developmental study of language behavior in retarded children. *Neuropsychologia, 6,* 301–320.

Leonard, L., Bolders, J., & Miller, J. A. (1976). An examination of the semantic relations reflected in the language usage of normal and language-disordered children. *Journal of Speech and Hearing Research, 19,* 371–392.

Morehead, D. M., & Ingram, D. (1973). The development of base syntax in normal and linguistically deviant children. *Journal of Speech and Hearing Research, 16,* 330–352.

7

Identifying Children With a Language Disorder

As pointed out in the previous chapter, the objectives of initial language assessment are (1) to determine the existence of a language problem; (2) given the existence of a language problem, to plan goals of intervention; (3) given the goals of intervention, to plan the procedures for an intervention program; and (4) to try to determine prognosis. Each objective requires different kinds of data, and different techniques are often necessary in order to obtain the different kinds of data that are needed. In order to provide a *plan* for assessment with a focus on these objectives, the chapters on assessment will discuss procedures as they relate to specific objectives and to the kinds of information needed to reach these objectives. The current chapter deals with the first objective of assessment—determining whether a child has a problem with learning or using the conventional system of signals as a code for representing ideas about the world for the purpose of communication.

It is often possible to determine that a child has a language problem after brief informal observation. The child's language skills may be either so severely delayed or so different from the language skills of peers that even the most unsophisticated observer would know that there is something wrong. The children who can be readily identified as having a language disorder are often referred for professional assessment by their families. In such a situation, confirmation of the language disorder may take only a short observation; elaborate assessment procedures or standardized language tests may not be necessary to achieve this first objective. When a language problem has been identified, the objective of assessment shifts to determining the goals and procedures for an intervention program that will best meet this child's needs (see Chapters 8–13).

On the other hand, there are children whose families suspect a language problem and bring the child for assessment, but brief observations do not readily verify the suspicion. Their language behaviors are not so obviously different from age peers, nor so clearly similar. Often standardized norm-referenced comparisons are helpful in determining whether there is a problem with language learning and use when the problems are not obvious but are suspected.

Furthermore, some children are referred for assessment to find out whether poor language skills might be related to, or account for, other behavioral differences that have been observed—for example, a failure to learn to read or otherwise to achieve in school. Language differences may not be so easily observed in children whose language development has not attracted attention until it was associated with difficulties in school language behaviors (e.g., reading, writing). Again, standardized norm-referenced descriptions may be helpful in determining the existence of a language problem in these cases, although such descriptions would not provide evidence of the relationship between language skills and other performance.

Before a battery of tests is administered to any child, school and medical records should be checked to see if any information is already available on language performance—information that was obtained as a part of another evaluation of the child. In addition, reported observations of the child's language and learning problems from those who are familiar with the child, and at least a short direct observation of the child's language behavior in a low-structured setting, should probably precede the administration of standardized instruments. The information that can be obtained from these reported and direct low-structured observations, in addition to whatever information might already be available from records, will aid in determining what further specific information is needed. By using these other sources of information, it may be possible to avoid wasting time in administering tests that provide unessential or redundant information. For example, if a child has been given a language test that includes vocabulary production as a subtest, another vocabulary production test may not be needed, unless there is reason to believe that the child might respond differently to the different tasks used on each test (e.g., naming pictures versus objects, naming objects within a category, telling what a word means) or to the domain of words tested (e.g., Spanish versus English, or verbs versus nouns).

Thus, before subjecting a child to a battery of tests, the evaluator should have the purpose of the assessment clearly in mind in order to be assured of obtaining the data that are needed to achieve this purpose. Where valid and reliable data are already available from other sources, they need not be duplicated. When there is insufficient evidence to confirm or reject the existence of a language problem, it will be necessary to obtain information about a child's language skills as compared with those of peers. The techniques that can be used to obtain this information are presented and are discussed in terms of the degree of structure they impose on the observation setting.

Low-Structured Observations

The techniques reported here can be used to examine the language performance of children in settings that are familiar and comfortable and that involve as little intrusion on their communicative efforts as possible. Data can be obtained indirectly from reports by those who have observed the child and from the persons who interact with the child frequently; data can also be obtained from direct observation of the child.

Reported Observations

Reported information comes from two sources: (1) other professional persons who have seen the child during other assessment or intervention procedures and (2) persons who are closely associated with the child in everyday environments, such as the child's parents, caregivers, or teachers. Both sources, if properly utilized, can supply a wealth of information that is pertinent to many of the objectives of language assessment. (See Table 7-1.)

When looking at what other professionals have reported about the child's behavior, one can search for communication-referenced descriptions. If the child's communicative interactions are different from those expected of peers, this will usually evoke some comment in psychological, medical, or educational reports. Such comments provide information that might be useful in helping to determine the existence of a problem, and they provide some information that may be useful in describing the child's content/form/use interactions for the purpose of planning intervention.

Information reported by persons who are with the child daily, either in school or at home, is potentially even richer than that provided by other professionals. By interviewing parents and teachers, one can often obtain descriptions of the child's communicative patterns in relaxed and familiar everyday environments. I have found it most useful to begin interviews with general questions that promote spontaneous descriptions, thereby encouraging parents and teachers to describe

TABLE 7-1   Information to Be Obtained from Reported Naturalistic Observations, and the Relevance of Reported Information to the Objectives of Language Assessment

Information to Be Obtained	Objective of Assessment: To Determine		
	Existence of Language Problem	Goals of Intervention	Procedures for Intervention
Historical			
Age at which language milestones reached	X		
Age at which other developmental milestones reached			X
Changes that have occurred in language behavior in the past, and correlated environmental or physical factors			X
Description of current language behaviors			
General comparison with peers	X		
Amount of verbalizations—how much the child talks	X	X	
Intelligibility of speech—how well the child is understood	X	X	
Comprehension of the language of others—how much the child understands of what others say with accompanying context and without relevant context	X	X	X
Use			
Functions for which language is used (demand, comment, question, tell stories, etc.)	X	X	X
Contexts o referents talked about (here and now, self-actions, etc.)	X	X	X
Form			
Kinds of words used (e.g., nouns, pronouns) and the variety of different words used	X	X	
Typical length of utterances	X	X	
Relative completeness of sentences	X	X	
Variety of sentence structures (e.g., statements, questions)	X	X	
Variety and appropriateness of morphological endings	X	X	
Other forms of communication (e.g., gestures and manual signs)	X	X	X
Content—what the child communicates			
Kinds of objects	X	X	X
Kinds of events	X	X	X
Kinds of states and feelings	X	X	X
Kinds of relationships between objects	X	X	X
Kinds of relationships between people, or people and objects	X	X	X
Kinds of relationships between events	X	X	X

Description of nonlinguistic behaviors

Social interactions with:

Children . . . . X . . . .

Adults . . . . X . . . .

Preferred activities, foods, etc. . . . . X . . . .

Medical history

Current medication, contraindications to

activities, possibilities of seizures, etc. . . . . X . . . .

Motor skills (coordination for running,

catching, drawing, etc.) . . . . X . . . .

Attention to sound, both verbal and nonverbal . . . . X . . . .

Span of attention to preferred and

nonpreferred activities . . . . X . . . .

Factors that interfere with attention . . . . X . . . .

Description of environment

Availability of others to assist in intervention . . . . X . . . .

Factors that may be interfering with language

growth (e.g., lack of peers, lack of

stimulation, bilingualism) . . . . X . . . .

Home setting . . . . X . . . .

School setting . . . . X . . . .

the child's communicative behaviors in their own words and from their own point of view. After a broad picture has been presented, questions can be more specific in order to obtain information about particular behaviors. These specific questions will best be derived from the general report that was given initially (or from the reported observations of others) and can be used to clarify, with examples, the information that was reported spontaneously. After a direct observation has been made by the evaluator, a follow-up interview can be used to try to determine if the behaviors observed were representative of the child's behavior generally and to obtain information on behaviors that were expected but not actually observed.

In addition to the assessment interviews, parents can be asked to keep a diary or log of certain communication behaviors that take place in the home. For example, parents can be asked to observe and report examples of the forms the child typically produces to talk about action events or possession, or they can be asked to report examples of the child's use of language or other communicative means to obtain objects in the environment. When requesting such examples, it helps to specify clearly the kind of information that is required and to stress the need for descriptions of the child's utterances and the contexts of these utterances instead of evaluations of the child's behaviors. To solicit information about how the child uses language to obtain objects, one might present a number of possible contexts and ask how the child would typically respond to each. For example, if the child wants a cracker or item of food that is not within reach and not in sight, what might the child do and say? If the child wants an object that another child or adult is holding and the object is readily visible, what might the child do and say? Do these response patterns ever vary? If so, how? Are the responses described prompted in any way by an adult or another child? These reported examples complement the data that are obtained from direct observation of the child's behavior in unstructured settings, as well as the information gained from more structured elicitations. (See Chapter 13 for further comments about diaries.)

Parents are a rich and important source of information if they are willing and able to cooperate. Unquestionably, some cannot, or will not, report reliable descriptions; fortunately, they are not the majority. (Reliability can often be checked by asking for similar information in different ways at different times during the interview.) The cooperation of a parent or teacher and the usefulness of the information that they can provide will depend in large part on the sensitivity and care with which the interview is conducted. For instance, more accurate descriptions are likely to be given if the persons who are reporting do not feel guilty about their role in the problem. Some of these feelings may need to be dealt with before inquiring about specific responses that the child makes.

Although there is, necessarily, some question about the accuracy of information reported by even the most cooperative informant, the majority report meaningful observations if the instructions and information requested are clearly specified. In any case, reported observations can only be used to supplement direct observations of the child. While reported information cannot be the sole source of data about the child, it provides some account of the child's behavior in a wider variety of settings than can be observed in direct assessment procedures and in the type of settings that are most natural to the child. Thus, reported observations can enrich and supplement direct observation, but major decisions about the goals and procedures of intervention are not made on the basis of information from this source alone.

Direct Observations

Naturalistic observations allow the evaluator to view a sample of the child's communicative behavior in order to compare the child's behavior with the communicative behavior of children of the same age. A naturalistic setting with relaxed structure can provide the context for observing interactions of content, form, and use that may not be as obvious in a situation where the observer imposes a high degree of structure. Observations of the child in a relaxed structure will provide information that is helpful in confirming or negating the existence of a problem, while also providing information relevant to determining the goals of intervention. (See Chapter 12 for information on the use of low-structured settings for obtaining a language sample.) Certainly, direct observation in a low-structured setting provides the opportunity to verify comments made by parents or teachers about the child's communication patterns.

If during the first part of the observation it is obvious that a problem exists, the remainder of the session should be used to obtain descriptive information that will be relevant to determining the goals of intervention. Moreover, even if it appears that there is not a language disorder, it is often important to pursue a description of the child's language behaviors if parents or teachers are concerned about the child's language development. The information about what the child does know about language and the hypotheses about what the child will most probably learn next are important for parent counseling; they aid in establishing realistic expectations for the child's development and in facilitating the learning process. Most parents are reassured when they have something positive to do to facilitate language development, when they have information on what aspects of language are probably going to emerge next, and when information is presented about what the child *does* do and apparently *does* know about language. Parents are less often reassured when they are only given a test score (particularly if it is low normal) or told that the child will eventually talk normally.

The situation is somewhat different when a child is referred (e.g., as a part of a general team evaluation) for assessment of language behavior and the presenting complaint is a problem with behavior, hearing, or learning, or some problem other than language. If a short observation of such a child does not suggest language behaviors that are obviously different from those of peers in the language community, one might want to terminate, temporarily, the naturalistic session and begin some standardized norm-referenced observations. When there is no need to calm a concerned parent, detailed descriptions of the child's behavior may be less relevant than standardized comparisons. In addition, evaluation teams that must make decisions regarding the child's need for special services are more often interested in norm-referenced descriptions than in criterion-referenced descriptions.

A number of analyses and indices that may aid in determining the existence of a problem allow for some norm-referenced descriptions of low-structured observations. Behaviors can be compared with developmental milestones as noted on many developmental scales such as the *Early Language Milestone Scale (ELM)* (Coplan, 1983), the *Receptive-Expressive Emergent Language Scale (REEL)* (Bzoch & League, 1971), the *Denver Developmental Screening Test* (Frankenburg & Dodd, 1969), or the *Cattell Infant Intelligence Scale* (Cattell, 1947). (For examples of some developmental language milestones, see McCarthy, 1954; Lenneberg 1967; and charts in Berry, 1969.) A number of measures of *form* have been normed on children's utterances obtained in low-structured observations. These measures were, in fact, one of the primary ways in which children were compared with their peers in the 1950s and 1960s when the only high-structured standardized language tests available were vocabulary tests (see Launer & Lahey, 1981). Most of these measures of form were based on 50 (not necessarily consecutive) hand-recorded utterances obtained in free play with a child.

An example of one such measure is found in Table 7-2. It summarizes the average number of words in children's utterances as reported in a number of studies. This is the type of data from which developmental milestones and age-equivalent scores are obtained. They might be interpreted in the following fashion. Using the information from column 1, a child with an average of 5.4 words per utterance in a sample could be said to have a language age of 4.0, or stated in reverse, a child of 4.0 is expected to have an average utterance length of 5.4 words. However, such comparisons are difficult to interpret when one does not know the range of scores and the variability within an age range and when the age-equivalent description is only slightly below the child's chronological age (see the discussion later in this chapter on the problems with using age-equivalent scores as a means of determining the existence of a problem).

It is easier to compare a child with peers when descriptions of language behav-

TABLE 7-2 Mean Number of Words in Oral Responses

Age	Templin (1957) (N = 60 per age level)	McCarthy (1930) (N = 20 per age level)
2.0		1.8
3.0	4.1	3.4
4.0	5.4	4.4
5.0	5.7	
6.0	6.6	
7.0	7.3	
8.0	7.6	

Note: Adapted from W. Johnson, Darley, & Spriestersbach, 1963, p. 188.

These data are based on 50 utterances obtained in an adult-child interaction using a prescribed set of books and toys. Intelligence, sex, socioeconomic status, and context were comparable in both studies.

Problems with utilizing such data for identifying a language disorder include the lack of variability information and the instability of such measures after the early stages.

iors are quantified and presented with some measure of the variability that is found in the population (such as standard deviation) for each age group as well as the usual measures of central tendency (e.g., means or medians). Such norms are found in a number of sources, particularly Templin (1957). As an example, Table 7-3 presents the number of different words used in a sample of 50 utterances. In addition, means and standard deviations for mean length of utterance in morphemes have more recently been compiled from a number of studies by J. Miller and Chapman (1981) and are summarized in Table 7-4. In contrast to Table 7-2, the data in Table 7-4 make apparent that a wide range of scores surrounded the mean and considerable overlap existed among scores for the different age groups. Such variability in scores is lost when only average scores are presented. (Further interpretation of this type of information is presented under the Measurement section later in this chapter.) Another procedure for obtaining similar-type norm-referenced scores from low-structured settings is offered by Lee (1974) and is based on an analysis of eight different grammatical categories (e.g., verbs, questions, pronouns) in 50 utterances.

The very strength of low-structured observations (i.e., their flexibility and opportunity for the individual child to display his or her uniqueness), however, makes them difficult contexts for comparing children. For example, the average length of utterance for children in conversation with an adult is different from that when narrating (J. Miller, 1986). When context is not controlled, differences in language behavior between children may be partially related to the differences in the context of the observation rather than differences in the children's language knowledge. However, the data from low-structured observations are at times helpful in the task of determining the existence of a problem. They are particularly relevant (1) when the evaluator is most interested in obtaining a language sample for descriptive purposes, but also needs quantitative verification of a language problem (thus, the same data can be used for both); or (2) when quantitative verification of a language problem is needed and the child will not respond in a formal standardized situation.

TABLE 7-3   Mean Number of Different Words Used in 50 Oral Remarks by Boys and Girls, Upper (USES) and Lower (LSES) Socioeconomic Status Groups

Age Yrs.	Boys (N = 30)		Girls (N = 30)		USES (N = 18)		LSES (N = 42)		Total (N = 60)	
	Mean	SD	Mean	SD	Mean	SD	Mean	SD	Mean	SD
3	94.3	29.9	90.7	21.4	102.4	26.7	88.3	24.6	92.5	26.1
3.5	100.6	20.5	109.0	19.4	115.0	17.9	100.4	19.8	104.8	20.4
4	115.7	28.9	125.2	25.3	127.8	27.1	117.3	27.2	120.4	27.6
4.5	128.6	28.3	125.4	16.5	136.2	17.4	123.0	28.1	127.0	23.9
5	125.8	26.5	139.1	26.1	141.3	25.6	128.6	26.9	132.4	27.2
6	155.2	25.8	138.8	27.0	151.0	23.9	138.6	42.2	147.0	27.6
7	156.0	29.1	159.4	24.9	164.1	22.6	145.8	42.3	157.7	27.2
8	164.7	28.1	168.4	30.6	173.8	30.1	163.4	28.4	166.5	29.5

Note: From Templin, 1957, p. 119.

Data were based on 50 utterances obtained in adult-child interactions. Note that the mean number of words increases with age, but that the standard deviations (SD) indicate considerable overlap between ages.

Summary

Both reported and direct observations of a child in low-structured context provide information that can be useful in determining the existence of a problem. With the use of the information from these observations, comparisons can be made with the language behaviors of similarly aged children. When differences among children are marked, short observations often confirm the existence of a problem and further norm-referenced observations are not necessary. Evaluators usually turn to standardized measures when (1) the differences are more subtle, (2) the evaluator has not had a lot of experience with both normal and language-impaired children, or (3) the referring source would like more quantitative comparisons.

Standardized Elicitations

Formal elicitation techniques that provide norm-referenced results generally have standardized administration procedures. In order to effectively use the information that can be obtained with such techniques (whether from currently available tests or from instruments that will be published in the future), it is important to know how to interpret the information about the child's language that results from each.

Are Tests Dangerous?

The dangers that can be associated with testing have been emphasized by many (e.g., Danwitz, 1981; Duchan, 1982; Muma, 1978; G. Siegel & Broen, 1976). The

TABLE 7-4   Predicted MLU Ranges of Children within One Predicted Standard Deviation of Predicted Mean

Age ± 1 mo.	Predicted MLU[a]	Predicted SD[b]	Predicted MLU ± 1 SD (middle 68%)
18	1.31	.325	.99–1.64
21	1.62	.386	1.23–2.01
24	1.92	.448	1.47–2.37
27	2.23	.510	1.72–2.74
30	2.54	.571	1.97–3.11
33	2.85	.633	2.22–3.48
36	3.16	.694	2.47–3.85
39	3.47	.756	2.71–4.23
42	3.78	.817	2.96–4.60
45	4.09	.879	3.21–4.97
48	4.40	.940	3.46–5.34
51	4.71	1.002	3.71–5.71
54	5.02	1.064	3.96–6.08
57	5.32	1.125	4.20–6.45
60	5.63	1.187	4.44–6.82

Note: From J. Miller and Chapman, 1981, p. 158.

[a] MLU is predicted from the equation MLU = −.548 + .103 (AGE).

[b] SD is predicted from the equation SD MLU = −.0446 + .0205 (AGE).

These data were obtained from 123 children interacting with their mothers. Observations were approximately 15 minutes long.

dangers lie primarily in the reliance on one measure of language for making decisions about the existence of a problem, in the use of tests as a means of describing what a child knows about language rather than as a gross comparison with other children, and in the misinterpretation and misunderstanding of tests and the information that they provide. It is the latter problem that this chapter dwells upon—how should tests be selected, and how should the information be interpreted? The problem of reliance on only one instrument for determining the existence of a problem is a related issue—one who understands testing has a healthy respect for what tests do *not* tell us. The solution to this problem is not to administer every test on the shelf to every child, but rather to use tests in conjunction with other types of direct observation—observation of communicative performance by an evaluator who is knowledgeable about language learning and the effects of context on language performance. It is hoped that reading other sections of this book (e.g., Chapters 1, 6, and 9–15) will help to increase your knowledge of language learning and improve your observational skills. The second problem, the utilization of tests to describe what a child knows about language, rather than only for gross comparisons, has been dealt with in the previous chapter and is, of course, related to the above. One who understands language as the interaction of content, form, and use should be aware of the influence of context;

one who understands testing is aware that comparison of performance with a general population in a limited context is the purpose of norm-referenced instruments, not description of what is known or performance in other contexts. Certainly, it is important to be aware of the dangers of testing, but we should also be aware of the advantages of testing and learn to use tests appropriately when necessary. Tests, like other assessment techniques, are dangerous only when they are *misused.*

At times children will come for assessment with records of test scores that were obtained previously or that were obtained in another context. As mentioned previously, sometimes these test scores can be useful in determining the existence of a language problem as well in reaching other goals of assessment. But at other times, the evaluator will be searching for a standardized test that will provide information relevant to determining the existence of a problem. What kind of information will best supplement the information obtained from observations in low-structured settings? Which instruments will provide that type of information? In the next sections some means of evaluating current tests and scales are discussed in relation to the information that they provide about the content, form, and use of language. Such evaluations should enable clinicians and educators (1) to decide *whether* to use such instruments and (2) to determine *how* to use the information that the instruments provide. Before discussing the information about language that is available from different standardized measurement instruments, it is necessary to consider some general principles of testing that are prerequisites to appropriate use of any test information.

Many of the language tests and scales available are normed on only small samples of children, they have little evidence of validity except a comment about scores increasing with age, and reliability information is limited and rarely presented in terms of standard error of measurement (Launer & Lahey, 1981; McCauley & Swisher, 1984a, 1984b). In the past few years there has been some improvement; this will continue only if the purchasers of these instruments demand it. The availability of standardized tests is relatively recent in the area of language (and in speech-language pathology in general); prior to the late 1960s vocabulary comprehension tests were the only standardized language tests published for children. Perhaps because of this, and because of the increased interest in identifying children with language problems (and, thus, immediate need for instruments), evaluators have not been sufficiently critical and demanding of the publishers and authors of tests. Choices are now increasing, and there is a need for more discrimination in the choice of instruments. To be discriminating requires some knowledge of measurement.

Measurement

To interpret norm-referenced standardized tests, one should be familiar with the science and practice of *measurement.* One should have an understanding of norming procedures, measures of central tendency (mean, median, and mode), measures of variability (standard deviation), concepts of reliability (including standard error of measurement), and concepts of validity (whether the tests provide the desired information).[*] In addition to this information on measurement, the evalua-tor must consider the relevance of the normative population to the individual being tested (e.g., a test normed on a population that speaks black dialect may not help in identifying a language disorder in a child whose native language is not that black dialect but standard English dialect, and vice versa). Such discussions are beyond the scope of this textbook. If you are not familiar with information on testing and will be using standardized test scores, you should consider reading a textbook about such information (e.g., Anastasi, 1982; Cronbach, 1984; Lyman, 1986; Salvia & Ysseldyke, 1981). If you are involved in the assessment of children who are bicultural or bilingual so that there is question about the relevance of the normative population to that child, you should consider reading books written about assessment of such populations (e.g., Mattes & Omark, 1984; O. Taylor, 1985).

Type of Norm Reference.   One consideration in the interpretation of any stan-dardized test information is the type of norm reference used to report results (e.g., equivalent scores versus standard scores). The raw score in a test, usually repre-senting the number of correct responses, has no meaning by itself. With norm-ref-erenced reports the raw score is described in relation to the raw scores obtained by other people who have taken the test. The raw score can be compared with the scores of other children who are in the *same* population as the child being tested (e.g., children of the same age or in the same grade) and is then referred to as a *standard score* (if only a rank, as a rank score); or the raw score can be classified or given a level status (as age or grade) depending upon others who have obtained the same score and is referred to as an *equivalent* score.

A standard score tells us how a child responded in relation to other children of the same population. If the child and the population with which the child is to be compared are the same (e.g., 5 years of age), and if the group of 5-year-old children is representative of all 5-year-old children, the scores can be converted in terms of a standard score. Standard scores relate directly to a theoretical distribu-tion of scores on a normal curve, and may be reported as stanines, deviation, or other scaled scores. Each can be described in terms of the number of standard deviations (*SD*) from the mean of the normative population and provides a mea-sure of the variability of scores within that population. The mean, median, and mode are simply measures of central tendency—clearly, not all children who score below such a measure have a language disorder and not all children who score above it have superior language skills. The standard deviation of the scores informs us of how scores were distributed around the mean.

The relationship of the various scores to the theoretical distribution of scores as represented by the normal curve is presented in Figure 7-1. Note that the mid-point on the chart represents the mean, or average, score—the 50th percentile and the 5th stanine. On the *Wechsler Scales of Intelligence*, this score is reported as 10, if it is based upon a subtest, or 100, if it is based upon an entire scale. Tracing a score from the bottom of Figure 7-1, you will find that a child with a 70 IQ on the

---

[*] It should be noted that reliability and validity concepts are important when any observational tech-nique is used whether standardized or not.

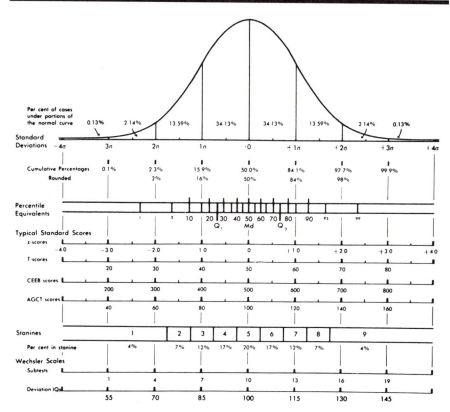

FIGURE 7-1   Standard Scores, Percentiles, and Areas Under the Normal Curve (From Test Service Bulletin No. 48. Reproduced by permission by The Psychological Corporation, San Antonio, Texas).

entire Wechsler, or a score of 4 on one of its subtests, has scored below the 5th percentile. That is, roughly 95% of children the same age who took the test as a part of the original normative population achieved higher scores. Each of the scores is based upon the relationship of a score to the mean, and the other scores of the children who were a part of the original normative population. In the above example, the child's score was 2 standard deviations below the mean—hence a z score of −2. The percent of a normally distributed population that scores between the mean and either 1 standard deviation above or below the mean is 34.13%. Thus, approximately 68% of the population fall within 1 standard deviation of the mean.

The important difference between standard scores and equivalent scores is that test results that are reported in standard scores can be described relative to the distribution of scores around the mean. If the child is below the mean, the evaluator can estimate what proportion of the normative population also received that score and is better able to estimate whether the child's performance was *suffi-*

ciently different from the mean to consider further observation. In contrast, equivalent scores do not compare raw scores with those of other children of the same age (or, in fact, with any population of which the child is a member unless the child's score is equivalent to the mean for peers). They cannot, therefore, so easily be used to identify children with a language disorder. Equivalent scores transform raw scores to a status (such as language age, mental age, or grade equivalency), which represents a measure of central tendency for that age or grade. Using Table 7-3, one could compute language ages in terms of the number of different words used in 50 oral utterances. For example, a 7-year-old child who had an average of 158 different words would be assigned a language age of 7 since that was the mean score for 7-year-old children; a 7-year-old child with an average of 132 different words would be assigned a language age of 5 (or less) since that was approximately the average number of different words found in the sample of 5-year-old children; and a 7-year-old child with 167 different words would be assigned a language age of 8, etc. Thus, only the first child was compared with a population of age peers (i.e., other 7-year-olds); the others were compared with children of different ages—one with a 5-year-old group and the other with an 8-year-old group.

Given such age-equivalent scores, the problem is whether Child 2, with a language age 2 years below chronological age, has a language disorder. Two years below grade or age level has often been a magic number used for determining the existence of a problem. But wait—how many other 7-year-olds (the population that this child should be compared with) obtained that score? Since standard deviations are reported here, we can determine whether the child fell within 1 standard deviation of the mean. If we subtract the reported *SD* of 27.2 from the reported mean of 157.7, we see that scores as low as 130.5 were still within 1 standard deviation of the mean for 7-year-olds in this normative population. Thus, when the child is compared with age peers (rather than with another age group), performance is below the mean, but certainly within the range considered normal (often called low normal).

Since the purpose of norm-referenced descriptions is to identify children who are not learning or using language as well as their peers, it follows that the type of score that is most applicable for this purpose is the standard score, which directly compares the child with a peer group. Therefore, measures that report standard scores are more useful than measures that report only age-equivalent scores; and when there is a choice between both types of reporting for an instrument, standard scores should be utilized. One consideration in selecting a norm-referenced instrument for use in assessment should be the availability of standard scores, or at least standard deviations for mean scores.

Interpreting Standard Scores. If we accept that what 68% of a population does is "normal," we can use scores that are not within 1 standard deviation of the mean as evidence of deviant or not-normal performance. Children who score above (+) 1 *SD* will be considered as having superior language skills; those who score below (−) 1 *SD* will be considered as having below-average or poor language skills. Alternatively, one could expand the definition of "normal" to include what 95% of the population does and identify deviant language by scores that are not within 2 *SD* of the mean. This latter standard (−2 *SD*) is used to identify mental retardation on the basis of intelligence test results (Grossman, 1973). With the first definition of normality, 16% of all children could theoretically be identified as having difficulty learning language; with the second definition, 2.5% of all children could be so identified.

Obtaining a score is only one step in assessment—a step that is followed by other direct and reported observations; decisions about intervention are not made on a test score alone. Taking the narrow view of normal (within 1 *SD*) may bring some children for further assessment for whom no recommendation is made about improving language skills. On the other hand, the broader definition of normal (within 2 *SD*) may mean that some children, who could benefit from recommendations or direct help, will be missed. If a score is being used as a screening device to identify children who need further observation (it is hoped, supplemented with some sort of reported observation about communication behaviors in general), the narrow definition of "normal" may be the safest. However, a score that is only 1 standard deviation below the mean should not be used automatically to suggest intervention—we do not expect 16% of the population to be needing special language services.

Another consideration in interpreting scores is a measure of the likelihood that any person's score will vary if similar information were elicited a number of times—that is, the standard error of measurement. It is a measure of reliability in terms of score units rather than coefficients. Given this measure, the evaluator can estimate the range in which the child's "true" score lies. For some tests, as the *Peabody Picture Vocabulary Test* (Dunn & Dunn, 1981), this is reported on the test form (referred to as the *true score confidence band*). See Figure 7-2. By shading the appropriate area on the score sheet, the evaluator is easily able to see the range in which the child's actual score probably lies. For example, if the child obtained a standard score equivalent of 85 (which is approximately 1 standard deviation below the mean), the probability that the true score is somewhere between 79 and 93 is 68 in 100. If one wished to increase that probability to 95 in 100, the standard error of measurement reported here would be doubled, and thus the range would be increased to about 73 to 101. On other tests, such as the *Illinois Test of Psycholinguistic Abilities* (Kirk, McCarthy, & Kirk, 1968), the standard of error of measurement is found in the manual (pp. 115–116) and is reported for each subtest at different age ranges. For example, if a 7-year-old child obtained a scaled score of 24 (which is 1 standard deviation below the mean of 30 on the test) on the Auditory Sequential Memory subtest, the probability that the true score lies somewhere between 13 (or -2 *SD*) and 33 (slightly above the mean) is 95%. Thus, it should be clear that test scores can only be interpreted in terms of a range of scores and that range is estimated by the standard error of measurement. If such information is not available in the manual, it can be computed using means, standard deviations, and reliability coefficients provided in the test manual. (Standard error of measurement is equal to the square root of 1 minus the reliability coefficient multiplied by the standard deviation see, for example, Lyman, 1986.)

Information about Language in Standardized Tests

Tests must also be evaluated in terms of the information they provide about language. By virtue of the fact that language necessarily involves the interdepen-

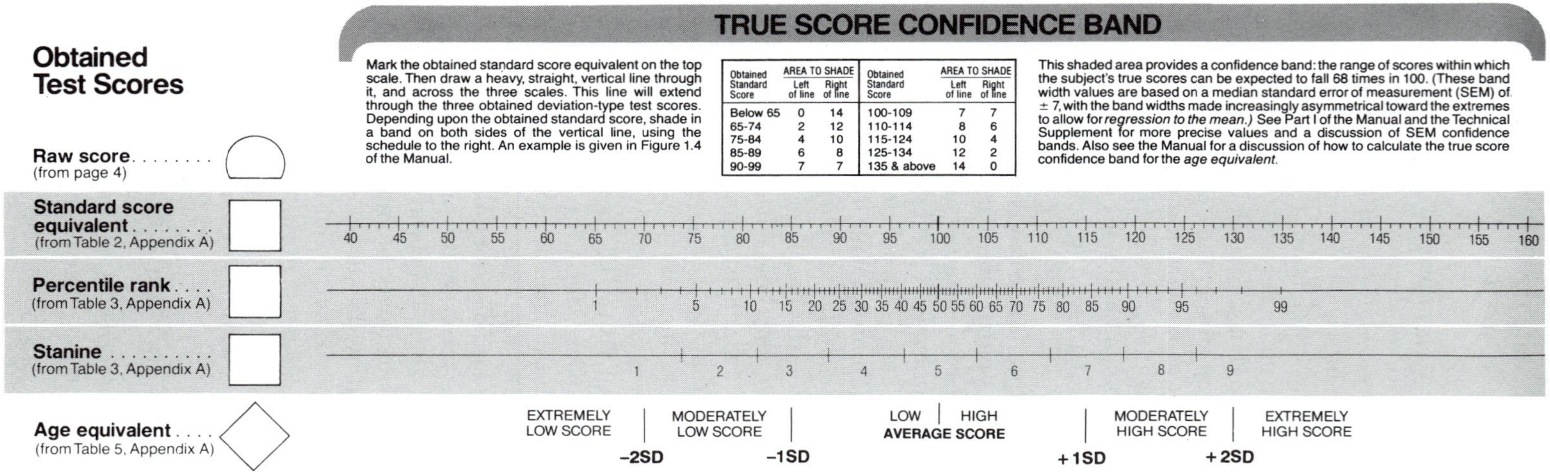

TRUE SCORE CONFIDENCE BAND

This shaded area provides a confidence band: the range of scores within which the subject's true scores can be expected to fall 68 times in 100. (These band width values are based on a median standard error of measurement (SEM) of ± 7, with the band widths made increasingly asymmetrical toward the extremes to allow for *regression to the mean*.) See Part I of the Manual and the Technical Supplement for more precise values and a discussion of SEM confidence bands. Also see the Manual for a discussion of how to calculate the true score confidence band for the age equivalent.

Mark the obtained standard score equivalent on the top scale. Then draw a heavy, straight, vertical line through it, and across the three scales. This line will extend through the three obtained deviation-type test scores. Depending upon the obtained standard score, shade in a band on both sides of the vertical line, using the schedule to the right. An example is given in Figure 1.4 of the Manual.

Obtained Standard Score	AREA TO SHADE		Obtained Standard Score	AREA TO SHADE	
	Left of line	Right of line		Left of line	Right of line
Below 65	0	14	100-109	7	7
65-74	2	12	110-114	8	6
75-84	4	10	115-124	10	4
85-89	6	8	125-134	12	2
90-99	7	7	135 & above	14	0

Obtained Test Scores

Raw score . . . .
(from page 4)

40 45 50 55 60 65 70 75 80 85 90 95 100 105 110 115 120 125 130 135 140 145 150 155 160

Standard score equivalent . . . .
(from Table 2, Appendix A)

Percentile rank . . . .
(from Table 3, Appendix A)

1 5 10 15 20 25 30 35 40 45 50 55 60 65 70 75 80 85 90 95 99

Stanine . . . .
(from Table 3, Appendix A)

1 2 3 4 5 6 7 8 9

Age equivalent . . . . .
(from Table 5, Appendix A)

EXTREMELY LOW SCORE	MODERATELY LOW SCORE	LOW | HIGH AVERAGE SCORE	MODERATELY HIGH SCORE	EXTREMELY HIGH SCORE
-2SD	-1SD		+1SD	+2SD

FIGURE 7-2 This figure is taken from the Individual Test Record of the Peabody Picture Vocabulary Test—Revised (Dunn & Dunn, 1981). It illustrates the use of the standard error of measurement in interpreting an individual score. (Standard deviations were added. Tables, figures, and appendix mentioned refer to the Manual that accompanies the Test).

dence among content, form, and use, instruments that measure language skills cover more than one dimension of language. But many tests focus on a particular dimension. From scores obtained on tests one can make comparisons among children in terms of aspects of form (general linguistic skills having to do with syntactic and phonological performance) and in terms of concepts that make up the content of language (i.e., knowledge about objects and events in the world) or of skills necessary to develop such concepts (e.g., representational thinking). More recently, some instruments have been developed to compare children on some aspects of language use (their adaptations of language according to different contexts or the production of form/content interactions for different purposes). In Table 7-5 examples of tests or subtests have been grouped according to the principal focus of each (further information about many of them can be found in Aram & Nation, 1982; Darley, 1979; N. J. Lund & Duchan, 1983; Mitchell, 1985; A. H. Peterson & Marquardt, 1981; see also Appendix B). The purpose of the table and the following discussion is to enable persons selecting tests or interpreting test scores to understand what dimensions of language are the focus of such instruments so that they may be better able to evaluate test scores. There is no attempt to make an exhaustive coverage of standardized tests; new ones will continually appear. Moreover, no attempt is made here to evaluate each instrument (in terms of reliability, validity, normative population, etc.). For an evaluation of some of these instruments see, for example, Mitchell (1985), McCauley and Swisher (1984a), and Darley (1979) as well as reviews of new instruments in *Asha,* or apply your own knowledge of measurement and language to a thorough reading of the test manual.

Assessment of General Language Skills

The first category listed in Table 7-5 includes instruments that cover a number of language skills and aim to answer the general question: Is the language performance of the child comparable to that of age peers? The developmental language scales have been compiled from more general developmental scales and profiles, and behaviors are often categorized according to age; age-equivalent scores are the result. The usual procedure is for the evaluator to interview a person who is familiar with the child or to observe the child directly and check for the presence or absence of each behavior. In most cases, the norms consist of a point count, where a total number of points is based on the number of behaviors that are either reported or observed. The behaviors that have been tapped are varied and cover linguistic responses as well as nonlinguistic behaviors (such as block building, drawing, or motor responses). Although some of these instruments attempt to separate different components of language and give age-equivalent scores for each, rarely is there enough depth of coverage of any particular aspect to allow for more than a comment on the child's overall language performance.

A last source of information on general language performance is the verbal portions of intelligence tests. Low verbal intelligence scores can be used to support the hypothesis that a child's language behavior is not comparable to that of peers. While it is not suggested that one administer an intelligence test in order to determine if there is a language problem, the information from intelligence testing

TABLE 7-5 Examples of Published Norm-Referenced Measures for Evaluating Language Behavior, Presented According to Information Each Provides about Language[a]

Information Available	Measures with Norms	Type of Norm Reference	
		Equivalent Score	Standard Score
GENERAL LANGUAGE PERFORMANCE	*Developmental scales* (solicited reported observation)		
	Verbal Language Development Scale (Mecham, 1958, 1971)	×	
	REEL—Receptive-Expressive Emergent Language Scale (Bzoch & League, 1971)	×	
	Communicative Evaluation Chart from Infancy to Five Years (Anderson, Miles, & Matheny, 1963)	×	
	Tests (direct observation and elicitations)		
	Preschool Language Scale (I. L. Zimmerman, Steiner, & Evatt, 1969)	×	
	Utah Test of Language Development (Mecham, Joy, & Jones, 1967)	×	
	Houston Test of Language Development (Crabtree, 1958)	×	
	Bankson Language Screening Test (Bankson, 1977)		×
	Sequenced Inventory of Communication Development (Hedrick, Prather, & Tobin, 1975)		×
	Intelligence Tests		
	McCarthy Scale of Children's Ability—Verbal (McCarthy, 1974)		×
	Wechsler Intelligence Scale for Children—Verbal (Wechsler, 1949, 1974)		×
	Wechsler PreSchool and Primary Scale of Intelligence—Verbal (Wechsler, 1967)		×
CONTENT/FORM Lexicon and Syntax Receptive	Test for Auditory Comprehension of Language (Carrow, 1973)		×
Lexicon Receptive	Peabody Picture Vocabulary Test—Revised (Dunn & Dunn, 1981)		×
	Full Range Picture Vocabulary Test (Ammons & Ammons, 1948)	×	
	Stanford-Binet Vocabulary Subtest (Terman & Merrill, 1960)	×	
	ITPA Auditory Reception Subtest (Kirk, McCarthy, & Kirk, 1968)		×
	Boehm Test of Basic Concepts (Boehm, 1969, 1986)		×

Category	Test		
	Test of Language Development (TOLD) Picture Vocabulary Subtest (Newcomer & Hammill, 1982)		×
Lexicon Expressive	Wechsler Vocabulary Subtest (Wechsler, 1949, 1974)		×
	ITPA Verbal Expression Subtest (Kirk et al., 1968)		×
	Clinical Evaluation of Language Function Producing Word Associations Subtest (CELF) (Semel & Wiig, 1980)	×	
	(Update II & IV, Merrill, 1982, 1984)		×
	(CELF-R, Semel & Wiig, 1987)		×
	One-Word Expressive Vocabulary Test (Gardner, 1979)		×
	Language Processing Test (Richard & Hanner, 1985)		×
	TOLD Oral Vocabulary Subtest (Newcomer & Hammill, 1982)		×
	Test of Word Finding (German, 1986)		×
Syntax Receptive	Northwestern Syntax Screening Test (Lee, 1971)		×
	Assessment of Children's Language Comprehension (Foster, Giddan, & Stark, 1973)	×	
	TOLD Grammatic Understanding Subtest (Newcomer & Hammill, 1982)		×
	Miller-Yoder Test of Grammatial Language Comprehension (J. Miller & Yoder, 1984)		×
Syntax Expressive	Berry-Talbot Exploratory Test of Grammar (Berry, 1966)	×	
	Northwestern Syntax Screening Test (Lee, 1971)		×
	ITPA-Grammatical Closure (Kirk et al., 1968)		×
	CELF-Producing Formulated Sentences Subtest (Semel & Wiig, 1980)	×	
	(Update II & IV, Merrill, 1982, 1984)		×
	(CELF-R, Semel & Wiig, 1987)		×
	TOLD Grammatic Completion Subtest (Newcomer & Hammill, 1982)		×
Phonology Receptive	Auditory Discrimination Test (Wepman, 1958)	×	
	Goldman-Fristoe-Woodcock Test of Auditory Discrimination (Goldman, Fristoe, & Woodcock, 1969, 1972)		×
	CELF-Processing Speech Sounds Subtest (Semel & Wiig, 1980)	×	
	(Update II & IV, Merrill, 1982, 1984)		×

(continued)

Information Avail- able	Measures with Norms	Type of Norm Reference	
		Equivalent Score	Standard Score
	TOLD Word Discrimination Subtest (Newcomer & Hammill, 1982)		×
Phonology Expressive	Developmental Articulation Test (Hejna, 1959)	×	
	Templin-Darley Screening Test (Templin & Darley, 1969)		×
	CELF-Producing Speech Sounds Subtest (Semel & Wiig, 1980)	×	
	(Update II & IV, Merrill, 1982, 1984)		×
	TOLD Word Articulation Subtest (New- comer & Hammill, 1982)		×
	Kahn-Lewis Phonological Analysis: For use with the Goldman-Fristoe Test of Articulation (Kahn & Lewis, 1986)		×
CONTENT-Related	ITPA: (Kirk et al., 1968)		
	Visual Reception		×
	Visual Association		×
	Manual Expression		×
	Goodenough-Harris Drawing Test (D. B. Harris, 1963)		×
	Leiter International Performance Scale (Arthur, 1952)	×	
	Wechsler Performance Intelligence Scale (Wechsler, 1949, 1967, 1974)		×
	Picture Arrangement		×
	Picture Completion		×
	Object Assembly		×
	Piagetian Sensori-Motor Scale (Corman & Escalona, 1969; Uzgiris & Hunt, 1975)	×	
USE General or Mixed	Pragmatics Screening Test (PST) (Prinz & Weiner, in press)		
	Test of Language Competence for Children (TLC-C) (Wiig & Secord, 1987)		×
	Interpersonal Language Skills Assess- ment (ILSA) (Blagden & McConnell, 1985)		×
Function	Let's Talk Inventory for Children (Bray & Wiig, 1987)		×
	Test of Pragmatic Skills—Revised (Shul- man, 1986)		×
Context-Linguistic	Preschool Language Assessment Inven- tory (PLAI) (Blank, Rose, & Berlin, 1978)		×

Note: The listing here is not exhaustive, nor does it represent any recommendation for the instruments included.

[a] These and other instruments are referenced in Appendix B.

is often available to the language specialist and might be used to support or question other data.

A measure of general language performance is most useful when there is some uncertainty about how the general language behavior of the child compares with peers. A norm-referenced description of the child's language might be in order if the comparative question could not be answered during direct observation in a low-structured setting, and there is some question that the child's language behavior might be inadequate and related to other problems. A general measure of language performance is least useful if it is already known that there is a general problem with language, and it is necessary to determine which aspects of language are affected or how the problem relates to some other problem the child presents. If one already knows that there is a language problem, but needs to know which components of language are affected with respect to norm-referenced standards, then instruments under content/form, content, or use assessment might be considered.

Content/Form Assessment

The second category in Table 7-5 lists some of the available instruments that measure responses based on content/form interactions of language. Many of the instruments differ in their emphasis, with some focusing on lexicon, others on syntax, and still others on phonology; in each case there can be a subdivision depending on whether the emphasis is on receptive or expressive skills. A test has been included as a vocabulary test in Table 7-5 if the response that is expected from the child is primarily dependent on the understanding or the use of a single word. A test has been included as a syntactic test in the table if the responses that are expected from the child are primarily dependent on the understanding and use of syntactic structures that present linguistic items in one or another relation to each other. For example, a test is a measure of syntax when each item used in the sentence stimuli is also pictured or otherwise presented to the child, so that the task is not to recognize the appropriate referents for the words but, instead, to demonstrate the *relationships* among the referents. A test has been included as a phonological test in the table if it measures the child's knowledge of the sound system more than it tests knowledge of word meaning or syntax.

Important differences exist among the tests within each of these categories—differences that probably account for the fact that dissimilar results may be obtained when two tests within the same subcategory are administered to a child. The tasks used to measure performance can be diverse. For example, the stimuli used to elicit responses may vary—they may be visual, auditory, or motor stimuli, or some combination of the three. Furthermore, certain tests have only a limited or closed set of responses from which the child can choose, while other tests are more open-ended. Other differences relate to the variety of language behaviors that are sampled within a category. For example, some vocabulary tests are concerned mostly with nouns (e.g., *Peabody Picture Vocabulary Test—Revised,* Dunn & Dunn, 1981), while others are composed of relational words (e.g., *Boehm Test of Basic Concepts,* Boehm, 1969) or test verbs and the semantic features of words that can be used with them (e.g., the ITPA Auditory Reception Subtest, Kirk et al.,

1968). Still other tests are concerned with rapid naming (e.g., *Test of Word Finding*, German, 1986) or with the semantic organization of the lexicon through word associations or other tasks (e.g., Producing Word Associations Subtest of the CELF, Semel & Wiig, 1980; the *Language Processing Test*, Richard & Hanner, 1985). The grammatical closure subtests on the ITPA and on the TOLD (Newcomer & Hammill, 1982) consider only grammatical morphemes, while the *Northwestern Syntax Screening Test* (Lee, 1971) covers grammatical morphemes as well as other syntactic structures, but usually includes only one instance of each. Consequently, different norm-referenced scores can result from tests listed under the same category in Table 7-5, because of either the different behaviors tested or the different tasks used to test the behavior.

Standardized elicitations of the types listed here are most relevant (1) when a child has not said very much during a low-structured observation, (2) when it is necessary to have a norm-referenced description of receptive performance in these areas, or (3) when a general language deficit has been reported and one is interested in determining whether the deficit involves all or only some of the components of language. Comparative information about receptive language is difficult to obtain in naturalistic settings. Most descriptions of children's understanding of content/form interactions in language have been based on controlled elicitations. There are more alternatives for production, for, as noted earlier in the chapter, there are norms both for lexical diversity as a measure of lexical development and for mean length of utterance or complexity indices as gross measures of early syntactic development. However, if comparative information about content/form interactions is *all* that is needed, it is often more efficient to administer a standardized measure than to obtain and transcribe a language sample. Norm-referenced observations reported in standard scores are helpful in confirming or rejecting hypotheses about the existence of a problem in this area, but they are not a substitute for describing *what* the child knows about language content/form in order to plan for intervention.

Content-Related Assessment

The third category of tests listed in Table 7-5 includes tests that tap the concepts that language codes (i.e., the ideas that make up the content of language) or skills necessary for developing such concepts. It is possible to obtain certain information about the child's cognitive development without directly testing language skills. A test is included in this category if (1) it gives information about the child's capacities for representational thought and ability to act on represented information (i.e., information in the mind) as opposed to empirical information (i.e., information in the context); (2) it does not require that the child respond to much verbal instruction, nor that the child interact verbally with the examiner in order to complete the task; and (3) completion of the tasks does not require that the child verbalize the answers, but, instead, the scoring reflects nonverbal solutions. If most of these tasks are successfully completed by the child, then it is possible to conclude that the child is able mentally to represent aspects of the world that are not also perceptually present in the situation, and to perform actions that are contingent on these mental representations. Although the tasks in such tests are not direct measures of the content that is coded by language, age-appropriate scores with these measures can suggest that the child's concepts of the world, and the ideas that are coded by language, are most likely intact. However, low scores do not also indicate that the reverse is true; task variables, motivation, and many other factors can account for negative results with the use of any measure of behavior.

Norm-referenced information obtained from the tests that fit into this category can assist in determining if the child has the concepts that language codes. The assessment of cognition is usually the responsibility of those trained in psychometrics. However, the ITPA (Kirk et al., 1968), the McCarthy Scales (McCarthy, 1974), and Piagetian scales (e.g., Uzgiris & Hunt, 1975) are commonly administered by the speech-language pathologist or learning disabilities specialist and include information relevant to language content. When the results of these tests or of intelligence tests are available, the evaluator should know the relevance of the various subtest scores to hypotheses about language learning.

Although a description of what the child does or does not know about language is more interesting and relevant than intelligence test scores, there are times when one wishes to determine the relative strength or weakness of the child's concepts as a component in relation to content/form interactions. Norm-referenced descriptions based on intelligence tests can do this more efficiently than criterion- or communication-referenced descriptions, and results of such tests are also often necessary for placing a child in one or another educational program. Assessment for planning remediation, however, is best geared to criterion- and communication-referenced descriptions that can be related to goals of intervention such as those outlined in Chapter 8.

Use Assessment

Determining the existence of a problem with language use is particularly difficult using standardized norm-referenced descriptions, because use is automatically constrained in any highly structured situation. A use of language that is commonly measured by standardized tests is the ability to manipulate verbal symbols in order to solve problems, to analyze relationships between symbols (e.g., as represented by analogies), or to talk about or operate on linguistic forms (as in word analysis). In addition, tests that require information that has had to be learned through verbal interaction [such as the question about the number of miles from New York to Chicago which is asked on the Information subtest of the WISC (Wechsler, 1949)] tell us something about the child's ability to learn through language (if it can be assumed that the child has been exposed to this information). Finally, tests of children's skills with inferences, metaphors, and ambiguity have also been developed (e.g., TLC, Wiig & Secord, 1987). A child who does poorly on such standardized measures of language use might, on the other hand, use language effectively for interacting socially and for solving problems about familiar things.

More recently a few standardized measures have been developed that attempt to measure a child's ability to adapt language to various contexts (e.g., *Let's Talk Inventory for Children*, Bray & Wiig, 1987), including some discourse strategies (e.g., *Pragmatics Screening Test*, Prinz & Weiner, in press), and to use language for various functions (e.g., *Test of Pragmatic Skills—Revised*, Shulman, 1986). Experimental contexts have been devised for a number of aspects of use (such as shifting reference with deictic terms, politeness, understanding and producing indirect versus direct requests, ellipsis, coding of new versus old information), and in the future more published standardized measures will most likely be devised.

Standardized observations and norm-referenced descriptions are, for many, unsatisfactory as a measure of a child's ability to use language for the exchange of information and ideas with another person; current instruments are relatively new, and their usefulness is yet to be established. Critics of such instruments suggest that any measure of use would have to be multidimensional and cover factors such as diversity (e.g., the number of different forms per function), efficiency (e.g., the effort required to communicate an idea), effectiveness (the success of the effort), and appropriateness (Kirchner, personal communication). At present, use is most often assessed through criterion- and communication-referenced descriptions of behavior in low-structured settings (see, for example, Prutting & Kirchner, 1987). Further comparisons of performance in low-structured versus standardized contexts are needed.

For screening large groups of children, an evaluator might well consider a short questionnaire that could be given to those who are familiar with the child. Teachers can be particularly helpful since they are able to observe the child's communicative pattern in relation to age peers. Certainly gross problems with use would be easily identified by even the most naive observer—a questionnaire coupled with the evaluator's observation during the administration of other measures of language would probably identify children in need of further assessment. More complete observations in many contexts would be necessary for planning goals of intervention.

Considerations in Test Selection

Among the many factors to be considered when selecting a test to be used in the assessment of a particular child's language, a number have been considered at length in this and the previous chapter.

1. If the purpose of description is identification, is it to identify overall language knowledge or knowledge of a particular aspect of language?
2. Does the test provide information about (*a*) overall language knowledge, (*b*) content/form interactions (vocabulary, morphological inflections, function words, word order, complex sentences, etc.), or (*c*) the ideas that language codes (i.e., content-related)? Is this information relevant to the purpose of description?
3. If the purpose is not identification, will the test provide information leading to goals or procedures of intervention?
4. Is the information supplied necessary?
5. Is the population on which the test was normed representative of the population of which the child is a member? That is, are the norms appropriate for the child? For example,
   a. Some tests are normed on children from a restricted geographical area,

such as a small midwestern city, a particular social class, a particular dialect pattern, or a narrow range of intelligence. Is the population relevant to the child?

b. Some tests tell only what the average score is for children of different ages or grades (equivalent scores) and not the distribution of scores for children of the same population (standard scores). Which is most relevant to the purpose of description?

6. How reliable is the test? What is the range of scores within which the obtained score most likely lies—that is, what is the standard error of measurement for the child's obtained score?

In addition, there are other considerations that each clinician must take into account. A few are listed here (see also Cronbach, 1984; Emerick & Hatten, 1974; Emerick & Haynes, 1986; Lyman, 1986; McCauley & Swisher, 1984a, 1984b).

1. Has the test been validated—that is, is there evidence that the test achieves your goal? Are the reports of validity appropriate to the purpose of assessment and the information needed for this particular child?

2. Can the information supplied by the test be obtained in any other way? If so, is the test the best means of obtaining it, considering the stress on the child, the time it takes, and the quality of the information that is obtained?

3. Will the test cause the child or parent to feel badly about the problem, and possibly create further problems?

4. Is the evaluator familiar with the test? Will it be easy to administer, score, and interpret?

5. Is the test material appropriate in terms of level, range of difficulty, directions, and tasks for the child's age, intelligence, interests, motor ability, behavior patterns, and the like?

Much of the information needed to consider these points can come only from a careful study of the test manuals, items, and materials. No one test or set of tests is right for all children or for all professionals. Each of us must be aware of instruments that are available and must choose among them or reject them according to considerations such as those listed above.

Bilingual and Bicultural Children. The problem of identifying a language disorder in a bilingual or bicultural child has not been dealt with in this chapter and is beyond the scope of this text. It is, however, a problem that plagues many of us, particularly if we do not share the native language or culture of the child in question. The tests discussed so far in this chapter, and most tests used by the speech-language pathologist, are normed on monolingual English-speaking children. It is obvious that if a bilingual child obtains a low score on such a test, that score cannot be used to indicate a language disorder. The child may have good language skills in his or her native language; the low score may reflect difficulty in learning (or insufficient exposure to) English as a second language. Similar problems in interpretation arise when tests are administered to children from different cultures even though their native language may be some dialect of English. Ideally, we would have available to us instruments that are normed on populations of which the child is a member (e.g., bilingual children with Mexican or Puerto Rican

Spanish dialect who have been in an English-speaking environment for specified periods of time). These tests should measure a child's skills in both the first and second language or dialect. While some instruments have been developed for bilingual and bicultural populations (see, for example, L. Cole & Campbell-Calloway, 1983; Deal & Yan, 1985), they are limited in both number and quality (Rupp, 1985). Some tests have been normed on populations outside of this country. For example, the Spanish version of the Peabody Picture Vocabulary Test (Dunn, Padilla, Lugo, & Dunn, 1986) is normed on monolingual Spanish-speaking children in Puerto Rico and Mexico.

Recommendations for overcoming the paucity of standardized measures and the problem of monolingual English-speaking speech-language pathologists often include use of low-structured observations (e.g., Mattes & Omark, 1984) with the aid of bilingual adults from a culture similar to the child's. Obviously comparisons among children are more difficult in this context (as discussed earlier). In addition to the use of such low-structured observations, clinicians working in school districts where large populations of multicultural children reside have an excellent opportunity to develop local norms on currently available instruments and to estimate predictive validity based on school success within that system. It behooves any clinician who is working with bicultural and bilingual children to learn as much as possible about the development of communication skills in the culture of those children. (See also O. Taylor, 1986.)

Comparing Norm-Referenced Tests of Content, Form, and Use

It is possible to compare test scores by plotting the scores in terms of their standard deviations from the mean. For clinical purposes, such an equation may seem useful, but it should be kept in mind that each test was normed on a different population and the comparisons are only as good as the degree to which these populations resemble each other. Comparisons are best made among subtests that have been normed on the same population. If normative populations are very different, comparisons should not be made.

It is rarely possible to make any fine comparisons between scores on different tests or even among subtest scores on the same test. To assume that differences between tests or subtests are "real" differences, the standard error of measurement of the difference needs to be computed (McCauley & Swisher, 1984a). Recall, this is an estimate of the range of differences that is likely to exist if the two tests were repeated a number of times—a *band of confidence* for the true difference between scores. Unfortunately, this can be computed only if information is available on the intercorrelation among the tests or subtests (in fact, such intercorrelations among subtests are often embedded within the statistical manual of tests). Thus, while test, or subtest, comparisons can be made in a dichotomous manner (i.e., whether or not each test suggested a problem in an area), they cannot be interpreted to indicate degrees of difference within such a dichotomy (see McCauley & Swisher, 1984a, for further discussion of this point). It is hoped that publishers will begin to provide data on the standard error of measurement of the differences between subtests along with test forms that take into account bands of confidence relevant to profiling scores.

What is needed after identification of low functioning in some component of language is data that will help to determine what it is this child is ready to learn and lead to the goals of intervention. Such information is not available from standardized assessment instruments. Just as the speech-language pathologist needs more than a cutoff score on an articulation screening test to plan which speech sounds should be immediate goals of articulation therapy, so the speech-language pathologist and teacher need more than norm-referenced language scores to plan which language behaviors should be goals of language intervention. To plan articulation goals, an inventory of a child's production of phonemes in various contexts is needed; to plan language goals the speech-language pathologist needs an inventory of language skills in various contexts. Only with such a description is it possible to know *what* to teach the child.

Summary

If the objective of assessment is to identify a language disorder, then descriptions that compare a child's communicative performance with those expected of similar-age children (i.e, norm-referenced descriptions) are relevant. The observation settings that are used can vary from low to high structure, depending on the child's reaction to each and the degree and type of deviation from normal language that is suspected or first observed.

It is suggested that reported observations and direct observations in a relaxed, low-structured setting precede high-structured observations (e.g., the administration of standardized tests). This ordering of observations helps one to decide selectively what information is needed and thus, which, if any, standardized tests might be appropriate.

If standardized tests are to be administered, a number of factors should be considered; many of these factors are discussed in this chapter. First, the point is made that standard scores are better for identifying a language disorder than equivalent scores. Second, it is necessary to look at the standard error of measurement for a test in order to interpret the obtained score so that the range in which the child's true score probably falls can be estimated. Third, it is suggested that the information available in tests can be described in terms of the dimension of language that they emphasize (i.e., content, form, use, or some interaction among them) or as a general measure of language performance.

After a problem with language learning has been identified, the task is to plan intervention. Planning intervention involves describing a child's language instead of comparing a child's responses to language tasks with those of other children. Descriptions of a child's language are usually criterion-referenced in relation to some sequence or plan for language learning. Thus, a plan for language learning is presented next (in Chapters 8–11) before procedures of describing particular language behaviors are discussed (Chapters 12 and 13).

Suggested Readings

Anastasi, A. (1982). *Psychological testing. Fifth Edition.* New York: Macmillan.

Cronbach, L. (1984). *Essentials of psychological testing. Fourth Edition.* New York: Harper & Row.

Darley, F. L. (1979). *Evaluation of appraisal techniques in speech and language pathology.* Reading, MA: Addison-Wesley.

Lyman, H. (1986). *Test scores and what they mean. Fourth Edition.* Englewood Cliffs, NJ: Prentice-Hall.

McCauley, R., & Swisher, L. (1984). Psychometric review of language and articulation tests for preschool children. *Journal of Speech and Hearing Disorders, 49,* 34–42.

McCauley, R., & Swisher, L. (1984). Use and misuse of norm-referenced tests in clinical assessment: A hypothetical case. *Journal of Speech and Hearing Disorders, 49,* 338–348.

Salvia, J., & Ysseldyke, J. (1981). *Assessment in special and remedial education* (2nd ed.). Boston: Houghton Mifflin.

8

A Plan for Language Learning: Assumptions and Alternatives

Once it has been determined that a child is not learning or using language as well as children of the same age (i.e., once a language disorder has been identified), the next objective of assessment is to determine the goals of intervention. Goals of language intervention are the specific language behaviors the clinician or teacher expects that a child will demonstrate after selected intervention procedures. For example, a language goal might be to produce two-word utterances (form) about action events (content) by naming both the action and the object acted on (e.g., "eat cookie," "throw ball"), as the child asks someone else to perform the action (use). One might further specify the frequency with which these forms are to be used before the goal is considered to have been met, for example, 50% of the time that the child talks about action events.

The most general goal of an intervention program is the long-term goal—to communicate effectively with language in different daily situations. In the interim, in the course of a child's participation in an intervention program, there is a continuous process of (1) setting immediate, more specific goals, (2) evaluating progress toward the goal, and (3) revising the goal as progress and learning occur, or where progress does not occur.

The more immediate goals of an intervention program are the expectations that one has for the child within a specific period of time, perhaps one month at a time. The goals that are set for the child must be realistic—goals that relate to the child's current performance and abilities with language. Goals should not be determined by what is missing from the child's language in comparison with adult language as a model; what the child already knows should determine the goals.

In order to determine goals that are reasonable and suited to the needs of a particular child, one must have a plan that provides (1) a means of describing specific language behaviors that are part of language learning, (2) a sequence in which these specific language behaviors can best be learned, and (3) a means of determining which of these language behaviors are already a part of a particular child's language system.

Without a format for describing language, it is impossible to specify what behaviors are already a part of a child's system or what behaviors must be learned. The behaviors to be described include the content of children's language, the linguistic forms they produce, and the way in which they use these forms to talk about ideas of the world and to interact with other persons in different contexts. Without a sequence of the behaviors to be learned, one is left with random or intuitive guesses about which behaviors to teach first. Without a means of determining what a child already knows about language, it would be impossible to utilize a plan efficiently. This plan is based on a set of assumptions about language and about facilitating language learning in the language-disordered child. A Content/Form/Use (C/F/U) Goal Plan for Language Learning is presented here and is discussed more fully in the chapters that follow. The present chapter concludes with a discussion of alternative plans, based on different assumptions.

Assumptions That Underlie the C/F/U Goal Plan for Language Learning

The basic assumptions that underlie this plan for language learning have to do, first, with the notion that language involves interactions among the three components of content, form, and use; second, with an emphasis on language and other communicative behaviors regardless of the cause of the disorder; third, with the use of information about normal language development as the basis for the sequence of the goals of intervention; and fourth, with the expression of goals in terms of language production explicitly and language comprehension only implicitly.

A Three-Dimensional Approach

A first basic assumption is that the form of utterances—words and syntactic structures—is only one of the important components of language. Cognitive notions underlie utterances; that is, children talk because they have something to say. Form alone, apart from the underlying meaning it codes, is empty. The semantic intentions or meanings of children's utterances recur with great frequency; that is, they underlie many utterances. These intentions originate in the child's experience—in the conceptual representation of the world of objects and events. In early language development it seems clear the child does not learn sounds, words, and syntactic structures and then find meanings for these forms; instead, it appears that children learn about objects and events and then search for the forms to code various aspects of their experience. Therefore the plan does not present forms before or in isolation from the meanings the forms represent. Learning a language depends on prior conceptual representations of experience. In addition learning a language involves more than learning a code; it involves learning to use that code in varying contexts and for varying purposes. Goals of intervention and assessment must include information about the interactions among content, form, and use.

A Communication-Language Approach

The second assumption is that a plan for language intervention should provide information about language as the basis for evaluating and facilitating a child's progress in the development of language—information about content/form/use interactions—regardless of the cause of the language disorder. The language that the child needs to learn is determined by the child's language performance, and not by the underlying emotional, intellectual, or physiological bases of the language disorder. Some, who view a language disorder as a symptom of one or another kind of pathology, would argue that the goal of assessment and the content of an intervention program should be directly related to the underlying basis of the language problem before being concerned with the language behavior itself. One might respond that language may well be the underlying basis of certain emotional and intellectual problems and should be considered prior to or concurrent with consideration of these other problems. Such rhetoric obscures the basic problem that cause-effect relations between two correlated behaviors are often impossible to determine.

The current view of most professional persons concerned with special education and communication disorders is that any remediable problem a child presents should receive attention; no one problem should wait upon remediation of another problem unless strong evidence exists that one cannot be remediated in the presence of the other. Usually help can be given in several areas simultaneously by one or several professional persons with different kinds of competence. For the speech-language pathologist, information about behaviors other than language behaviors may aid in determining *how* a child can be taught, but it is the information about language behavior that determines *what* needs to be learned. The plan presented here is thus oriented to the language code and to language use as the basis of a language intervention program. It is concerned with the *learning* and the *use* of a conventional system of arbitrary signals to code ideas about the world and is thus a *communication-language* approach.

A Developmental Approach

The third basic assumption is that the most reasonable and practical hypotheses on which to base intervention goals are to be derived from what is known about normal language development. Both conceptual development and linguistic development have built-in systems of priorities; what happens at any point in the development of either is important in influencing subsequent development. Knowledge of one part of either system will predict information about other parts, and one cannot ignore such sequential dependencies in progressing from one stage to another in language development. With respect to form, children will characteristically learn and use certain, particular words that will relate in an important way to the phrase structures they can be expected to learn and use subsequently. In turn, certain early two- and three-word phrases will be necessary antecedents to the more complex sentence structures that will be used subsequently. What may appear to be the simplest and most fundamental phrase structure in adult sentences may not necessarily be the first structure learned by children. For example, it is less conceptually complex for children to know and code the relations between agent, action, and object than to know and code notions such as causality or the relative size or color of objects. It is suggested, therefore, that success in teaching the language system will depend on respect for certain priorities—both linguistic and cognitive priorities—in the course of development. The plan suggested here takes such priorities into account and is thus a *developmental* approach.

It can be argued that information on normal development is not appropriate for planning intervention programs for the child with a language disorder. Since the child is, by definition, not learning language as a normal child would, it is in fact the normal learning process that has failed. Does not a developmental approach just provide the child with more of the same experience, and does not the child need something different from the normal model? To be sure, the child with a language disorder has not learned language as the normal child has, but the use of developmental information does not imply that the experiences provided will be the same experiences with which the child has already failed. However, some children may indeed need *more* of just the same experience with which they have difficulty. It is reasonable that more of the same input that is received by the 2-year-old learning language would help the older child who is performing with the language skills of a 2-year-old.

Another objection to a developmental approach is that precisely because the child with a language disorder is older than the normal child learning language, his or her ideas about the world are probably not the same. Therefore the older child should not be expected to use language with the same content, form, and use as is represented in the language behavior of a younger child. However, as discussed in Chapter 1, the content of a linguistic code has to do with meaning relations that can be considered independent from specific topics or situations. Older children talk about the existence, nonexistence, and recurrence (language content) of baseball cards and pizza (specific topics of content), just as younger children talk about the same content with respect to topics such as choo-choo trains. Similarly, with respect to other content categories such as action, location, possession, and attribution, the topics can vary with age level, but the linguistic content is the same, regardless of topic. Indeed, nonexistence, recurrence, action, location, state, possession, and so forth are the content categories represented in adult speech as well. (See Chapter 1 as well as Chafe, 1971; Fillmore, 1968; and Leach, 1970.)

The current choice for planning a program for assessment and intervention is between the available information about *normal language development* and *adult intuitions* about which linguistic forms (words and structures) are simplest, easiest to learn, easiest to teach, and most important. The use of clinical intuition for planning assessment and intervention has resulted in several easily recognized clichés in programs for children with language disorders. One such cliché is the widespread practice of teaching children to label objects and then teaching children to combine words. This procedure is contradicted by data on language development. At even the single-word level, children talk about *relations* between objects and events in their environment instead of only labeling objects. Indeed, not only the presyntax child, but also older children and adults, talk about *relations* between objects and events more often than identifying the names of objects.

A second cliché in language intervention programs that has resulted from reliance on adult intuition instead of on information about language and language development has been the emphasis on coding attribution and plurality. Children with language disorders had been, typically, taught names of objects such as "ball" and "book" and then taught "balls," "books," "big ball," "red ball," "new book," and "two books." Such phrases *seem* simple, but the evidence suggests that they are cognitively and linguistically more complex than action and locative relations, which appear earlier and more frequently in normal language development.

Consideration of developmental information indicates that the normal child learning to talk is efficient in terms of both the information selected to code and the forms selected for representing this information. Not only does the coding of action relations ("throw ball," "push car") more closely approximate the basic structure of English sentences (subject-verb-complement) than attribution ("red ball"), but it appears to be the kind of information more often communicated by adults and older children as well. Many factors may account for the normal sequence of development—cognitive development is only one factor. Thus, the plan certainly recognizes that the older child is cognitively and emotionally different from the 2-year-old learning to talk, and such differences will be important in influencing the topics ("balls" or "baseball cards") that the child chooses to talk about. At the same time, the child needs to learn the linguistic code for representing the common properties and relations that many different objects share. Thus, information about normal language development can provide the most reasonable hypotheses for language assessment and intervention, until evidence to the contrary is available. (See Lahey, 1978, and Ruder, & Smith, 1974, for further discussion of this issue.)

A Production Approach

The goals to be presented here relate to the production of linguistic forms to code meanings for different functions and in different contexts. The reason for listing goals for production instead of or along with goals for comprehension is simply because more is known about the development of children's production of content/form/use interactions than is known about the development of children's comprehension of these interactions. Contrary to the expectations of many, comprehension does not always precede production. A sequence of development related to comprehension cannot yet be even approximated. Moreover, production deficits in preschool years appear to be a better predictor of later difficulties in language learning than comprehension deficits that exist without problems with production (Silva, 1980). The absence of comprehension goals is *not* to be interpreted to mean that comprehension is unimportant or ignored in the C/F/U Goal Plan. In intervention, all content/form interactions are presented in a context that represents the meaning relation being coded. Input is stressed throughout. Thus, comprehension is being facilitated at the same time as production. Production, however, is used as the measure of progress and as the behavior by which the sequence of goals is determined.

A C/F/U Goal Plan for Language Learning: Goals of Content/Form

The goals of content/form will be discussed here; the goals of use interacting with content/form will be presented in the sections that follow. The content/form goals of language intervention consist of categories of linguistic forms that code the ideas that children have of certain regularities in the world. Those ideas are not the only knowledge that children have of the world, but these are the ideas that are coded with the earliest linguistic forms.°

Content of Different Forms

The meaning categories that are presented in the plan were derived from the spontaneous speech of children with normal language development. The categories include the relationships among objects and events and are not topic specific. (See Chapter 1 for a review of this distinction between topic and content.) These categories are presented in the tree diagram in Figure 8-1, according to the kind of knowledge they include: knowledge of objects and classes of objects; knowledge about relations of objects of the same class (intraclass relations), and of objects of different classes (interclass relations); and knowledge of event relations between two events (interevent relations). All of the categories presented in the plan are defined in Appendix B, and examples are included in Chapters 9 and 10.

It is important to remember that the categories represent regularities between content and form and are not intended to represent all that the child actually

---

° For some children some goals of content (which deal with learning about regularities in the world), some goals of use (which deal with encouraging interpersonal communication), and some goals of form (which deal with actually making linguistic forms, either signs or vocalizations) may need to precede the plan. Some of these behaviors that are precursors of content/form/use interactions in normal language c/f/u goal development are outlined in Chapter 9.

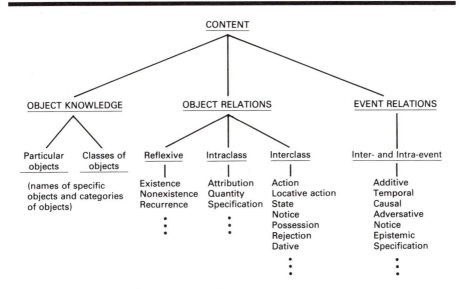

FIGURE 8-1   Examples of Categories of Content

means. Thus, when a child locates an object and says "sweater chair," the utterance is categorized as locative action, but when the child points to the sweater that is on the chair and says the same words, "sweater chair," the utterance is categorized as locative state. It is not possible to know whether the child meant action in one instance and state in the other, but it is possible to categorize regularities between context and form (in this case action versus state events).

There are certainly alternative ways of categorizing what children talk about; the categories presented as language goals have evolved out of research in language development that has described the content of children's utterances. Certain additional kinds of utterances have been noted, as vocatives (calling someone), instrument (one object used to act on another object, as "He cut the cake with a *knife*"), affirmation ("yes," "OK"), comparatives ("more than," "bigger," etc.), greetings ("Hi," "Good morning"), routines and stereotypes ("Thank you," etc.), and comitive ("Go with me"), but these have not been included in the chart. These were not included in the plan for language intervention because they either:

1. Have not been reported in the speech of most children before the age of 3 years.
2. Did not manifest systematic developmental change.
3. Did not represent meaningful relations (e.g., they appear to be routines and stereotypes).

Form in Relation to Content

Some of the descriptions of form included in the plan have evolved from research in language development, such as the distinction between relational and substan-

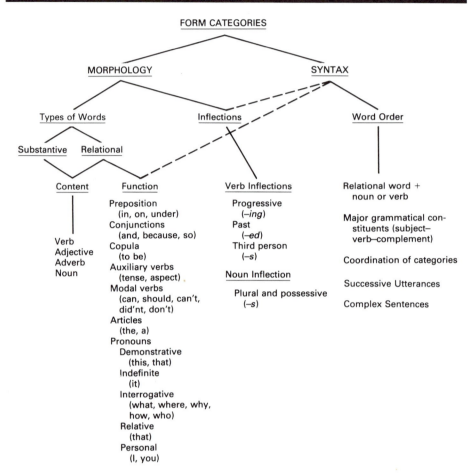

FIGURE 8-2   Examples of Categories of Form and Some Specific Forms

tive words. Other descriptions of form, such as words for parts of speech, have been borrowed from the adult model for convenience of description. The C/F/U Goal Plan describes form both in terms of these descriptive categories and in terms of specific lexical items or inflections such as *can't* or *-ing*. The categories and lexical items that are used are presented in Figure 8-2 according to the superordinate categories of morphology and syntax.

Phases of Content/Form Interaction

The interaction of language content (meaning) with linguistic form (words and structures) has been presented as successive phases of development. The phases present a developmental sequence of the way children code ideas of the world with linguistic forms. The sequence has been derived from a number of sources, but primarily from the data of Lois Bloom and her associates (e.g., 1970, 1973, 1980, 1982).

The boundaries of the first five phases were determined by mean length of utterance (MLU) values. (See Appendix D for directions for computing MLU.) This measure has been found to be a convenient index of linguistic development in the early stages of language development—until MLU of 3.0. It is also the measure that was used to equate subjects in the studies of normal children on which the developmental sequence was based. Behaviors in each phase represent the interactions found in samples of normal child language with the following MLU values: less than 1.2 in Phase 1, less than 1.5 in Phase 2, less than 2.0 in Phase 3, less than 2.5 in Phase 4, and less than 3.0 in Phase 5.

After MLU of 3.0, Bloom and her associates found there was less regularity in the relation between MLU and language behaviors among the children studied (i.e., Eric, Gia, Kathryn, and Peter). For this reason, the samples of language behavior data were used in a different way in order to determine phase levels 6 to 8. The language behaviors presented in Phase 6 represent the interactions found in the first two samples from Eric, Gia, Kathryn, and Peter after each had reached an MLU of 3.0. For example, for Gia, the samples of Phase 6 behaviors were obtained when Gia was 28 months, 1 week, and 29 months, 3 weeks old, and her MLU was 3.07 and 3.64, respectively. The language behaviors presented in Phase 7 were obtained from the next two samples, that is, the third and fourth samples after MLU reached 3.0, and the behaviors presented in Phase 8 were obtained from all the remaining samples, after MLU reached 3.0.

The information about order relations, grammatical morphemes, and complex sentences represents a consensus in the early child language literature. In contrast, other aspects of development have not received the same attention in research, and the corresponding information that is presented in the plan is necessarily more tentative. The coordination of categories that begins in Phase 3, for example, has not been studied in depth, and the sequence suggested here is the result of preliminary analyses of the original transcriptions of the language samples from Eric, Gia, Kathryn, and Peter. Post Phase 8 considers narrative development and was derived from reports in the literature.

Each phase presents the appearance of new language skills—that is, the *productive* use (five different utterances) of a specified form for talking about particular ideas; it was *not* based on the children's *mastery* of these interactions. Thus the increased use of these interactions continues to be a goal in succeeding phases. Information about the expected sequence of eventual mastery is available only for grammatical morphemes (Brown, 1973; J. de Villiers & de Villiers, 1973), but even that is not specified by content category. Thus, complete mastery is not a part of the plan, and all of the phases should be viewed as a flow of behavior.

The phase boundaries are arbitrary and are used to help focus thinking and organize the material; they are not demarcations or entities that exist within the child, nor do they represent clear-cut differences in behavior. Although behaviors listed as new interactions in one phase are developing, those behaviors in a previous phase are continuing to be used, and behaviors in a following phase may begin to appear.

In the C/F/U Goal plan outlined in Box 8-1 the content categories (defined in Appendix E) are represented by columns. The number and type of content catego-

(For prelinguistic goals, see Chapter 10)

Function	Context	PHASE	EXISTENCE	NONEXISTENCE	RECURRENCE	REJECTION	DENIAL	ATTRIBUTION	POSSESSION	ACTION	LOCATIVE ACTION	LOCATIVE STATE	STATE
		1	sw	sw	sw	sw	(sw)	(sw)	(sw)	sw	sw		
1,2 3,4 5,6 7,8,9	10, 11, 12, 13, 14	2	R + S	Neg + C C + Neg	R + S S + R			(Adj + N)	(N or P + N)	2 Constit.	2 Constit. V + Prep Prep + N		
		3	(+ATTRIB.)					(+EXIST.)		3 Constit.	3 Constit.	2–3 Constit.	2–3 Constit. V="want"
above plus 15, 16	17, 18, 19, 20, 21, 22, 23	4	+RECURR. +POSSESS. "a" What Q	+Action	+EXIST +ACTION	(Neg + C)		+ACTION	+EXIST.	+ATTRIB.* +PLACE +NONEXIST* +RECURR.* +VOL/INT −ing irreg. past	VOL/INT V + s	+Prep "in" "on" Where Q	VOL/INT V − c + VP V = "want" "go"
		5	+Copula Who Q (+LOC. ACT.)	"can't" "didn't" "not"	(+STATE)	"don't" ACTION	Neg + C "not"	(+STATE)	N + s +ACTION +LOC. ACT.	+POSSESSION* +REJECTION* Multiple-Coordination	V + Prep.* +POSSESSION* (+NONEXIST.*) −ing		(+ATTRIB.) (+RECURR.) VOL/INT V+"to"+VP V="want" "like" "have"
above plus 24 25, 26	27, 28, 29, 30, 31, 32, 33, 34, 35	6			(+LOC. ACT.)			+LOC. ACT.	(+STATE)		+ATTRIB.* (+RECURR.*)		(+POSS.)
		7								"What""How" Q			VOL/INT V+NP−"to"+VP V="want" POSSIBILITY "can"
		8											VOL/INT V+NP+"to"+VP V="want" OBLIGATION "should"
Chapter 11		8+											

*Numbers refer to number preceding each goal of USE in Chapter 8 pages 192–193.

Box 8-1   A Content/Form/Use Goal Plan for Language Development Goals

KEY

R = Relational word	Inflect = Inflection
S = Substantive word	Dur = Durative
C = Content word	irreg. pst = irregular past
N = Noun	Habit = Habitual
V = Verb	Prep = Preposition
VP = Verb Phrase	Constit = major grammatical constituents
NP = Noun Phrase	(subject-verb-complement)
Dem = Demonstrative	( ) = optional goal–can be postponed
Neg = Negative word	* = first productions may be with two
c = Connective	instead of three constituents
P = Pronoun	+ = plus
sw = single word	Rel Cl = Relative Clause
sent. = sentence	Cx = Context
F = Function	Int = Intention
Vol = Volition	EXIST. = Existence
	LOC.ACT. = Locative Action
	RECURR. = Recurrence
	POSSES. = Possession
	ATTRIB. = Attribution
	Coord. = Coordination

QUANTITY (−s) (numbers)	NOTICE PERCEPTION	TEMPORAL	ADDITIVE	CAUSAL	SPECIFICATION	DATIVE	EPISTEMIC	ADVERSATIVE	COMMUNICATION
"some" "many" "all"	2–3 Constit.	ASPECT V Inflect. +Dur −ing −Dur ireg. pst +Habit. −s	VP+/−c+VP NP+/−c+NP c="and"	VP−c+VP	Dem+N Dem="this" vs "that"	N+N			
		"now" SEQUENCE VP+/−c+VP c="and"		OBJECTIVE VP+c+VP c="so" "and" "because"	"the"	+Prep "to" "for"			
	V−c+NP+VP V="see" "look"	VP+c+VP SEQUENCE c="then" SIMULTANEOUS c="when"		SUBJECTIVE VP+c+VP c="so" "and" "because"	(Dem+(is)+c+VP) c="what" "where" (VP+c+VP) c="and"		V+c+NP+VP V+c="know what" "know where" V−c+NP+VP V−c="think"	VP+c+NP+VP c="and" "but"	
	V−c+NP+VP (V−c="watch") ("show") V+c+NP+VP V+c="see what" "see if" "look what"	("When" Q) +TENSE−Aux= "is" "was" ("will") "-ed"		"Why" Q	(VP+c+Rel Cl) c="that"				(V+c+NP+VP) V="tell" "say" "ask"
		(Sent+Sent+++)	Sent+Sent+++	(Sent+Sent+++)					

ries follow a developmental sequence. Although only 9 categories are needed to describe the content of utterances in Phases 1 and 2, at least 21 categories are needed to represent the content of children's language in Phases 7 and 8. This increase in categories is schematically represented by the steplike increase in the number of columns. The rows represent the sequence of development from first interactions of content and form in Phase 1, at the top of the chart, to later developments in Phase 8. The first column indicates the goals of use that interact with content/form at the various phases. The numbers refer to goals in Box 8-2.

The forms used to code the categories are described in the boxes at the intersections of the columns and rows. Thus the description of form listed in a box represents the type of form that has become productive to code the content listed at the top of the column. The changes in form within a column from row to row represent developmental change in how children talk about the same ideas.

In addition to noting the use of a single-word or multiword combination to code a content category, the use of specific forms (such as certain lexical items, grammatical morphemes, or question words) is noted at the appropriate phase. The language development of children includes more than the coding of particular content categories; it also includes the coordination of one or more categories in a single utterance; for example, the utterance "read my book" includes the coordination of action with possession. Such coordinations are marked by the sign "+" and the category that is embedded. For example, in Phase 3, in the column marked "Existence," the entry "+ Attribution" indicates that attribution, such as "dirty ball," is coordinated with existence, such as "that ball," to form utterances such as "that dirty ball." Empty boxes do not mean that the child has ceased to code a particular content category but, instead, that *no new forms* are used; the child codes the category with the same forms used in previous phases.

There is an important limitation (by design) in the plan that needs to be pointed out and underlined at the outset, and then again as the plan is used. The interactions represented here have to do with only the meaning of the actual linguistic elements and the relations between linguistic elements that are used by the child. In a particular situation, there will often be many different aspects and nuances of an event that will be communicated in various ways—through voice tone, gesture, facial expression, and eye gaze. However, the focus on the interaction of form with content has to do with only the meaning of linguistic elements in relation to one another. The major issue is how children use linguistic form to represent or code meaning. Any meanings that are conveyed by other mechanisms are certainly important, but do not contribute to an understanding of what children know about the linguistic code for representing information about objects and events in the world. For example, if a child says, "go outside," it may be quite clear that the child has the *intention* to go outside (the child might get a coat, run to the door, etc.). However, with the utterance "go outside" only the relation between a locative action and place has been coded, and not any of the accompanying aspects of the event—such as *intending* to go outside, or *who* will go outside. Similarly, if the child says "sweater chair" while carrying a sweater to the chair, only the relation between an object (sweater) and a place (chair) has been coded in a locative action event. The event is a locative action event because the relation between "sweater" and "chair" is dynamic (includes movement) and involves a change in location (to the chair). But the child has *not coded* the actual movement (putting or carrying) and has not coded intention, any more than the facts that the sweater is green and handknitted by grandmother, or that the chair is mommy's usual reading chair.

Although the utterance may be categorized as a locative-action utterance because it includes two major grammatical constituents of locative-action utterances (object-place) in a locative-action event, the child is not given credit for coding the locative action itself. Likewise, if two utterances are juxtaposed and the relationship between them is temporal (e.g., the child says "put here/sit down" while putting the sweater on the chair and sitting on it), she or he will be credited with talking *about* sequential events with successive utterances, but not with coding the temporal sequence, as with "and" or "and then." The C/F/U Goal Plan, then, quite literally presents the interaction between form and content. The issue at question has to do with how much of the child's semantic intention actually gets translated (represented or coded) by the child's knowledge of language, in an actual utterance.

It is also important to reiterate that a goal represents the productive use of an interaction and not complete learning. A goal may be considered attained if the child is able spontaneously to use a form to code a particular content category without prompting and in a few contexts that were not used in training. It is not expected that the child will immediately use the content/form interaction in all possible contexts. Increasing the frequency of the interactions is an ongoing goal. Thus, while the child is expected to use two-word utterances to code action relations before completing Phase 2, it is expected that single-word utterances will still be used to code the same relations. Plural -*s* is presented in Phase 3, but it is expected that the child will continue to omit this morpheme in many contexts until well into Phase 4. [Note that the plural morpheme is not used in obligatory contexts 90% of the time until an MLU of 2.25 (Brown, 1973).] Thus a goal does not mean that complete learning of that interaction should occur in a phase, but that productive use of the new interaction should be established before moving to a new phase. Goals from previous phases continue to remain as goals until complete learning is accomplished. Such a pattern reflects the normal course of language learning.

Certain behaviors have been placed in parentheses to indicate either their infrequent use or variability among children in the sequence of acquisition. Such behaviors should be considered as optional in their phase placement; that is, they may be delayed until a later phase.

With the exception of connectives, question words, some verbs, and a few grammatical morphemes, actual lexical items are not listed because the items selected will vary with topic, and appropriate topics will differ greatly among children. Some criteria for selection are discussed in Chapter 15. Growth in vocabulary is a continual goal. Although it is not represented on the chart, it is expected that new lexical items will be gradually and continually incorporated into the program. The rate at which new items are added and specific lexical items selected will vary with the individual child's rate of learning, interests, and the context.

Verb categories (e.g., action, locative action, notice, state) in many phases are marked by the number of constituents included in the utterance—constituents defined as the major grammatical constituents of subject-verb-complement. (Note that complement can include two constituents, object and place, in locative categories.) Embeddings within a verb category, marked with a + and the name of the category (e.g., possession), indicate the presence of at least two constituents plus the embedded category; when an embedding is marked with an asterisk, it indicates that the inclusion of this complexity within the utterance may result in a reduction of the full three-term constituent structure (subject-verb-complement) to two terms—usually by omission of the subject. (This reduction of constituent structure is also likely to occur with the introduction of new lexical items. See Chapter 10 for a discussion of factors influencing reduction.) The development at each phase is discussed with examples in Chapters 9–11. (Careful reading of Chapters 9–11 is essential before implementing this C/F/U Goal Plan.)

It is particularly important to stress that the C/F/U Goal Plan is a clinical tool—a plan for the goals of language learning—and was not designed as a means for determining qualitative differences between normal and deviant language. The sequence is based on the study of normal development, both research reported and in progress, but there is variability both within and among children, some of which is noted on the chart by either parentheses, brackets, or asterisks. The C/F/U Goal Plan is a *hypothesis* about the sequence in which content/form/use interactions can best be learned through intervention, and not a list of behaviors that are the correct behaviors for a particular MLU. If a language-disordered child with an MLU of 2.75 is missing behaviors that are listed in Phases 3 and 4 but has some behaviors that are listed in Phase 6, this suggests only that those missing behaviors in Phases 3 and 4 should be goals of intervention before other behaviors listed in later phases. The plan should *not* be used to describe the child's language as qualitatively different. If the intent of describing the child's language is to determine if qualitative differences exist, comparisons should be made with the original research on which the plan was based.

A Plan for Language Learning: Goals of Content, Form, and Use

Knowledge of the language code has been described as content/form interactions, while skills involved in using the language code have been referred to as content/form/use interactions. Goals for facilitating language learning must take into consideration both the contexts in which the content/form interactions are used, that is, the situations in which children speak or sign, and the purpose or functions for which they speak or sign.

The use of language can be considered from a number of perspectives. For the purpose of outlining some developmental aspects of use that can serve as goals, two factors are considered: the context of the speech event and the function of the utterance (i.e., the desired result). Each of these factors can be further dichotomized. Contexts are dichotomized into linguistic and nonlinguistic contexts, and functions can be dichotomized into personal and social functions. Some of the elements of each are schematized in Figure 8-3. These distinctions are important because they change developmentally. Nonlinguistic context also includes the child's growing awareness of the need to adapt messages to the listener—eventually through the use of alternative forms to code the same content for the same use, depending upon shared information, status relations, and so forth—as well as techniques for regulating social interactions.

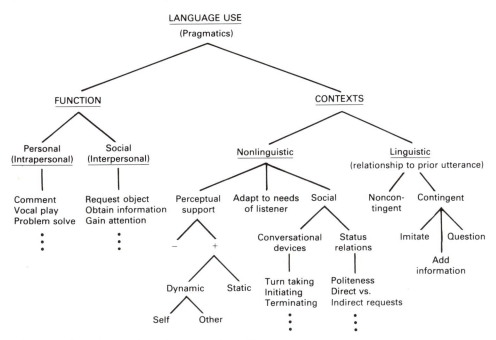

FIGURE 8-3   *Examples of Categories of Use*

Observations of children learning language without difficulty suggest that there are developmental aspects of learning to use messages that parallel the learning of content/form interactions presented earlier. A summary of certain aspects of use are outlined on the use chart (Box 8-2) according to the phases of development presented in the section on goals related to content/form interactions. Earlier phases are located at the top of the box. Phases have been grouped when differences in use have not been found among the phases. The columns refer to the contexts in which, and the functions for which, messages are produced. The first column concerns the functions of language—the purpose for which the child produces the language he or she knows. Considered under context are both the nonlinguistic and the linguistic contexts in which language is sed. Nonlinguistic contexts include the child's growing ability to talk about objects that are not within the perceptual field and about events in which the child is not a participant. Last, nonlinguistic context includes the growing adaptation to the different needs of different listeners. Linguistic context, on the other hand, includes the child's changing responses to the linguistic input of others—the development of discourse.

The information in these two presentations of goals for language learning, one with the goals of content/form and the other with the goals of content/form/use, is further described, with examples, in the next three chapters. In Chapters 12 and 13, procedures for determining which of these behaviors a child already knows are discussed.

BOX 8-2   A Plan for Language Development Goals: Use Interacting With Content/Form   (Numbers do not imply sequence, but are used for reference)

USE

FUNCTION	CONTEXT		LINGUISTIC
	Nonlinguistic		Linguistic
	Perceptual Support	Other	

PHASES 1, 2, AND 3

1. Comment (most frequent including interactive & noninteractive, label, indicative etc.)
Regulate:
2. Direct action
3. Call-focus attention
4. Protest/reject
5. Obtain object
6. Obtain response
7. Respond
8. Vocal play
9. Routines (e.g., greet, transfer objects, etc.)
	10. Communicates about events and objects that are present (+here +now)	11. Most Utterances about
		  a. What child is about to do
		  b. What child is doing
		  c. What child wants others to do
		12. Awareness of listener
		  May talk less to strangers
		13. Listener adaptation
		  May repair, upon request, with phonetic recoding
			14. Most utterances follow (adjacent to) those of others; if contingent may be by
			  a. Imitation (may be frequent)
			  b. Adding a related word (less frequent)
			  c. Contextually related (because both focus on the same topic) rather than linguistically related

PHASES 4 AND 5

As above plus 15. Obtain information (Many questions are asked that are not to obtain information, but as routines or as requests for confirmation, etc.) 16. Greater variety of forms for all functions	17. Increasing number of utterances about immediate past and imminent future	18. Increasing number of utterances about what others are doing 19. Speaks more utterances/unit of time 20. Listener adaptation: Repair, upon request, with phonetic recoding and deletions	21. Number of nonadjacent utterances increases, but still adjacent are most frequent 22. More contingent utterances that add to prior utterance of another (with word or phrase) plus some that repeat a part of prior utterance and add to it. 23. Recoding of prior utterance, mainly pronominalization of object and change of agent (I/you)

PHASES 6, 7, AND 8

24. Obtain information about what someone else has said
25. Increase in frequency of social functions
26. Inform or report
	27. Increased distancing of utterances from referent (−here −now)	28. Deictic forms used (I/you, this/that, here/there, a/the)
		29. Listener adaptations:
		    Politeness markers to strangers
		    More explicit information
		    Get attention before requests
		    Repair, upon request, with phonetic recoding, deletions, and substitutions
			30. The number of nonadjacent is now greater than the number of adjacent utterances
			31. Imitation is rare, but other contingent utterances have increased and convey new information usually by repeat/recode/add
			32. More utterances of child are related to and add information to prior child utterance
			33. Some anaphoric ellipsis is used
			34. An increase in questions that are contingent on prior utterances

Alternative Plans

Alternative plans exist for facilitating language learning. Since 1978 most of these plans have included not only form but some aspects of content and/or use, have been based on developmental information, and have focused on production. However, differences exist: in the sequencing of behaviors; in the taxonomies used to describe language; and in the degree to which content, form, and use are covered and integrated.

The Sequencing of Language Behaviors

As mentioned earlier, before the 1970s the sequence of language goals within most language programs was determined primarily by adult intuition. Those forms that adults (clinicians, teachers, parents) felt were most important for the child to learn, or easiest for the child to learn, were taught first. It is now apparent that the intuitions that adults may have about the relative simplicity or importance of different words or syntactic structures do not agree with the kinds of words and sentence relations that young children normally use when they first learn to talk.

Adult intuitions about language learning similarly resulted in prescriptions for teaching the correct adult model of a sentence instead of approximations to that model, for fear of allowing incorrect productions to become established. Thus, when teaching sentences like "The boy is chasing the cow," each morpheme (as *the, is, -ing*) was given equal weight. A child might have been taught to imitate the entire sentence, often by chaining the words in sequence ("the—the boy—the boy is," etc.) or backward ("cow—the cow—chasing the cow," etc.). However, in the normal process of learning language, the basic grammatical relations (such as between *boy* and *chase* and between *chase* and *cow* are expressed long before the articles (*the*), auxiliaries (*is*), or morphological inflections (*-ing*) are added. The normal child learning language is most likely to say "chase cow" and then "boy chase cow" before learning "chasing cow" or "the boy is chasing." It would seem reasonable that the more appropriate hypotheses to use in planning the goals of an intervention program ought to come from the information that is available about sequential development in normal language acquisition. It is certainly conceivable that the use of adult intuitions to prescribe a sequence of treatment goals may have partly accounted for the fact that spontaneous and creative use of language was not often reported as a result of intervention programs.

Since the 1970s, developmental data have been a frequent source of information for sequencing goals of language intervention programs, but the resulting sequences are not exactly the same in all plans. In some cases this is because of the different data base from which the developmental information was drawn. For example, Lee (1974) places the conjunctions *but* and *so* before *because*, while the C/F/U Goal Plan contained within this book places the conjunctions *so* and *because* at the same level and places *but* at a later level. This difference may be related to Lee's inclusion of only utterances that contain a subject and predicate, in contrast to the use of all utterances in the data utilized in this plan (as reported by Bloom, Lahey, Hood, Lifter, and Feiss, 1980). Other differences among plans may also relate to data bases, but in different ways. For example, some plans state that their developmental data were obtained from the literature, without specifying which studies (e.g., Crystal, 1982; Hubbell, 1981). Taking information from a number of studies and drawing conclusions about comparable levels of performance may lead to different findings than conclusions drawn from cross-sectional data collected by the same investigators (e.g., Lee, 1974; Tyack & Gottsleben, 1974) or longitudinal data on the same children as in the present plan.

Such differences should serve to convince clinicians and educators that any plan is but a suggested sequence. Unfortunately, there is little empirical evidence to support any sequence with any child, much less to generalize to all language-impaired children. Consequently (as noted before), any sequence that is used to determine goals of intervention is but a *hypothesis* about the sequence to be tried, and clinicians must not adhere to a plan in such a rigid fashion as to preclude adaptations that may benefit a particular child, especially when progress is not being made. While most professionals would now agree that plans for language intervention goals should be based on developmental data, few would argue that such a sequence is anything but a guideline to suggest what the child is likely to learn most easily.

Consideration of the Three Dimensions of Language

Alternative plans also vary in the extent to which they emphasize form alone, content alone, linguistic forms in interaction with content, or aspects of use.

Research on language development has repeatedly emphasized the importance of both semantics and pragmatics in language learning. As a result, the emphasis on both content and use in language-teaching programs has become more apparent. Before 1978, two programs talked of content and form in early single and two-word utterances—those of J. Miller and Yoder (1974) and MacDonald and Blott (1974). The year 1978 brought forth a number of publications that stressed the importance of all three components in language intervention programs—content, form, and use (though not always using those terms). Beginning with the publication of Bloom and Lahey, early in 1978, there followed in 1978 (in alphabetical order) Kretschmer and Kretschmer, McClean and Snyder-McLean, Muma, and Waryas and Stremel-Campbell. In the following years a number of other publications stressed the importance of incorporating content, form, and use in both assessment and intervention (e.g., Aram & Nation, 1982; Bangs, 1982; Carrow-Woolfolk & Lynch, 1982; P. Cole, 1982; Fey, 1986), and some have developed plans for sequencing intervention goals (e.g., Crystal, 1982; J. Miller, 1981; Prutting, 1979).

While the importance of incorporating all three dimensions into both assessment and intervention has been generally accepted, the various plans for intervention goals differ in the extent to which the three components are covered and to which they are integrated (see Appendix C). For syntactic utterances, many plans analyze the various concatenations of grammatical categories, such as subject-verb-object, and lexical categories, such as preposition-adjective-noun (e.g., Crystal, 1982; Tyack & Gottsleben, 1974), while others analyze some combination of grammatical categories such as questions, negatives, conjunctions, or pronouns (e.g., Lee, 1974; J. Miller, 1981).

Most plans that concern themselves with content have integrated at least content and form in single-word utterances and in early two-word utterances (usually referencing Bloom, 1970, and Brown, 1973), for this is the period that has been most studied. Few have integrated content beyond two-word utterances. Many have separated content from form and use and have listed a taxonomy of semantic relations that are expressed by children.

Despite considerable attention within the past decade, use continues to be the least well understood component in terms of its integration with content and form and even in terms of its development. Certainly, the importance of use has been discussed and suggestions have been made for assessing it (e.g., Geller & Wollner, 1976; N. J. Lund & Duchan, 1983; L. Miller, 1978; Prutting, 1979; Prutting & Kirchner, 1983; Roth & Spekman, 1984a, 1984b), and some have reviewed the literature on the development of use and related it to age and cognitive level (e.g., Chapman, 1981). Bloom and Lahey (1978), the present C/F/U Goal Plan (which is a revision of the one in Bloom & Lahey), and Prutting (1979) have attempted to integrate its development with what is known about content and form beyond two-word utterances. Despite the attempt in the present plan and by Prutting to integrate use with content/form, this integration can only be done by phases and rarely by particular content/form interactions; this is how the study of the development of use has been structured. Perhaps within the next decade this pattern will change and more evidence will be available on the interactions of aspects of use with form (as studied by Bloom, Miller, & Hood, 1975; Gerber, 1987; Longtin,

1984) and the interactions of use with content/form (as that by Bloom & Capatides, in press, for causality).

Extent of Coverage

Finally, plans differ in the span of coverage. Some plans (such as the present plan) begin sequences with precursors to language development; others begin with single words (e.g., Crystal, 1982; Lee, 1974). While most plans end with complex sentence productions (e.g., Bloom & Lahey, 1978; J. Miller, 1981), some plans end before this period (e.g., MacDonald & Blott, 1974), and a few plans cover some aspects of form (e.g., Lee, 1974) or form/content/use interactions beyond the emergence of complex sentences (e.g., the present plan).

Summary

Thus, the goals in plans for language intervention have shifted away from sequences determined by adult intuitions and toward those based on what is known about the normal sequence of development. Since the early 1970s, a corresponding shift (which was also influenced by information about normal development) has occurred from considerations of linguistic *form* alone to an increasing emphasis on the ideas coded by (or the *content* of) linguistic forms. Since the late 1970s, an even greater emphasis has been placed on the *use* of the language code, with an awareness that if use is not considered, resulting linguistic productions may be stereotypic, may be limited to specific situations, and may not lead to communicative competence.

Despite the inclusion of these three components of language in recent plans, there are differences in sequences and in coverage of the components. (See Table 8-1.) The ultimate goal of any language program is to develop language skills that will enable a child to be linguistically creative and to use language as a means of representing and exchanging ideas. Although most language programs have achieved some success toward reaching these goals, the past decade has brought an expanding interest and enthusiasm for more refined application of developmental data on content/form/use interactions in order to bring even greater success.

Any program is but a first hypothesis about the language behaviors that are goals and about the sequence in which they can be expected to develop. Further information about normal development, the facilitating of language learning, and the influence of environmental and physical factors on language learning will need to be incorporated into any sequence of goals for language learning. The plan proposed here is, thus, a hypothesis based on currently available data about normal language development. The assumptions and overall design of this plan have not changed since Bloom and Lahey (1978), and may not change in the future, but the specifics of the plan have been, and must continue to be, adapted to new information.

Summary

The plan for language learning presented in this chapter is based on four assumptions—assumptions about language in general and about facilitating language de-

TABLE 8-1 Some Alternative Plans for Determining Developmentally Sequenced Language Inervention Goals Presented With Components of Language Considered and Degree of Interaction Among Components (See Appendix C for further information.)

Reference	What Analyzed
Precursory Behaviors	
*Bloom and Lahey, 1978, Lahey (this volume)	
*Crystal, 1982	C/F − U
Kretschmer and Kretschmer, 1978	C − F
*Miller, 1981	C − F − U
McLean and Snyder-McLean, 1978	C − F − U
Prutting, 1979	C − F − U
Single Word Utterances	
*Bloom and Lahey, 1978, Lahey (this volume)	C/F − U
*Crystal, 1982	C F
Kretchmer and Kretschmer, 1978	C − F
McLean and Snyder-McLean, 1978	C/F U
*Miller, 1981	C − F − U
Prutting, 1979	C − F − U
Early Word Combinations	
*Bloom and Lahey, 1978, Lahey (this volume)	C/F − U
*Crystal, 1982	(C) − F
Hubbell, 1981	F
Kretschmer and Kretschmer, 1978	C − F
*Lee, 1974	F
MacDonald and Blott, 1974	(C) −(F)
McLean and Snyder-McLean, 1978	(C) −(F)
*Miller, 1981	F
Prutting, 1979	[C − F − U]
*Tyack and Gottsleben, 1974	F
Complex Sentences	
*Bloom and Lahey, 1978, Lahey (this volume)	C/F − U
*Crystal, 1982	C/F
Hubbell, 1981	F
Kretschmer and Kretschmer, 1978	F
*Lee, 1974	F
*Miller, 1981	F
*Tyack and Gottsleben, 1974	F
Narratives	
*Lahey (this volume)	C/F F/U
Other Aspects of Later Development	
*Lee, 1974	F

Note: Other taxonomies are presented by the following but they are not presented as a Plan or they are not presented by developmental level.

Miller, 1981 C U; McLean and Snyder-McLean, 1978 U; Prutting and Kirchner 1983 U; Kretschmer and Kretschmer, 1978 U; Lund and Duchan, 1983 C F U.

Key—C = Content; F = Form; U = Use; / = interaction; − information presented for similar level, but not interaction. ( ) = minimal developmental sequence within period. [ ] = taxonomies or indices very general. * = Plans which include procedures for determining goals of intervention.

velopment in the language-disordered child in particular. These assumptions are that (1) language is three-dimensional and includes content/form/use interactions; (2) the goals of language intervention should be based first on linguistic behavior and not on etiology or correlates of the language disorder; (3) the best hypotheses for determining the goals of an intervention program currently come from information about normal development; and (4) goals are best described in terms of the child's productions, since developmental sequences of language comprehension are not yet available for the early stages of language learning.

The C/F/U Goal Plan is presented in two parts. The first part outlines the goals related to the interactions of content with form sequenced into eight arbitrary phases; the second part outlines the goals related to the interactions of use with the development (as indicated by phases) of content/form. Differences among alternative plans and the C/F/U Goal Plan presented here are discussed, including the sequencing of behaviors as well as the degree to which content, form, and use and the interactions among them are covered.

In the next three chapters (9, 10, and 11) the C/F/U Goal Plan is detailed with descriptions and examples of the behaviors at each level of development. Following that (in Chapters 12 and 13), procedures are discussed for determining where a child is within this sequence.

Suggested Readings

Become familiar with some alternative plans. See Appendix C for summaries of other plans and for references.

9

Language Development: Goals Precursory to Language Learning and Goals of Early Language Learning

The goals of early language learning presented in this chapter are relevant to Phases 1, 2, and 3 of the C/F/U Goal Plan for Language Learning that was outlined in the previous chapter. In addition, certain nonlanguage behaviors are considered as goals that should either precede or co-occur with the content/form/use goals of Phase 1.

In normal language development, children demonstrate evidence of having categorized some of the regularities in their linguistic and nonlinguistic environment before they show evidence of having induced the conventional interactions among language content, form, and use. Certain of these behaviors are listed here as goals of early language learning. It is not clear that each of these behaviors must be established *before* Phase 1 behaviors are learned—that is, it is not clear that each is prerequisite to learning about the interactions of content, form, and use. However, the behaviors are directly related to later communication with content/form/use interactions. For example, precursory goals of use include skills at turn taking that are necessary for carrying on a conversation; precursory goals of content include evidence of how objects can relate to one another, necessary knowledge if one is to communicate about relations among objects; and precursory goals of form include the production of the sound patterns that are a part of the phonology of the child's native language. The behaviors listed here as precursory continue to develop throughout the early stages of language learning. The emphasis that is placed on precursory goals in an intervention program would vary with different children according to their individual readiness to learn Phase 1 goals.

Precursory Goals of Language Use

Children communicate with others throughout their first year of life. However, it is not until the latter part of the first year that the communication becomes intentional. Behaviors that occur before the interaction of content, form, and use include communicating by reciprocal gaze, focusing on an object through joint attention, taking turns, making reference to or calling attention to objects and events, and regulating the behaviors of others. (For more information about these behaviors, see Bates, 1976, 1979; Bloom, 1984; Bruner, 1983; Halliday, 1975; Lifter, 1982; Lifter & Bloom, 1986; Piaget, 1954; Stern, 1977.)

Using Reciprocal Gaze Patterns

Reciprocal gaze is an early form of interpersonal communication between care-givers and children. Such gazing usually takes place in a context of interpersonal exchange such as smiling, touching, feeding, and vocalizing. To say that reciprocal gaze is expected is not to say that a child will sit still and maintain eye contact in the absence of other activity (as has been suggested in some language intervention programs). Rather, the goal is for the child:

GOAL 1°

Gaze   To make frequent exchanges of gaze in the context of other interpersonal activities (such as when being fed, when playing peekaboo, when someone enters, when playing ball, etc.).

Focusing through Joint Attention

The infant is able to follow another's gaze to an object; focus on an object when directed by gesture, intonation, or other cues; and in general attend to an object that another has focused upon. If this behavior cannot be elicited, the goal is for the child:

GOAL 2

Joint Attention   To focus on an object when directed to do so by gesture, vocalization, and gaze shift of another person (for example, the child will look at a toy that the adult looks at, points to, or moves into the child's space).

Taking Turns and Exchanging Roles

Turn-taking behavior is evidenced during exchange of prelinguistic vocalizations with the young infant and in routines and games such as peekaboo, give-and-take exchanges, hiding and finding objects, and book reading (see Bruner, 1983; Stern 1977). If such behavior has not been observed or reported, the goal is for the child:

GOAL 3

Turn-taking   To partake in one or two routine sequences in which turn taking is a part of the sequence and eventually to take either role (e.g., the hiding and the finding)

Making Reference to and Calling Attention to Objects and Events

At first, infants attend to either objects or people. It is only in the latter half of the first year that the infant is able to attend to both (Sugarman, 1973). This dual focus is demonstrated by gaze that shifts between object and another person and has

---

° The goals are numbered for ease of reference, but the numbers do *not* imply developmental sequence nor order in which they should be facilitated.

been described as having a referential function. Further evidence of the dual focus is demonstrated as infants show and give objects to another person and eventually point out an object to another (Bates, 1976). Each of these behaviors could be considered referencing without linguistic labels; referencing that is not in the service of some concrete end is a hallmark of human language (see Terrace, 1985, for a discussion of referencing in humans and apes). This pointing out, or indicative function, is well documented as a frequent and early communicative function—one that occurs before the use of conventional words (e.g., Dore, 1975, 1986; Flax, 1986; Greenfield & Smith, 1976; Halliday, 1975; Longtin, 1984) and continues to be frequent in the single-word-utterance period (Bloom, 1973; Flax, 1986; Gerber, 1987; Longtin, 1984). If a child does not focus alternately on persons and objects and point out or otherwise draw another's attention to an object, the goals (in essentially the order presented) are for the child:

GOAL 4
Making Reference

a. To show objects to another
b. To give objects to another
c. To point out objects to another
d. To vocalize while pointing or otherwise indicating an object of interest

Regulating the Behavior of Others

In the latter part of the first year of life, infants attempt (and generally successfully) to manipulate the behavior of others. The infant requests attention, assistance, and objects by using gesture, facial expression, and nonlinguistic vocalization (e.g., Flax, 1986; Halliday, 1975; Longtin, 1984). If there is not evidence that the child requests or attempts to intentionally regulate the behavior of others, the goals are for the child:

GOAL 5
Regulating Others

a. To reach toward objects desired (perhaps with fretting sounds)
b. To reach toward desired object with nonfretting vocalization while gazing toward the possessor of the object
c. To request assistance with activities that the child cannot complete alone by gazing toward the adult and vocalizing
d. To request actions (e.g., to be picked up) by gesture, gaze, and possibly vocalizations
e. To protest or reject the behavior of another with gesture and vocalization

Summary

Thus, the child usually comes to the task of learning the interactions of content, form, and use with considerable skill in communicating with others through nonlinguistic means. These goals, which represent some of the normal child's behaviors that precede the learning of conventional forms for communication, are suggested as goals that precede and co-occur with Phase 1 goals. However, they are behaviors that continue to develop throughout the preschool years and can be encouraged along with all language-learning activities in the contexts of an intervention program.

Precursory Goals of Language Content

Other nonverbal behaviors that precede the onset of linguistic behaviors reflect the development of the cognitive skills that are prerequisite to language development. The ability to represent something in mind when it is not present (i.e., representational thinking) is important for the development of language (see, e.g., Bloom, 1973, 1987; Bloom & Beckwith, 1986; Piaget, 1954). As noted in Chapter 1 of this book, language codes ideas of the world, not external reality. A noun, for example, refers not only to a particular object, but to a class of objects that come together as a class because of certain properties and functions that they share. It is necessary to have some sort of mental schema or representation of the relevant objects that were experienced in the past so that a linguistic form can be learned in relation to such a class. In addition, in order to learn the conventional word associated with a concept, the child must be able to represent the phonetic form of that word from past experience; in order to use the word appropriately, the child must be able to represent the contexts for its use. Representational thought continues to develop after the child's first words; the child becomes increasingly able to hold in mind complex relationships that are not directly cued by the context.

Some of the behaviors that give evidence of developing representational thought are presented below with the contexts in which their development might be observed and encouraged in the course of an intervention program. Play behavior will continue to become more sophisticated than what is described here as the child's representational skills continue to develop. For further information on this aspect of development, see Bates (1976); Bloom and Beckwith (1986); Bloom, Lifter, and Broughton (1985); Lifter (1982); Piaget (1954); Sinclair (1970); and Uzgiris and Hunt, (1975).

Searching for Objects

In early infancy, the disappearance of an object causes no more than a fleeting glance in the direction it moved. The child acts as though the object does not exist unless it is within the perceptual field. A more prolonged search by the child requires that the object be mentally represented, and there are several activities that can be directed toward that goal. The first requirement is to have an object or person that has strong interest value for the child, such as a favorite toy or food (see Box 9-1).

An object may be removed from sight slowly so that the child can follow its path. Initially the object or person can be only partially hidden, generally in the same location. As the child is successful in such search activities, the process of hiding can gradually become more complex with complete disappearance, more rapid rate of disappearance, and new locations. Ultimately, other objects may be

---

BOX 9-1   An Example of Facilitation in an Exchange Between the Nineteenth-Century Teacher Jean-Marc-Gaspard Itard and His Pupil, Victor, "The Wild Boy of Aveyron." Itard Used Tasks Related to Object Permanence as a Means of Encouraging Social Interactions with Victor, When Games More Appropriate For His Age Failed to Hold His Attention. This Illustrates How Different Goals Can Be Facilitated Simultaneously With Similar Activities

Here is one, for example, which I often arranged for him at the end of the meal when I took him to dine with me in town. I placed before him without any symmetrical order, and upside down, several little silver cups, under one of which was placed a chestnut. Quite sure of having attracted his attention, I raised them one after the other excepting that which covered the nut. After having thus shown him that they contained nothing, and having replaced them in the same order, I invited him by signs to seek in his turn. The first cup under which he searched was precisely the one under which I had hidden the little reward due to him. Thus far, there was only a feeble effort of memory. But I made the game insensibly more complicated. Thus after having by the same procedure hidden another chestnut, I changed the order of all the cups, slowly, however, so that in this general inversion he was able, although with difficulty, to follow with his eyes and with his attention the one which hid the precious object. I did more; I placed nuts under two or three of the cups and his attention, although divided between these three objects, still followed them none the less in their respective changes, and directed his first searches towards them. Moreover, I had a further aim in mind. This judgment was after all only a calculation of greediness. To render his attention in some measure less like an animal's, I took away from this amusement everything which had connection with his appetite, and put under the cups only such objects as could not be eaten. The result was almost as satisfactory and this exercise became no more than a simple game of cups, not without advantage in provoking attention, judgment, and steadiness in his gaze.

Note: From Itard, 1962, p. 21.

---

placed as obstacles in the search, such that the child will have to displace the obstacle object in order to reach the hidden one.

The subgoals presented below were derived from the descriptions of the development of object permanence by Piaget (1954). If a child does not already search for hidden objects, the goals are (in essentially the order as presented and with objects of interest) for the child:

GOAL 1
Object Search

    a. To gaze in the direction of a moving object, visually tracking its movements
    b. To gaze at a moving object and look for its reappearance after it disappears behind an obstacle (such as a screen)

    c. To gaze at a moving object that is then partially hidden by a stationary object (or screen) and actively search for it when it fails to reappear from behind the stationary object

    d. To gaze at a moving object that is then entirely hidden by a stationary object (or screen) and actively search for it when it fails to reappear from behind the screen

    e. To watch as an object is first hidden behind one obstacle and then a second obstacle (i.e., visibly displaced), and then actively search for the object behind the second obstacle

    f. To search actively for an object behind a second obstacle, where the child has not seen the object hidden (i.e., invisible displacement) the second time

While the above contexts can be embedded in free-play sessions, they are essentially contrived by an adult. In addition to such contrived searching contexts, children occasionally search during free play for objects that have recently been in their possession. At first, the found object is merely examined, but later the search appears to be for the purpose of joining with other objects (to be discussed later). On the basis of this more naturalistic context, the goals are for the child:

    g. To search actively for an object that was recently the focus of attention in free play

    h. To search actively for an object that was recently the focus of attention in order to relate it to another object

Causing Objects to Disappear

The child comes to discover that objects exist even after they have disappeared. First the child watches them reappear and then actively searches for them, after they have disappeared, in order to cause them to reappear. Causing the objects to disappear and then reappear again affirms for the child that objects are permanent events. Activities where this behavior is quite obvious are in two of the most popular of infant play behaviors: playing peekaboo and playing with a jack-in-the-box. (Note that these are also parts of routines previously discussed in the section on Precursory Goals of Use.)

If a child does not cause objects to disappear, the following subgoals should be considered in the sequence presented. With each, the child first watches someone else perform the action—perhaps a number of times—and then the child attempts the action. The goals are for the child:

GOAL 2
Disappearance

    a. To drop objects into a box and cover the box
    b. To hide an object under a screen of some type
    c. To hide several objects in the same place
    d. To hide several different objects in different places

Acting on Different Objects

These goals of finding objects and causing objects to disappear are related to the content categories of *existence, disappearance, nonexistence,* and *recurrence* that the child will eventually learn to code with conventional linguistic forms. Each refers to a relation between an object and the child more so than one object to another object. Other goals relate more to objects in relation to other objects. A predominant relation between objects that forms a major content or meaning category in the subsequent development of language is the action relation.

Acting on Different Objects in Similar Ways (Nonspecific Play). Certain actions can be performed on objects regardless of the different perceptual properties or different functions that different objects might have. For example, children learn that objects with different tastes and textures can, nevertheless, be mouthed and many objects can be eaten. Many kinds of objects can be dropped, thrown, or banged. This kind of play with objects, where different objects are manipulated in the same way, was described by Sinclair (1970) as an important step in children's development of play in the second year. Before children demonstrate object-specific play, they watch different objects as they are moved or touched. Then they themselves perform the same movements on different objects. If a child does not manipulate objects early, goals are for the child:

GOAL 3
Action on an Object

   a. To attend to adult manipulation of objects

Acting on Different Objects in Prescribed Ways (Object-Specific Play). There are other actions that can be performed with only certain objects, depending on the perceptual properties of different objects and the way children have observed others use different objects. For example, children learn that a ball can be rolled, but a book or a hat cannot; a hat goes on a head, but a ball or a book does not; a piece of paper can be crumpled, but a ball or shoe cannot; a crayon can make marks on paper, but a ball or a shoe cannot (Box 9-2). If a child does not demonstrate object-specific play, the subgoals would be (in the following sequence) for the child:

   b. To imitate object-specific actions with a few familiar objects
   c. To evidence appropriate actions with a few familiar objects without an immediately prior model
   d. To evidence appropriate actions more frequently with a wider variety of familiar objects

Acting on Two Objects in Relation to Each Other. Actions discussed thus far have consisted of movements by the child to affect a single object in a particular way. In addition, children act upon objects such that objects are separated or moved apart from other objects and placed together in constructing activities (including actions of objects on other objects) (Lifter, 1982; Lifter & Bloom, 1986). For the child who does not demonstrate the following behaviors the subgoals (in sequence) are for the child:

BOX 9-2

The distinction between object-specific play, where the child's manipulation of an object is different according to the properties of the object, and nonspecific play, where the child treats objects in similar ways regardless of the differences among them, was described by Sinclair (1970) in her description of the normal development of patterns of play in the second year of life. The same distinction has also been made by W. A. Bricker and Bricker (1974) in an early language intervention program that has stressed the importance of learning the nonlinguistic behaviors that are preliminary to learning language behaviors in development. They reported a comparison between two groups of 2-year-old children playing with objects, one a group of mentally retarded children and the other a group of children developing normally. The retarded children used more nonspecific play behaviors, while the normally developing children used more object-specific play.

GOAL 3
Object-to-Object Relations

a. To separate objects (e.g., take nesting blocks apart, take peg people out of seesaw)
b. To join objects as they were originally presented (e.g., put nesting blocks together, put peg people back in seesaw)
c. To join objects in a new relation that is not necessarily taking into account the specific properties of the objects (e.g., put peg people in the nesting blocks)
d. To join objects in a relation (not just seen) that takes into account the specific properties of the objects, such as feeding a doll with a spoon or putting beads on a string.°

Children learn such things about objects without knowing how such objects or object relations are coded with language. The interaction of content and form is the knowledge of the words and the linguistic structures that represent such objects and object relations.

Precursory Goals of Language Form

Before learning the words and the linguistic structures that code or represent the content of language, most children also display evidence of some knowledge of form. Infants, for example, vocalize frequently, and their later vocalizations include some of the segmental and suprasegmental features of the adult language. Thus, production of the linguistic signal should be a goal related to early language learning. It is again stressed, however, that while the child is not expected to have learned words or signs at this point, the context of facilitating these goals should involve input that is meaningful.

° Later play behaviors that tend to co-occur with Phase 2 language behaviors include searching for an object in order to relate it to another object (Lifter & Bloom, 1986; McCune-Nicholich, 1981).

Imitating Movement and Vocalization

The imitation of body movement and sound vocalization can eventually lead to the movements and sounds that provide the forms of language. The goals of imitation not only are goals of form, but are also related to both content and use. In order to imitate, the child must attend to and respond to another person—an aspect of use. The movements and sounds that the child imitates are often meaningful to the child and to the context in which they occur—aspects of content.

At first, one may be able to instigate behavior by the child, either motor or vocal behavior, by copying the child immediately after the behavior has been produced. When this can be accomplished, then the time delay between the child's original action and the adult's copying can be carefully increased. In time it should be relatively easy to stimulate the child to imitate any action that is a part of the usual repertoire, even if it has not occurred for a long period of time. Eventually some of the child's behaviors can be combined in ways in which they have not been combined before—so that it is possible to form a novel pattern made up of behaviors already familiar to the child. At the same time, new behaviors that are somewhat similar to old behaviors might be attempted. The following subgoals were derived from the descriptions of the development of imitation by Piaget (1962). If the child does not demonstrate imitative behavior, the following subgoals for the child should be, in approximately the sequence presented:

GOAL 1
Imitation

  a. To imitate body movements of an adult that are imitations of the child's own prior movements
  b. To imitate vocalizations of an adult that are similar to those the child has previously produced
  c. To imitate vocalizations and body movements that the child has not made but are movements that the child can see herself (or himself) make
  d. To imitate new models that the child has not made and where the movements are those that the child cannot see himself (or herself) make (e.g., move tongue from side to side)

Producing the Linguistic Signal in Varying Degrees of Approximation to the Adult Model

Before the interaction of form with content or use, the child will usually demonstrate reduplicated babbling (i.e., the repetition of syllables such as /ba ba/) and will have produced many of the segmental and suprasegmental features of the adult model in vocal play (see, e.g., Oller, Wieman, Doyle, & Ross, 1976; R. Stark, 1979). Following this, nonreduplicated babbling will appear (i.e., the production of different syllables in succession, such as /ba da ma/ (R. Stark, 1979). Furthermore, many children begin to simulate the prosodic features of the adult model by producing stress and rhythm patterns that sound sentential. If the child does not do the above, the goals of intervention would be:

GOAL 2
Approximating the Forms of the Adult Model

a. To produce sequences of similar syllables (reduplicated babbling)
b. To produce sequences of dissimilar syllables (nonreduplicated babbling)
c. To produce sequences of sounds with the suprasegmental features of the adult model

Early Nonconventional Interactions of Form with Content or Use

As form interacts with content and use, only gradually does the child approximate the features of the model utterance (i.e., say a word or make a sign precisely like the adult target). At first the child produces a consistent form in relation to some meaning—either a function or a referent. Early interactions may be cued by suprasegmental features of the adult target (Flax, 1986; Halliday, 1975; Menn, 1971) or by segmental features (Carter, 1979). In either case the child has a consistent phonetic form (Dore, Franklin, Miller, & Ramer, 1976) to communicate meaning. If the child does not have consistent phonetic forms, the goal of intervention following those above would be:

GOAL 1
Nonconventional Interactions of Form with Content or Use   To produce consistent (but not necessarily conventional) phonetic forms for particular objects and/or functions (e.g., /a/ for "watch me" or /aba/ for a favorite toy; such forms do not need to approximate the adult model in any way).

Later Developments of Form in Interaction with Content and Use

More conventional productions follow this use of consistent phonetic forms. However, exact reproductions of the segmental features of the adult target are not expected until the child has achieved the behaviors listed in the eight phases of the C/F/U Goal Plan for Language Learning. Just how phonological, syntactic, and lexical developments correlate with one another in normal development is not known. However, many normal children have not mastered the phonemes of the adult language until the age of 7 years (Poole, 1934; Templin, 1957) when their other linguistic skills are well beyond the skills described in Phase 8. Accurate articulation of words is not a goal in these early phases.

A phenomenon may occur which at first seems surprising. A child may initially produce words rather accurately (particularly in the single-word-utterance period) only to have this production degenerate at a later time. Such behavior is commonly reported in the literature on normal language learning (see, e.g., Ingram, 1976; Leopold, 1939). It has been suggested that early productions are not yet part of a phonological rule system and that the change in these productions often reflects the child's development of such a system. In addition, there may be a synergistic relationship between the production of a word and the structure in which it is embedded such that increased complexity in sentence structure may result in decreased complexity in phonetic output (e.g., Panagos, Quine, & Klich, 1979). Thus, it is not expected that the child will always maintain the same level of approximation. In all situations, facilitation of this goal should be carried out in meaningful contexts—that is, for most children the production of forms should be encouraged in the context of related content and use.

Summary of Precursory Goals

Table 9-1 lists the precursory goals of language learning. These include behaviors related to use, content, and form and to some beginning interactions, but the goals do not include the use of conventional forms to represent ideas for the purpose of communication. See Chapter 12 for assessment of precursory behaviors. The first content/form/use interactions are discussed in the next section and begin the plan for language learning.

Goals of Content, Form, and Use: Phases 1, 2, and 3

The first phases of language learning that are presented here represent the behaviors that have been described for non-language-disordered children with a mean length of utterance (MLU) less than 2.0. Presented first are the goals of use that interact with content and form in Phases 1, 2, and 3.

Goals of Use that Interact with Content and Form: Phases 1, 2, and 3

When most children begin to use a conventional system of forms to code ideas, they typically talk about objects and events that are in the immediate environment. As with each of us, children talk about what is in their consciousness (i.e., their Intentional states—see Bloom & Beckwith, 1986, for a discussion of Intentional states). In early childhood, the ideas in consciousness seem constrained by what the child can see, hear, and touch—that is, by data from perception. Early in the single-word-utterance period children talk about what they see, hold, or are in the process of doing; later in this period of development there is an increase in their expression of anticipated events (Bloom, 1987). Thus, we would not expect children in the early stages of language development to talk of objects and events that are not perceptually present (although some language-impaired children with well-developed representational abilities may do so). Moreover, events talked about tend to be events in which the child is a participant or in which the child wishes someone else to participate; the child rarely talks about what others are doing.

While many utterances in these phases follow, or are adjacent to, those of another, they are often not related to the previous utterance. When utterances are related to the prior utterance, they may be related by the nonlinguistic context both speakers are sharing (that is, they are both talking about the same object or event), by the repeating of part of the prior utterance (i.e., imitation), or by a response to a question which adds or replaces a word in the prior message (Bloom, Rocissano, & Hood, 1976). Imitations of prior utterances are very frequent (15–40% of all utterances) for some children at this level, while other children rarely imitate the utterances of others (Bloom, Hood, & Lightbown, 1974). When imitation is frequent, it may be motivated, at this point in development, by the

TABLE 9-1   Summary of Precursory Goals

Precursory Goals Related to *Use*

1. *Gaze*—To make frequent exchanges of gaze in the context of other interpersonal activities
2. *Joint Attention*—To focus on an object when directed to do so by gesture, vocalization, and gaze shift of another from child to object
3. *Turn-Taking*—To partake in one or two routine sequences in which turn taking is a part of the sequence and eventually to take either role
4. *Making Reference*—To show and give objects to another and eventually to point out objects and vocalize while pointing or otherwise indicating an object of interest
5. *Regulate*—To reach toward objects desired (perhaps with fretting sounds) and eventually reach with nonfretting vocalization while gazing toward the possessor of the object, to request assistance or action or to protest or reject an object or action

Precursory Goals Related to *Content*

1. *Object Search*
   1-1. To gaze in the direction of a moving object, visually tracking its movements
   1-2. To gaze at a moving object and look for its reappearance after it disappears behind an obstacle (such as a screen)
   1-3. To gaze at a moving object that is then partially hidden by a stationary object (or screen) and actively search for it when it fails to reappear from behind the stationary object
   1-4. To gaze at a moving object that is then entirely hidden by a stationary object (or screen) and actively search for it when it fails to reappear from behind the screen
   1-5. To watch as an object is first hidden behind one obstacle and then a second obstacle, and then actively search for the object behind the second obstacle
   1-6. To search actively for an object behind a second obstacle, where the child has not seen the object hidden the second time
   1-7. To search actively for an object that has just been the focus of attention in free play
   1-8. To search actively for an object in order to relate it to another object
2. *Disappearance*
   2-1. To drop objects into a box and cover the box
   2-2. To hide an object under a screen of some type
   2-3. To hide several objects in the same place
   2-4. To hide several different objects in different places
3. *Action on an Object*
   3-1. To attend to adult manipulation of objects
   3-2. To imitate object-specific actions with a few familiar objects
   3-3. To evidence appropriate actions with a few familiar objects without an immediately prior model
   3-4. To evidence appropriate actions more frequently with a wider variety of familiar objects
4. *Object-to-Object Relations*
   4-1. To separate objects
   4-2. To join objects as they were originally presented
   4-3. To join objects in a new relation that is not necessarily taking into account the specific properties of the objects
   4-4. To join objects in a relation (not just seen) that takes into account the specific properties of the objects

Precursory Goals Related to *Form*

1. *Imitation*
   1-1. To imitate body movements of an adult that are imitations of the child's own prior movements

(continued)

TABLE 9-1   Precursory Goals (continued)

Precursory Goals Related to *Form* (continued)

1-2. To imitate vocalizations of an adult that are similar to those the child has previously produced

1-3. To imitate vocalizations and body movements of another that the child has not made but are movements that the child can see herself (or himself) make

1-4. To imitate new models that the child has not made and where the movements are those that the child cannot see himself (or herself) make

2. *Approximating the Forms* of the Adult Model

   2-1. To produce sequences of similar syllables (reduplicated babbling)

   2-2. To produce sequences of dissimilar syllables (nonreduplicated babbling)

   2-3. To produce sequences of sounds with the suprasegmental features of the adult model

Nonconventional Interactions of *form* with *content* or *use*

1. To produce consistent (but not necessarily conventional) phonetic forms for particular objects and/or functions

---

adult's use of structures or lexical items that the child is in the process of learning (Bloom et al., 1974). Children are more likely to imitate if the prior adult utterance is a repetition or expansion of the child's previous utterance (Folger & Chapman, 1978). Children's imitation of adult utterances decreases with increasing language development (Bloom et al., 1976). While decreasing the frequency of imitation (or echolalia) should probably never be a goal of intervention, it certainly should never be considered until at least Phase 7 or 8. Perhaps the best way to decrease what may appear to be excessive imitations is to help the child learn developmentally appropriate content/form/use interactions.

One reason why linguistically contingent responses are limited in the early phases of language learning may be because it is difficult for the child to create a mental representation based on the utterance of another. If the adult utterance does not refer to the context, it means the child must process the linguistic message and draw information from long-term memory in order to mentally represent what another is talking about. Such mental representation is necessary for the child to respond contingently (see Bloom, 1974; Bloom & Lahey, 1978; Bloom et al., 1976). Thus, it is not expected (though with some language-impaired children it may occur) that children in the early phases of content/form interactions will respond contingently to the utterances of another, particularly when the utterances of others are not about the current shared context. Linguistically contingent responses, which are not imitations of prior utterances, await linguistic as well as nonlinguistic development; nonresponses or inappropriate responses need to be considered in regard to development in each area.

Adaptation to the listener may be evident in the amount of talking to strangers in contrast to familiar persons and in responses to questions for repair. At this point children will often respond to a request for clarification with a phonetic recoding of the original utterance (see Gallagher, 1977, 1981).

Conventional words are rarely used to code feelings (such as happiness, sadness, fear etc.) until at least Phase 7 or 8; children's early expressions of feelings are in the form of nonlinguistic vocalizations, gestures, and facial expressions. In fact, most early productions of conventional words are spoken in states of rather neutral or low *positive* affect in the single-word-utterance period and even the low positive affect occurs most often on words that are well known to the child rather than new words (Bloom, in press; Bloom & Capatides, in press).

While many of the functions expressed prelinguistically by the infant are requests for actions or objects, the production of *conventional words* early in the single-word-utterance period serves more often to comment (to another as well as to themselves [Gerber, 1987]) on objects and events rather than to regulate or manipulate the actions of another (e.g., Flax, 1986; Halliday, 1975; Longtin, 1984; Sachs, 1983). That is, children talk about what *they* are doing or what *they* want to do more often than they talk about what they want others to do; words are not used primarily as tools for manipulating the actions of others (Bloom, 1987). The use of conventional words to regulate others increases during Phase 1. Thus, early goals regarding the functions for which conventional words are used would include a variety of types (as suggested below). We would, however, expect that commenting (both comments that are directed to another, that is, interactive comments, as well as non-interactive comments) would be coded with conventional words earlier and more frequently than some of the regulating functions.

The goals as presented in the C/F/U Goal Plan for this period are outlined below (with no sequence of development implied in the order of presentation).

FUNCTION
To produce utterances for the purpose of:

1. Commenting about objects and ongoing events in an interactive or noninteractive fashion including indicating and labeling
2. Directing others to act
3. Calling or getting attention
4. Protesting
5. Obtaining an object
6. Getting someone to respond (i.e., to say something)
7. Responding to the utterances of others (not necessarily contingently)
8. Playing with sounds
9. Greeting, transferring objects, or carrying out other social routines

CONTEXT—NONLINGUISTIC
To produce utterances

10. About objects and events that are ongoing or present.
11. About the child's dynamic interaction with the environment: at first about what the child is doing and with increasing frequency about what the child is about to do and what the child wants others to do
12. That indicate awareness of differences among listeners (e.g., by differences in amount of talk, loudness of speech, etc., to strangers versus known listeners)
13. Upon request that attempt to clarify the listener's understanding of the child's prior utterance by phonetic recoding

CONTEXT—LINGUISTIC
To produce utterances

14. Following the utterances of other persons that:
    a. Are exact imitations
    b. Add a related word (usually following a question)
    c. Are related to the same nonlinguistic context

Goals of Content and Form: Phases 1, 2, and 3

The content/form interactions that characterize the early phases of language learning are elaborated on in this section. Each phase is presented separately, and each goal within the phase is listed, followed by examples.

Phase 1: Coding Object and Relational Knowledge with Single-Word Utterances

The point when children use single-word utterances has long been recognized as the first of the linguistic "developmental milestones." In the past, this period was often considered one of learning the names for things. Consequently, clinicians and educators concentrated on teaching children to label static objects—to acquire a vocabulary of nouns. It is now apparent that naming is only a small part of what young children are doing in this period when they are able to say only one word at a time. In fact, for many children the words that are used most often and most consistently in this period are not names of objects (e.g., Bloom, 1973; Lifter, 1982; Rocissano, 1979) but words that code relations (e.g., *no, gone*). More important, the view of single-word utterances as primarily and simply naming behavior ignores the different underlying meanings represented by single words that come to be expressed with more and more elaborate forms in later phases as well as the communicative competence and interactional skills that the child is learning. Early words are produced for a variety of functions in this period (e.g., Gerber, 1987; Longtin, 1984).

Although a child may have a vocabulary of 20 or 50 words, a small core of these words will be produced frequently, while the others will appear infrequently. For many children, the most frequently used words are relational words (Bloom, 1973; Gopnik, 1981; Lifter, 1982). Relational words are not names for things but words that refer to the relations between objects—relations that exist across objects of different classes. For example, some words (e.g., *this, that*) are used by children to refer to the fact that objects exist, while others (e.g., *all gone, no, away*) refer to the fact that objects have disappeared or do not exist. Still other relational words can be used to reject or deny (*no*); to note the recurrence of some object or action (*more*); to refer to locating objects (e.g., *up, out*); or to attributes of objects (e.g., *hot*). Relational words are, therefore, among the earliest words learned and are often produced more frequently than object names. In addition, they combine syntactically with object names in Phase 2.

In addition to relational words, the child also learns substantive words (i.e., words that name things of substance—or nounlike words). Nouns are produced in contexts that are similar to the contexts that elicit relational words. Thus, the child might be looking for an object that has disappeared and name the object "ball" (or use the relational word *gone*); or the child might point to one ball and say "ball" (or use the relational word *that*) and then point to a second ball and say "ball" (or use the relational word *more*). Children at this phase of development also reject objects by naming them, often accompanied by a negative headshake or whine, instead of negating them with the relational word *no.* Furthermore, nouns are used to label objects as they are acted upon (e.g., taken out of a box, given or shown to another).

The first nouns used are often about things that move (persons, animals) or things that the child can move (balls, food) and not about stationary objects. Moreover, nouns that appear among the child's first words often make reference to one instance of an object rather than to a class of objects. For example, a child might use the word *dog* to refer to only one dog in one context and not to other dogs (i.e., an example of underextension of the term). Some of these words are dropped from the child's productive repertoire when that particular instance (e.g., the dog in our example) is no longer available although other exemplars of the class (e.g., dogs) are present (Bloom, 1973). Other words may be tied to sensorimotor schemata, particular interpersonal situations, or particular contexts (Bloom, 1973; Dore, 1986).

Likewise, comprehension of early words is often limited to certain contexts. Although comprehension vocabulary is usually larger than productive vocabulary, the words comprehended are not necessarily the words produced (Bloom, 1974; Bloom & Lahey, 1978). For example, in a study by Benedict (1979), more action-related words were found in the children's comprehension vocabulary than were found in their production vocabulary, and the action words spoken were different from those comprehended. In English, names of actions (i.e., verbs) are rare early in Phase 1; they tend to appear late in Phase 1 or with the emergence of word combinations in Phase 2 (Bates, Bretherton, & Snyder, in press; Bloom, 1973, Goldin-Meadow, Seligman, & Gelman, 1976). [In American Sign Language when both the action and the object of the action are marked with one sign, verbs emerge earlier (Launer, 1982).]

Toward the end of Phase 1, a marked increase in vocabulary occurs as children seem to realize that everything has a name. This vocabulary spurt co-occurs with the more denotative use of words [i.e., words are less tied to sensorimotor schemata (Bloom, 1973)] and is followed by an increase in the child's ability to locate objects that are out of sight in order to relate these objects to other objects such as putting peg people in the bus (Lifter, 1982).

For some children, the end of Phase 1 is also marked with the production of successive single-word utterances; that is, a series of words relates to an event where the ordering of the words is not consistent and not syntactic (see Bloom, 1973, for examples and discussion). Early examples of saying more than one word about an event are often chained to the child's actions. For example, the child might say "truck" as it is picked up, "go" as it is pushed, and "stop" as it is stopped. Later the successive words are not chained to actions and appear to relate to a mental representation that the child has in mind. For example, the child might say "mommy/ baby/ truck/" in an attempt to get her mother to make the doll sit in the truck. In other cases, the series of words may be interspersed with adult comments or questions. For example, the child may say "more" and an adult might follow with "more what?" which elicits "cookie" from the child. These types of successive utterances have been labeled vertical constructions by Scollon (1976).

The single-word utterances that the child produces express certain basic ideas about the environment. At this phase, linguistic *form* first intersects with *content*. The content expressed includes the categories of existence, nonexistence, recurrence, rejection, denial, attribution, possession, action, and locative action. Some content categories are notably absent in this early period—for example children do not talk about their internal states or feelings. While certainly the children have such feelings, talking about feelings appears to be a late development (Bloom, in press; Bretherton & Beeghly, 1982). This may be because it is difficult for the child to match words with such feelings (see Lahey & Bloom, 1977, for a discussion of this point). Contexts that are coded in Phase 1 are described below—see also Appendix E.

Existence   The child attends to an object (by looking, picking up, pointing, touching, etc.) and either names the object or uses a relational word (such as *there, that,* or *this,*) to indicate the object.

Nonexistence or Disappearance   The child expects an object to be in the context but does not see it, or the child expects an action to occur, but it does not happen, and the child produces a relational word to code the nonexistence of the expected object or action (e.g., *gone, away, no, bye-bye*). While nouns may be used in this context, they do not *code* nonexistence.

Recurrence   The child produces a relational word such as *more, another,* or *again* to refer to the recurrence of an event, the reappearance of an object, or another instance of an object. The naming of the action or object would not be considered coding of recurrence.

Rejection   The child opposes an action or object and produces the relational word *no.* A noun and a headshake may also be used in this context, but such expression would not be counted as linguistic coding of rejection.

Denial   Denial is not coded by all children at this point of development and thus is an optional goal in Phase 1. When it is coded, the child negates the truthfulness of a prior utterance with a relational form such as *no.*

Attribution   Attribution is not coded by all children in this period, and so it is an optional goal in Phases 1 and 2. When it is coded, the child mentions an attribute of an object by the use of a relational word (e.g., an adjective like *hot* or *dirty*). However, in early child language, attributes are not used in a contrastive way—that is, to distinguish the object from similar objects (big hats versus small hats). Early attribution is used in a more nominal way—"party hat" is the name of the hat, and "hot stove" is the name of the stove. While color words may be used, they are often incorrect or, again, are assigned in a nominal manner (e.g., there are "red pajamas" and "yellow pajamas"). Some of these nominal-type codings of attribution expressed in two-word utterances may, in fact, have been learned as a unit. In any case, the use of attribution through Phase 3 is infrequent and rarely used in a contrastive manner (see Bloom & Lahey, 1978).

Possession   Possession is not coded by all children in the period and so is optional in Phases 1 and 2. For the young child, certain objects are associated with particular people, and the child may name the person when he or she sees the object. Since names are not relational and cannot code a relation such as possession, we do not give the child credit for coding *possession* in these instances. In assessment (see Chapter 12), however, we do note that the child uses names of persons associated with objects (what might be called a context for possessive coding). Other children may, in the single-word-utterance period, use the relational pronoun as *mine* to directly code possession. By Phase 2 the child may combine the name of the object possessed and the name of the possessor ("mommy pen") with consistent word order, thus coding the relationship of possession. Early coding and understanding of possessive relationships involve inalienable (or intrinsic) relationships—that is, relationships that could only belong to that person, such as parts of the body ("baby's ear") (Brown, 1973; Golinkoff & Markessini, 1980). Coding of possessive relations for objects that could belong to anyone is a later development. Thus, early goals for coding possession should focus on the coding of inalienable relations.

Action   When children begin to combine words, talking about agents acting on objects is one of the most frequent categories coded. In the single-word-utterance period, children refer to action events by naming the agent of an action or the object of an action, but these are nouns and do not *code* the action relation. Again, the use of these nouns in action contexts is important and should be noted. Relational words that code action are verbs that name the action, and these are infrequently used as single-word utterances (Goldin-Meadow et al., 1976) but tend to emerge in syntactic utterances. A few relational words describing action do, however, appear *late* in Phase 1. These may not all be verbs in the adult model. Some such relational words that describe actions and that have been reported in the single-word-utterance period (e.g., Bloom 1973) include *help, stop; back,* to refer to the action of moving something back; *open; go,* to refer to moving an object; *ride; wipe;* and *run.*

Locative Action   Another type of action event is one that involves changing the location of objects—here referred to as locative action. As children are in the process of moving an object, they often describe this locating action in the single-word-utterance period with relational words that are prepositions (such as *in, out, up, down*), verbs (such as *sit, lie down*), or adverbs (such as *here* or *there*). The static location of objects (such as *sit* to refer to a doll that's been sitting for a long time, or *in* to refer to an object that has been in a box for a long time) is not talked about until Phase 3.

As children first begin to use conventional forms to code ideas for the purpose of communication, we find individual differences among them in the forms they choose and in the way they use these forms. In a study of two infants, Dore (1975) found that one child had a larger vocabulary but used the words for fewer functions than the second child, who had a smaller vocabulary but used the words for many functions by varying intonation patterns. It was as if one child had focused on the form/content interactions and the other, on the form/use interactions of language. Differences in the types of words learned have also been described by K. Nelson (1973). She reported that the first 50 words of some children consist of over 50% nounlike words (she referred to these children as *referential* children), while for others over 50% consist of relational-type words, with many being social words such as *hi* and *thank you* (she referred to these children as *expressive* children).

Some relationship exists between the type of word used and the function of that word—for example, nouns are frequently used as comments or labels (Gerber, 1987; Longtin, 1984). But children produce similar word types (e.g., nouns) as well as identical lexical items for different functions. Furthermore, different children are apt to have different form/function preferences (Gerber, 1987; Longtin, 1984).

Examples of content/form interactions that appear in Phase 1 are presented in Box 9-3. See Chapters 12 and 13 for procedures that can be used to determine which should be goals of intervention for a particular child.

Phase 2: Coding Relations between Objects with Emerging Syntax

Once the child has begun to express many basic notions in the form of single words, he or she progresses to an elaboration of the form in which these very same notions are expressed. The distinguishing feature of Phase 2 is the elaboration of the linguistic representation—increased complexity of utterances. This is the phase familiarly referred to as the "two-word stage," and, indeed, this is a true description of the form of the utterances; children now combine two words in one utterance.

It is not the case, however, that the child has simply matured to the point where he or she can actually produce two words together and so simply joins together any two words that he or she has often heard expressed together in the speech of others. If that were the case, then language learning would be a matter of learning sequences of words that are commonly heard together without particular motivation for the sequence. Considerable argument has been advanced against this view. The intersection of particular words and the *order* in which these words occur is motivated by the *relationship* between the words that code the conceptual notion or meaning the child intends to express. The child's two-word utterances at this point are, for the most part, syntactic. Order of words is now used to code the relationship between the words, but there appears to be a limit to only two words at a time. This limit holds even though the child is able to code a number of different and often intersecting relationships (such as action-object, agent-action, agent-object).

Two elaborations in form develop during this phase. One that has been discussed is the combination of words into ordered relationship—the use of word order as the first expression of syntax. A second elaboration is the increase in the number of different words to express the same relationships—more topics are coded within a relationship—that is, more objects and actions are talked about. Thus the child uses longer utterances and more words to talk about the same content categories that were talked about in Phase 1. However, the same notions are still often expressed in single-word utterances or in a series of single words.

A number of individual differences that have relevance for establishing goals of language intervention are evident at this point of development. For one, children in this phase may show a preference for nominal or pronominal forms for agent and object of action or locative action (e.g., "eat it" versus "eat cookie," or "you go" versus "mommy go"), place in locative action (e.g., "put there" versus "put table"), and for possessor (e.g., "my car" versus "Peggy car") (Bloom, Lightbown, & Hood, 1975; K. Nelson, 1975). If such individual preferences are noted, they

BOX 9-3   Goals of Content/Form Interactions
Introduced in Phase 1

Content Category	by	Form
To code:		
Existence		Single-word utterances; relational words and later object names
Examples:		
(*Allison showing a picture to someone*)		*there*
(*Allison pointing toward the photographer*)		*man*
Nonexistence[a,b]		Single-word utterances; relational words
Examples:		
(*Gia reads book; closing it*)		*no more*
(*Gia sees a fly land on Lois's leg; flies away*)		*leg/all gone*
(*Allison looks at picture of girl; turns picture over so she can't see girl*)		*no*
Recurrence[a]		Single-word utterances; relational words
Examples:		
(*Peter drinks all the milk in his glass*)		*more*
(*Allison takes broken cookie from bag; puts it down; reaching in bag for another cookie*)		*more*
Rejection[a,b]		Single-word utterances; relational words
Examples:		
(*Lois starts to put blocks away; Gia stopping her*)		*no*
(*Eric is playing with his toy vacuum cleaner; mother wants him to show Lois his new truck which makes noise*) *Make noise with the truck*		*no*
(Denial)[a,b,c]		Single-word utterances; relational words (used less frequently than previous categories)
Examples:		
(*Allison puts calf on floor*) *Is that the lamb?*		*no*
(*Eric has his toy telephone*) *Is that Lois's telephone?*		*no*

(continued)

BOX 9-3   Phase 1 (*continued*)

Content Category	by	Form
(Attribution)[d]		Single-word utterances; relational words as adjectives (frequency of use is variable—less frequent with some children than others)
Examples:		
(*Peter eating lunch; touching his spoon which is warm*)		*hot*
(*Mommy and Allison give doll a "bath" in a paper cup; Allison takes doll from mommy; looking at it*)		*clean*
(Possession)[a]		Single-word utterances; name of possessor or pronoun (use in this phase variable among children; if coded, it may be by naming the person associated with an object, or by a pronoun)
Examples:		
(*Gia holding up mommy's telephone book*)		*də mommy*
(*Peter picks up blocks; holding them to his chest*)		*mine*
Action[a]		Single-word utterances; relational words as verbs
Examples:		
(*Peter opening flap of tape recorder case*)		*open*
(*Allison turning book over from front cover to back cover*)		*turn*
(*Allison trying to put horse on chair and can't do it; giving it to mommy*)		*help/horse/help*
Locative Action[a]		Single-word utterances; relational words as verbs or prepositions
Examples:		
(*Allison trying to get on chair*)		*up*
(*Peter reaching out to his stool*)		*sit*
(*Allison stepping out of truck*)		*out*

[a] In addition to the behaviors listed here, object names are used in many situations: for example, naming the object acted on, located, possessed, noticed, wanted, etc. They are not listed under content because the relational meaning of such words is not clear. Their use in these contexts should, however, be encouraged.
[b] Some children do not have negation utterances early in this phase.
[c] Parentheses indicate that goal is optional in this phase.
[d] Attributes rarely refer to color or shape.

should be followed during this phase. It is not until Phase 5 that goals should be concerned with using both nouns and pronouns.

Another source of individual differences that has been reported in this phase is a preference for either transitive or intransitive verbs (e.g., the children studied by Bloom, Lightbown, & Hood, 1975, and Brown, 1973, used verbs that took an object, while those studied by Bowerman, 1973, tended to use verbs that did not take an object). Again, it seems wise to stay with a child's preference, if there is one, at this stage of development. The coding of action with intransitive verbs would be agent + action (e.g., "baby run"), while with transitive verbs it is most likely to be action + object (e.g., "eat cookie"), but could be agent + action (e.g., "baby eat") or agent + object (e.g., "baby cookie").

Locative-action relations (i.e., those that talk of moving objects to places) may be of three types (Bloom, Miller, & Hood, 1975). In one, the agent of the locating action is also the object being moved—that is, the child is talking about an agent that moved itself (e.g., "I sit in the chair")—referred to as mover–locative action. Such utterances have two or three major constituents—agent, locating action, and usually (but not always) place. Place in locative-action utterances refers to the goal of the locating action. In a second type, referred to as agent–locative action, an agent moves an object, other than self, to a location (e.g., "I put the pencil on the table"). Agent–locative-action relations involve four major obligatory constituents—agent, locating action, object moved, and place. In this phase any two of these could be named, but the agent is least likely to be included. Finally, in some locative-action utterances an agent moves an object to a location, but the agent is not mentioned in the utterance and the preverbal noun is the located object (e.g., "the pencil goes on the table"). These are referred to as patient–locative action. In these latter utterances there are three major constituents—the object being moved (i.e., the patient), the locating action, and the place. In this phase only two of these constituents are coded (e.g., object + place; action + place; action + object), and often the action constituent is coded with a preposition (e.g., "in box" —as the child places a toy in the box).

Verbs that were most frequently used, by the children studied by Bloom and her associates (see Bloom & Lahey, 1978), in action and locative-action utterances were general verbs describing actions that could involve many different objects (such as *do*, *make*, or *go*) rather than descriptive verbs that described actions that were more specific to particular objects (such as *bounce* or *tear*). The most frequently used verbs are listed in the discussion of Phase 3.

Other changes occur in form coding within Phase 2. For example, existence utterances are generally coded with a demonstrative pronoun (e.g., *this* or *that*) or the schwa /ə/ plus a substantive word. Nonexistence is coded with *no* or *no more* plus a content word (i.e., a noun, adjective, verb), while recurrence is coded with a relational word (such as *more*) plus a content word. Possession and attribution are still optional. No new content categories are coded in this phase. Examples of new behaviors that become productive in Phase 2 are found in Box 9-4. Procedures for assessment are found in Chapters 12 and 13.

Phase 3: Coding Relations between Objects with Further Semantic-Syntactic Development

During this phase there is continued development in the use of word order to express semantic relations. Three constituents are used to code action relations;

BOX 9-4 Goals of Content/Form Interactions Introduced in Phase 2

Content Category	by	Form
To code: **Existence**		Two-word utterances—relational word plus object name
Examples: (*Lois just put microphone on Kathryn*)		*this necklace*
(*Gia pointing to picture of rabbit*)		*ə rabbit*
Nonexistence		Two-word utterances—relational word plus object name
Examples: (*Kathryn searching for pocket in mommy's skirt; there is no pocket*)		*no pocket*
(*Kathryn picking up clean sock; then picking up dirty sock*)		*no dirty/this dirty*
(*Eric heard an airplane outside a few minutes previous*)		*no more airplane*
Recurrence		Two-word utterances—relational word plus object name
Examples: (*Mommy is giving Kathryn a bath; finishes lathering her*)		*more soap*
(*Peter pointing out window at street light; pointing at another one*)		*light/more light*
(*Eric twists wheels; stops; twisting wheels again*)		*no more noise/more noise*
Rejection		No new behaviors (still use of single word as in Phase 1)
Denial		No new behaviors (still use of single word as in Phase 1)
(Attribution)[a]		Two-word utterances—adjective plus noun (used infrequently by some children—generally is a small proportion of syntactic utterances at this phase)

(continued)

BOX 9-4 Phase 2 (*continued*)		
Content Category	**by**	**Form**
Examples:		
(*Mommy is about to put freshly washed overalls on Kathryn; Kathryn had spilled something on them the day before*)		*dirty pants*
(*Peter looking at tape recorder buttons*)		*tape recorder button*
(Possession)		Two-word utterances—noun plus noun, pronoun plus noun (used infrequently in this phase by most children)
Examples:		
(*Kathryn has pair of mommy's socks*)		*mommy sock*
(*Gia pointing to hat on her doll*)		*dolly hat*
Action (agent-action-object relations)		Two-word utterances—verb plus noun or pronoun, and pronoun or noun plus verb are most common (preference for either nouns or pronouns is likely)
Examples:		
(*Eric reaching for cup of juice*)		*ə eat juice*
(*Gia riding her trike bike*)		*ride this*
(*Gia carrying book to mommy*)		*read ə book*
Locative Action (agent-action-object-place relations)		Two-word utterances—verb plus noun or pronoun, and pronoun or noun plus verb—are most common (most often the object is named with either the place or the action; noun or pronoun preference is likely)
Examples:		
(*Gia takes handful of snapshots to desk*)		*away picture*
(*Kathryn trying to climb on chair*)		*up Kathryn*
(*Kathryn putting sweater on chair*)		*sweater chair*

[a] Parentheses indicate that goal is optional in the phase.

that is, the basic form of the sentence, subject-verb-complement, becomes productive to express agent-action-object relations. Three of the four terms of agent–locative-action relations (agent-action-object-place) or the three terms of other locative-action relations (patient-action-place; mover-action-place) also become productive. As mentioned in Phase 2, the most frequent verbs used tend to be general verbs. Verbs that were used most frequently for locative action and action by the children studied by Bloom, Miller, and Hood (1975) are listed in Box 9-5.

While the production of three constituents becomes productive in Phase 3, it is not achieved (i.e., used in most obligatory contexts); the children frequently produce two-constituent utterances. When only two constituents are produced, they are usually the verb and object in action and agent–locative-action utterances, the verb and mover in mover–locative action, and the verb and place or patient in patient–locative-action utterances (Bloom, Miller, & Hood, 1975). In this same study, the children were more likely to produce the full three-constituent structure when the utterances included familiar verbs than when more recently learned verbs were used. Furthermore, the full three-constituent structure was more likely to occur after the child had just produced two of the constituents. In the data reported by Bloom and her colleagues, three constituents were often produced in a sequence where the child produced two constituents followed by the adult saying "hum?" or "what?" or repeating the two constituents spoken by the child with an intonation pattern that invited a response. From the point of view of goals and techniques of intervention, this is an interesting finding. So often clinicians and educators attempting to facilitate three-constituent utterances do not give the

---

BOX 9-5   Frequently Used Verbs for Action and Locative-Action Utterances Presented According to Frequency of Use

Action	Agent–Locative Action	Mover–Locative Action	Patient–Locative Action
get	put	go	go
do	take	sit	fit
make	away	go bye-bye	sit
read	turn	come	fall
play	out	get	bye-bye
find	get	fall	stand
eat	fit	stand	
fix	do	climb	
draw	dump	jump	
		move	

Note: Adapted from Bloom and Lahey, 1978, and Bloom, Miller, and Hood, 1975.
Action verbs came from the samples of four children with MLUs of about 2.5. They represent verbs used greater than 50 times.
Locative–action verbs were used less frequently and represent occurrences of a verb over 5 times in all of the samples of the same 4 children when MLUs were between 1 and 3.0.

BOX 9-6 Goals of Content/Form Interactions Introduced in Phase 3[a]		
Content Category	**by**	**Form**
To code:		
Existence		Two- and three-word utterances generally coding the two constituents, subject-complement; coordinated with attribution for some; frequent use of /ə/ as an apparent article; occasional use of contracted copula but not productive with most children
Examples: *(Kathryn pointing to picture in magazine)*		*that ə funny man*
(Eric holding yellow disc)		*that's yellow one*
Nonexistence		Two-word utterances; no new behaviors (same as Phase 2)
Recurrence		Two-word utterances; no new behaviors (same as Phase 2)
Rejection		Single-word utterances (some children start to use two-word utterances, but single-word utterances more common, as in Phase 1)
Denial		No new behaviors; single-word utterances (same as Phase 1)
(Attribution)[b]		Two- and three-word utterances; *coordinated* with existence; simple attribution is most common (see Existence for examples)
Possession		Two-word utterances; no new behaviors (same as Phase 2)
Action		Three constituents: subject-verb-complement; generally the most frequent relation expressed; pronominal/nominal preferences still exist (either nouns or pronouns can occur)

(continued)

BOX 9-6	Phase 3[a] (*continued*)	
Content Category	**by**	**Form**
Examples:		
(*Eric stacking blocks*)		*I do it*
(*Gia holding book out to mommy*)		*Mommy open that*
(*Kathryn opening book to first page*)		*Kathryn read this*
Locative Action		Three constituents: subject-verb-complement (object and/or place); used frequently; pronominal/nominal preferences still exist (either nouns or pronouns can occur)
Examples:		
(*Eric putting man on train*)		*man sit train*
(*Gia putting lamb on toy car*)		*lamb ə go car*
(*Kathryn pushing lamb through windows of dollhouse*)		*lamb go in there*
Locative state[c]		Two- and three-word utterances often including two constituents of the subject-verb-complement (usually object and place are mentioned); pronominal/nominal preference may exist
Examples:		
(*Eric points to toys on shelf*)		*ə dolly up here*
(*Gia points to picture of a baby in a basket*)		*baby basket*
(*Gia pointing to baby figure on form board*)		*baby in*
State[c]		Two or three constituents of the subject-verb-complement; pronominal/nominal preference may exist
Examples:		
(*Eric tries to take book from Lois; whines*)		*I want book*
(*Eric pointing to photograph of himself sleeping*)		*baby sleep*
(*Gia reaching for daddy figure*)		*Gia want daddy*
		(continued)

BOX 9-6   Phase 3[a] (*continued*)

Content Category	by	Form
(Quantity)[c]		Plural -*s* and/or a number word, such as *two*
Examples:		
(*Peter looking out window; to one then another chimney*)		*two buildings*
(*Kathryn pointing to library books on piano*)		*Mommy library books*
(*Eric pointing to two calves*)		*two cow*

[a] The greatest proportion of utterances are about action and locative action. Utterances about state, locative state, and possession are a small proportion of the total utterances. The proportion of utterances about attribution varies among individual children.
[b] Parentheses indicate that goal is optional in this phase.
[c] New category.

---

child the opportunity to build upon a prior statement; they are apt to jump in with "good boy (or girl)," with "say the whole thing," or with a model of the "whole thing." Although "hums" and "whats" and repetitions can be carried to an extreme, judicious use of responses that give the turn back to the child without demands and without added information may be worth trying as a means of facilitating three-constituent structures.

As an optional goal for those children who are coding attribution, the first coordinating of content categories occurs in Phase 3 with attribution + existence. The grammatical morpheme −*s* becomes productive to code *quantity*, or the notion of more than one, but it is not yet used in most instances that are considered obligatory in the adult model. Number words may also be used to code quantity, usually the number *two* to refer to more than one. Other number words may be used, but they are often inaccurate in referring to actual number.

In addition to the new coding of quantity, two other new content categories become productive—locative state and internal state. Each of these refers to static rather than dynamic events. In child language, syntactic coding of dynamic events, as actions and locating actions, precedes the coding of static events, as locative states and internal states—that is, the syntactic coding of static events emerges later than the syntactic coding of dynamic events and occurs less frequently than the syntactic coding of dynamic events (Bloom, Lightbown, & Hood, 1975).

Locative-state   Locative-state utterances can be formally similar to locative-action utterances. For example, the utterance "she is sitting down" can refer to the act of sitting (locative action), or, if she has been sitting for awhile, to the state of affairs (referred to as locative state)—On the other hand, descriptions of dynamic events such as "coming, going, putting" cannot be considered locative state at any time, for they do not describe static events. What happens in Phase 3 is that the child now talks about objects that are not being moved and describes their location—place in these instances is location and not the goal of movement, as it is in locative action (e.g., "sweater chair" referring to the location of the sweater and not to the placement of the sweater; or "daddy work" referring to daddy's present location, or where he is now located; or "blouse on" referring to the fact that mommy has a blouse on at this moment).

State State, which is productive at this phase for most children, is usually the coding of internal state with the verb *want* plus the object desired. In some cases early use of *want* seems more like an action verb than an internal state, for it is often used in the sense of "give me." However, children do begin to code the internal state of wish or volition at this phase. Coding is limited to desired objects in Phase 3 (e.g., "want cookie"); desired events (e.g., "want eat cookie") are *not* coded until Phase 4. The coding of other states may appear in Phase 3 (e.g., external state as, "it's dark"; attributive state as, "it's red"; or possessive state as, "it's mine"); however, information is not available on the developmental sequence of such productions, and so they are not listed as goals. Other children may talk about epistemic states or notice states in this phase, but these categories are considered as later goals since they generally are productive at later phases when the children code event relations; those states are given status as separate content categories in later phases.

Examples of the behaviors that become productive in Phase 3 are presented in Box 9-6. The new behaviors described in this and each phase have just become productive (i.e., used a few times with a variety of lexical items) and are not well established. Behaviors that became productive in prior phases are continuing to develop and probably mark the majority of utterances found at this time. Although not specified on the chart in Chapter 8 or in the boxes in Chapters 9 and 10, continued development of more lexical items to express the same meaning categories presented in earlier phases is a part of this and every succeeding phase.

Summary

In normal language learning, certain behaviors precede the interaction of language content, form, and use. Some of these behaviors that are precursory goals for the development of language use include using reciprocal gaze, regulating the behaviors of others, and calling attention to objects and events. Other precursory goals are related to development of content—behaviors that demonstrate an increased ability to represent something in mind when it is not present. Certain other behaviors are precursory goals for the development of language form—primarily the behaviors that are involved in the ability to imitate movements and vocalizations that are related to the form of linguistic signals. These early behaviors are suggested as early goals of language learning that should precede or be concurrent with Phase 1 of the plan.

The early phases of the plan for language learning are presented as goals for language learning. Phase 1 marks the first intersection between content, form, and use—the single-word utterance stage; Phases 2 and 3 represent the emergence of syntax—the use of word order to code meaning relations. In this period children talk about objects and events that are present and that they themselves are involved in. Many utterances are comments; others are used to regulate the environment.

Suggested Readings

Bates, E. (1976). *Language in context.* New York: Academic Press.

Bates, E., Bretherton, I., & Snyder, L. (in press). *From first words to grammar.* New York: Cambridge University Press.

Bloom, L. (1973). *One word at a time: The use of single-word utterances before syntax.* The Hague: Mouton.

Bloom, L. (in press). Development in expression: Affect and speech. In *Proceedings in the psychological and biological development of emotions, University of Chicago 1986.* Hillsdale, New Jersey.

Bloom, L., Lightbown, P., & Hood, L. (1975). Structure and variation in child language. *Monographs of the Society for Research in Child Development, 40* (Serial No. 160).

Dore, J. (1986). The development of communicative competence. In R. Schiefelbusch (Ed.), *Language competence: Assessment and intervention.* San Diego: College-Hill Press.

Halliday, M. A. K. (1975). *Learning how to mean—Explorations in the development of language.* London: Edward Arnold.

Piaget, J. (1954). *The construction of reality in the child.* New York: Basic Books.

10

Language Development: Goals of Later Language Learning

The goals of later language learning presented in this chapter relate to Phases 4 to 8 of the C/F/U Goal Plan for Language Learning that was outlined in Chapter 8. New goals of use that interact with content/form include an increase in the number of utterances that are produced without perceptual support from the nonlinguistic context, an increase in the number of utterances that are linguistically related to the utterances of others, an increase in the number of utterances that are adapted to the needs of the listener, and an increase in the number of utterances that serve to obtain information. New content/form goals include the emergence of morphological inflections to code aspect (and eventually tense), the embedding of certain content categories in verb relations, and the development of complex sentences to code event relations.

These developmental changes are presented in two parts. Those that occur in Phases 4 and 5 are presented first, followed by those that occur in Phases 6, 7, and 8.

Goals of Use that Interact with Content/Form: Phases 4 and 5

In Phases 4 and 5, an increasing number of utterances are about objects and events that are not present in the nonlinguistic context. Although the child is beginning to talk about objects and events without immediate perceptual support, it is important to note that the child is rarely talking about events that have occurred days or weeks ago or that will occur days or weeks in the future. Instead, when children are not talking about the "here and now," they are usually talking about something that has just been experienced, perhaps minutes before, or that they are planning to do or want to happen in the next few minutes, or about "scripted events" (i.e., events that frequently reoccur; see K. Nelson, 1986). In contrast to the earlier phases, the children are also beginning to talk about the actions of others and not only about their own actions or what they want others to do. The use of language in these new nonlinguistic contexts (i.e., without immediate perceptual support and about others' actions) increases in later phases.

Accompanying the changed use of language in nonlinguistic contexts is a changing response to linguistic contexts. First, there is an increase in the number of utterances that do not follow the utterances of another (i.e., utterances that are nonadjacent). The number of these spontaneous utterances increases in comparison with the earlier phases, but they still number less than half of the total number of utterances produced by children at this point in development. The adjacent utterances are now, however, more often likely to be linguistically contingent on the prior utterance. Many of these linguistically contingent utterances that add information are appropriate answers to questions.°

Although they are more likely to be contingent, the contingency does not come from only an imitation of the prior utterance. Most linguistically contingent utterances either add information or repeat a part of the adult utterance with an addition or replacement of a word or phrase (e.g., *Adult:* "Want a cookie?" *Child:* "Want a *chocolate* cookie"). Additions, as in the earlier period, may be in the form of an additional constituent or the replacement of a constituent (e.g., *Adult:* "What do you want?" *Child:* "Cookie"), and now occasionally in this period may be an added sentence (e.g., *Adult:* "You're gonna carry the doll?" *Child:* "Cuz she's tired"). But most frequently, linguistic contingency is in the form of repeat + add, with the verb from the prior utterance most frequently repeated and a lexical item

---

° Note that the content of questions asked of children varies over time and appears to depend on the content the children themselves talk about; thus children are rarely asked questions about causality until they themselves begin to talk about causality. Linguistically contingent responses may not occur to questions about content the child is not talking about in other situations.

or phrase (as in the first cookie example) added. Most of the linguistically contingent utterances are in response to questions (Bloom, Rocissano, & Hood, 1976).

When the adults' questions are requests for confirmation of a previous child utterance, the child usually gives an affirmative response at this point in development even when a negative response would have been appropriate (see Gallagher, 1981). General requests for repair (such as "what?" following a child utterance) are responded to by a change in the phonetic shape of the elements or by deletion of one of the elements that was in the original utterance (Gallagher, 1977).

Not only are children beginning to relate their utterances to the prior utterance of another, but they are also beginning to produce utterances that are related to their own prior utterance. In Phase 5 we see evidence of the child talking about two events (or states) that are related by time and space (additive relations) or causally related (with some temporal and adversative relations). Such productions are usually independent of the utterances of others; that is, the two events (or states) are coded by the child (Bloom, Lahey, Hood, Lifter, & Fiess, 1980).

At this point in development children begin to ask an increasing number of questions primarily about identity and location (e.g., "What's that?" or "Where is X?"). Not all of these questions function as a means of obtaining information; the child often already knows the information requested. However, a gradual increase in the use of questions to obtain new information occurs. Almost all questions are related to context and not to the prior utterance of another (i.e., children rarely respond to the utterances of another with a contingent question) (Bloom, Rocissano, & Hood, 1976). If a contingent question is asked, it is usually a request for confirmation (Gallagher, 1981).

The goals of use that interact with content and form in these phases relate to function, nonlinguistic context, and linguistic context:

GOALS
Related to function

1. To increase the number of utterances that serve the social (or interpersonal) functions listed for Phases 1, 2, and 3 (e.g., regulate, respond)
2. To produce utterances in order to obtain information about identity or location of objects related to present context
3. To utilize a greater variety of forms for all functions

GOALS
Related to nonlinguistic context

4. To produce utterances about objects that are not present and about events that have just happened or are about to happen
5. To increase the number of utterances about what others are doing
6. To increase the amount of talking (e.g., the number of utterances per unit of time)
7. To clarify utterances, upon request, through phonetic recoding and deletions

GOALS

Related to linguistic context

8. To increase the number of nonadjacent utterances
9. To increase the number of contingent utterances by adding a word (or occasionally a phrase or clause) to a prior utterance, often in addition to repeating a part of the prior utterance
10. When repeating a part of prior utterance, to recode a part of it (primarily by pronominalizing the object and shifting pronouns in the subject)

Each of these goals of use is an important part of development within these phases and should co-occur with the goals of content/form interactions.

Goals of Content/Form Interactions: Phases 4 and 5

Phase 4: Coordinating Content Categories with Embedded Relations

In Phases 1, 2, and 3 the child learned the first intersections of content/form in the single-word-utterance period (Phase 1) and then moved to the first syntactic coding of semantic relations with the use of word order (Phases 2 and 3). Each of these achievements continues to develop in later phases—the variety of lexical items used, the number of utterances spoken per unit of time, and the number of utterances that use word order as a means of expressing semantic relations increase.

While behaviors learned in Phases 1, 2, and 3 continue to develop, new behaviors emerge and mark this fourth phase. For one, new content categories emerge —notice and temporal. *Notice* forms a major verb category (along with existence, action, locative action, locative state, and state). Notice verbs code the perception of an event or state (e.g., *see, look, hear, listen, watch, show*), and coding with a single word may be found in some children earlier than this phase (particularly with the verbs *see* and *look*). However, by Phase 4, notice is generally coded syntactically with two or three constituents where the complement of the notice verb is a perceived object (e.g., "I see bird"; "look at me"). It is only in the later phases that children code the perception of events where the complement of the notice verb is a clause (e.g., "watch me jump").

Another verb category that may appear at this time is *epistemic*, which codes mental states of mind. At this period of development children may code epistemic with the verb *know*, particularly with routine utterances (such as "I don't know"; "I know it"). It is not included as a goal at this phase because coding is so often limited to these routines; it will become a goal in Phase 7 when it is coded with more varied verbs (e.g., *think, remember*) and complements (usually in the form of another verb relation, such as "think it fits"). It will be further discussed at that time.

Another new content category that *is* considered as a goal at this time is *temporal*. The temporal category includes coding of aspect, sequence, simultaneity, and tense. Sequence and simultaneity refer to the relation between events (or states) and do not emerge until Phase 5 or later. Tense, on the other hand, is the relation between the time when an event occurs and the time when the utterance refers to that event; that is, I can tell you about an event before it happens, while it is going on, or after it happens. The coding of tense in the English language is confounded with the coding of aspect, but it appears that tense is coded developmentally later than aspect.

In contrast to tense, aspect refers to the temporal contour of the event itself rather than to the relationship between when an event happens and when it is talked about (as is the case for tense)—that is, some events last over time and are durative events (e.g., playing), while others are momentary, or nondurative (as to drop something and have it break); some events have a clear result and can be called completive (e.g., the broken glass), while other events are noncompletive (such as playing); and some events are habitual (e.g., the person who jogs daily), while others are not (e.g., the occasional jogger). We can see some distinction in the coding of aspect and tense. For example, -ing often codes durative (where there is no definite period of time) noncompletive events in both the past and present with the tense distinction marked by the auxiliary ("he *is* eating breakfast" versus "he *was* eating breakfast"). Habitual can be coded by the present tense form of the verb with inflection -s if the subject is third person singular (e.g., "he eats breakfast," which implies that he usually does so; or "it goes here," which implies that this is its habitual location). However, the adult model of the English language does not mark the distinction between tense and aspect as clearly as many other languages. The use of irregular past and -ed marks past, completed, and nondurative actions (where there was a definite period of time—e.g., "he ate breakfast"), but it can also mark tense for durative noncompletive events (e.g., "he played").

Observations of children learning the inflectional system of verbs suggest, however, that the early use of these inflections is more related to aspect than to tense (Antinucci & Miller, 1976; Bloom, Lifter, & Hafitz, 1980; Bronkart & Sinclair, 1973; Feintuck, 1985). The verb inflections (-ing, -s, and irregular past) emerge at about the same time (Phase 4) and are used in contexts that relate to aspectual meaning—that is, -ing is first used to code durative noncompletive events; irregular past and -ed are first used to refer to completive punctual events; and -s is used to code habitual contexts.

When first learned, the inflections are added to pro-verbs (i.e., verbs that stand for many events, such as do, make, go) or to verbs that themselves code aspectual meaning. Thus, break is a verb that is inherently completive and nondurative and is inflected with irregular past before -ing; write, on the other hand, is a verb that (for children and sometimes for authors) is inherently more durative and noncompletive and is inflected with -ing before the irregular past. During Phase 4, -ing and irregular past are produced primarily with pro-verbs coding action (such as do, make, go), and -ing is used on some descriptive verbs (such as eat, hide, write, ride, dance, wash, cook). The inflection -s is added to some action verbs, but primarily it is added to locative-action verbs (go, fit) as the child places objects in their habitual location (e.g., puzzle pieces in the puzzle, furniture in the dollhouse). Contrastive production of inflections (i.e., different inflections on the same verb stem) emerges first on pro-verbs in the contexts where the aspectual coding is appropriate (e.g., *doing* to refer to continuative noncompletive events and *did* to refer to nondurative completive events). As the children advance in language development, more verbs are inflected and the inflections occur contrastively on the same verb stems. Examples of verbs that are used with the verb inflections through Phase 5 are found in the next section (Box 10-2).

The point at which the inflections are well achieved (i.e., reach the criterion of 80–90% correct application in obligatory contexts) varies with children (see differences in Bloom, Lifter, & Hafitz, 1980; Brown, 1973; J. de Villiers & de Villiers, 1973; and Feintuck, 1985). Achievement relative to inflections is not a goal for any of the inflections during Phase 4 or 5. One might expect between 20 and 60% use in obligatory contexts for *-ing*, irregular past, and *-s*, but contexts may be few and the variety of verbs that are inflected may be quite limited. The use of *-ed* is more variable, with lower proportions of correct application by most children and perhaps no production by many children until Phase 5. Goals in later phases should include increases in proportional use and increases in the variety of verbs inflected.

In addition to the emergence of the verb inflections, the grammatical morpheme *a* plus the demonstrative pronoun (i.e., *this* or *that*) appears in existence utterances (e.g., "that a boat"). Previously one or the other had been combined with nouns to code existence, but rarely both together. In addition, the prepositions *in* and *on* are used in utterances coding locative state as well as in utterances coding locative action.

The previously established category of rejection is now syntactically coded (e.g., "no soap") and a number of previously established nonverb content categories are coordinated with verb relations. Recurrence and possession are coordinated with existence at this time. Categories coordinated with action include attribution, nonexistence, recurrence, and place (which was previously expressed mainly as a constituent of locative relations). This coordination is accomplished by the embedding of a nonverb relation into the constituent structure of a verb relation. When this embedding intervenes between the major constituents of action (e.g., the placement of an attribute between the action and the object of the action, as in "ride red bike"), it is likely that only two of the constituents will be produced at this phase—usually the verb and the complement (Bloom, Miller, & Hood, 1975). Thus, goals of intervention that involve such embedding should reflect this possible reduction of the constituent structure by expecting the production of only two constituents when coordinations are first produced. Recall from the previous chapter that the production of three constituents is facilitated by the use of familiar lexical items and discourse support (i.e., the prior production of two constituents by the child or a contingent query by the adult).

Two *wh*-question forms appear as goals in Phase 4; "what" is produced in order to question identity (and is placed in the category of existence), while "where" is produced to question location (and is placed in the locative-state category when questioning static location, such as "where is X?" or in the locative-action category when, at a later time, questioning place of a locating action, such as "where is X going?"). Each emerges within copula sentence structure (e.g., "what's that?" or "where's ___?") although the copula may or may not be present (Bloom,

Merkin, & Wooten, 1982; Brown, 1968). Some children seem to learn the contracted copula as a part of the *wh* form, while others omit it at first or use it
variably. (For more information on the development of questions read the above
references as well as Labov & Labov, 1977; Lewis, 1938; M. Smith, 1933; and
Tyack & Ingram, 1977.)

Finally, utterances with two verbs emerge in Phase 4. The first verb in such
utterances is usually *want* or *go* followed by a complement that includes an action
or locative-action verb. The first verb in the utterance acts as a modal verb coding
volition (wish) or intention about an event, and thus these first multiverb utterances are placed in the category of state. The complements of the modal verbs
produced in this phase include a verb phrase whose subject is coreferential with
the subject of the modal verb and is, thus, redundant and deleted (e.g., in "I want
eat" the subject of both *want* and *eat* is *I,* and so it is not repeated before the verb
eat). Such structures can be referred to as infinitival complement structures. Generally, at this period, the children omit the word *to* before the infinitive although
they may include the schwa as a part of the modal (e.g., *wanna, gonna*). It appears
that these concatenated modal forms are learned as a unit and do not represent a
contraction of *to* as they may in the adult model. Thus, the form of these infinitival
complements coding state may be described as (subject) + verb − connective *to*
+ verb phrase (where parentheses indicate optional elements). For further information see Bloom, Tackeff, and Lahey (1983); Brown (1973); Limber (1973); Paul
(1981); and Tyack & Gottsleben (1986).

Box 10-1 includes specific examples of the new behaviors that become productive in Phase 4.

Phase 5: Coding Relations between Events with Successive Related Utterances

Phase 5 is marked by the coding of four new categories of content—dative, specification, additive, and causal. *Dative* refers to the indirect object of recipient and is
here coded with noun plus noun (e.g., "give sweater daddy"). *Specification* serves
to point out or describe a particular object or event in contrast to another. In Phase
5 we find the use of the demonstrative pronouns *this* and *that* used with a noun or
pronoun (e.g., "this one"; "that book") to specify which referent is intended. [The
use of the demonstrative as subject or object (e.g., "I want that") may also refer to
specification if stress and gesture are used to mark the contrast, but it is only the
demonstrative + noun that is a goal in Phase 5.] The other categories of additive
and causal refer to relations between events.

Additive refers to the co-occurrence of events and/or states in time and space.
No dependency relation exists between the events (or states), and the order of
mention could be reversed without changing the meaning. The combination of the
two clauses did not create a meaning that was anything other than the meaning of
the two clauses separately. This category includes sequential events if the child
codes the two actions as they are carried out—that is, the utterances are chained
to the actions much in the way that early successive single-word utterances are
chained to actions. In many instances, both clauses have the same verb; different
verbs in each clause are more likely to appear when the clauses are chained to
actions.

BOX 10-1 Goals of Content/Form Interactions Introduced in Phase 4

Content Category	by	Form
To code:		
Existence		Coordinated with possession and recurrence; inclusion of demonstrative pronoun and *a*; *wh* questions for identity with or without copula.

Examples:
Possession and existence
(*Gia sitting on her bike*)   *this ə my bike*

(*Peter looking at Patsy's pen on floor*)   *that's ə Patsy's pen*

Recurrence and existence
(*Gia takes clown from toy bag; taking
out second one*)   *this another clown*

Wh question
(*Eric holding out piece of puzzle to Lois*)   *what's this*

Content Category	Form
Nonexistence	Coordinated with action (see Action for examples)
Recurrence	Coordinated with existence and action (see Existence and Action for examples)
(Rejection)[a]	Two- and three-word utterances; not frequently used and not productive yet by all children

Examples:
(*Kathryn finds bear book; puts it down;*   *no bear book*
picking up slide)

(*Gia has been holding lamb; throwing it*
on the floor)   *no want that*

Content Category	Form
Denial	No new behaviors; single-word utterances (same as Phase 1)
Attribution	Coordinated with action (see Action for examples)
Possession	Coordinated with existence (see Existence for examples)
State	Increased use of two- and three-word utterances; coding of volition/intention with action and locative action using infinitival complement constructions and with the matrix verb *want* or *go* plus a verb phrase without the infinitive *to* but often with [ə] (e.g., *wanna*).

(continued)

BOX 10-1 Phase 4 (*continued*)		
Content Category	**by**	**Form**
Examples:		
Volition/Intention		
(*Allison turning to M.*)		*want eat my snack*
(*Gia pointing out window*)		*I wanna go outside*
(*Peter drawing*)		*gonna make it man/ house*
(*Gia going to door*)		*I'm open door*
(*Peter pointing to screws on wheel of car; then starts to unscrew tire*)		*gonna take wheel out*
Locative Action		Increased use of three constituents; agent–locative action coordinated with intention/volition (see State for examples); patient–locative action coordinated with third person -*s* (see Temporal for examples).
Temporal[c]		Some verbs inflected with -*ing*, -*s*, and irregular past in about 20% of obligatory contexts to code aspect; coding intention with modal verbs could also be considered temporal—here it is placed under State (see Examples).
Examples:		
Third person -*s* (habitual)		
(*putting lamb in barn*)		*this one goes in there*
(*attaching trains*)		*that goes here*
Durative with -*ing*		
(*Peter drawing*)		*I writing circles*
(*Gia looking at a book*)		*man making muffins*
Irregular past (nondurative-completive)		
(*Gia closing book*)		*Gia did book*
Action		Coordinated with place, attribution, recurrence, nonexistence, intention (see State for examples); irregular past and -*ing* (see Temporal for examples); increased use of three constituents, but subject may be deleted with coordinations marked with symbol [b].
		(*continued*)

BOX 10-1 Phase 4 (*continued*)		
Content Category	**by**	**Form**
Examples:		
Action and nonexistence[b]		
(*Gia tries to put lamb in block; can't*)		can't do it
Action and recurrence[b]		
(*Gia bringing a man to Lois*)		man read another book
(*Peter draws circle, which he calls "hole," drawing another one*)		write it nother hole
Action and attribution[b]		
(*Peter tries to draw a tree*)		make ə big tree
(*Gia painting with black paint*)		I draw red man/ I draw black man
Action and place		
(*Gia scribbles on toy pan*)		I write my pan
(*Peter holding box of recording tape; pointing to tape recorder*)		there's ə tape go round right there
Locative State		Use of prepositions *in, on; wh* questions; this category is less frequently coded than action and locative acion
Examples:		
(*Peter noticing piece of masking tape on car*)		tape on truck
Locative state and *wh* questions		
(*Peter noticing train car is missing a plastic disc*)		where is it
(*Gia looking around for car driver*)		where man go
Quantity		Plural *-s* used most of time when required
Notice—Reception[c]		Two- and three-constituent utterances
Examples:		
(*child shouts in hall outside; Gia listens*)		I hear Kevin
(*Gia pointing to rabbit in a picture*)		ooh look at the rabbit
(*Lois drew a screwdriver on Peter's paper; Peter gets toy screwdriver and puts it on paper next to drawing*)		look at that

[a] When a content category is in parentheses, it indicates the goal is optional in this phase.
[b] May result in omission of the subject.
[c] New category.

During this phase, the child may simply produce in succession two utterances that are related in an additive manner, or the child may use the conjunction *and* to join clauses or phrases. Phrasal coordination (e.g., "eat cake and cookie") and clausal coordination (e.g., "I sit here and you sit there") emerge at about the same time with *and*. These early clausal coordinations do not usually remention coreferential items (i.e., we find "I kiss doll and hug teddy" and not "I kiss doll and I hug teddy"), but they do include two complete clauses when subject and object are not coreferential (e.g., "that is mine and that is mine" referring to two different objects) (Bloom, Lahey, Hood, Lifter, & Fiess, 1980). The conjunction *and* is also used to chain an utterance to context, as, for example, when a child is taking a lot of toys out of a bag without saying anything and then, while taking out a car, says "and a car."

Some of the successive utterances produced by the child at this level of development have a causal relation between them. In *causal* relations, one clause refers to a state or event that is a necessary (but perhaps not a sufficient) condition for the state or event referred to in the other clause to exist. The two clauses may have been spoken one after another or may have had an intervening utterance from an adult. Intervening utterances can include those with no new content, such as "oh" or a repetition of the child's utterance, as well as those that ask "why." Some children have a preference for ordering the clauses—using either cause and then effect or effect and then cause—and this order continues into the next phase and influences whether the conjunction *because* or *so* is learned first (Hood & Bloom, 1979).

Different types of causal relations can be identified—for example, some relations refer to *objective* relations that are evident in the physical world (e.g., consequences, such as rain causing puddles; means-end, such as getting a stick to reach the apples). Other relations are more *subjective* and depend on personal or sociocultural judgment (for example, stopping because the light is red or crying because the fish died). Both types of causal meanings are found in juxtaposed utterances during this phase, but in later phases we will see that the type of meaning interacts with the early inclusion or omission of a conjunction (Bloom & Capatides, in press a). Most of the utterances are spoken in interactive environments—either in conversational exchanges where an adult utterance intervenes or in negotiations where the child is directing, prohibiting, or requesting; most were not elicited by "why" questions, nor was the causal relation connected to the utterance of another (Bloom & Capatides, 1983; Hood & Bloom, 1979).

As just noted with causal utterances, children do not usually add a clause to the clause of another speaker to code any event relations at this point, nor is the second clause usually prompted by an adult question. Thus, the successive clauses are both uttered by the child although an adult comment may intervene.

As with Phase 4, nonverb content categories continue to be coordinated with verb categories. Possession is now coordinated with both action and locative action, while rejection is coordinated with action. Optional goals include the coordination of nonexistence with locative action and the coordination of attribution and recurrence with state. As in Phase 4, the subject of the sentence may be omitted when coordinations are first embedded within the constituent structure. Other changes within verb categories include productivity, but not achievement, in the use of the copula with existence and the inclusion of both the verb and the preposition in locative-action utterances. Questions are now asked about existence using the forms *who* as well as *what* (Bloom et al., 1982), and *to* is now productively used in the infinitival complement structures coding state (Bloom, Tackeff, & Lahey, 1983). Finally, verb inflections are used more frequently and with a greater variety of descriptive-type action verbs as well as with state and locative-action verbs. The regular past inflection *-ed* is now occasionally used with action verbs (e.g., *comb, jump, fix*), but such use is not a goal in this phase. However, in this phase, inflections begin to be used contrastively across a number of verb stems (Bloom, Lifter, & Hafitz, 1980; Feintuck, 1985). See Box 10-2 for examples of verbs that Bloom, Lifter, and Hafitz found inflected at this period.

Changes within the nonverb categories include the emergence of *'s* to mark possession, the syntactic coding of denial with *no* or *not* plus a content word (e.g., noun, verb, adjective), and new relational words for coding some of the nonverb categories. The new relational words code quantity (*some, many, all*), nonexistence (*can't, didn't, not*), rejection (*can't*), and denial (*not*).

Behaviors that became productive earlier are used more frequently; the number of syntactic utterances with three constituents is more frequent; the production of grammatical morphemes in obligatory context increases; children talk more per unit of time; and vocabulary continues to expand.

It is also at this point that pronominal/nominal preferences begin to disappear; pronouns are used by children who have not yet used them, and nouns are used more frequently by children who had preferred pronouns. Thus, the child who has used only person names for agent begins to say the personal pronouns (first *I* and *you*, then *he* and *she*); the child who has used only nouns for spatial locations now uses *there*. In contrast, the child who has depended heavily on such pronominal forms now uses the nominal form (as person, object, or place name), particularly

---

BOX 10-2   Examples of Verbs Used With Various Verb Inflections by Children with MLU <3.0

Inflection

-ing		Irreg./ ed		-s
do	get	do	have	go
make	cry	find	jump	fit
go	look	get	buy	come
eat	put	come	comb	
play	work	say		
write	fix	break		
ride	sit	fall		
hold	take	go		
dance	drive	make		
read	cook	bring		
fly	hide			
blow				

Note: From Bloom, Lifter, and Hafitz, 1980.

when the form is a part of the complement—as the object of an action or a location. (See Bloom, Hood, & Lightbown, 1974).

Examples of new behaviors that become productive within this phase are in Box 10-3. Information on assessment of these behaviors is presented in Chapters 12 and 13.

Goals of Use that Interact with Content/Form: Phases 6, 7, and 8

As children become proficient with more sophisticated forms to code ideas, they also use the code in a wider variety of contexts. Increasing reference is made to the activities of others, and to objects and events that are further removed in time from the context of the utterance. Adaptations to listeners are evidenced by a number of behaviors. By the end of this period children change voice and sentence structure when speaking with younger infants (Shatz & Gelman, 1973). When they perceive that they are misunderstood, they revise their messages by substituting linguistic elements as well as deleting and/or changing the phonetic shape of elements (Gallagher, 1977). Regulatory utterances are more often preceded by attempts to gain attention if the hearer is preoccupied (Ervin-Tripp & Gordon, 1986). Regulatory utterances are more specific; they are more likely to state the agent, action, and goal than only the problem or desired object or action (Ervin-Tripp & Gordon, 1986, citing Newcombe & Zaslow, 1981, and Read & Cherry, 1978). Furthermore, adaptations to the listener are evident in the use of politeness markers (more are used with strangers than with mothers). The markers at this level are primarily the use of *please* and different intonation (Ervin-Tripp & Gordon, 1986).

Some alternative forms (e.g., *here* versus *there*, *this* versus *that*, *a* versus *the*) are used appropriately late in this period, but it is not clear that these are always adaptations to the listener. For example, while the articles *a* and *the* code definite and indefinite reference (Maratsos, 1974), children do not take into account information that is, or is not, shared with the listener until the school years (Warden, 1976). Thus, it seems that the child makes adaptations to different listeners from an early age, but using language to adapt to the listener's *perspective* is a slower process. (See Geller, in press, for a review of perspective-taking skills.) Later in this period some adaptation to listener perspective is evident in the explicitness of information presented depending on whether or not the listeners have shared an experience with the child or whether they can see what the child is talking about (e.g., Maratsos, 1974; Menig-Peterson, 1975). However, it is quite a while before children can be explicit in complex tasks like describing abstract objects to someone on the other side of a screen (Glucksberg, Krauss, & Higgens, 1975).

Ellipsis, or the deletion of redundant items, is one form of text cohesion (Halliday & Hasan, 1975). The deletion of elements in utterances is of course a hallmark of early language development. The deleted information is more likely given or known information, and is thus redundant (Greenfield & Smith, 1976; MacWhinney & Bates, 1978). However, early deletion in child language is not the textual cohesive device talked about by Halliday and Hasan (1975). Textual cohesion is usually formed by anaphoric ellipsis where the referents deleted can be recovered from the prior *linguistic* context. With deletions in early child language, the refer-

---

BOX 10-3   Goals of Content/Form Interactions
Introduced in Phase 5

Content Category	by	Form
To code:		
Existence		Copula, generally in the contracted form; *wh* questions include *who*
Examples:		
(*Kathryn picks up her new book*)		*that's a book*
(*pointing to picture*)		*who that*
Nonexistence		*Not, can't, didn't;* [coordinated with locative action (see Locative Action for examples)]
Examples:		
(*Gia trying to get a toy*)		*I can't reach*
(*Gia looking in the bag*)		*it's not in the bag*
(Recurrence)[a]		Coordinated with state (see State for examples)
Rejection		*Don't;* coordinated with action (see Action for examples)
Denial		Two- and three-word utterances; at first with *no* and later using *not*
Examples:		
(*Peter pointing to barrels*) Barrels		*there's the bolt* / *barrels/ not bolts*
(*mommy to Kathryn*) You're just tired		*I not tired*
(Attribution)[a]		Coordinated with state (see State for examples)
Action		Coordinated with rejection, possession; some multiple-category coordination, usually with intention/volition; verb inflections used with more descriptive verbs.
Examples:		
Action and irregular past (used with descriptive verbs as *find, get, say, break* for completed punctual events and rarely about events in the distant past).		
(*knocking down blocks*)		*I broke a bridge*
(*looking in box of toys and holding up train*)		*I found choo choo train there*

(continued)

BOX 10-3 Phase 5 (*continued*)		
Content Category	**by**	**Form**
(*Eric went to the zoo yesterday; he is telling Lois about it*)		I fed ə ducky
Action and rejection[b]		
(*Lois scatters Gia's blocks*)		don't touch my blocks
(*mommy to Kathryn*) Do you want to go to the bathroom?		no/ I not go in bathroom/ I did tinkle
Action and possession[b]		
(*Kathryn and Lois are reading a book; referring to picture*)		
daddy's hanging up the clothes.		mommy hangs my socks up
Multiple coordinations:		
Action and intention and possession[b]		
(*Gia has washcloth; then pretends to wash hands*)		I going wash my hands
Action and intention and place		
(*Peter has train*)		I wanna write the choo choo train
(*Gia reaching for microphone*)		I want touch here
Possession		Coordinated with action, locative action (see Action and Locative Action for examples); also, *-s* inflection becomes productive but is not always used
Examples:		
(*Kathryn pointing to gifts for daddy*)		that's daddy's birthday
(*Lois picks u one of Gia's blocks; Gia reaching for it*)		that's my's
Locative Action		Verb plus *in*, verb plus *on*[b]; coordinated with nonexistence (rare but productive with some children)[b]; coordinated with possession[b]; plus *-ing*; irregular past
Examples:		
Verb plus preposition[b]		
(*Kathryn putting discs on her lap*)		put this on my lap
(*Patsy is holding Peter's baby sister Jenny; Jenny begins to cry*)		put her down in the cradle
(*Locative action and nonexistence*)[b]		
(*daddy left; mommy stayed*)		not going away
(*Eric tries to sit on high stack of blocks*)		and ə no sit down

(continued)

BOX 10-3   Phase 5 (*continued*)

Content Category	by	Form
Locative action and possession[b] (*Peter trying to put Patsy's barette in his* *hair*)		*put in my hair my* *barette/ I put on ə* *Patsy barette*
(*Lois takes her sweater off*)		*you putting your sweater on*
Mover–locative action and - ing (*Eric opening door*)		*I going*
(*Gia going to door*) *I'll see ya later/ where're* *you going?*		*I going out to playground.*
Locative action and irregular past		
(*knocking tower over*)		*it fell down*
(*mother had just left*)		*mommy went bye bye*
Temporal		Verb inflections now used with more descriptive verbs (see Action, Locative Action, and State for examples) and occur in about 30– 50% of obligatory contexts.
State		Coordinated with attribution and recurrence; *to* more likely to appear with infinitival complements; new verbs used to code volition/ intention (e.g., *like* and *have*).
Volition/Intention with *to*		
(*getting up and starting for next room*)		*I have to get your hat*
(*opening box*)		*I want to look*
(*getting ball*)		*hafta play ball*
(*listening to noise*) (State and recurrence)		*want to see that noise*
(*Lois and Kathryn are pretending to have* *lunch*)		*I want some more egg*
(*Peter had eaten some pretzels; running* *back to kitchen*)		*I want some more pretzels,* *mommy*
(State and attribution) (*Gia gets her new sand pail and shovel;* *showing it to Lois*)		*I got new pail*
(*Kathryn holding red disc*)		*Kathryn want red one*

(*continued*)

BOX 10-3 Phase 5 (*continued*)

Content Category	by	Form
Locative State		No new behaviors
Additive[c]		Successive utterances with and without the form *and* to join clauses or phrases

Examples:
Without *and*
(Kathryn pretending to have stove— utterances said as she acts) — *that be the stove/ want cook it/ I dump out this way/ stir it*

Phrases joined with *and*
(Peter telling Lois about trip) — *going to see Nanna and Bill and Jack*

Clauses with *and*
(Gia looking at a book) — *look/ there's a bear having a birthday party and there's a buzz*

(Eric taking girl out) — *and the little girl goes out the bathtub*

(putting girl in dining room) — *and eats*

Content Category	by	Form
Quantity		*Some, many, all*

Examples:
(Eric pointing to pieces of clay) — *look/ see/ see clay/ two clay/ many clay/ 1-2-3-4/ 2-3-3-3/ look*

(Kathryn pretending to drink) — *I have some orange juice*

(Kathryn looking at picture of moths) — *all these in there*

Content Category	by	Form
Notice		No new behaviors; same as Phase 4
Causal[c]		Successive utterances with an implicit causal relationship between them; they may occasionally be conjoined with *and*

Examples:
(Peter gets ink on this hands) — *dirty hands/ hafta wash əm*

(Eric's train is stopped by a pile of blocks) — *choo choo train can't go anyplace/ fix dat*

(Gia trying to unbutton pocket of doll's dress; there is a handkerchief inside the pocket) — *I want ə handkerchief/ unbutton it*

Content Category	by	Form
Dative[c]		Three- and four-word utterances; prepositions are usually missing

(continued)

BOX 10-3 Phase 5 (*continued*)		
Content Category	**by**	**Form**
Examples:		
(*Lois arrives at front door; Eric runs to open it*)		open door Mrs. Bloom
(*Lois pretends to eat*)		you get some Kathryn
Specification[c]		This and that used contrastively to specify which object; commonly used with state
Examples:		
(*Gia pointing to her brush on shelf*)		I want that brush
(*Eric standing in front of chest under which discs had rolled*)		I need that blue

[a] When a content category is in parentheses, it indicates that goal is optional in this phase.
[b] May result in omission of the subject.
[c] New category.

ents can usually be found in the nonlinguistic context (exophoric ellipsis) or are understood because of shared experiences with the hearer. With the exception of yes/no responses, deletions are rarely related to prior messages. Anaphoric ellipsis, or deletion based on redundancy with a prior utterance, begins to appear at this point in development (see L. Bernstein, 1981; Bloom et al., 1982; Bloom, Miller, & Hood, 1975).

Children's utterances are now more frequently related to prior utterances of their own as well as to those of another. They begin to juxtapose clauses as well as string series of utterances together which are semantically related and which are more than self-repetitions or self-expansions.

In addition, a marked increase is found in the number of utterances that do not follow those of another (sometimes referred to as *nonadjacent* or *spontaneous*), so that now these nonadjacent utterances are more frequent than utterances that are adjacent to those of another (Bloom et al., 1976). The adjacent utterances that do occur are now primarily contingent on both the linguistic form and the semantic content of the prior utterance, and few are contingent based only on imitation (which has declined markedly in those children who did imitate). Linguistic contingency in this period continues to involve adding information with more frequent addition of clauses (rather than just words and phrases) to the prior utterance. In addition, recoding of the prior utterance includes dietic shifts for objects (*this* and *that*) and place (*here* and *there*) as well as the earlier recoding of agents (*you* and *I*) and pronominal recoding of nominal objects (Bloom et al., 1976). While contingent utterances remain more frequent following a prior question than a nonquestion, there is a marked increase in the proportion of contingent utterances following nonquestions.

For the first time, questions (other than those for confirmation) asked by children are now occasionally contingent on the prior utterance of another. This late emergence of contingent questions suggests that asking contingent questions is more difficult than asking noncontingent questions or making contingent statements (Bloom et al., 1976). Questions are asked more frequently and with a greater variety of content/form interactions (e.g., new forms are added, such as *why*, *when*, and *how*, to code different meanings). Furthermore, they increase in complexity (e.g., they include verbs other than the copula and pro-verbs) (Bloom et al., 1982).

In general, the proportion of utterances that serve social (or interpersonal) functions (e.g., regulatory) increases; however, it seems that at least some new content/form interactions first appear in less social utterances (i.e., utterances that do not require a response by another). For example, while most causal utterances are produced for interpersonal, or social, functions (e.g., as a part of a conversational exchange or a negotiation), causal conjunctions appear to emerge in comments about ongoing or intended activity (Bloom & Capatides, 1983). This suggests that some new content/form interactions might first be facilitated in contexts where need for social interactions is relatively low. Further research is needed to support this hypothesis.

The goals of use, then, that interact with content/form in these phases relate to function and nonlinguistic and linguistic contexts:

GOALS
Related to function

1. To further increase the number of utterances that serve social (or interpersonal) functions.
2. To obtain information about a prior utterance of another.
3. To inform.

GOALS
Related to nonlinguistic context

4. To increase the number of utterances that refer to nonpresent objects and events.
5. To use deictic forms according to context (e.g., *here/there*, *this/that*, *a/the*, *I/you*).
6. To adapt to different listeners
   a. To use politeness markers (intonation and *please*) with strangers.
   b. To gain the attention of a preoccupied hearer prior to regulatory tterances.
   c. To begin to take into account knowledge of another by giving more explicit information when necessary in simple contexts.
   d. To repair, upon request, with substitutions as well as deletions and phonetic changes.

GOALS
Related to linguistic context

7. To increase the number of nonadjacent utterances.
8. To reduce the number of utterances that are exact (or reduced) repetitions of the prior utterance.

9. To respond to the utterances of others with contingent utterances that add to and recode information from the prior utterance of another using clauses as well as lexical items and phrases. Such utterances may also repeat a part of the prior utterance (i.e., repeat/recode/add).
10. To increase the number of utterances that the child produces which are semantically related to the utterance just produced by the child.
11. To reduce redundancy based on prior messages—that is, to begin the anaphoric use of ellipsis late within the period.
12. To increase the number of questions that are contingent on prior utterances.

Goals of Content/Form Interaction: Phases 6, 7, and 8

Phase 6: Coding Event Relations—Emerging Use of Conjunctions

The production of successive clauses that just emerged in Phase 5 develops more fully in this phase. Additive relations (described in Phase 5) are more likely to be connected with a conjunction (generally *and*). As in Phase 5, many of these utterances include the same verb in both clauses (e.g., pointing to two different chairs, "you sit here and I sit here"); the conjoining of different verb relations most often co-occurs with actions chained to the utterances (e.g., putting a book on the shelf, "I gonna put it here," and then picking up another book, "and read this"). However, coding of sequential temporal relations, where at least one of the events is not chained to the utterance (e.g., as putting a book on a shelf and before picking out another book, "I gonna put it here and read another one"), emerges in this phase either by successive utterances without a conjunction or by conjoining with the conjunction *and* (Bloom, Lahey, Hood, Lifter, & Fiess, 1980).

In addition, the use of conjunctions *and*, *so*, and *because* now emerges with utterances that refer to objective causal relations (i.e., relations that are perceptible in the world, such as getting wet when you step in a puddle). Subjective causal relations (i.e., relations that are personally determined, such as loneliness when no one is around, or relations that are determined by society, such as stopping when lights are red) are still more likely to be successive utterances without a conjunction (Bloom & Capatides, 1983, in press a). At this phase, causal relations are least frequently coded and are the last to emerge with a connective. Connectives used in this period are most frequently *and*, although *because* or *so* may be productive for some children. However, the proportion of utterances coded with conjunctions is very low (under 10%) (Bloom, Lahey, Hood, Lifter & Fiess, 1980; Paul, 1981). In addition to the inclusion of connectives in some utterances, the number of successive utterances without connectives also increases.

New grammatical morphemes become productive—*the* to code specific or definite referents under the category of specification and *to* to code dative. Attribution is coordinated within locative-action utterances. Listed as optional goals (because of their variable use among children) are recurrence coordinated with locative action, and possession coordinated with utterances coding internal state (e.g., "I want my car," which is different from the coding of possessive state, such as "The car is mine"). Examples are presented in Box 10-4.

BOX 10-4 Goals of Content/Form Interactions Introduced in Phase 6

Content Category	by	Form
To code:		
Existence		No new behaviors (same as Phase 5)
Nonexistence		No new behaviors (same as Phase 5)
(Recurrence)[a]		Coordinated with locative action (see Locative Action for examples)
Rejection		No new behaviors (same as Phase 5)
Denial		No new behaviors (same as Phase 5)
Attribution[b]		Coordinated with locative action (see Locative Action for examples)
(Possession)		Coordinated with state— infrequently used (see State for examples)
Action		No new behaviors (same as Phase 5)
Locative Action		Coordinated with attribution[b]; coordinated with recurrence[b]; (both are rarely used)

Examples:
Locative action and attribution[b]
(*Gia sliding wheels down a slide*)   *here goes a green wheel/ there goes a green wheel*

(*Eric looking for something to put in a dump car*)
What are you looking for?   *I put a little thing in it*
(Locative action and recurrence)[b]
(*Eric putting lambs on the train*)   *I get more lamb in the train*

| **Temporal** | | Sequential relations between events with or without *and; now.* |

Examples:
With *now*
(*Kathryn can't tie the shoe; gives it to Lois*)   *now/ your turn*

(*Lois starts*)   *now my turn*
Sequential relations with *and*
(*what are you gonna do?*)   *let's go get a cup for them ok/*

ok
(*K leaving room*)   *and they gonna have some cereal*

(*continued*)

Content Category	by	Form
BOX 10-4 Phase 6 (*continued*)		
(*talking about a visit*)		*Jocelyn's going home and take her sweater off*
Causal		Use of *and, so,* or *because* in about 30% of causal utterances. Connectives are most often used in utterances that are comments and code causal relations that are objective—that is, perceptible or given in the physical world (versus personal or cultural judgments)
Objective causal relations with connectives		
Examples:		
(*Gia talking to Lois*)		*I gonna step in puddle with sandals on and get it all wet*
(*tiny barrel is inside other barrel*)		*You can't see it cause it's way inside*
Locative State		No new behaviors (same as Phase 4)
(State)		Coordinated with possession; rarely used
Examples:		
(*mother asks Eric if he wants supper*)		*yeh*
(*to Lois he says*)		*you come back/ you come next year/ I want my supper*
(*mother returning from store; Gia expected her to buy furniture*)		*I wan · I wan my table and chair*
(*Kathryn speaking of her mother*)		*she has a Band-Aid on her toe*
Quantity		No new behaviors (same as Phase 5)
Notice		No new behaviors (same as Phase 4)
Dative	*To, for*	
Examples:		
(*Gia gets stool for Lois*)		*this is a stool for you*
(*Eric takes form board in case from toy bag; handing it to Lois*)		*will you open these for me*
Specification		*The* used to indicate specificity
Example:		
(*Kathryn picking up crayon box*)		*let's put these in the box*

[a] When a content category is in parentheses, it indicates the goal is optional in this phase.
[b] May result in omission of the subject.

Phase 7: Coding Event Relations with Coordination, Complementation, and Modal Verbs

In this phase we find an increase in the number of utterances coding event relations, in the types of meaning relations coded between clauses, and in the forms used to code the meaning relations.

One new form that is used, sentential complements, is best illustrated with the developmental change that occurs within the category of state from Phase 3. State verbs such as *want* were used in Phase 3 to code wish for an object (e.g., "I want cookie"). In Phase 4 the first inclusion of two verbs within one utterance emerged in state (volition/intention) with verbs such as *want* and *go* as matrix verbs and the coding of action or locative-action relations in the complement (e.g., "I want eat cookie"); in Phase 5 a greater variety of verbs coding volition/intention was evident, and the word *to* was included in the infinitive (e.g., "I like to eat cookie"). However, in Phases 4 and 5 the subject of the second verb was always coreferential with (i.e., the same as) the subject of the state verb (e.g., in the above example, *I* is the subject of both *like* and *eat*). These complements were referred to as infinitival complements. In Phase 7, the complements of these state verbs of volition/intention include subjects that are not coreferential (i.e., not the same) as the state verb in the first clause (e.g., "I want mommy eat cookie"). Thus, these complements include a subject noun phrase as well as a verb phrase and are referred to as *sentential complements.*° The developmental sequence in the use of complement constructions is, therefore, infinitival complements with coreferential subjects before sentential complements with noncoreferential subjects (Bloom, Tackeff, & Lahey, 1983; Paul, 1981; Tyack & Gottsleben, 1986).

In the case of state, the first use of each type of construction occurs minus the connective *to;* the inclusion of *to* follows in the next phase (Bloom et al., 1983). In Phase 7, when sentential complements first emerge to code volition/intention, the connective *to* is again often omitted in the sentential complements although it continues to be used when volition/intention is coded with infinitival complements.

Sentential complements are also used for the coding of a number of other interclausal meaning relations in Phase 7—notice, epistemic, and specification. Notice referring to the perception of objects was coded in Phase 4 with two or three constituents. If the complement was included, it was a noun phrase (e.g., "watch me"). Now, in Phase 7, notice of events and states is coded with sentential complements where the complement includes a verb phrase (e.g., "watch me jump"). In the sentential complement construction the complement of the notice verb contains a verb relation with a noncoreferential subject (i.e., a subject that is different from the subject of the notice verb). While verbs in the complement vary (e.g., children code notice of different static states as well as of different dynamic events), the notice verbs used in this type of structure are limited. They generally occur without a connective form until Phase 8 (e.g., "look I do" where *what* is omitted). Examples of verbs that take complements and are used in this period of development (as reported by Bloom, 1981; Bloom, Rispoli, Gartner, & Hafitz,

---

° Verb phrases may also substitute for the subject of a sentence (e.g., "running to school is fun"), but such constructions are rarely found in the speech of young children.

> **BOX 10-5   Complement-taking Verbs Used by Children in Phases 7 and/or 8**
>
> | Notice | Epistemic | State Volition/Intention | Specification | Causal |
> |--------|-----------|--------------------------|---------------|--------|
> | | | (Used most frequently) | | |
> | see | think | want | to be | let |
> | look | know | go | | make |
> | | | (Used less frequently) | | |
> | watch | | like | | |
> | show | | have | | |
> | | | got | | |
> | | | try | | |
> | | | (Used least frequently) | | |
> | | forget | need | | help |
> | | wonder | | | get |
> | | remember | | | |
> | | bet | | | |
> | | mean | | | |
> | | afraid | | | |
> | | decide | | | |
>
> The verbs in the second clause (the complement) include many of the verb categories (e.g., existence, action, locative action, state).
> *Note:* From Bloom, 1981; Bloom, Lahey, Hood, Lifter, and Fiess, 1980; Bloom, Rispoli, Gartner, and Hafitz, 1987; Hafitz, Gartner, and Bloom, 1980; Limber, 1973.

1987; Limber, 1973) are listed in Box 10-5. These verbs are listed according to the meaning relation of the first verb (i.e., the complement-taking verbs like *look*).

The function of utterances that use notice verbs of *see* and *look* is not always (as one might suppose) to attract the attention of another person. In an analysis of interactions when these verbs were used by the children, Bloom and her colleagues found that the verb *see* was most often used with shared adult attention to the topic, while *look* (as well as *know*, to be discussed under the category of epistemic) was more often used in contexts where the child was directing the adult's attention to a new topic. *Look* tended to be used in utterances that initiated a conversational exchange rather than in utterances that responded to those of another. Such contexts provide hypotheses for facilitating the early use of these content/form interactions.

A new content category that becomes productive in this phase, epistemic, also involves coding event relations. The first verb in *epistemic* utterances codes a mental state of affairs about the event or state described in the complement. Some children have coded epistemic earlier with three constituents and the verb *know*. However, these earlier codings are often stereotypic (e.g., "I don't know," "I know it"), and if a complement is included, it is a noun phrase and not another verb relation. As with notice, only a small set of epistemic verbs is consistently used to code this category (see Box 10-5). When the verb *know* is used, it generally occurs with the connective form *what* or *where* (i.e., "know what" or "know where"). In contrast, the epistemic verb *think* rarely occurs with any connective even through Phase 8. While, as mentioned above, *know* is often used to direct an adult's attention to a new topic, *think* is not used in this way. In the analyses by Bloom, Rispoli, Gartner, and Hafitz (1987) the verb *think* was used most frequently when adult and child were focused on the same topic and when it followed the utterance of an adult that also included the verb *think*. Thus, it appears that discourse support facilitated the production of *think*, but was not necessary for *know* or for the notice verbs. These findings provide hypotheses for the contexts of facilitation as well as expectations for the contexts of production.

Finally, specification now includes specification of events as well as objects and persons. In the interclausal meaning relation of *specification*, the second clause describes an object or person mentioned in the first clause, with the most common description being that of function, place, or activity. In this phase, the first clause often simply identifies the object or person, while the second describes its function or activity (e.g., "it's a chair and you sit on it"). The specification of events or states can be coded with a number of syntactic structures. Sentential complements as well as coordinate structures are found. When specification is coded with sentential complements, the first verb is usually the copula (present or deleted) preceded by a demonstrative pronoun and followed by the connective *what* or *where* (e.g., "that's where it belongs"). In coordinate structures, the first clause is often an identity statement (e.g., "that's a top and it spins").

The variability found in the number of children who code specification of states or events causes this to be an optional goal. (The information presented above on sentential complements has been taken from Bloom et al., 1987; and Hafitz, Gartner, & Bloom, 1980. Further information on the development of forms of complex sentences can be found in other references in this section and in sections on Phases 5 and 6 as well as Bowerman, 1979; E. Clark, 1973; Flores d'Arcais, 1978; and Lust & Mervis, 1980).

In this phase, causal relationships are now more commonly coded by *because* or *so* for both subjective causal connections (e.g., those connections made on the basis of personal or sociocultural belief) as well as the objective connections that began to be coded with conjunctions in the prior phase (Bloom & Capatides, 1983, 1987). Conjunctions are appropriately used, with *because* coding effect-cause order and *so* coding cause-effect order. Errors are rare; if found, they are usually patterned (e.g., *because* used for *therefore*) (Hood & Bloom, 1979). Sequential temporal relations are often coded with *then* or *and then*. Simultaneous relations (where the two events overlap in time, as "when he sleeps he snores," rather than occurring in succession) are now coded. If a conjunction is used, it is usually *when* (Bloom, Lahey, Hood, Lifter, & Fiess, 1980).

Another new interclausal relation, adversative, is expressed with conjoined clauses with the connective forms of *and* or *but*. In utterances coding *adversative*, the relation between two events and/or states is one of contrast, where most often one clause opposes or negates the other or where one clause qualifies or limits the other. Some children juxtapose clauses that have an adversative relation between them in earlier phases, but it is about this phase that most children are productively coding the relation with a connective form. Both adversative and causal are categories that are occasionally used wit dependent cohesion—that is, they are the two content categories where the child's utterance is, at times, connected to that of another person rather than to a prior self-utterance (as are most of these interclausal relations). This tie to another's utterance (referred to as *dependent cohesion*) is minimal at first, but increases with development (Bloom, Lahey, Hood, Lifter, & Fiess, 1980).

Questions are now asked about action—the agent of an action, the objects of an action, or the action itself. These questions may be in the form of *how* or *what*. *How* questions include both descriptive verbs and pro-verbs, while *what* questions include primarily pro-verbs (including *do, go, happen*) and the copula (Bloom, Merkin, & Wooten, 1982).

In addition to the use of sentential complements to code relations between events, children code other attitudes, or moods, about events besides volition/intention. The mood of possibility or certainty (and, for some children, permission) is coded with the modal verb *can*. This has been considered as a type of internal state and has been placed under the category of state. [Prior to this the negative form *can't* has been used to code the nonexistence (and probably the impossibility) of expected actions.] See Box 10-6 for examples of new behaviors in Phase 7.

Phase 8: Coding Event Relations with Relative Clauses and Increased Use of Complement Connectives

In Phase 8 children are producing more complex sentences, and these sentences increasingly include more than two verb relations (e.g., Bloom, Lahey, Hood, Lifter, & Fiess, 1980; Paul, 1981). While the children are producing many complex sentences, these sentences still make up a small proportion of their total utterances. In the data of Bloom, Lahey, Hood, Lifter, and Fiess (1980), less than 15% of the children's utterances included connectives in this phase of development (with highest MLU = <4.5). Two cross-sectional studies since that time have found similar results. The proportion of utterances that were categorized as complex sentences in these studies did not exceed 20% of all utterances until MLU reached 5.0, and then the maximum reported was <30% (Paul, 1981; Tyack & Gottsleben, 1986). These data suggest that complex sentences should not be expected frequently at this time in development. Such infrequent use of complex sentences makes assessment, reassessment, and intervention difficult because any one type of content/form interaction may occur very infrequently. Throughout this period, state remains among the more frequently coded event relations. A shift occurs in the frequency of coding additive and causal relations. While additive is coded proportionally more often than causal in Phases 5 and 6, by Phase 8 causal is proportionally greater than additive (Bloom, Lahey, Hood, Lifter, & Fiess, 1980). Of course, all relations are coded more frequently in absolute numbers as the child produces more utterances per hour than in earlier phases. A number of new interactions mark this phase; connective forms are more likely to be used with complement constructions; a new content category, communication, emerges; some children produce relative clauses for specification; some children

BOX 10-6   Goals of Content/Form Interactions Introduced in Phase 7

Content Category	by	Form
		No new behaviors in any categories except:
To code: (**Action**)[a]		*Wh* questions used infrequently and not by all children to question agent, or object of an action, or the action itself
Examples:		
(*Peter takes broken airplane from toy bag and brings it to Patsy*)		*who broke it*
(*Peter rolls discs down slide*)		*now what should we do with əm*
(*Lois puts train together; Gia watching*)		*what you doing*
(*Kathryn and Lois looking at picture of boy feeding elephant peanuts*)		*what's the boy feeding*
Temporal		*Then* and *and then* used to code sequential relations; *when* used to code simultaneous relations
Examples: Simultaneous		
(*Gia showing Lois her bedroom*)		*that's a __/ and this is my bed/ even--- pajamas/ I can only have the nightie when I go to sleep*
Sequential		
Examples:		
(*Lois and Eric pretending it's lunchtime for the children*)		*let the mommy into the frigerator and get some pineapple yogurt and then she come out*
Causal		*Because* and *so* used more frequently with objective relations and also now with subjective relations
Subjective relations (*Lois and Patsy are ready to leave*)		*I wanna come with you/ cause I got shoes on and I'm ready to go*

(continued)

BOX 10-6 Phase 7 (continued)		
Content Category	**by**	**Form**
(*Lois follows Kathryn into bathroom*)		*you stay away cause I hafta go in there*
Objective relations (*Gia at her bookcase*)		*let's all take all the books out so we can read them*
(*Kathryn giving bendable girl to Lois*)		*you bend her over okay/ so I can put her on this rocking chair so she can rock*
Epistemic[b]		Complement constructions with *know what, know where,* and *think*
Examples:		
(*Putting sugar in her mother's coffee*)		*I think I put some lot of sugar in here*
(*Gia selecting crayon*)		*I think draw pink first*
(*Kathryn offering Lois a ride*) *you think you can pull me?* *you do?*		*you can go on this train* *yes* *I think I can pull---/ it's broke*
(*Peter getting another crayon out*)		*look at this one*
What color is that?		*I don't know what color*
State		Use of sentential complements with verb *want* and without the connective *to; can* is used to code possibility
Examples: Volition/Intention (*Rejecting Lois's offer*)		*I want mommy get it*
(*trying to stand doll*)		*want the man stand up*
Possibility (*Kathryn dragging bag*) *I'll come help you*		*I can do it*
Notice-Perception[b]		Complement constructions with matrix verbs *see* and *look,* usually without connective forms.
Examples: (*leaving the room*)		*I gon see there's more tape*
(*holding up a toy just taken from a box*)		*look I found*
(Specification)[a]		Demonstrative pronoun plus optional *is* followed by a complement with connective *what* or *where;* conjoined clauses with *and*
		(*continued*)

BOX 10-6 Phase 7 (*continued*)		
Content Category	**by**	**Form**
Examples:		
(*pointing to a picture*)		looks like a fishing thing and you fish with it
(*showing Lois a box on the counter*)		and that's where the cake goes
(*pointing to her blouse*)		this what I got in New York
Adversative[b]		
Example:		
(*Eric looking at a book*)		the butterflies saw the bumble bees here · but they ə not coming out.

[a] When a content category is in parentheses, it indicates the goal is optional in this phase.
[b] New category.

use the auxiliary *will*; verb inflections are more commonly produced; *why* questions are frequent; and children begin to conjoin sequences of sentences.

The increased use of connective forms in complement constructions appears to be related to particular matrix verbs. It is not that children learn a connective and apply it to all complement-taking verbs. For example, *see* is used primarily with *what* and *if* and rarely with *how* or *where* at this point in development, while *know* might be used with *where* and not with *if* (Bloom et al., 1987). Thus, it should not be expected that a connective form will necessarily transfer to all complement-taking verbs because it has been learned with one. It may well be that the complement-taking verbs are each independently learned with particular connective forms.

In this phase connectives are more likely to be used with notice (e.g., "look what," "see if," "see what") than in the prior phase. Two new verbs may appear to code notice; these verbs, *show* and *watch*, often occur at first without a connective. The variation among children in the use of these particular verbs makes their inclusion as goals optional. (As noted earlier, hypotheses about goals relative to notice complements come from the data in Bloom et al., 1987; and Hafitz et al., 1980.)

In state, the connective *to* becomes productive in sentential complements as well as in infinitival complements (Bloom, Tackeff, & Lahey, 1983). Infinitival complements are also used to code categories other than volition/intention (e.g., epistemic, "I forgot to get the machine"). Within state, the mood of obligation is coded with the modal verb *should* as well as *have to*.

One new event relation, communication, emerges for some children and is usually coded with *tell* or *say* (and occasionally *mean*). (Such talk about talking can be seen as evidence of early metalinguistic skills.) This category is an optional goal in Phase 8 since not all children code the category at this point in development.

Another optional goal involves a new structure for coding specification. Some children code specification with right-branching relative clauses. The relative clause usually describes function, place, or activity of the object noun phrase that is identified in the first clause (e.g., "it's the train that goes in the roundhouse"). The connective *that* or *who* may be used (Bloom, Lahey, Hood, Lifter, & Fiess, 1980).

Optional goals are also found in the coding of temporal relations. While *when* has been produced as a conjunction since Phase 7, it is still rarely used as a question form. For some children the question *when* becomes productive at about this level of development, but even for these children it occurs rarely at this time (Bloom et al., 1982). It is included in the plan as an optional goal for Phase 8.

Another optional goal is the auxiliary *will*, which becomes productive for some children in Phase 8. According to research by Gee and Savasir (1985), the early production of *will* not only coded future time, but was often a social commitment to carry out the activity described; in contrast, *gonna* carried no such commitment. *Will* was more likely to occur in social exchanges than *gonna*.

Phase 8 is also marked by further productions of verb inflections; aspectual distinctions are less apparent since a wide variety of verbs is now inflected with each. By this period, the regular past tense inflection *-ed* is productive for many children (Bloom, Lifter, & Hafitz, 1980), and the auxiliary is productive in both past (e.g., *was*) and present (e.g., *is*) form. However, neither auxiliary nor *-ed* has reached levels of achievement—that is, neither is used in 80 to 90% of obligatory contexts. In fact, for many children, none of the verb inflections has reached this level of achievement. In the Bloom, Lifter, and Hafitz (1980) data, verb inflections of *-ing, -s,* and irregular past were produced in about 40% of the obligatory contexts; in other studies, achievement was reached on a few of the inflections by this level (see, for example, Brown, 1973; J. de Villiers & de Villiers, 1973). It appears that considerable variability exists in rate of achievement for verb inflections. Given this variability, goals for the language-impaired child should probably not be set for achievement (80 to 90% use in obligatory contexts) until after Phase 8; goals should, however, continue to be set for increased production of these inflections.

A new behavior that becomes productive in Phase 8 and appears quite frequently is the question form *why* to ask about causal relations (Hood & Bloom, 1979). *Why* is more often contingent on a prior statement than other question forms, and often these contingent questions use the same descriptive verb as the prior adult utterance (Bloom et al., 1982).

In addition to the above behaviors, we find scattered constructions that are not productive within particular children's language samples or with particular content categories, but that are found in large samples of data. For example, the complementizer *-ing* appears in some sentences during this phase (e.g., "mommy's busy eating her grapes"; "are you having trouble getting all done"; "this one's tired of lying down"). These should probably not be goals at Phase 8, but could be considered when Phase 8 behaviors are productive.

Finally, we see children talking about relations among a number of events. For

BOX 10-7 Examples of Sequences of Utterances Produced by Kathryn in One of the Last Samples Used to Derive Phase 8 Goals.

Telling a Story with a Picture Book

once upon a time there was a little elephant/ and he lives in a zoo—mouse/ and once upon a time there was a little baby one holding on to the mommy's tail/ and then he came another zoo feed the birds/ again once upon a time there was another elephant/ and there was a rhinoceros/ a once upon a time/ there was/ what's those three/ what's those eating/

. . .

what's this an another rhinoceros/

   adult: yes/ what is he doing?

he's smelling some flowers/ no/ he's smelling a red flower/ he's smelling lots a flowers/ but here's a big tiger/ and dere's/ here's mommy/ doing—/ she's taking a bath/

(closes book)   *dat's all/ bye bye elephant.*

(The above story was interspersed with the adult periodically repeating part of the child's utterances.)

Describing a Past Event

You have a good time this morning?

                           yes

what'd you do?

                           I paint

yes

                           and I plays/ London Bridge fall down/ and I play the box/

you played what?

                           in a box in a box

the box in the box?

                           no no the Jack and---

oh Jack in the box

                           and we played/ we played ball/ --- and we had a good time

you had a good time

Chained to Actions (Setting Up a Pretend Party)

.

.

                           here's your plate/ here's the plate

(bringing plate to Lois)

                           here plate

(going back to table, picking up plate)

                           havta get another plate/ this plate

(bringing it to Lois)

                                    (continued)

BOX 10-7 Phase 8 (*continued*)		
Content Category	**by**	**Form**
		here's another plate
(*going back to table*)		here's spoon and here's a cup
(*bringing them to Lois, putting on floor*)		
		now dat's/ dat's right down there
hm?		
(*picks up plate*)		
		there/ and that's where the cake goes
ok		
(*taking knives & forks off table*)		
		I'll bring this and this/ I got some somethin
(*going around side of closet*)		
		I have to go around here
(*bringing things to Lois*)		
		take these out of my hand
etc.		

quite awhile, this is simply a set of successive sentences with no hierarchical structure (although local cohesive ties may appear through reiterations of particular lexical items or use of the conjunction *and* or *and then*). Frequently these sentences are chained to actions or occur in the context of book reading where the child pretends to tell the story. Others may be elicited by questions from an adult. Some examples are illustrated in Box 10-7.

Developmentally, causal and temporal relations become more frequent in such sequences of sentences, and the events are less likely to be chained with the utterances. This development is discussed further in the next chapter under the development of narratives. The development of longer cohesive and coherent units of texts, such as narratives, is considered a goal for Post Phase 8. Examples of the behaviors that are to be goals of intervention in Phase 8 are presented in Box 10-8.

Summary

This chapter is concerned with the goals of later language learning—with elaborating the behaviors outlined in Chapter 8 as the goals of content, form, and use in Phases 4 to 8. Goals of use that interact with content and form include an increasing number of utterances that (1) are produced without the perceptual support of nonlinguistic context or the child's own activities; (2) are nonadjacent (i.e., do not follow the utterance of another); (3) use alternative forms that require adaptation to the listener; and (4) are used to obtain information.

There is concurrent growth in the number of content categories that are coded with linguistic form. In Phase 4, 14 content categories account for most of the

---

BOX 10-8   Goals of Content/Form Interactions
Introduced in Phase 8

Content Category	by	Form
		No changes in any categories except:

To code:

Notice — Complement constructions

Examples:

(*Kathryn jumping on a board*)	*watch what I'm doing*
(*Kathryn running*)	*see how fast I can run*

Temporal — Third person -*s*; regular past -*ed* applied to more different verbs; auxiliary *to be*; (*when* used as question late in phase by some)

Examples:

Third person -*s*

(*Kathryn trying to put girl doll on chair*)	*you try to put that girl on here because she keeps falling off/ okay*
(*Lois to Gia*) What does mommy do when Daddy goes to work?	*she sweeps*

Regular past

(*Lois picking up Kathryn's blocks*)	*well I dumped all these blocks out and made a big big mess*
(*Eric looking at a book*) This animal you can't see/ why?	*because is all covered up*
Why?	*because the zookeeper closed it*

Auxiliary *to be* and -*ing*

(*Eric looking at a book*)	*and the bunny rabbits are sleeping and everybody's sleeping*
(*Kathryn looking at a book*) What are the others doing?	*oh, they're eating/ and this little girl is having milk/*
How about that dog?	*he isn't having any food*
(*Kathryn scratched her head*) What is the trouble?	*I was scratching my head*

(Auxiliary *will*)

(*playing with dolls in tub*)	*maybe the mommy will go/ maybe the mommy will wash the boy and the girl*
	(*continued*)

BOX 10-8	Phase 8 (*continued*)	
Content Category	**by**	**Form**
(See also next example under *Wh* Question)		
Wh question (*to Lois*)		when will you go home
Causal		*Wh* questions
Examples:		
(*Kathryn pointing to Lois's shoes*)		why'd you bring these shoes
To cover my feet		Why
Cause they were cold		Why
Cause it's cold outside		
(*Patsy playing with Peter moves microphone*)		why are you putting it right there
Notice-Perception		Complement constructions with matrix verbs *watch* and *show,* often without a connective; *see* and *look* are more likely to have connectives such as *what* or *if*
Examples:		
(*Gia showing Lois some clothes*)		look what my mommy got me
(*Lois playing with Kathryn's toy*)		now let me try to see if I could hit
(Optional verbs) (*trying to do a somersault*)		would you help me show you how to do a somersault
(*directing Lois to the kitchen*)		you go in there and watch me eat Lois
(Specification)		Occasional use of relative clause, sometimes with *that*
Examples:		
(*Kathryn talking about a scoop*)		it's just a thing that I hold
(*Gia using toy telephone*) Mom: Who'd you call?		the man who fixes the door
(*playing with toy beds*)		just like that little bed/ this is the big one that goes over here
		(*continued*)

	BOX 10-8 Phase 8 (*continued*)	
Content Category	**by**	**Form**
State		A variety of modal verbs used for obligatory mood and occasionally permission; sentential complements used with connective *to*
Examples: Sentential complements with *to* (*eating lunch, turns to Lois*)		*want something to eat*
(*requesting that Lois leave her doll when she goes home*)		*I want this doll to stay here/ I want · I want Lois' doll to stay/ I want this doll to stay there/ I want · I want Lois' doll to stay*
Obligatory mood (*Kathryn taking a hot dish from oven, then putting it down*)		*I better get a pot holder because I might burn my hands*
(*Eric wants dolls to sit in chair*)		*they should sit down in a chair*
(*Kathryn and Lois having a tea party*)		*well I hafta get that knife so I can cut the cake*
(Communication)[a]		Complement constructions using verbs such as *say*, *tell*, and *ask*
(*Gia to her mother*)		*and I wan · l · l · l asked you to buy more cereal*
(*telling Lois*)		*Mommy said I can have it*

[a] When a content category is in parentheses, it is optional at this phase.

content expressed by forms, while in Phase 8, at least 21 categories are needed to describe what children talk about.

Finally, there are changes in the forms used to code other content categories. Phases 4, 5, and 6 include the embedding of two content categories within one utterance—such as the embedding of attribution within utterances coding action relations. Phase 5 marks the appearance of many juxtaposed successive sentences that, while meaningfully related to each other, are not usually connected syntactically. In Phase 6 some of these successive sentences are connected with *and* to form complex sentences; and in the last two phases there is further use of syntactic connectives to form other complex sentences, with more specification of the semantic relationships between the clauses. There is continued development of grammatical morphemes in Phase 8.

Certainly there are other developments that occur during this period—developments that have not yet been described in a manner that is useful for a C/F/U Goal Plan for Language Learning, but that could be incorporated in such a plan as additional information becomes available.

Suggested Readings

Bloom, L., Lahey, M., Hood, L., Lifter, K., & Fiess, K. (1980). Complex sentences: Acquisition of syntactic connectives and the semantic relations they encode. *Journal of Child Language, 7*, 235–261.

Bloom, L., Lifter, K., & Hafitz, J. (1980). Semantics of verbs and the development of verb inflection in child language. *Language, 56*, 386–412.

Bloom, L., Merkin, S., & Wooten, J. (1982). Wh-questions: Linguistic factors that contribute to the sequence of acquisition. *Child Development, 53*, 1084–1092.

Bloom, L., Rocissano, L., & Hood, L. (1976). Adult-child discourse: Developmental interaction between information processing and linguistic knowledge. *Cognitive Psychology, 8*, 521–552.

Bowerman, M. (1979). The acquisition of complex sentences. In P. Fletcher and M. Garman (Eds.), *Language acquisition*. London: Cambridge University Press.

Ervin-Tripp, S., & Gordon, D. (1986). The development of requests. In R. Schiefelbusch (Ed.), *Language competence assessment and intervention*. San Diego: College-Hill Press.

Gallagher, T. (1977). Revision behaviors in the speech of normal children developing language. *Journal of Speech and Hearing Research, 20*, 303–318.

Tyack, D., & Gottsleben, R. (1986). Acquisition of complex sentences. *Language Speech and Hearing Services in Schools, 17*, 160–174.

11

Language Development into the School Years: Further Goals

Just as children move from communicating with more than one word at a time, eventually they move beyond communicating with one sentence at a time. Beginning around Phase 8, we see children producing sequences of sentences. Eventually (Post Phase 8), these sequences form a connected unit, and thus they can be considered a form of discourse, or text (i.e., a unit of connected language that is larger than a sentence). A sequence is evident in the ways that the connectedness develops within such units, much as there is a developmental sequence in the ways that other units of language are connected (i.e., words to clauses and clauses to complex sentences).

This chapter presents information on developmental changes in the expression of one type of text, or discourse—the narrative. Narratives are a report of "what happened"; they can be real or imaginary (the latter are often called stories). Much of the available data concern children's productions (or reproductions) of imaginary narratives. However, some data are available on the production of personal experience narratives. In this chapter, we will see that the structures of real and imaginary narratives follow similar developmental trends, although differences between the two may occur in a given child at a given point in time. Development entails both an increase in the length and complexity of narratives related by children and a change in the means by which the propositions within the narrative are connected to form a whole. Narrative development can be examined from at least two levels: a macrolevel and a microlevel. Some developmental trends at each level will be presented in the following sections.

The information presented in the previous two chapters was based primarily on longitudinal data; the developmental sequences presented here are based on cross-sectional data. Since cross-sectional studies involve different children, it is not always possible to know when some of the Post Phase 8 skills overlap and co-occur. However, given changes in proportional usage across age groups, we can hypothesize some developmental sequences.

Developmental Sequence of Narrative Productions: Logical-Temporal Structure (Content/Form)

At one level of description, we might examine how each proposition or subsection of the narrative relates to the narrative as a whole. One such macroanalysis would describe the meaning relation between propositions and the whole text. This might be considered a content/form analysis. For example, at the two-word level we examined how one word related to another, and we derived content categories such as possession, attribution, and rejection. At the complex-sentence level, we examined how one clause related to another and derived content categories such as additive, temporal, and causal. Similarly, at the level of the narrative, we can look at how one sentence is related to the other sentences within the unit, and we can derive categories to describe these relations. (In this case, we are interested not only in how the sentence is related to preceding and succeeding sentences, but in how the sentence meaning relates to the entire report of what happened.) When the use of these categories emerges in a developmental sequence, we have a description of the acquisition of narrative production.

The developmental sequence is presented here in terms of four levels of increasing complexity that vary in the ways that sentences (or propositions) within a narrative are related to the whole. The developmental data come from a number of sources (Applebee, 1978; Botvin & Sutton-Smith, 1977; Lahey, 1986; C. Peterson & McCabe, 1983; Stein, 1986; Stein & Glenn, 1982; Stein & Policastro, 1984; Sutton-Smith, 1981; and Trabasso, Secco, & van den Broek, 1984). The description of the chains comes from the work on complex sentences (Bloom, Lahey, Hood, Lifter, & Fiess, 1980) which was discussed in the preceding chapter.

The first units that children produce are sequences of sentences (or phrases or clauses) that could be arranged in any order. In this sense they resemble the early complex sentences that we described in the last chapter as additive; such sequences of sentences are here referred to as *additive chains*. In additive chains, utterances have no dependency relations among themselves; that is, each could be moved anywhere in the text and the meaning of the entire text would not change. (See Box 11-1 for examples.) The additive chains do not contain any temporal or causal dependencies among the sentences as we see in later narrations. While there is no causal or temporal connection among the sentences, there is often some sense of unity; it may come from the repetition of actions or from a central theme or topic (see Applebee, 1978; C. Peterson & McCabe, 1983; Stein, 1986; Sutton-Smith, 1981). Early exemplars may be simply listings, such as the story by Adam in Box 11-1. Later, some structure and cohesion are achieved by the repetition of actions by either the same or different agents (e.g., the continual eating of the monster in the story by Farrah in Box 11-1). Finally, an additive chain may be a description of some scene, such as the story by Ephra in Box 11-1. Descriptive sequences describe a setting or person with few, if any, actions (unless they are habitual actions). These three types form subtypes of additive chains, as noted in Table 11-1 and Box 11-1.

The second level of narrative development proposed here is the *temporal chain*, which is usually a sequence of events without causal relations among the events. The utterances refer to actions that occurred in a temporal sequence, and so the order of utterances is important. Such chains might also contain additive relations among the sentences, but the most advanced content/form connection is temporal sequence. (See Applebee, 1978; C. Peterson & McCabe, 1983; Stein, 1986; Sutton-Smith, 1981.) In the story by Watson in Box 11-1, the sequence is clear—the dog went to the doctor, got a shot, and went home. While it is possible that the dog went to the doctor in order to get a shot, such a causal relation is not coded nor is it implied. Thus, this was called a temporal chain.

TABLE 11-1   A Proposed Developmental Sequence of Content/Form Interactions in Self-Generated Narratives

Level 1 Additive chains
  A. Listings
  B. Repeated actions
  C. Descriptive sequences

Level 2 Temporal chains

Level 3 Causal chains
  A1. Abbreviated causal chains
  A2. Reactive or automatic causal chains
  B. Goal-based causal chains without obstacle
  C. Goal-based causal chains with obstacle

Level 4 Multiple causal chains
  A. Conjoined causal chains
  B. Embedded causal chains

BOX 11-1   Goals for Content/Form Interactions in Self-Generated Narratives

(At the bottom of each example is the first name or initial of the child if known, and the source of the narrative.) To code relations among events as:

Level 1 Additive Chains

   A. Listing

      For example:

         A monkey/ a dog/ a book/ a fish/

         (Adam, from Sutton-Smith, 1981)

   B. Repeated Actions

      For example:

         The dog went on the puppet

         The puppet went on the house

         The house went on the pigeon

         (Alice, from Sutton-Smith, 1981)

         A monster

         the monster ate the house

         the monster ate the kids

         the monster ate the dad

         the monster ate the cat and also the dog

         he ate the furniture

         and then he went home to the zoo

         the end

         (Farrah, from Sutton-Smith, 1981)

   C. Descriptive Sequence

      For example:

         Once there was a horse

         and a little farm

         and some pigs were there

         and once there was a apple tree

         and there was a banana tree there

         there was a little farmer who gave hay to the horse

         and there was a little pond with little fish in it

         and a little house

         that's it.

         (Ephra, from Sutton-Smith, 1981)

         Once there was a big grey fox

         who lived in a cave;

         He was mean and scary, really scary.

         He had big giant eyes

         And a bushy tail that hit people in the face.

         And he ate little rabbits.

         (From Stein, 1986)

Level 2 Temporal Chains

     For example:

        About Noodle (his dog). He went to the doctor.

        He give a shot. He go home. He drink milk.

(continued)

BOX 11-1   Narrative Goals (*continued*)

He didn't drink his milk.
(Watson, 3:6, from Pitcher & Prelinger, 1963)

When I was at home I looked in the closet and I saw a big giant bear. I treated him like a nice little bear. We went to the park alot. We slept together and also we ate together. Next morning we looked at a book together and then we helped our father paint the house. Next winter it was Christmas and I got a new jacket. My teddy bear got a baby teddy bear, and they lived happily together. The end.
(Alan, from Sutton-Smith, 1981)

Level 3 Causal Chains

  A1. Abbreviated Causal Chain

      For example:

        Baby cried. The baby hurt his eyes.
        The baby broke his eye. Then he
        got it all fixed.
        (Watson, from Pitcher & Prelinger, 1963)

        Once there was a robber
        and then a girl was lost
        and the robber came and put her in jail
        and then the police came and got her out of jail
        and then the police put the robber in jail
        (Farrah, from Sutton-Smith, 1981)

        Once upon a time there lived a zebra
        and the zebra he went to the park
        and he got lost
        and he didn't know his way home
        so he had to try both ways
        and he had to tell the police which way to go
        that's the end
        he had to tell him what house was like
        the zebra telled the police
        and that's the end.
        (Alice, from Sutton-Smith, 1981)

  A2. Reactive or Automatic Causal Chain

      For example:

      Adult. What happened in the accident that you saw?
        L. Car got burned up.
      Adult. A car got burned up? Tell me about what
      happened when the car burned up.
        L. There was three kids in there. Everybody got
        out in time, and, and then, my Dad didn't keep
        his eyes on the road and we were almost *wrecked.*
      Adult. You were almost wrecked too?
        L. *Yeahhhh.* I wouldn't want that to happen.
        I'd be out of school about a *week.*
        (L, 6, from C. Peterson & McCabe, 1983)

(*continued*)

BOX 11-1   Narrative Goals (*continued*)

> Once there was a girl named Alice
> who lived down by the seashore.
> Alice was in the water,
> floating on her back,
> when along came a shark
> and GULP GULP
> That was the end of Alice.
> (From Stein, 1986)

B. Goal-Based Causal Chain without Obstacle
  For example:
> B: I remember when my brother got a sliver, a sliver.
>   Adult: Oh, tell me about it.
> B. We were playing outside. I don't know how it
> happened. We were playing outside and when we
> came in he had a sliver in his hand.
>   Adult: He had a sliver in his hand.
> B: Just before he took a bath my Dad came up
> and took it out, and he was *cry-ying, cry-y-ing,*
> *oow, ooh.* He cried for a little while. He
> started and he didn't want to get into the tub.
> (B, 4, from C. Peterson & McCabe, 1983)

> Once there was a big grey fox
> who lived in a cave near the woods.
> One day he decided that he was very hungry
> and that he need to catch something for dinner.
> So he went outide,
> spotted a baby rabbit
> caught him,
> and had him for dinner.
> (From Stein, 1986)

C. Goal-Based Causal Chain with Obstacle
  For example:
> Once there was a fox
> who lived in a cave near a forest.
> He wanted some food for dinner,
> and went out looking for something.
> He looked and looked, but nothing.
> Suddenly, he saw a rabbit hopping by,
> He ran really fast and tried to catch him,
> but he kept missing
> cause the rabbit was smarter than the fox
> So he didn't get any dinner.
> (From Stein, 1986)

> A few years ago Henry Tick lived in a hippie's hair, but he got a crew cut
> so Henry had to move. He went to the pet shop but it was closed too.
> Finally he found a nice basset hound. So he moved in. . . . (continued
> below, level 4A)
> (Olive, from Sutton-Smith, 1981)

(continued)

BOX 11-1 Narrative Goals (*continued*)

Level 4 Multiple Causal Chain (or Episode)

A. Conjoined Causal Chain (or Episode)
    For example:
    (continued from Olive, above, level 3D)
    . . . He got a good job at the circus jumping two inches in mid-air into a glass of water. One day he jumped but there was no water. He was rushed to the hospital. They put twelve stitches in his leg. Well, he never went there again. The end. . . . (additional chapters with further episodes)
    (Olive, from Sutton-Smith, 1981)

B. Embedded Causal Chain (or Episode)
    For example:
    A man named Mr. Dirt lived in the country all by himself and owned a farm. One calf got away and went into the woods and headed for the mountains. So Mr. Dirt went up the mountain after the calf. On the way a bear came after Mr. Dirt. He ran up a tree and the bear came after him. Mr. Dirt threw his ax at the bear and hit the bear in the head. Blood poured out of his head and the bear fell down and died. A few minutes later the calf ran over to Mr. Dirt and they went back to the farm.
    (From Botvin & Sutton-Smith, 1977)

At Level 3 we see the emergence of causal connections between events and states and, thus, *causal chains*. In causal chains individual utterances are related to the text by means of a causal dependency in that events (or states) enable or cause other events (or states). While other utterances that are related in only an additive or temporal manner may be included within the causal chain, the narrative concerns some problem or change of state that has consequences or is resolved. Causal chains are often referred to as plots (e.g., Botvin & Sutton-Smith, 1977) or episodes (e.g., Stein & Glenn, 1982) since they contain a problem and some resolution to that problem.

At first, causal chains are apt to be incomplete or very abbreviated (including only problems and consequences), and the results or consequences are unrelated to the planning of another animate being (i.e., they are automatic or out of the control of another). Each of the above forms a subtype of causal chain (see Table 11-1 and Box 11-1)—the first, called *abbreviated causal chains*, and the second, *reactive or automatic causal chains*. In the first example under Causal Chains in Box 11-1, Watson tells about a problem, the broken eye, and immediately follows with the resolution, it got fixed. This simple description of problem and resolution is an example of an abbreviated causal chain. A wonderful example of a reactive causal chain comes from Stein's (1986) data when Alice was gulped by a shark (see Box 11-1). Alice apparently had no time for plans to solve this problem. Both of these subtypes appear to emerge at the same time. Reactive causal chains continue to be used frequently throughout the school years (C. Peterson & McCabe, 1983), but the abbreviated causal chains are produced less frequently as children's narrative skills develop.

Causal chains become more elaborate with time and experience and do eventually include the goals and plans of other animate beings. When goals are first included, the narrative may contain no obstacles to the achievement of that goal. In this next subtype, *goal-based causal chain without obstacle*, the resolution of the problem is not automatic; it is related to the successful or unsuccessful goals and attempts of an animate being. For example, the fox in the story from Stein (1986), given as an example in Box 11-1 (Level 3B), had a plan to overcome his hunger; his attempts met with no obstacle, and he was successful in finding food and eating it.

Eventually, children are more likely to include obstacles in their stories and personal narratives. Adults rank the "goodness" of stories in a sequence that is similar to this developmental sequence, placing automatic consequences at the lowest level, followed by goals without obstacles and, at the highest level, goals with obstacles (Stein, 1986; Stein & Policastro, 1984). *Goal-based causal chains with obstacles*, the next subtype, are similar to the previously described subtype except that an obstacle needs to be overcome in order for the main character (i.e., the protagonist) to meet the goal. For example, in another fox example from Stein (1986) used as an illustration in Box 11-1 (Level 3C), the fox kept missing the rabbit and so his plan was not successful.

Finally, the most advanced level of narrative included here, Level 4, involves the joining of *multiple causal chains* (or *episodes*). In these chains, more than one plot (i.e., problem and resolution) is included. When multiple causal chains are first narrated, there is a tendency for children to conjoin the two or more plots in an additive or temporal fashion, referred to here as *conjoined causal chains.* In this subtype, one causal chain is not causally related to the other causal chains. For example, in Olive's story in Box 11-1, the problem described under Level 3C could have occurred before or after the problem illustrated in Level 4A. Moreover, neither problem was caused by the other.

Finally, in the second subtype of multiple causal chain, the *embedded causal chains*, different plots or episodes (i.e., causal chains) are causally related to one another, and one may be embedded in the other. In the final example in Box 11-1, the embedded problem is the bear chasing Mr. Dirt; this problem would not have occurred if Mr. Dirt was not out looking for his calf (i.e., his first problem).

For more information on the development of causal chains see Botvin and Sutton-Smith (1977), C. Peterson and McCabe (1983), Stein (1986), Trabasso et al., (1984), and Westby (1984). These developmental trends are proposed here as a sequence of content/form interaction goals for facilitating narrative development.

Preschool children produce narratives that generally fall into Levels 1 and 2. Children 7 and 8 years of age produce all levels, but they use Levels 3 and 4 more frequently than the earlier levels (with additive chains appearing least frequently). Each content category (i.e., additive chain, temporal chain, and causal chain) continues to appear in the discourse of adults in the same way that additive, temporal, and causal relations continue to relate clauses in the complex sentences of children and adults. That is, additive and temporal relations, while less complex in a developmental sense, are not discarded. We may, for example, describe scenery, weather, or people in a text using additive chains. Temporal chains are frequently used in descriptions of events recounted by adults. The type of chain selected for a narrative is influenced by the states and events to be described as well as the function and context of the discourse. Certain sublevels of the these chains, however, are less likely to appear in adult language (e.g., concatenated actions and abbreviated causal chains). It is not clear that this sequence can be generalized to cultures other than the mainstream culture of the United States, the culture of the children from which the data reported here were collected. Narrative styles vary with cultures, and it is important to understand the styles that are common in different cultures when assessing or working with children from minority cultures (see, for example, Heath, 1986).

The Development of Subcategories of Causal Chains

Causal chains can be described in terms of a number of subcategories (such as setting, complication, and resolution) (e.g., Stein & Glenn, 1982). Many of these subcategories are linked together in a causal fashion such that each is the result of at least one preceding subcategory while at the same time it is the cause of at least one subsequnt subcategory. For example, the causal chain includes a *complication* (or some form of disequilibrium in the current state of affairs) and a *resolution* (which may or may not be a successful resolution to the complication). Complication and resolution are two subcategories found in any complete causal chain. Further, most causal chains consist of a *setting* that is considered causally related to the complication and resolution in that it enables and constrains what can occur. Consider the influence of the setting "I was in my car." It would be hard to participate in a car accident if you were not in a car, and being located in a car would make it difficult to actively participate in a boat wreck or a ski race. Thus, settings enable the subsequent events as well as constrain them. Settings appear in early narratives and can be expected in all causal chains.

In addition to the setting, complication, and resolution, other categories may appear in the causal chain. For example, the narrator might describe an *internal response* to the complication, such as a goal and plan to overcome the complication—such goals and plans or other internal responses are caused by the complication and may further lead to *attempts* to carry out the plan. The attempts are, therefore, caused (or motivated) by the goals and plans, and they, in turn, lead to *consequences*. Note that consequences are then causally related not only to the complication, but also to the plan and to the attempts. Thus, a complex causal chain is formed, and this chain can be broken down into subcategories for analysis. (See Box 11-2.) These subcategories have been discussed in terms of story grammars (e.g., Rumelhart, 1975; Stein & Glenn, 1982) and in terms of "causal chains" (Trabasso et al., 1984).

Not all causal chains include each of the subcategories mentioned, even in adult narratives. Some development is found in the use of subcategories; Sutton-Smith (1981) reported that early productions of causal chains (plots) included only complication and resolution (the Abbreviated Causal Chain in Box 11-1) with no intervening actions; other information (i.e., subcategories) were added as the child's narrative skills developed. Sutton-Smith observed that the inclusion of actions between the complication and resolution is apt to disappear for a while when early multiple episodes are first produced (providing further evidence of synergy or trade-off in language development) (e.g., Bloom, 1976; Shriner, Holloway, & Daniloff, 1969).

**BOX 11-2   Subcategories of Goal-Based Causal
Chains and Their Causal Connections**

1. Setting—The internal, external, or habitual states that introduce the characters and the environment of the story.
   For example: "I was sailing my friend's boat. . ."
   (Enables 2, 3, 4, 5, 6)

2. Complication—The disequilibrium or change in the environment.
   For example: "A squall came out of nowhere and the boat almost went over. . ."
   (Enabled by 1; causes 3, 4, 5, 6)

3. Internal Response—The effects, plans, goals, and cognitions that result from the complication.
   For example: "I tried to steady the boat. . ."
   (Enabled by 1; result of 2; causes [or motivates] 4 and possibly 5)

4. Attempts—The actions that result from the goals and plans that are aimed at achieving the desired state (i.e., restoring or adapting to the disequilibrium).
   For example: "I pointed into the wind and dropped the jib. . ."
   (Enabled by 1; result of 2, 3; causes 5)

5. Consequence—The states or actions that are the result of the successful or unsuccessful attempts.
   For example: "The boat straightened out. . ."
   (Enabled by 1; result of 2, 3, 4; may Cause 6)

6. Reactions—Actions or states that are precipitated by the complication but do not cause or lead to other states or events.
   For example: "I was so scared. . ."
   (Enabled by 1; result of 2 and/or 5; dead end because it does not cause other events or states)

Note: Based on Rumelhart, 1975; Stein and Glenn, 1982; Trabasso et al., 1984.

There does not seem to be a great deal of differential development among the subcategories. Internal responses tend to be a bit less frequent in younger children's causal chains (C. Peterson & McCabe, 1983), but most causal chains do include goals (one type of internal response). Even the inclusion of goals, however, increases with age (Stein, 1986). Younger children are also likely to omit information about attempts to reach goals (C. Peterson & McCabe, 1983). In establishing goals of intervention for subcategories of causal chains the clinician must keep in mind that some of these subcategories may decrease when multiple causal chains first emerge.

These subcategories are used primarily with causal chains. They are not considered in the presence of additive chains since the additive chain has little structure that could be described by this type of analysis (however, the additive chain may contain cohesive relations, which will be discussed later). Temporal chains sometimes include a setting that describes the location and participants in the events, but the primary content/form structure entails sequencing of a chain of events. Other forms of structure and subcategorization can be found in each of the chains mentioned using a different type of analysis, such as the ones presented in the next section.

Summary

As children join propositions to form a unit of text, we see a developmental sequence in the meaning relations (i.e., content) among events: first additive, then temporal, and, finally, causal. (Causal chains within a narrative are often referred to as episodes or plots.) Eventually, these episodic (or plot) units are joined to other episodic (or plot) units to form longer and more complex narratives. At first, one episode is related to other episodes in an additive or temporal relationship; later, one episode is the cause and/or result of other episodes. The sequence of additive, temporal, causal is, therefore, common to the joining of clauses (to form complex sentences), to the joining of propositions (to form a simple narrative), and to the joining of episodes (to form more complex narratives). The sequence of additive, then temporal, and then causal appears to reflect an increase in complexity that is manifested in developmental sequence and in judgments of what makes a good story (Stein, 1986; Stein & Policastro, 1984) or what makes a good personal narrative (C. Peterson & McCabe, 1983).

Developmental Sequences in Narrators' Adaptations to the Listener: Goals of Use Interacting with Content/Form

"Narratives are concerned with more than making sense. They are also concerned with being appreciated, being amusing, being considered well done, and so on" (Kernan, 1977, p. 100). In addition to looking at the logical/temporal structure of the narrative in terms of the meaning relations among the sentences or subcategories, we can look at how well the narrator adapts to listener needs and successfully meets these other criteria. At the macrolevel, we can describe how the narrative helps the listener to understand what is happening and to get the point of the narration. Subcategories relating to this type of analysis were first suggested by Labov (Labov, 1972; Labov & Waletzky, 1967) and have since been applied to personal narratives of children (e.g., Kernan, 1977; C. Peterson & McCabe, 1983; Sleight & Prinz, 1985; Umiker-Sebeok, 1979). Children's fantasy narratives have less often been analyzed using such subcategories. Subcategories that show developmental change in personal narratives include orientations and evaluations. In addition, there are some changes in the way children begin and end their tales.

Orientations

Orientations serve to let the listener know who the participants are in the narration, as well as where, when, and why the events took place. This subcategory is similar to that of "setting" mentioned above in the content/form analysis, only here it is looked at in terms of the listener's need to understand the point of the narration.

Orientations are present in the narratives of some young preschool children, but the number of preschool children using orientations increases from 3 to 5 years of age (Umiker-Sebeok, 1979), and data suggest that the proportion of narrative devoted to orientations increases with age (Kernan, 1977). However, the most striking developmental change in the use of orientations is in the amount and type of information provided. For example, the young child tends to give only the names of participants and the place where the events took place (enough information for a setting, but perhaps limited in terms of understanding the point of the story). Older children are more likely to give information about participants' relationships to each other and the narrator as well as details about the personality characteristics of the participants and ongoing actions (Kernan, 1977; C. Peterson & McCabe, 1983). In fact, with development, children provide more and more information about the who, what, when, where, how, and why of their narratives. They provide more detail about moods, motivations, and circumstances. Older children are also more apt to place these orientations at the beginning of the narration rather than scattering them throughout as younger children do. It appears as if the older children are more aware that the appreciation of narrative events is dependent, in part, upon information that is different from a description of what happened.

Thus, goals of intervention (see the listing in the Summary of Goals of Use presented later in the chapter) include increasing the type of orientation information that would help the receiver appreciate the point of the narration. Obviously, the more information the listener and child share about the participants, location, etc., the less complete the orientation needs to be for that listener. The child has, then, two tasks. One is to determine how much information is shared with the listener, and the other is to decide which parts of the unshared information are necessary in order for the listener to understand the point of the narration.

Evaluations

Personal narratives express both referential information (i.e., information about what happened) and evaluative information (i.e., information about how the narrator felt about the events that took place) (Labov, 1972). While evaluations can occur anywhere in the narrative, they are generally concentrated after the complication so as to build a high point and create suspense and interest. An evaluation stops the action, or the recapitulation of events, and tends to emphasize that part of the narrative. Evaluations can include voice stress or changes in pronunciation, the insertion of an evaluative word or attention getter, and the inclusion of clauses that provide judgments, desires, causes, comparisons, or tangential information. The narrator's evaluations may be expressed directly by a statement of feelings (e.g., "I was so happy"); the evaluations may be implied in a report of what happened (e.g., "and I got the very dollhouse I had pleaded for"); or evaluations may be implied by means of a quote that indirectly conveys an attitude (e.g., "I said, 'I can't wait to show this to my friends' ").

A developmental increase has been reported in the number and variety of evaluations used. Older children are likely to express their feelings directly or to use a quote to imply feelings, while younger children imply an emotional state by reporting an action and using a considerable amount of repetition (Kernan, 1977; C. Peterson & McCabe, 1983). Thus goals of intervention focus on increasing the number and type of evaluative devices and increasing the number of direct statements of feelings. As with orientations, however, context (including the listener) and function (the reason the child is narrating an event) will markedly affect the use of evaluations. A narrative elicited from an uninvolved child may be devoid of evaluations; the child may, in fact, have no particular feelings about the events or any point to be made.

Appendages

Marking the narrative's beginning and end can be an assist to the listener and to the conversational flow. The beginning can be indicated by means of an attention getter or introducer that is a stylized way of letting the listener know that a narrative is to follow (e.g., "guess what," "once upon a time"). An abstract that summarizes the narration at the beginning (e.g., "I was in an accident") helps prepare the listener for what follows. The use of such introductory markers increases with development in the recounting of personal narratives as well in the generation of stories (e.g., Kernan, 1977; C. Peterson & McCabe, 1983; Sutton-Smith, 1981; Umiker-Sebeok, 1979). It is also possible that there are more subtle ways to inform the listener that a narrative is about to occur, such as with prosodic shifts (Michaels, 1986), but there is little developmental information on the use of this strategy.

Developmental changes in the marking of endings include both an increase in the number of children who use them and an increase in the sophistication of the ending (see, for example, Kernan, 1977; C. Peterson & McCabe, 1983; Stein, 1986; Sutton-Smith, 1981). Younger children's endings to stories and to personal recounting of experience tend to be in the form of "that's it" or "the end"; in this way the child successfully turns the floor back to the listener. As children get older, however, endings are used to tie the entire narrative together and to specify its lasting significance. Children are more likely to add statements like "they never fought again." Morals, however, are rarely provided by elementary school children (Stein, 1986).

Thus, goals of intervention (see the listing in the Summary of Goals of Use presented later in the chapter) would focus on an increase in the inclusion of boundary markers, and, eventually, an increase in the use of abstracts at the beginning and ending to tie the narrative together and talk about its current or lasting significance.

Summary

In general, when creating narratives, younger children focus on the events to be described and seem less concerned with the needs of the listener. They spend less time on orienting the listener with the appropriate background information and less time on directly stating their feelings about the events. Furthermore, younger children are less likely to mark the boundaries of their narratives. When they do mark boundaries, the markings are, at first, simple and stylized, with a gradual increase in the use of abstracts at the beginning and with endings that note the significance of the narrative. Appreciation of the narratives of younger children comes more from an understanding of the events themselves than from the elaboration presented by the narrator.

Goals of intervention might focus on increasing the elaboration of the events so that the point of the narrative is explicit. This would involve an increase in the sophistication of the orientations, an increase in the use of evaluations (particularly a direct statement of feelings), and an increase in the inclusion of boundary markers that not only mark the beginning and end, but also aid the listener's understanding of the point.

Finally, it has been suggested throughout this section that context may have a major effect on what is observed. Adaptations to the listener (i.e., the use interactions with content and form discussed here) are, by definition, influenced by the listener. Some data are available on the direct effects of listeners. Preschool children reportedly produce longer and more complex narratives to adults than to other children (Umiker-Sebeok, 1979), and even 4-year-olds provide more explicit descriptions to those who do not share similar information than to those who shared an event with them (Maratsos, 1973; Menig-Peterson, 1975). It is both obvious and logical that the shared information of listener and speaker should affect the use of each of these structural subcategories. To ignore this in an educational or clinical setting and insist on, for example, complete orientations when they are not necessary (because of shared information) is as inappropriate as insisting that a child produce a complete sentence in response to a question such as "What are you eating?" Thus, goals for increasing the sophistication of these categories (for example, orientations) should specify the prior knowledge of the listener. Additionally, the goals should include some awareness of the function for which the child is telling the narrative (e.g., to impress, amuse, fulfill teacher's request) and the logical influence of this function on the inclusion of such categories as evaluations. Unfortunately, developmental data are not available on such influences, but it is quite likely that an uninvolved or unmotivated child will use few evaluations.

Developmental Sequences in Narrators' Adaptations to Linguistic and Other Contexts: Goals of Use Interacting with Content/Form

The previous goals of content, form, and use were based on a global, or macrolevel of, analysis. Narratives also have structure at a microlevel, cohesive structure that ties the sentences together to form a connected unit. A number of linguistic devices (forms), called *cohesive devices*, can be used to tie a span of sentences together. These have been described by Halliday and Hasan (1975) and include reference (e.g., pronouns, demonstratives, comparatives); conjunction (forms such as *and, then, so, but, because*); lexical cohesion (e.g., repetition of a word or use of a related word); and ellipsis (i.e., the omission of an item that can be retrieved from elsewhere in the text). In addition to these devices, similar syntactic structure (parallelism) across utterances can serve as a tie (Bennett-Kastor, 1986). The developmental data on cohesive ties in oral narratives are primarily concerned with the cohesive devices of reference, conjunction, and parallelism; the developmental changes that have been reported are presented below.

Conjunction

The meaning relations between adjacent clauses within the narrative can be coded by a conjunction in the same way that meaning relations between clauses within a sentence were coded in complex sentences. This type of tie is the second most

---

BOX 11-3 Examples of Connective Forms That Might Be Used by Children to Code Semantic Relations between Clauses in Narratives

Additive—(*addition*) and; (*alternative*) or

Temporal—(*successive*) then, and then, next, just then, after that, before; (*simultaneous*) when, while

Causal—so, because, therefore, so that; (*conditional*) if (or then)

Adversative—but, although, only, however

Comparative—like, as, similarly

Note: Adapted from Halliday and Hasan, 1975; Martin, 1983, p. 21.

---

frequent type of cohesion found in the narratives of children 7 to 10 years old (Liles, 1985). (The most frequent type of cohesive tie reported by Liles was personal reference; following conjunction, the most frequent types were demonstrative reference and then lexical cohesion.) Some conjunctions serve to code both the semantic relations between sentences and the semantic relations between clauses within a sentence. Meaning relations found at both levels include additive, temporal, causal, and adversative (see Chapter 10 for full definitions). Other relations may also occur, such as continuative or comparative.

The developmental sequence in which conjunctions emerge in narrative productions is the same as that described for clauses outside the narrative; that is, additive and temporal are used first, followed by causal and adversative relations (e.g., Bennett-Kastor, 1986; Kernan, 1977; Martin, 1983). Children who are coding many causal relations in utterances that are not part of a narrative may still be coding only additive or temporal relations within the narrative structure. While children at the age of 3 code causal relations among clauses more frequently than additive or temporal relations (Bloom, Lahey, Hood, Lifter, & Fiess, 1980), the school-age children studied by Kernan (1977) and Martin (1983) were using mostly additive and temporal conjunctions within the narrative. Furthermore, the frequency of coding different conjunctive relations may vary even within the narrative depending upon the task and the topic (Martin, 1983).

Older children are also more likely than younger children to make connections between clauses within the narrative more explicit (Martin, 1983). Thus, goals of intervention (see the listing in the Summary of Goals of Use presented later in the chapter) would be to increase the explicit marking of semantic relations between clauses within the narrative with additive and temporal conjunctions before causal, adversative, and comparative conjunctions. (See Box 11-3 for examples of some forms that might be used.)

Reference

Reiteration of a referent by actual remention or by pronominalization is the most common type of textual cohesion (Bennett-Kastor, 1986). If a narrative has a theme (i.e., if it concerns a particular topic), then one would expect the noun phrases that refer to that theme (object, person, place, location, etc.) to be repeatedly mentioned throughout the narrative. For example, if a narrative is about a car accident, reference to the car and to the person involved should appear in more than one sentence. In preschool children, repeatedly mentioned noun phrases are usually subjects of sentences (Bennett-Kastor, 1983). With development, increments are found in the *frequency* with which a particular noun phrase is rementioned, in the *variety* of noun phrases that are rementioned, and in the *distance* (i.e., the number of clauses) between each mention (Bennett-Kastor, 1983).

Developmental changes also occur in the way in which a noun phrase is rementioned. One can identify a referent by presenting its name (e.g., "A boy was driving a car"). Note that in this case the referents are nominalized and preceded by the indefinite article *a*. However, when it is presumed that the referent is known to the listener, reference is usually made in a different fashion. The referent may again be nominalized, but the definite article *the* would be used (e.g., "The boy couldn't control the car"). In such a case, cohesion is provided by two means. Lexical cohesion is evident in the repetition of the words *boy* and *car*, and a form of reference appears in the use of the article *the*. Inclusion of the definite article presumes that the listener knows which car and which boy are the referents. Similarly, when we remention a referent, we could use a pronoun (e.g., "he jumped out of it"). Both definite articles and pronouns are forms of reference that tell the listener to search elsewhere for the specification of the referent. In the above examples, the search would bring the listener to a prior utterance.

Children use the *forms* of reference early. That is, during the second or third year of life children seem to learn content/form interactions relevant to reference, such as definite/indefinite or the fact that "it" equals object and "I" equals speaker (Bloom, Lightbown, & Hood, 1975; Brown, 1973; Karmiloff-Smith, 1979; Maratsos, 1973). However, in the early phases of language learning (e.g., Phases 1 through 8) children talk mostly in the "here and now," so the referents mentioned are usually shared in the immediate context. Moreover, at this early point in development, children do not talk in extended narratives, so cohesion among their utterances is not a concern. Even when narratives first appear, preschool children initially talk about events that have just been shared in the context; even at 5 years of age half of the personal narratives produced are still about events within the present context (Umiker-Sebeok, 1979). An early goal of narrative productions, if a child's narratives are primarily about the immediate context, would be gradually to increase the distancing of events the child recapitulates. This goal might well precede any goals related to listener needs (see also the listing in the Summary of Goals presented later in the chapter).

As utterances extend beyond the immediate present and as the child begins to produce longer stretches of discourse, the use of various forms of reference must include awareness of the information that is shared with the listener; that is, the child's utterance must reflect the interaction of use with content and form. Research suggests that the development of this content/form/use interaction is a slow process. To understand what needs to be learned, let us first look at how information may be shared between speaker and listener.

Box 11-4 presents a schematic representation of the means by which a referent can be known by the listener. We can presume (i.e., a phoric type of reference) that a referent is known to a listener because of our culture (referred to as *homo-*

BOX 11-4   REFERENCE: Establish Identity by PRESENTING a New Referent or REFERRING to a Referent PRESUMED to Be Known.

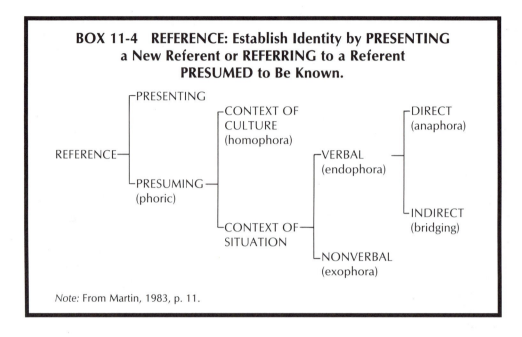

Note: From Martin, 1983, p. 11.

phora). For example, we assume everyone knows "the Cookie Monster" or "the moon," and we do not use indefinite articles even when first presenting such referents. In addition to shared culture, the present context makes information about referents available and is thus shared by speaker and listener. Such context includes both the nonlinguistic environment (i.e., those things present and observable by the participants) and the linguistic context (or the utterances produced by discourse participants). When the referent can be identified by means of the nonlinguistic context, we speak of *exophoric reference;* when the referent is to be found in other utterances (i.e., the linguistic context) we refer to it as *endophoric reference.* Assumptions based on the linguistic context (i.e., endophoric reference) can be related to indirect associations (i.e., bridging), as might be the case with a car door. If I told you that "I entered a car," I can follow with "I tried to close *the* door" since I can presume that you know which door I mean. More direct remention of an identical referent (i.e., the car door) can be made without renaming it. Thus, I might continue by saying "*It* wouldn't close." Remention of a previously stated referent is termed *anaphoric reference.* Developmental data have primarily focused on the use of exophoric reference and one type of endophoric reference —anaphoric reference.

Early use of reference appears to be unrelated to endophoric context; the referring expression is often appropriate because the child associates a given form with a particular content (e.g., *a* is associated with identity expressions) and because referents are generally shared through either context or past history (Karmiloff-Smith, 1979). From ages 6 through 9, there is an increase in the production of referring terms and a concurrent decrease in the expression of presenting terms (i.e., names of referents, and thus one would presume, a decrease in lexical cohesion). Similarly, there is an increase in the use of anaphoric reference and a decrease in the use of exophoric reference (see, e.g., Karmiloff-Smith, 1979,

1985; Martin, 1983; Warden, 1976). The use of bridging, where knowledge of the referent is inferred from other information in the text, is infrequent and increases with age (Martin, 1983). Use of references that can be taken for granted because of culture also increases with age (Bennett-Kastor, 1983; Martin, 1983).

When referring terms are produced, it is important that the referent be easily retrievable and not ambiguous. This can be a problem in certain contexts, such as when talking about a number of people of the same age and gender whose names are unknown (Bartlett, 1982). Children continue to become better at using referential terms through junior high school, with a developmental decrease in inappropriate and incomplete use of reference terms (Klecaen-Adler & Hedrick, 1985). Goals of intervention, therefore, involve increasing the use of referring terms in narrative productions, increasing the use of referring terms with anaphoric reference, and increasing the appropriate use of such terms (see also the listing in the Summary of Goals of Use presented later in the chapter).

Ellipsis

Deletion of words occurs from the very early stages of language learning; the deleted information is usually available from context, since children talk in the "here and now." According to some reports, the deleted information is generally the constant rather than the changing element in the situation (e.g., Greenfield & Smith, 1976). If one considers this deletion to be ellipsis, we could call it exophoric ellipsis, since the omitted information is available from the context. Such deletions decrease with age.

In another form of ellipsis the deleted information is available from the text or discourse (endophoric ellipsis) usually in a prior utterance (anaphoric ellipsis). If one excludes responses to questions and affirmative and negative responses to statements, anaphoric ellipsis increases with age (L. Bernstein, 1981; Bloom, Merkin, & Wooten, 1982; Bloom, Miller, & Hood, 1975). Furthermore, the use of anaphoric ellipsis decreases in language dissolution exhibited in written language samples (Lahey, 1984). I am not aware of data on the use of such ellipsis in the oral narratives of children but would speculate that the textual cohesive device of anaphoric ellipsis may increase with development in children's oral narratives and that deletion without anaphoric reference may decrease.

Parallel Structures

Finally, the recurrence of a grammatical structure throughout one or more successive clauses of a text serves as a cohesive device (Bennett-Kastor, 1986). Such parallel structures may or may not include the same lexical items. The developmental use of three types of parallel structures has been examined in the oral narratives of children aged 2 to 5 years of age by Bennett-Kastor (1986). One type, structural parallelism, is described as the repetition of a verb phrase structure with varying lexical content (e.g., "I rode my bike to the school and then brought my books to the library"); the second type, lexical parallelism, is where both lexical content of the verb phrase and its structure are repeated (e.g., "I ate a cookie and then Joe ate one"); and the third type, global parallelism, is where the structure and the lexical content of the entire clause is repeated (e.g., "this goes here, this goes here, and this goes here," where different objects are placed but lexical content and structure are similar). The results indicated a proportional increase in the use of structural parallelism and lexical parallelism, and a proportional decrease in the use of global parallelism in children from 2 to 5 years of age. If global parallelism is predominant, a goal of intervention might be to shift to more frequent use of lexical and structural parallelism. Beyond this point, we would expect more variety in structure with the use of more varied means of cohesion. (See the examples of structural parallelism among the first chains in Box 11-1.)

Summary of Goals of Use That Interact with Content/Form in Narrative Productions

Goals of use that interact with content/form for narrative productions are concerned with the adaptations that take place with regard to context. First, we find a decreasing reliance on perceptual support as children grow older and develop greater skill with language. Early narratives are about events that have just happened or events that occur frequently (i.e., scripted events); over time, children talk about events that have occurred in the more distant past and that will happen in the future. Another aspect of context is the listener. Adaptations to listener needs involve inclusion of content/form interactions that will orient the listener (by means of introducers, abstracts, and orientations) and help the listener understand the point of the narrative (e.g., by means of evaluations as well as orientations). Adaptations to linguistic context as well as listener needs are apparent in the development of cohesive devices.

Narratives become more cohesive as children expand the number of noun phrase reiterations within the narrative. Rementions are increasingly made with referring expressions rather than repetition of lexical items, and the referent can be found more often in prior utterances (anaphoric reference) than in the nonlinguistic context (exophoric reference). Semantic relations between clauses within narratives become more explicit, first by means of conjunctions that mark additive and temporal relations and then conjunctions that mark causal, adversative, and comparative relations. In preschool children there is a shift from use of global parallelism to more frequent use of structural and lexical parallelism.

Using this information about the development of narrative productions, we can derive goals of use that interact with content and form at this Post Phase 8 level of development.

GOALS
Related to nonlinguistic context:

1. To increase the number of narratives about events removed from the immediate context

GOALS
Related to linguistic context and perspective of the listener (cohesion):

2. To increase the number of rementions of the themes within the narrative
3. To increase the use of referring terms in narrative productions to use given information

4. To increase the use of anaphoric reference rather than exophoric reference
5. To shift from the use of global parallelism to the use of structural and lexical parallelism

GOALS
Related to listener needs:

6. To mark the boundaries of narratives, at first with stylized markers (e.g., "once upon a time" or "the end") and eventually with more sophisticated beginnings (such as an abstract of the events) and endings (such as those that relate the lasting significance of the tale)
7. To increase the amount of orienting information when it is necessary in order that the listener get the point of the narration
8. To increase the use of evaluators (such as repetition, stress) and to place these at the high point of the narration
9. To increase, gradually, the variety of types of evaluators used, including direct statements of feelings

Some caveats should be noted. These goals are very general because of the nature of the data from which they were derived. They should serve as a reminder that normal children have quite a bit of experience in telling stories before their narratives begin to sound like adult narratives. In addition, context and culture have a major effect on the narrative productions that are observed; what is appropriate and interesting in one context is not so in another.

Other Language Development into the School Years

Certainly, during the school years, children learn more about language than how to tell a tale. For example, in addition to the academic skills of reading and writing language, we know that they learn to adapt content/form interactions to varying contexts, to talk about language and treat it as an object of knowledge, to comprehend syntactic utterances based on only grammatical knowledge when necessary, to become better conversationalists (e.g., by providing more feedback to the speaker and by staying on topic for longer periods of time), and to break the rules of language for particular effects (e.g., humor). We are still learning about many of the accomplishments of young schoolchildren and about the sequences in which the learning takes place.

These later developments depend upon the early foundations of content/form/ use interactions (e.g., Phases 1–8 of the C/F/U Goal Plan). For example, it appears that some time after children have become productive with Phase 8 behaviors, they begin to reorganize their knowledge of content/form interactions so that for periods of time we see an apparent decline in adult-like performance (Bowerman, 1978, 1982; Karmiloff-Smith, 1985). This has been referred to as the U-shaped learning curve (e.g., Karmiloff-Smith, 1985); first we see apparent adult-like performance, then a decline, and finally adult-like performance again. However, this reorganization does not happen to all language behaviors at the same point in time. Rather, it occurs at different times with different aspects of content/form interactions. After children have learned the interactions at one level, they apparently are able to reorganize that knowledge to form another level of more abstract grammar. As yet, there is but limited information on such reorganization relative to syntax.

Similarly, comprehension strategies change with development, but it looks as though these shifts are also spread out over a period of time and are dependent on the child's knowledge of particular sentence types. The comprehension strategies of children without language-learning problems appear to be primarily context-bound or related to the probability of events at a time when their productive skills are within Phases 1 to 7 or 8 (Chapman, 1977). The first linguistic strategy to appear is one that involves the order of words. However, this word-order strategy overcomes a probable-event strategy for some sentence types before others. Word order is used on simple active declarative sentences before it is applied to passive sentences and passive sentences before cleft sentences (Stanton, 1986). This sequence follows the reported order of acquisition of the productive use of these sentence types (although the use of word order for comprehension of simple active declaratives is further removed from productive control than for the others). Thus, it does not seem that syntactic comprehension strategies should become goals of intervention until a child is well into, if not beyond, Phase 8; and if such strategies are goals, they should be related to some sentence types before others. Since information on this interaction is still limited, it is difficult to write such goals, and it is not clear whether such strategies need to be specifically facilitated.

The ability to talk about language and treat it as an object of knowledge (i.e., metalinguistic skill) also develops slowly and is often an important part of the language skills program in the school curriculum. Very early metalinguistic awareness is evident in Phase 8 as children begin to talk about talking. Recall that under the content category of communication, the verbs *say* and *tell* emerged. Furthermore, even in the early phases of development, young children self-correct (that is, they change their wording or pronunciation of words as they are talking), and they play with words and endings, at least when alone (e.g., Weir, 1964). Such behaviors demonstrate language awareness at some level (E. Clark & Andersen, 1979; Van Kleeck, 1984). Preschool children also correct or comment on the pronunciation of others, and they repair their own productions when so requested (Gallagher, 1977). All of these behaviors suggest that language awareness begins early, but in comparison to later behaviors, it is tied to meaning and communication. Operating on language apart from meaning (e.g., segmenting sentences into words or words into phonemes, judging grammaticality or ambiguity, and talking about sentences and parts of speech) appears to await further experience with language, as well as cognitive development, and, most likely, schooling. [However, McDaniel & Cairns (1986) report eliciting judgments of grammaticality from 4-year-olds following some training sessions; reliability of these judgments is yet to be determined. It may be that our attempts to elicit metalinguistic judgments have been limited by the tasks we use.]

Finally, the use of figurative language emerges in the early school years. Children's learning to tell a joke is a painful process for many parents as they must often listen to what seems to be a pointless recounting of a previously heard joke—a recounting that maintains the frame of the joke (e.g., "knock-knock") but suggests that the child never got the point to begin with. Levels of development in the retelling of jokes have been described for children 6 through 9 years of age

(Fowles & Glanz, 1977). Since much humor is based on ambiguity, the development of joke-telling skills may await a certain level of metalinguistic awareness in addition to certain levels of cognitive development, such as concrete operations (see D. Bernstein, 1986, for further information on the development of humor).

These and other language behaviors are the concern of the speech-language pathologist and the special educator. They have not been outlined as goals of intervention in this book for a number of reasons. First, for many aspects of language learning, developmental sequences are not yet available. The plan for language learning presented in these four chapters has been based on developmental information. Second, where developmental sequences are available, they have often been based on responses to elicitation tasks (e.g., recall of jokes). The plan of language learning presented here is concerned with the spontaneously generated language with which children communicate rather than with recall or task-specific behavior. Third, much of the language learning that takes place in the school years is directly taught (e.g., reading and writing). The C/F/U Goal Plan for Language Learning outlines development that occurs without apparent explicit instruction.

Until we have more empirical data on the sequences in which children can best facilitate nonacademically learned language skills, normal development remains our best first hypothesis for sequencing goals of intervention. Using developmental sequences, we are less likely to demand behaviors for which our language-disordered children do not have the prerequisite skills. The view expressed here is that caution is necessary in setting goals of intervention that are derived from taxonomies of language for which we have little, or no, developmental data. So many of the later language skills that we observe in children, including adaptations of language to context, are based on the children's knowledge of and experience with the earlier content/form/use interactions. It may well be that automaticity with earlier levels of language enables later developments to occur. We should not expect more from our language-impaired children than we observe in children without language-learning problems. The language-impaired child also needs a foundation on which to build later skills and an opportunity to develop some level of automaticity.

Summary

Goals of content/form/use interactions can be written for children's productions of narratives. These goals follow Phase 8 goals of language learning and extend well into the school years. Content/form interaction goals are related to the logical/temporal structure of the narrative, where we see a progression from additive to temporal and finally to causal chains. Goals of use that interact with content and form include adaptations to the listener through orientations, evaluations, abstracts, and endings. In addition, these goals involve the use of cohesive devices to tie sentences together. While other language behaviors are also learned at this time, developmental information on their production in spontaneous language is as yet too incomplete to write content/form/use goals into this C/F/U Goal Plan for Language Learning.

Suggested Readings

Halliday, M. A. K., & Hasan, R. (1975). *Cohesion in English.* London: Longman, 1975.

Heath, S. B. (1986, December). Taking a cross-cultural look at narratives. *Topics in Language Disorders,* 7:1, 84–95.

Martin, J. R. (1983). The development of register. In J. Fine and R. Freedle (Eds.), *Developmental issues in discourse.* Norwood, NJ: Ablex.

Peterson, C., & McCabe, A. (1983). *Developmental psycholinguistics: Three ways of looking at a child's narrative.* New York: Plenum.

Stein, N., & Policastro, M. (1984). The concept of a story: A comparison between children's and teacher's viewpoints. In H. Mandl, N. Stein, and T. Trabasso (Eds.), *Learning and comprehension of text.* Hillsdale, NJ: Erlbaum.

Sutton-Smith, B. (1986, December). The development of fictional narrative performances. *Topics in Language Disorders,* 7, 1–10.

Westby, C. (1984). Development of narrative language abilities. In G. Wallach and K. Butler (Eds.), *Language learning disabilities in school-age children.* Baltimore: Williams & Wilkins.

12

Determining Goals of Language Learning From a Language Sample

A description of language behaviors, in terms of content/form/use interactions, and a sequence for presenting these behaviors, based on normal development, were presented in Chapters 8, 9, 10, and 11. In order to select the behaviors that are the most appropriate goals for each child, some techniques for determining which content/form/use interactions the child already has established and which the child has yet to learn will be considered in this and the next chapter. Although the procedures discussed may be applied to alternative plans, they will be considered and applied here primarily in terms of the sequence of the C/F/U Goal Plan of Language Learning presented in Chapters 8–11.

Too often in assessment, there is a tendency to focus on what a child does not know—what a child must learn. In order to plan goals that are determined by a developmental model, it is equally important to describe what the child *does* know; only knowing what the child does know are we able to hypothesize what the child is ready to learn. To determine what behaviors are a part of a child's language system, it is necessary to observe the child's language behaviors, obtain a record of the observations, analyze the observed behaviors according to content/form/use interactions, and set a criterion for deciding that the observed behaviors are the result of the child's language system and are not unique utterances. This chapter includes discussion of each of these points as applied to direct low-structure observations. More highly structured observations are discussed in Chapter 13.

Using Low-Structure Observations

Following the identification of a language disorder, the clinician should directly observe the child in settings that are representative of his or her daily life, and reported observations should be obtained from people who are in contact with the child in normal everyday activities. These direct and reported observations provide the first bases for description of the child's language system—description that can be supplemented later with information obtained from some means of non-standardized elicitation. Thus, a sample of the child's language behaviors obtained in a low-structure setting can be used to generate hypotheses about the child's language system; elicitation tasks can then be used to test some of these hypotheses and fill in missing information. The combined use of information from low-structure observations and elicitation tasks provides the most complete picture of the child's content/form/use interactions.

The problems with using low-structure observations to obtain information about language behavior are primarily related to the time involved in obtaining and analyzing such samples, and the extent to which the sample of language can be considered representative of the child's language behavior in general. Critics of this method of obtaining evidence feel that the amount of time needed to obtain, record, and analyze a sample of language behavior is impractical for the average clinician. Certainly, the time involved in obtaining and analyzing language samples is not brief. However, traditional diagnostic procedures, which include the administration and scoring of numerous standardized measures, also take a considerable amount of time. What is more critical is that, while the administration and scoring of standardized tests of language behavior can take as much, or more, time as the analysis of a language sample, such standardized tests have not been able to provide the rich information that is potentially available in a representative language sample, that is, information about the kinds of ideas the child can code and the ways in which the child can use the linguistic code in interpersonal situations.

The second problem—whether the sampled behaviors are truly representative of what the child knows—is not unique to language samples (e.g., it is also a major source of error in standardized observations). Observing a child using language in a naturalistic setting seems to be far more representative of what the child actually *does* than is the highly constrained sample of behavior collected with formal elicitation techniques under unrealistic conditions (see Chapter 6, as well as Bersoff, 1971; Blau, Lahey, & Oleksiuk-Velez, 1984; Lahey, Launer, & Schiff-Myers, 1983; and Prutting, Gallagher, & Mulac, 1975). The flexibility available in the variety of contexts that can be sampled in low-structure observations enhances the possibility of obtaining a representative sample (see Gallagher, 1983). However, these two criticisms (the time it takes to obtain a sample of language behaviors, and the extent to which the sample is representative of the child's language behavior in general) have limited the use of language sampling to those clinicians who have been specifically trained in such procedures or who are particularly interested in a communication-language orientation to childhood language disorders. The recent interest in use (pragmatics) has increased the interest in and necessity for such observations. For those willing to devote the time and energy needed to take advantage of this potentially rich source of information, some advance preparation is necessary.

Planning direct low-structure observations involves consideration of a number of factors: context of the observation, length of observation, method of transcribing, and method of analysis. Each is discussed below.

Context of Observations

As pointed out in Chapter 6, the more varied the contexts in which the child is observed, the better the chance of obtaining information that is representative of the child's knowledge of language (see also Gallagher, 1983; Muma, 1978). When possible, therefore, the child should be observed in a number of situations. In school, a child might be observed in a classroom setting, playing with a friend, and in direct interaction with the evaluator; in a clinic, the direct observations might include interactions with the evaluator as well as interactions with a member of the family and with another child; and in the home, the child might be observed interacting with family and friends. If there is time for only one direct observation, care should be taken to arrange a setting that will allow for the largest and most representative sample possible. Since the goal of this observation is to find out what the child *does* (i.e., what language the child uses), adult intrusions and interactions should be as relaxed and as natural as possible and should not be designed to test the child or to elicit specific words or linguistic structures. There will be time after the direct low-structure observation to attempt to elicit behaviors that have not yet been observed.

The most frequently suggested sampling contexts have been focused on describing pictures, talking about toys, or responding to probes by an interviewer (Engler, Hannah, & Longhurst, 1973; Lee, 1974; J. Miller, 1981; Tyack & Gottsleben, 1974). Describing pictures seems to be a strain for many children, particularly young children who tend to label objects in a picture, thereby limiting the content/form/use interactions that can be observed. These same children respond more naturally and more spontaneously when simply presented with a few objects and activities.

Longhurst and Grubb (1974) and Longhurst and File (1977) investigated the effect of various contexts on the language sample obtained. They found that less structured conversational settings elicited more language and more complex language than structured, task-oriented settings or pictures, and that pictures were least effective. Lee (1974) also reported that younger normal children used more spontaneous speech when presented with toys than with pictures or stories. She noted that older normal children tended to talk more in response to pictures and the retelling of a familiar story than they did when presented with toys. It has been my experience that a greater number and variety of language behaviors may be obtained when conversation revolves around some concrete activity (e.g., toys, science experiments, or art projects) and the child is free to talk about the activities in any way. This is particularly important for children who are in the early stages of language development, regardless of age.

Although questions are a part of any adult-child interaction, they alone cannot be counted on to elicit the major portion of a language sample from children in the early stages of language development. This is especially true if the questions are not related to ongoing here-and-now activities. When questions are used, they should be open-ended and not yes/no or *wh* interrogatives which tend to elicit single-word responses. Since many children in the early stages of language learning do not comprehend the more complex question forms that elicit longer utterances (such as "how does," "what would happen if," or even directions such as "tell me about"), the usefulness of questions is limited even when they do refer to ongoing events. In adult-child interactions during normal language development, adults ordinarily ask children questions that are consistent with the child's level of development. For example, adults do not ask "where" or "why" questions until the time when children talk about location or causality in their own spontaneous speech (e.g., Hood & Bloom, 1979).

When children are beyond Phase 8 in the C/F/U Goal Plan for Language Learning, the evaluator can more safely use questions, but should be ready to paraphrase these questions if the child seems not to understand. Open-ended questions will help avoid the single-word response. Questions (even yes or no, followed with a request to "tell me") are often helpful in eliciting narratives of personal experience (e.g., Labov & Waletzky, 1967; C. Peterson & McCabe, 1983). For example, in a conversation the evaluators might mention a recent accident they observed or a popular TV show; children can then be asked, "Have you ever seen an accident?'' or "Did you see this week's (TV show)?'' If the answer is yes, a response of "Really, tell me about it" and in the case of the TV show "I missed that show, what happened?" might elicit a narrative in a naturalistic environment (see C. Peterson & McCabe, 1983). Multiple topics can be interspersed throughout the session. Topics prompted by Peterson and McCabe included fights, car accidents, pets, trips, breakages, parties, hospital and doctor visits, and experiences with bullies. Each concerned specific experiences (e.g., "Did you ever bring your pet to the doctor?") rather than generalized knowledge (such as, "What usually happens when . . . ?"). While the child was relating a narrative, the researchers attempted to maintain a conversational manner by using content-free feedback remarks such as "oh" or "uh hum" or by repeating a part of what child had said (see Bloom, Miller, & Hood, 1975, summarized in Chapter 10, for a discussion of the facilitating effect such comments can have on the use of three-constituent structures). In essence, the researchers set themselves up as interested listeners. Such a technique is readily adaptable to an assessment situation in either a clinic or a school. Shorter prompts could be presented (e.g., "Once I saw two cars in an accident") followed by a question (e.g., "Have you ever seen a car accident?"). If the child answers yes but does not relate the experience spontaneously, the evaluator can add "Tell me about the experience."

Fantasy narratives can sometimes be elicited by having the child tell a doll a story at bedtime, or make a book to bring home by dictating a story that the evaluator writes. The tape or video recorder motivates some children when used as a radio or TV show where real or imaginary events are broadcast. Sometimes children can be convinced to share the story read to them by the classroom teacher or a parent. Finally, observation (or recording) of "show and tell" presentations in the child's classroom is another source of narrative productions as well as observations of sociodramatic play (such as doctor-patient games) with other children. Since topic as well as motivation has such a great impact on the structural level of narratives (e.g., Stein, 1986), many topics and contexts should, again, be considered.

In order to plan for the contexts that will be most productive in terms of amount and variety of content/form/use interactions observed, Gallagher (1983) has suggested a preassessment questionnaire. She asks caregivers and teachers (by mail, phone, or interview) about the influence of various contexts on the child's communicative performance and about activities and toys that the child enjoys. This type of preplanning allows the evaluator to best utilize the relatively short periods of direct observation.

Observation of a child who is prelinguistic or in Phase 1 must involve very different context. A good deal of information can be obtained simply by observing the child interacting with a familiar adult. It is helpful, however, to include toys that tend to encourage particular behaviors. For example, including toys that can be separated and joined (e.g., nesting blocks, rings on a stick, people in a bus) would enable a child to demonstrate the ability to separate and join. Objects such as dolls, blankets, bottles, animals, or trucks might encourage both object-specific play and object-to-object play. As with any observation, the materials provided should be appropriate to the child's interests. To observe certain communicative functions, such as requests or protests, it may be necessary to manipulate the environment and create a context for certain behaviors (e.g., putting a desirable object slightly out of reach or deliberately providing the wrong item when a child indicates a desire for a particular object may elicit requests or protests). See Chapter 13 for further examples.

Length of Observations

The minimum duration of an observation and the minimum number of utterances that should be obtained in a clinical sample have not been agreed on. Many have suggested 50 to 100 different utterances as a sample for clinical analyses (Lee, 1974; Tyack & Gottsleben, 1974). Fifty utterances are necessary to obtain reliability on a measure of mean length of utterance within a sample (Darley & Moll, 1960; McCarthy, 1930). The length of a clinical sample is limited by time pressures imposed on busy clinicians and the difficulties involved in eliciting speech from the language-disordered child. Too few utterances, however, make it impossible to say much about the child's language in terms of content, form, and use. A sample of 200 or more different utterances would provide a better data base, although undoubtedly this number may be unrealistic for many children in a clinical situation. In reality, the time that is available probably sets the limit on size of sample. Most diagnostic sessions are limited to 1 hour per visit, both for purposes of scheduling and for reasons relating to a child's interest span. If a child does not use much spontaneous speech in $\frac{1}{4}$ to $\frac{1}{2}$ hour of observation, it is probably better to switch contexts than to continue the same observation for a longer time. With a very talkative child, a full 1-hour session may not be needed for the low-structure direct observation, and the extra time may be used for eliciting particular responses. In general, one should attempt to record a minimum of $\frac{1}{2}$ hour of direct observations. The $\frac{1}{2}$ hour may involve more than one context and can be obtained over a period of days if necessary. Larger samples and varied contexts enhance reliability (and, therefore, validity).

Recording and Transcribing Observations

The three widely used means of recording clinical language samples are videotaping, audiotaping, and handwritten notes. Many clinics and schools have ready access to videotape equipment and use it routinely to record both assessment and intervention sessions. This method of recording is ideal because it can provide a record of context, facial expressions, and body movement as well as speech. Videotape can be transcribed to include all speech, context, body movement, and the like and enhances the likelihood of valuable and accurate (i.e., reliable) descriptions (see also Dollaghan & Miller, 1986).[*]

Next in preference, after videotaping, is an audiotaped recording of direct observations. This method is far less expensive and is less obtrusive in the environment, and the equipment is generally more portable; but audio recordings only provide a record of vocal interactions. Many experimenters and clinicians have managed to overcome this limitation in a number of ways. Some record much

---

[*] The transcription conventions that have been developed by Bloom and her research assistants for transcribing audiotapes are included in Appendix A.

information about context in side comments that are spoken softly into the recorder, or by comments to the child that mention context (e.g., the child says "help me" and the clinician responds "help you? you can't get the toy box open?"). These methods of describing the context help in the recall of the situation during transcription. Most observers have found that handwritten notes during the observation are necessary in order to obtain useful contextual data. These notes are coordinated with the vocal utterances as the tapes are transcribed.

It is important to note that audiotapes should be transcribed soon after taping by someone who was present at the observation and is, therefore, able to recall context and coordinate context with utterances. Furthermore, it is usually necessary to replay the tape a number of times in order to get an accurate transcription.

In both audio and video recording, clinicians and experimenters have found it useful to repeat many of the child's comments during the interactions in order to clarify what may not be intelligible when listening to the tapes. However, caution is needed in using this technique; repeating children's utterances can be overdone. If repetitions make the diectic shift (as the "you/me" in the previous example) and are expanded in some way (as in the addition of the question illustrated in the previous example), the interaction is more like a usual adult-child discourse than a clinical parroting and is less likely to be disruptive. Adult imitations of the child are also likely to elicit imitations from the child (Folger & Chapman, 1978), so their overuse might distort the child's use of imitation.

A last recording method that is frequently used, but is less accurate, is the hand transcription of utterances and contexts as the interactions take place. This method is particularly useful in situations where it is difficult to audiotape or videotape (e.g., on the playground or in the cafeteria, and when background noise may be too great to obtain clear voice recordings with ordinary recording equipment). The method can be used with children who produce few utterances or with those who speak primarily in single-word utterances. Handwritten recordings are less effective with the child who uses more language, particularly the child who speaks in more than three-word utterances, because of the limitations in the amount of information that can be written in a period of time. (Two exceptions may be stories that are dictated by the child with the express purpose of having you hand-record them and ongoing assessment when only one or two behaviors are of interest.) If handwritten transcription is the only feasible method of recording, it is helpful to write down (in the interests of time and expedience) every third or fourth utterance. The major shortcoming with on-the-spot hand transcriptions is questionable accuracy (e.g., determining if there really was an -s inflection attached to a word) and the problem of recording form at the same time as recording context or making judgments relative to content and use.

With practice in carefully transcribing many audiotapes and videotapes, some clinicians have found direct on-site hand transcription an effective way of obtaining information that otherwise would be lost—because of either time constraints or of situational limitations. Some speech-language pathologists perform their entire assessment in the classroom (e.g., Taenzer, Harris, & Bass, 1975; Taenzer, Bass, & Kise, 1974) by following the child, writing down as many utterances as possible, and coding some aspects of context in order to determine content and use. Obviously, much information is lost by this technique, but by collecting hundreds of utterances in continual assessment, some clinicians (e.g., Taenzer,

Harris, & Bass, 1975) have been able to describe children's language effectively in terms of the goals outlined in the previous chapters.

Hand notes may provide supplemental information for a language sample. For example, the evaluator may record utterances and their surrounding contexts from *show and tell* or *free play* activities in the classroom or from hallway conversations. When observations are geared to a specific question, such as a particular content/ form interaction or a certain aspect of use, recorded information is particularly useful. Given a specific category or utterance type to record, the observer does not have to take notes on *all* utterances and contexts. Belkin (1975) found that trained observers agreed well with transcriptions of audiotapes when they were asked to hand-record children's negation utterances in direct, low-structure observations. In an unpublished pilot project,° trained observers were able to hand-record examples of action utterances that correlated highly with the action utterances transcribed from a videotape of the same observation.

Thus, the use of handwritten notes as a method of recording behavior does offer possibilities to the overscheduled clinician who feels that tape-recorded observations are an extreme burden and therefore, language samples are an impossible assessment procedure. Videotaped or audiotaped observations are the preferred methods of recording language samples, but a record of utterances and context provided by on-site hand notes is better than no sample at all and is worthy of consideration if the limitations are fully recognized. Certainly for the student and the clinician who are inexperienced in language sampling and analysis techniques, practice with tape recording and careful transcription of language samples should precede reliance on hand notes. Audio or video recordings are also a necessity for the child who is not readily intelligible.

Preparing to Analyze Transcriptions of Direct Observations

Most clinical techniques used to analyze language samples are comparative analyses that describe the behaviors of the language-disordered child in relation to a predetermined taxonomy of language behaviors (i.e., an etic-type analysis). The taxonomy may have been derived from the adult model or from a child model (see Chapter 6). The disadvantage of comparative, or etic, analyses is that behaviors that are unique to a particular child's language system may be missed (see Lund & Duchan, 1983). This becomes more of a problem as the language system of the child deviates more from that of the comparative model.

The alternative to a comparative analysis is to derive categories for each child from the language samples available (an emic-type analysis). This was, in fact, the means by which the taxonomies presented in the C/F/U Goal Plan for Language Learning (Phases 1–8) were derived, using 6 to 8 hours of longitudinal observation of children who were developing language normally. It is the procedure that should lead to better understanding of language-learning problems. However, deriving new categories demands more data than comparative analyses and takes considerably more time and experience (see Chapter 2 of Bloom & Lahey, 1978, for further discussion of this type of analysis). Thus, it is not likely to be the

° Carried out in collaboration with S. Gozenbach at Montclair State College in 1975.

procedure used by clinicians with the majority of their language-disordered children. More important, the resultant information may or may not be useful for planning goals of intervention—describing a deviant system at one point in time does not automatically lead to a sequence for improving that system. At present, comparative (or etic) analyses based on developmental information are a useful clinical tool for planning goals of intervention. However, clinicians should keep in mind that for some children they may need to go beyond the etic analysis to obtain supplemental data with a more emic-type analysis of at least some aspects of language.

The comparative analysis described below is based on taxonomies of content, form, and use as well as interactions among these components. No matter what aspect of language is the focus of the taxonomies or how the taxonomies are obtained, the evaluator must have a criterion for deciding how many examples of a particular behavior will be necessary to make the judgment that a particular language behavior is a productive part of the child's language system.

Criteria of Productivity and Achievement

Goals of learning need to include criteria of acquisition as well as descriptions of the behaviors to be learned. In terms of language behaviors, a criterion can be one of productivity or one of achievement. Meeting a criterion of *productivity* would provide evidence that a behavior is systematic and is the product of the child's language system. Meeting a criterion of *achievement* would provide evidence that a behavior is used most of the time that it is expected to be used according to some standard, usually adult language usage, which is the ultimate goal of language learning.

Several different examples of a particular language behavior (e.g., two constituents to code a content category) can be taken as evidence that a content/form interaction has been established and is part of the child's productive language system. A stronger case is made for the induction of a rule if the different examples of each interaction combine lexically free words, that is, words that appear alone or in other multiword combinations, and if a variety of verbs are used to code verb relations (see Leonard, Steckol, & Panther, 1983). A specified number of different utterances can be used as a criterion reference (see Chapter 6), that is, a standard of performance that can be used in describing the child's performance in relation to the C/F/U Goal Plan for Language Learning. For example, if a child produces over five different utterances using more than one verb and lexically free nouns in verb-object word order to code action as a comment, it is assumed that the utterances are derived from knowledge of a rule. One could not be as confident that a rule for this content/form/use interaction was established if only one or two different utterances were produced, if the same token (such as "hit it") was uttered five times, if the utterances obtained were exactly the utterances taught in the same situation, or if they did not contain at least one lexically free word.

A criterion of five different utterance types was arbitrarily set by Lois Bloom and her associates (1970, 1975) as a criterion for assuming that a content/form interaction was productive. This criterion was based on 5 to 8 hours of data obtained from each child observed in the course of normal language development.

[Post hoc analysis (Bloom, Lightbown, & Hood, 1975) suggested the criterion was a reasonable one based on the increased frequency of use of behaviors after they met the productivity criterion.] Since samples used for clinical assessment are generally $\frac{1}{2}$ hour to 1 hour long, the criterion must be set at a lower number. It would seem that four *different* examples or utterance types in 1 hour may be taken as strong evidence (and three different examples as, perhaps, weak evidence) that a content/form/use interaction is established. Of course, if there are fewer occurrences of a behavior or none at all, there is still the possibility that the behavior would have occurred if the assessment sample had been longer or the context had been different.

The fact that an interaction is productive and, therefore, assumed established does not mean that it has been mastered or achieved. One way of estimating the achievement, or mastery, of a productive behavior is to compute the frequency of its use in contexts where its use is obligatory in the adult model. For example, when describing the sequence in which some children achieved control of morphological inflections, Brown (1973) used a criterion of 90% use in obligatory contexts for two consecutive samples. Thus, for productive behaviors, proportional measures can be used as an estimate of *achievement.* In clinical language samples 80 to 90% use of productive behaviors in obligatory contexts can be used to assume full achievement or mastery of a content/form/use interaction. Ideally, this level of achievement would occur in more than one sample.

To compute level of achievement, the number of utterances that include a particular content/form interaction (such as subject-verb-complement to code action) can be compared with the total number of utterances in which this interaction would be expected in the adult model (in our example, the utterances coding action where three constituents were obligatory). For example, if a child said "eat cookie," "mommy make cookie," "get pan," "me help mommy," in contexts where a subject was obligatory in the adult model, level of achievement regarding the use of three constituents to code action is 50% (i.e., two occurrences divided by four contexts). Although an interaction may be considered systematic, or productive, based on the production of four different utterances, low proportional frequency may suggest that the interaction should continue to be monitored or be included as a minor goal in order to increase the frequency of production. It is difficult to determine where on the C/F/U Goal Plan different levels of achievement should be expected for behaviors other than morphological inflections: the data available on the sequence of development relative to achievement are primarily limited to morphological inflections.

Unfortunately, not all language behaviors can be examined in terms of a criterion of achievement. It is not always possible to determine the *expected* number. For example, in collecting a naturalistic sample it is difficult to determine the number of expected instances of attribution coordinated with action utterances. Only given a context of alternatives (i.e., other similar objects) is attribution *expected* in an utterance. However, when feasible, a measure of achievement is useful for determining how well-established a behavior is in a child's system. Thus, it is suggested that, when possible, both frequency counts and proportional measures be used in analyzing a language sample.

Determining Which Level of Analysis to Use

Since the C/F/U Goal Plan for Language Learning spans development from pre-linguistic behaviors to complex narratives, it is obvious that the analysis will not be the same for each language sample. In the following sections, five levels of analysis will be described. The level of entry into the data can usually be estimated while listening to the child or when scanning the transcript. If analysis indicates that the chosen level is inappropriate, then further analyses will be needed.

The first level of analysis is a set of questions regarding nonverbal behaviors that are usually precursors to or concomitants of single-word utterances. This *Level 1* analysis would be important for the nonverbal child and the child who is producing only single-word utterances. The second level of analysis concerns early content/form/use interactions when form comprises mostly single words rather than syntactic combinations of words (i.e., the child is functioning at Phase 1). If the child in question produces words but few, if any, syntactic combinations of words, *Level 1* and *Level 2* are the preferred levels of analysis. *Level 3* focuses on the early syntactic combinations of words; it includes two-word syntactic utterances as well as simple sentences with embeddings (primarily Phases 2 through 5, with some interactions through Phase 8). When most of the child's utterances are multi-word-syntactic utterances, but few, if any, have more than one verb, this is the appropriate level of analysis. *Level 4* is concerned with joining clauses to form complex sentences (primarily Phases 5 through 8, with some interactions at Phase 4). When a child is producing more than four or five utterances that include at least two verbs or is sequencing clauses that are related, this level of analysis should be selected. Finally, *Level 5* entails production of narratives (Post Phase 8). When a child is sequencing many related clauses, this type of analysis might be attempted. Using these brief descriptions of the predominant forms a child used, the clinician can determine the level of analysis that seems most appropriate as an entry into the data. After completing assessment at that level, the clinician may consider another level as well. In most cases, no more than two levels of analysis will be necessary in order to plan immediate goals of intervention. These levels are summarized in Box 12-1.

Analyzing Direct Observations, Level 1: Co-occuring and Precursory Nonlinguistic Behaviors

The first level of analysis is concerned with the nonlinguistic behaviors that are relevant to the development of language content, form, and use and that are generally found in normal infants before or about the same time as they begin to speak one word at a time (see Chapter 9). It is unusual for clinicians to have transcribed observations of precursory nonlinguistic behaviors; descriptions are most often made as the evaluator interacts with the child or observes the child interacting with another person. It is helpful in such contexts to have a checklist of such behaviors and to note their presence or absence in particular time segments of an observation, or to judge their frequency of occurrence over the entire observation. One can simply list the behaviors of interest with spaces for noting their occurrence. An example of such a form is presented in Box 12-2.

BOX 12-1　Levels of Analysis

Level 1—Co-occurring and precursory nonlinguistic behaviors: To be used with prelinguistic children or children with a limited number of single-word utterances.

Level 2—Early coding of object and relational knowledge: To be used with children who use single-word utterances but few, if any, multiword-syntactic utterances. (Phase 1.)

Level 3—Coding of relations between objects: To be used with children who are producing more than five different multiword-syntactic utterances but few, if any, multiverb utterances. (Phases 2–5 with some behaviors through Phase 8.)

Level 4—Coding event relations: To be used with children who are producing more than five multiverb-syntactic utterances or are juxtaposing related clauses. (Phases 5–8 with some behaviors at Phase 4.)

Level 5—Coding relations among events with narratives: To be used when a child is sequencing many related clauses. (Post Phase 8.)

Since many of these behaviors may not occur in a single observation, multiple observations are desirable. When this is impractical, reported observations may be used. That is, the care givers may be asked whether or not the child ever shows evidence of particular behaviors (e.g., joining or separating objects, nonreduplicated babbling). On the recording sheet, distinctions should be made between evidence obtained through direct versus reported observations.

On the basis of such a worksheet as well as other information about the early social, cognitive, and physiological status of the child, hypotheses about precursory goals of intervention can be formulated. *Behaviors* that are not observed or reported and, therefore, appear not to be established are targeted as goals for further assessment or for intervention. For example, if direct observation and report indicate that a child has little interpersonal gaze and that it is possible but difficult to establish joint attention with the child, then these behaviors may become goals of intervention.

General Comments about Level 2 through Level 4 Analyses

In the following sections procedures for analyzing language samples will be presented. Box 12-3 (page 303) outlines some of the procedures that are common to each level. Box 12-4 (pages 304–305) provides a key for coding certain aspects of use at each level. Illustrations of the analyses at each level are presented in some detail in Appendix G based on data obtained from a language-impaired child, Bill, as he progressed through the various phases of the C/F/U Goal Plan. In Appendix G, worksheets for analyses are completed for this child, and goals of intervention are determined based on the information presented in the forms. Furthermore, some more general descriptions of the child's language are included. Appendix G should be referred to as you proceed through the rest of this chapter.

BOX 12-2 Level 1: Worksheet for Describing Precursory Goals of Content, Form, and Use

	Observation Number or Time Segment					
	1	2	3	4	5	6

Use

1. Gazing interpersonally
2. Focusing using joint attention
3. Taking turns
4. Making Reference
   a. Show object
   b. Give object
   c. Point out object
5. Regulating
   a. Reach toward
   b. Reach for object + vocalize
   c. Gesture to request help
   d. Gesture to request action
   e. Protest or reject
6. Other (specify)

Comments Regarding Use:

Goals of Use:

Content

1. Object search
   a. Gaze at moving object
   b. Look for reappearance
   c. Search for partially hidden object
   d. Search for object visibly displaced
   e. Search for invisibly displaced object
   f. Search for object during free play
   g. Search to relate one object to another
2. Disappearance—Hide objects
3. Action on an object
   a. Attend to adult action on object
   b. Imitate object—specific actions
   c. Limited object—specific actions
   d. Wide repertoire of object-specific actions
4. Object-to-object relations
   a. Separate objects
   b. Join object as presented
   c. Join objects, new Nonspecific way
   d. Join objects, new specific way

Other

(continued)

BOX 12-2   Level 1 (*continued*)

	Observation Number or Time Segment					
	1	**2**	**3**	**4**	**5**	**6**

Comments Regarding Content:

<u>Form</u>
1. Imitate
   a. Copies of child motor behavior
   b. Copies of child vocal behavior
   c. New behaviors can observe on self
   d. New behaviors cannot observe on self
2. Approximating adult linguistic forms
   a. Reduplicated CV sequences
   b. Nonreduplicated CV sequences
   c. Nonsegmental features

Comments Regarding Form:

<u>Nonconventional Interactions</u>
1. Consistent phonetic forms for contexts or functions

Overall Comments and Other Behaviors

Goals:

Key:
N = never   F = frequently
O = occasionally   No = no occasion for the behavior
XX = not clear, further observation necessary
R = reported by others, but not observed

Analyzing Direct Observations, Level 2: Coding Object Knowledge and Relational Knowledge with Single-Word Utterances

When a child is producing primarily single-word utterances, we are interested in knowing how many, if any, of the Phase 1 goals have been reached. To determine this, we will look at each utterance and describe the words used, the meanings coded with those words, the contexts in which the words are spoken, and the functions that they appear to serve.

Analysis 1

This first analysis of single-word-utterance development involves the use of conventional forms to denote adult-like semantic domains for various communicative

---

BOX 12-3   General Procedures for Analyzing a Language Sample

1. Transcribe the sample of language (see conventions for transcription in Appendix A).
2. Number each child utterance in the sample.
3. Determine level of first analysis (see Box 12-1).
4. Review relevant information on goals for that level (e.g., Chapter 9, 10, or 11).
5. Select appropriate worksheets for level of analysis (e.g., from Appendix G and H).
6. Review procedures for appropriate level (e.g., this chapter and Appendix G).
7. Select a key for abbreviating descriptions of different behaviors (see Box 12-4).
8. Complete coding on worksheets suggested for desired level (see sections that follow).
9. Review completed worksheets in terms of the C/F/U Goal Plan and criteria for productivity and achievement (see earlier section on criteria).
10. Note goals that are productive by filling in a summary sheet (e.g., Box 12-14) or by marking on an abstract of the plan (e.g., the chart presented in Chapter 8), as illustrated in Figure 12-1.
11. Select behaviors where further information is needed (see Chapter 13).
12. Select behaviors to become goals of intervention—behaviors that were not productive but that are expected at earlier levels, or adjacent levels to the productive goals.
13. Proceed to plan procedures for facilitating language learning relative to those goals.

---

functions. Development includes an expanded use of established words for different communicative functions (Gerber, 1987) as well as an increase in the number of words produced and understood. (Reread Chapter 9 for a review). Following our earlier discussion of *productivity*, we will look to see if our data include three or four different examples of behaviors for each goal specified in the C/F/U Goal Plan discussed in Chapter 8 and further elaborated on in Chapter 9.

In carrying out such an analysis, nouns cannot be placed into most relational content categories on the C/F/U Goal Plan since nouns alone do not code a relationship. The only category in which they are included is existence, and then *only* if it appears that the child is calling attention to or naming an object. Other instances of nouns should be categorized separately (e.g. under "other"), and the context of their use should be described. These contexts are important. The child who uses nouns in various contexts (such as naming an object that has disappeared), and also uses relational words in these same contexts (e.g., *gone*), appears more likely to move into two-word utterances coding these same relations than the child who uses nouns in limited contexts, or not at all, or the child who does not use relational words. Some utterances will not fit into any of the categories in the C/F/U Goal Plan. A number of potential categories were not included in the plan because, in the data on which the plan was based, these categories did not appear frequently at these levels of development, or because there was little developmental change in their use throughout the span of the plan. Such utterances can be

BOX 12-4   Abbreviations That Can Be Used
to Code Some Aspects of Use

LINGUISTIC CONTEXT

0		None. Prior utterance was too far removed to have been an impetus for the utterance under consideration.
FS		Child utterance follows (i.e., is adjacent to) another utterance.
	FSnc	Utterance is not contingent on prior statement.
	FSc	Utterance is contingent on prior statement
	FSc self	Utterance is contingent on prior utterance of child.
FQ		Child utterance follows question of another. Above subcategories of nc, c, and self are also added.
IPU		A large proportion of child utterance includes words that occurred in the preceding utterance.
	IPUr	In addition some recoding of prior utterance has taken place (e.g., changing of a noun to a pronoun, or deictic shift).
	IPUa	Information is added to the prior utterance —it could be words, phrases, or clauses. If there are many, these types of addition can be distinguished.
	IPUra	Child utterance includes words from prior utterance, recoding of some words in prior utterance, and additions to the prior uterance.

FUNCTION (see Appendix F for more complete definitions). Note that more than one function may be applied to an utterance.

Comment	Utterances identify or describe objects, persons, states, or events with no apparent function. Subcategories may, or may not, be necessary. Some that can be used include:
	Comment—Other (Interactive)
	When utterance appears directed to another.
	Comment—Self (Noninteractive)
	When utterance appears directed to no one.
	Comment—Label
	When function is to provide name.
Regulate	Utterances serve to regulate others and require a response.
	Focus Attention
	Draw attention to self, others, objects, or events.
	Direct Action
	Express a desire for some action to continue or to take place.
	Obtain Object
	Express a desire for some object.
	Obtain Response
	Requires a linguistic response from another (questions fit this description if they are not asking for information—that is, questions for affirmation, permission, etc.).

(continued)

BOX 12-4   Abbreviations (*continued*)

Obtain Information

> Require a linguistic response from another, as above, but with goal of obtaining information.

Protest/Negate — Utterances express objection or refusal of object or action.

Emote — Utterances express some emotion, such as joy or sadness.

Routine — This category includes stereotyped utterances used for greeting, for transferring objects, and in accompanying play (e.g., telephone); noises made with vehicles or animals and the like; songs and poems; vocal play; and repeated utterances that appear to serve no other function.

Discourse — Utterances serve to regulate and maintain conversation.

Acknowledge — Agree with or indicate one has heard the utterance of another.

Negate — Disagree with a prior utterance and perhaps offer an alternative.

Repair — Respond to evidence that a prior utterance was not understood.

Initiate — Attempt to get a turn in a conversational exchange or to start such an exchange.

Respond — Express utterances that are obliged by the utterance of another if they do not serve any other apparent function.

Imitate — Repeat the utterances of others, where the repetitions appear to serve no other function.

Pretend — Utterances involve pretend interactions (e.g., talking for the doll). These utterances may also be coded with another function.

Inform — Utterances about nonpresent events are intended to provide the listener with nonshared information.

Other — Categories are derived as necessary to describe particular children. With older children beyond Phase 8 many more categories will be essential.

Note: Categories have been adapted from a number of sources (e.g., Bloom, 1970; Bloom, Rocissano, & Hood, 1976; Dore, 1977, 1986; Gerber, 1987; Flax, 1986; Halliday, 1975; Longtin, 1984; McShane, 1980; Prutting & Kirchner, 1983).

described separately (e.g. under an "other" category) or can be ignored if they do not provide information that will influence goals of intervention. An illustration of the coding of single-word utterances can be found in Appendix G with a listing of derived goals; a sample of that analysis is included in Box 12-5. In Box 12-5 only the category of existence is illustrated, but the procedure would be the same for each of the Phase 1 categories. Note that under Form, the actual lexical items are written with the frequency of occurrence; under Use, both linguistic context and function are coded as well as a notation regarding whether or not there was perceptual support (i.e., the utterance was about the here and now).

BOX 12-5   Level 2

Sample of Analysis 1—Content/Form/Use Interactions in Single-Word Utterances

Child's Name <u>Bill</u>   Date <u>Sample-1</u>

Content	Form		Use		
Category	Item	Fre-quency	Linguistic Context	Perceptual Support	Function
Existence	I		0	+	Regulate—focus atten.
	I		FSc	+	Discourse—negate
	me	2	0	+	Comment—label
	baby	3	IPU	+	Acknowledge
	ma	2	0	+	Comment—label
	fish		IPU	+	Comment—label
	fish		0	+	Regulate—focus atten.
Nonexistence		·			
		·			
		·			

Analyses of other categories can be found in Appendix G.

On the basis of such an analysis, Phase 1 goals that are productive and goals of intervention for Phase 1 can be determined. For example, on the basis of the data in Box 12-5, it is apparent that coding of existence is productive in Phase 1. The child used five different lexical items to code the category. One might want to set a goal of increasing the variety of lexical items used to code this category (e.g., using relational words such as *this* or *that*). If few nouns are used in other contexts, one might want to increase the variety of nouns produced in many contexts including existence. Further information may be needed in some categories before goals can be determined. (See Appendix G for analysis of further information obtained from this child, and see Chapter 13 for more general suggestions.)

Analysis 2

If the child produces a limited number of conventional words, we may be interested in other behaviors that often occur early in the single-word-utterance period, and we may need to do two more analyses. Even though they do not directly lead to goals on the C/F/U Goal Plan, these analyses may help us in understanding what inductions the child has made about language content, form, and use and may lead to intermediary goals. For example, when a child is using only a few conventional forms, it would be interesting to see if these forms are broad or limited in their domain of reference in comparison with the adult model (i.e., overextended chained or holistic associations as described, for example, by Bloom, 1973, and Bloom & Lahey, 1978). No doubt this distinction will be difficult to make in a brief direct observation, but supplemental information from a caregiver may be helpful. Any overextended words can be analyzed separately and may provide specific contexts and goals for intervention (e.g., to limit or extend the domain of reference). See form in Appendix H.

Analysis 3

A last analysis is an elaboration of what was referred to under Level 1 as nonconventional interactions of form with content or use—that is, the production of consistent (but not conventional) phonetic forms (Dore, Franklin, Miller, & Ramer, 1976) in predictable contexts or for particular functions. While the presence or absence of such forms was noted in the Level 1 descriptions, the interactions are specified here in terms of their form, context, and function. Recognition of such interactions provides us with contexts, topics, and functions that can be used to facilitate inductions of conventional interactions. In the analysis illustrated in Appendix G, Bill did not use many conventional forms to request an object or action. The transcript was scanned to see if any vocalizations were associated with requests. It was found that a consistent phonetic form, the vowel [æ], was often associated with the category regulate—requests. Thus, intervention did not need to facilitate requesting behavior, but rather the goal was to code requests with conventional forms that were a part of his vocabulary. See form in Appendix H.

Play

In addition to the above descriptions, a short description of play behaviors should be obtained. It is particularly important when Level 1 analysis (of precursory behaviors) has not been carried out, but is useful in any event. Of particular interest as the child moves to Phase 2 is object-to-object play. On the basis of the available literature, we would expect children to show evidence of relations between objects through play and gesture at about the same time as, or even before, coding those relations with language. Thus, a description of this play behavior would help us to determine readiness for Phase 2 interactions of content, form, and use and to set goals for nonlinguistic behaviors.

Summary

In summary, the description of single-word utterances can involve three types of analysis. At first, all of the conventional forms are examined in relation to Phase 1 of the C/F/U Goal Plan for Language Learning. When the child has only a few conventional forms, the second level of analysis may be appropriate if the information is available. In this situation, the forms are examined to analyze their domain of reference and to determine whether they are associated with particular contexts or sensorimotor schemata rather than with content/use interactions. Finally, one might look for consistencies in form and context that are not conven-

---

BOX 12-6   Procedures for Level 2 Analyses

ANALYSIS 1: Content/Form/Use Interactions

1. Categorize all conventional words in terms of:
   1.1. Content categories coded in Phase 1—write the lexical item and its frequency of occurrence under the appropriate category.
   1.2. Discourse context (see Box 12-4 for categories and abbreviations).
   1.3. Perceptual support—(+) if present, (−) if not present.
   1.4. Function (see Box 12-4 for examples of categories).
2. List other nonrelational words (e.g., nouns not coding existence) under "Other," and describe context (see Appendix G).
3. Determine which categories of content and function are productive.
4. Summarize overall patterns and determine whether Analysis 2 and/or 3 is necessary.
5. If necessary, complete Analysis 2 and/or 3.
6. Write goals of intervention.

ANALYSIS 2: Overextended Forms

1. Interview parent for examples of word use for extended or limited domains of reference.

ANALYSIS 3: Consistent Phonetic Forms

1. Search data for repeated use of similar vocalizations that are not conventional words.
2. Examine context to determine if there is any consistent association of forms with context.
3. List any patterns on worksheet.

---

tional codings of content or use. This is particularly important when the child is using few if any conventional forms. See Box 12-6.

Children using only single-word utterances may not produce many words during one observation period. Supplemental reported observations together with supplemental direct observations are usually needed to fill in gaps of information. Moreover, the child's play behavior should be noted in terms of some of the precursory goals mentioned in Level 1 if that checklist has not been completed. Based on the combined information, goals of intervention can be derived. Continued observations (in the form of additional language samples, reported information, or observations directed at only particular behaviors) are used to modify and change these goals over time. When the child begins to produce more than five or six multiword syntactic utterances, the next level of analysis is appropriate.

Analyzing Direct Observations, Level 3: Coding of Relations between Objects with Early Syntactic Utterances

When a language sample consists of many multiword syntactic utterances but few utterances that include more than one verb, the content/form interactions are most likely similar to the behaviors described in Phases 2–5 of the C/F/U Goal

Plan for Language Learning. A method for analyzing these utterances is presented below.

As with Level 2, the goal of the analyses is to determine which content/form/use interactions are productive in the language sample and from that information to infer which behaviors the child is ready to learn. Analysis 1 at this level involves categorizing all utterances that include a verb relation (whether or not the verb is omitted). The focus is on the verb relations because eventually other categories are coordinated with these verb relations (e.g., eventually the child coordinates nonverb categories such as attribution with verb categories such as action: "I eat chocolate cookies").

Analysis 1: Verb Relations

The major verb relations coded with early syntactic utterances include *action, locative action, state, locative state, notice,* and *existence.*° The first step in analysis is to determine the appropriate content category for each utterance with a verb relation. Definitions of these categories are provided in Appendix E as well as Chapter 9.† Utterances coding each of the above verb relations are placed together for further analysis (as is shown for state utterances in Box 12-7 and for all categories in Appendix G).

Goals for each verb category are listed in the Summary of the C/F/U Goal Plan in Chapter 8 and elaborated on in Chapters 9 and 10. The objective of this assessment is to determine which of the behaviors in each verb category column is productive. Development within each category involves the number of major grammatical constituents (e.g., subject-verb-complement) that the child uses in coding the various relations as well as the number and type of other content categories (e.g., nonexistence, attribution, possession, quantity) that are included within utterances that code a verb relation. Certainly, developmental information should be reviewed (e.g., by rereading Chapters 9 and 10) before attempting to determine whether a child is productive with such goals.

To determine productivity of the goals listed under each verb category, all utterances coding the above-mentioned verb content categories are described in terms of their form (in this case, the number of constituents included in relation to those that are expected) and in terms of their coordinated content categories (that is, the coding of other content beyond the major subject-verb-complement relations). Whenever you find three or four unique productions of a behavior (e.g., two or three constituents coding some content category, or the coordination of other content categories within two or three constituent codings of a verb relation), the relevant goals are considered productive. A sample of Bill's coding of state is illustrated in Box 12-7 to demonstrate how such analysis might be handled (see Appendix G for a similar analysis of the entire sample).

Describing Use. In describing use, two factors are considered: the context in

---

° Epistemic is sometimes coded with early syntactic utterances, but usually it is not coded until multiverb relations are prevalent.

† Chapter 9 also includes both samples of the verbs used to code the categories and examples of children's utterances that code each category in Phases 2 and 3 (see Chapter 10 for examples in later phases). Furthermore, more explicit instructions and examples are presented in Appendix G with the illustration of a Level 3 analysis of data obtained from a language-impaired child, Bill.

which the utterance was spoken and the apparent function of the utterance. As noted in Chapters 1 and 8, this includes the nonlinguistic context (the degree of perceptual support, and the adaptation to the listener) as well as linguistic context (how the utterance related to prior utterances). Few utterances at this level are spoken without perceptual support or *use* alternative linguistic devices to adapt to the listener; if either occurs, the frequency of such use should be determined for each category.

BOX 12-7

Level 3

Language Sample Analysis Worksheet—Verb Relations

Content Category <u>State</u>   Child's Name <u>Bill</u>   Date <u>Sample-3</u>

Utterances[a]	Form Analysis					Use Analysis	
	S-V-C Constituents						
	Include		Expect				
	2	3	2	3	Comments	Linguistic Context	Function
Internal State							
97 oh no . want ani- mal out <u>my</u> truck	2		2		—subj. + talk for doll	0	Pretend— comment
200 want <u>yellow</u> one	2			3		FSnc	Obtain infor- mation
Further information from other data							
a. him fraid	2			3	—copula	FSc self	Comment
Attributive State							
92 all fill up <u>now</u>	2		2			FSc self	Comment
134 him crazy	2			3	—copula	FQc	Respond
137 mine's dead		3		3	talk for doll	FSc self	?
Frequency	5	1			4 = 2 constituents productive		
		↓		↓			
Proportion with 3 expected		1	÷	4	= 25% level of achieve- ment for 3 constituents		

(continued)

BOX 12-7   Level 3 Verb Relations-State (*continued*)

Coordinated categories (utterances that include 2 constituents plus another
category) =

Nonexistence	Recurrence	Rejection	Denial	Attribution	Possession	Quantity	Temporal	Specification	Other

200 (yellow)	97 (my)	92 (now)

COMMENTS: Weak evidence of productivity; increase coding internal state
with *want*.

PRODUCTIVE AT: Phase 3 (with 2 constituents)

GOALS: Phase 3 To: Increase coding with 2 or 3 constituents for
                      internal state (e.g., *want*)
                4 To productively code volition/intention (*want, go*)
                      plus action and/or locative action

*Numbers in front of utterances refer to the number of the utterance in the transcript.
Analysis of other verb relation can be found in Appendix G.

A judgment is made of the apparent function each utterance serves as well as
the linguistic context. Definitions of some functions and contexts can be found in
Box 12-4. Other descriptions can be used (see, for example, Chapman, 1981;
Gerber, 1987; Roth & Spekman, 1984a, 1984b). Comments should also be made
about the variety of lexical items (with emphasis on verbs) included within each
verb content category. It is sometimes apparent, when looking at a list of utterances that code a particular category, that the child has a limited repertoire and
that many of the utterances appear to contain unanalyzed chunks. Such observations should be recorded under Comments. Finally, the behaviors from the C/F/U
Goal Plan which are productive, based on this analysis, are listed, as are the goals
of intervention that follow from the productive behaviors; results of other analysis
may lead to goals not listed on this plan.

Following this analysis of verb relations, goals can be written for the verb categories of existence, action, locative action, locative state, notice, and, possibly, epistemic. However, it is not always clear which, if any, goals should be written for the
nonverb categories (i.e., nonexistence, rejection, denial, recurrence, attribution,
possession, quantity, time, and dative). In order to determine goals for these
categories, the data need to be reexamined in terms of each of these nonverb
categories.

Analysis 2: Nonverb Relations

The goal of this analysis is to determine the productivity of the following: Phase 2
goals for nonexistence, recurrence, attribution, and possession; Phase 3 goals for
quantity; Phase 4 goals for time and rejection; Phase 5 goals for denial, quantity,
and dative; and for time, Phase 6 goal for *now* and Phase 8 goal for *will*. Beyond

---

BOX 12-8

Level 3

Worksheet for Nonverb Category Analysis

Child's Name <u>Bill</u>   Date <u>5-3</u>

Content		Form		Use	
Category	No. of Times Coordinated	Other Examples[a]	Comments	Linguistic Context	Function
Nonexistence	3	10 no think	(2 times)	FSc	comment
		68 no head		0	comment

Types: *no* <u>4</u> ; *can't* <u>   </u> ; *didn't* <u>   </u> ; *not* <u>   </u>; other <u>1</u>

COMMENTS: He talked of nonexistence in relation to action, states, and objects.

PRODUCTIVE AT: Phase 2
GOALS: Coordinate nonexistence with action

[a] Number before utterances refers to the number of the utterance in the transcript.

---

these phases, goals for these categories are related to coordinations with verb relations or to relations between and among clauses. Box 12-8 illustrates an analysis of two of the nonverb categories, nonexistence and recurrence, for Bill's language sample (for the complete analysis, see Appendix G).

The first procedure for analyzing the productivity of nonverb categories is to count the number of times each category was coordinated with a verb category. If three or four unique examples of the coordination of any category are found, no further analysis is necessary; multiple coordinated examples would certainly indicate productivity for two-word utterances coding the category. However, for some categories (e.g., specification, quantity, and time), it will be necessary to specify the particular lexical items (i.e., *this/that, the, now, will*) or morphological inflections included in the C/F/U Goal Plan. If that particular lexical item or inflection is coordinated within the verb relation analyses in at least three or four different utterances, then that interaction would be considered productive at the appropriate phase (e.g., if the child used *now* with two different action utterances and with two different locative-action utterances, then Phase 6 coding of temporal with *now* would be considered productive).

When four coordinated examples are not found, the transcript must be searched for other instances of coding. Many of these nonverb content categories may have been coded in phrases that did not include two constituents of a verb relation. At first, one would look for syntactic coding (e.g., phrases like "more cookie" for recurrence), but if three or four unique instances are not found in syntactic utterances, single-word utterances would be need to be examined to discover whether the relation was coded at all.

BOX 12-9   A Sample Summary of Some Aspects of Use

In general, Bill's use of language was appropriate to his level of content/form interactions and in some cases was more advanced. For example, many of his utterances were contingent upon those of his mother. Bill used language to comment, regulate, and maintain the flow of discourse. These functions did not seem to be restricted to particular forms given his level of content/form development. Prosodic patterns appropriately stressed new or contrastive information as well as signaled yes/no questions and certainty versus uncertainty. A different register was produced for vocalizations that were a part of play with dolls and were not interactive with other persons; such utterances were less intelligible and were often spoken in a higher-pitched voice. Bill talked about the here and now—mainly about what he was doing, was about to do, or wanted others to do. With prompting he was able to answer questions about nonpresent events such as school and breakfast. He did not talk about the actions of others. Given these observations, a goal of use might be to increase the number of utterances about the actions of others.

Summarizing the Observations and Analyses

Worksheets should not *constrain* descriptions of a child. At the completion of any analysis, the clinician should make notes that help to summarize not only the formal analyses, but other *regularities* in behavior that have been observed. For a sample of such a description of use, see Box 12-9; for summaries on the Level 2 analysis of the entire sample, see Appendix G. Upon completion of these analyses, the goals for content/form can be plotted on the chart of the plan presented in Chapter 8, as represented in Figure 12-1. The chart provides a graphic illustration of where the child is functioning, and it can be used to illustrate progress. The analyses can also be summarized in a table such as the one presented in the next section (Boxes 12-13 and 12-14).

Ongoing Reassessment

In order to determine when particular goals have been reached and to plan new goals of intervention, reassessment continues as intervention proceeds. Ongoing assessment may be accomplished by periodically collecting language samples and repeating the analysis illustrated above. While complete periodic analyses of language samples provide extensive information, time constraints render such procedures impractical. In fact, such continuous sampling is not usually necessary. As with testing, complete transcription and analysis of a language sample is most important for initial planning and perhaps before decisions are made about terminating intervention. It may also be necessary to collect a new sample when moving from one level of analysis to another—for example, when moving from analysis of simple syntactic utterances to analysis of multiverb relations or to narratives. An alternative to a complete analysis would be to record and analyze only the behaviors that are of particular interest at the time. For example, continued observations of Bill would focus on those behaviors that have been goals of intervention, and if

USE — Goal Numbers* (Function / Context)	PHASE	EXISTENCE	NONEXISTENCE	RECURRENCE	REJECTION	DENIAL	ATTRIBUTION	POSSESSION	ACTION	LOCATIVE ACTION	LOCATIVE STATE	STATE
(For prelinguistic goals, see Chapter 10)	1	sw	sw	sw	(sw)	(sw)	(sw)	(sw)	sw	sw		
1,2 / 10, 3,4 / 11, 5,6 / 12, 7,8,9 / 13, 14	2	R + S	Neg + C, C + Neg	R + S, S + R			(Adj + N)	(N or P + N)	2 Constit.	2 Constit. V + Prep, Prep + N		
	3	(+ATTRIB.)					(+EXIST.)		3 Constit.	3 Constit.	2–3 Constit.	2–3 Constit. V="want"
above plus 15, 16 / 17, (18), 19, 20, 21, 22, 23	4	+RECURR. +POSSESS. "a" What Q	+Action	+EXIST +ACTION	(Neg + C)		+ACTION	+EXIST.	+ATTRIB.* +PLACE +NONEXIST* +RECURR.* +VOL/INT –ing irreg. past	VOL/INT V + s	+Prep "in" "on" Where Q	VOL/INT V–c+VP V = "want" "go"
	5	+Copula Who Q	"can't" "didn't" "not" (+LOC. ACT.)	(+STATE)	"don't" ACTION	Neg + C "not"	(+STATE)	N+s +ACTION +LOC. ACT.	+POSSESSION* +REJECTION* Multiple-Coord.	V +Prep.* +POSSESSION* (+NONEXIST.*) –ing		(+ATTRIB.) (+RECURR.) VOL/INT V+"to"+VP V="want" "like" "have"
above plus 24, 25, (26) / 27, 28, 29, 30, 31, 32, 33, 34, 35	6			(+LOC. ACT.)			(+LOC. ACT.)	(+STATE)	+ATTRIB.* (+RECURR.*)			(+POSS.)
	7							"What""How" Q				VOL/INT V+NP–"to"+VP V="want" POSSIBILITY "can"
	8											VOL/INT V+NP+"to"+VP V="want" OBLIGATION "should"
Chapter 11	8+											

*Numbers refer to number preceding each goal of USE in Chapter 8, pages 192–193.

FIGURE 12-1   A Summary of Level 2, 3, and 4 Analysis of Content/Form/Use of a Language-Impaired Child Based on Three Samples (see Appendix G)

KEY

R = Relational word	Inflect = Inflection
S = Substantive word	Dur = Durative
C = Content word	irreg. pst = irregular past
N = Noun	Habit = Habitual
V = Verb	Prep = Preposition
VP = Verb Phrase	Constit = major-grammatical constituents (subject-verb-complement)
NP = Noun Phrase	( ) = optional goal–can be postponed
Dem = Demonstrative	* = first productions may be with two instead of three constituents
Neg = Negative word	+ = plus
c = Connective	Rel Cl = Relative Clause
P = Pronoun	Cx = Context
sw = single word	Int = Intention
sent. = sentence	EXIST. = Existence
F = Function	LOC.ACT. = Locative Action
Vol = Volition	RECURR. = Recurrence
	POSSES. = Possession
	ATTRIB. = Attribution
	Coord. = Coordination

○ = Immediate goal
↗ = Increase frequency
⫽ = Partial evidence
▭ = Productive
? = Unclear information

QUANTITY (–s) (numbers)	NOTICE PERCEPTION	TEMPORAL	ADDITIVE	CAUSAL	SPECIFICATION	DATIVE	EPISTEMIC	ADVERSATIVE	COMMUNICATION
	2–3 Constit.	ASPECT V Inflect. +Dur –ing –Dur ireg. pst +Habit. –s							
"some" "many" "all"			VP+/–c+VP NP+/–c+NP c="and"	VP–c+VP	Dem+N Dem="this" vs "that"	N+N			
		"now" SEQUENCE VP+/–c+VP c="and"		OBJECTIVE VP+c+VP c="so""and" "because"	"the"	+Prep "to" "for"			
	V–c+NP+VP V="see""look"	VP+c+VP SEQUENCE c="then" SIMULTANEOUS c="when"		SUBJECTIVE VP+c+VP c="so""and" "because"	(Dem+(is)+c+VP) c="what" "where" (VP+c+VP) c="and"		V+c+NP+VP V+c="know what" "know where" V–c+NP+VP V–c="think"	VP+c+NP+VP c="and""but"	
	V–c+NP+VP (V–c="watch") ("show") V+c+NP+VP V+c="see what" "see if" "look what"	("When" Q) +TENSE - Aux= "is" "was" ("will") "-ed"		"Why" Q	(VP+c+Rel Cl) c="that"				(V+c+NP+VP) V="tell" "say" "ask"
		(Sent+Sent+++)	Sent+Sent+++	(Sent+Sent+++)					

they are productive, attention would shift to the next expected behaviors on the C/F/U Goal Plan.

For reassessment, the language sample need not be transcribed entirely; rather, it can be scanned for the behaviors in question, and only those relevant behaviors need to be transcribed and analyzed. Or the data could be hand-recorded during the observation with inclusion of the contexts necessary for categorizing content and use. It is not always easy to record while interacting with a child; such on-line recording is easier when observing others interacting.

These continued observations can be made in the child's classroom, in the lunchroom, during recess, or, if necessary, during a free-play period at the beginning or end of an intervention session. It is important to look for examples that provide evidence of productive use and not routines that have been a consistent part of the intervention process. Reported evidence of the production of particular behaviors in other contexts can often be obtained from the caregiver or from school personnel. For an example of reassessment using a later language sample, see Appendix G. Based on new data, the new productive behaviors and new goals could be marked on the chart (as had originally been done in Figure 12-1) or on the summary sheet, as is shown in the next section in Boxes 12-13 and 12-14.

This completes the Level 3 analysis (see an outline of procedures for Level 3 in Box 12-10). In the next level of analysis we will be looking at utterances that contain more than one verb.

Analyzing Direct Observations, Level 4: Coding Relations between Events with Complex Sentences

When a language sample contains more than five or six utterances with multiple verbs, or more than five or six successive utterances that are semantically related, an analysis of how these verbs are related to one another should be completed. The fourth and last videotaped sample of Bill was used to illustrate this type of analysis in Appendix G, and a part of the analysis is shown in Box 12-11.

The content categories of interest now are those that describe the meaning relation between the verbs (or propositions coded by a clause) in the child's utterances. These categories include volition/intention (under the state category), additive, temporal, causal, epistemic, specification, adversative, communication, and notice (see Appendix E and Chapter 10 for definitions and examples of these categories). The child may utter two related clauses within one utterance, as in utterance 3 in Box 12-11, or two clauses may be produced in separate utterances, as in utterances 62 and 63 in Box 12-11. Some utterances may include more than two verb relations. Separating the verbs (and their related arguments) and then bracketing them to note what other propositions (or verb relations) they are related to helps to sort out multiple verb relations.

In addition to knowing the content of the multiverb meaning relations that the child codes, we are interested in knowing the forms that the child uses. First, we can describe what, if any, connective forms (e.g., conjunctions, complementizers) that the child produces to code each content category. Second, we can describe the syntactic structures used to code the various relations (e.g., coordination, subordination, complementation, relativization, or successive utterances). These

---

BOX 12-10   Procedures for a Level 3 Analysis

ANALYSIS 1: Verb Relations

1. Set aside a sheet of paper (or worksheet) for each verb category: existence, action, locative action, state, locative state, and notice (and, if needed, epistemic).
2. Select all utterances with a verb relation and place each on the appropriate verb category sheet.
3. Describe the form of each utterance in terms of the number of major grammatical constituents (i.e., subject-verb-complement) included and the number expected given the contexts.
4. Describe the use of each utterance in terms of:
    4.1. Linguistic context (see Box 12-4 for categories and abbreviations)
    4.2. Function (see Box 12-4 for categories)
5. Describe additional relations coordinated with each:
    5.1. Underline any extra relations coded—that is, content categories present in *addition* to those coded by the subject, verb, and direct object (and place in locative action).
    5.2. Categorize underlined relations (i.e., the coordinated categories).
    5.3. List the coordinated categories for each verb relation with the number of examples.
6. Examine utterances for patterns: Consider variety of lexical items, variety of functions, linguistic contingency, etc., and comment on findings.
7. Determine and list goals that are productive for each verb category (as in Figure 12-1 or Boxes 12-13 and 12-14).
8. Determine goals of intervention and list these for each verb category.

ANALYSIS 2: Nonverb Relations

1. List all nonverb categories (i.e., nonexistence, recurrence, rejection, denial, possession, attribution, quantity, specification, temporal, dative)
2. List under each nonverb category the number of times it was coordinated with any verb relation.
3. If that number does not equal three unique examples, look in the data for other examples of the nonverb categories that were coded syntactically.
4. If coordinated examples plus additional examples of syntactic coding do not total three or four unique examples, mark syntactic coding as a potential goal of intervention and look for single-word coding of the relations (with the exception of specification and dative, which need multiword coding).
5. On the basis of the above, note which behaviors are productive and which should be goals of intervention.

Note: Goals of intervention are usually those nonproductive behaviors that are adjacent to or in earlier phases than productive goals.

---

need to be considered for each content category (see the comments at the end of the analysis in Appendix G). Finally, we are interested in describing how the child uses the utterances. In addition to the categories described earlier in this chapter, we are interested in whether the relations are always between two child utterances or whether they are sometimes between a child utterance and an utterance

BOX 12-11

Level 4

Worksheet for Multi-Verb Relations: Content/Form

Child's Name Bill _____   Date Sample 4 _____

Context of Sample Free-play with mother _____

Utterance[a]	V/I	Add.	Temp.	Caus.	Epi.	Spec.	Adv.	Comm.	Not.	Comments
3 I think / it fit up here					X					
4 I wanna / see / this happen	X								0	
6 can't race							0			
7 this one can										
20 see / how it rolls down									how	
62 you do it, mommy										
63 you took them out				X						
75 I go				X						
76 who crash on side / go again						X				
77 I go again				0						

	V/I	Add.	Temp.	Caus.	Epi.	Spec.	Adv.	Comm.	Not.	Comments
Totals	1	0	0	3	1	1	1		2	
− Obligatory connective (0)				1			1		1 how	
+ connective									1	

Key:

0 = missing obligatory connective
X = missing nonobligatory connective
V/I = volition/intention
Add. = additive
Temp. = temporal
Caus. = causal

Epi. = epistemic
Spec. = specification
Adv. = adversative
Comm. = communication
Not. = notice

[a] Number before each utterance refers to the number of the utterance on the transcript.

BOX 12-12 Procedures for Level 4 Analysis

1. Identify all utterances where one verb (and its arguments) is related to another verb (and its arguments).
2. List these utterances with each verb relation on a different line.
3. Bracket these lines to indicate which verbs are related.
4. Determine the content category that best describes each bracketed relation.
5. Write the connective form used for each relation. If no form was used, note whether a connective form was obligatory. (See Key in Box 12-11.)
6. Total the exemplars of each content category as well as the use of connective forms for that category.
7. Note the syntactic structure used to code the relations (e.g., complementation, coordination, subordination, relativization, or successive clauses) for each category. (This can be noted in the comments column or separately. The exact count beyond 4 or 5 is not necessary.)
8. Summarize descriptions and determine content/form goals that are productive and that should be goals of intervention.
9. Examine utterances relative to use as done in Level 3 if this has not been done for other data or if use appears different with these utterances. Adapt goals of use interacting with content and form accordingly.
10. Look for other patterns (e.g., aspects of content/form/use interactions in these multiverb relations in contrast to utterances with only one verb relation).

---

of another (a later developmental phenomenon). Of course, each verb relation within these utterances can also be described using Level 3 analysis procedures. This may, in fact, be necessary if other utterances have not indicated that goals relevant to Level 3 analysis are productive. A summary of procedures for Level 4 is presented in Box 12-12.

On the basis of the information obtained from this Level 4 analysis, the evaluator can determine which of the goals of the C/F/U Goal Plan are productive. The results of all of these analyses can also be summarized in a chart (see Figure 12-1) or listed in a table (see Boxes 12-13 on pages 320–322 and 12-14 on pages 323–324). The tables presented here summarize the analyses in Appendix G, noting in which sample (or it could be on what date) each goal was productive (P—) and when each was set as a goal (G—). For clinical purposes, such a chart could be used to indicate the history of a child's progression through the C/F/U Goal Plan.

Analyzing Transcriptions of Direct Observation, Level 5—Narratives

If a child's language behaviors are productive through Phase 8, it is time to consider goals for narrative development. When analyzing narratives (a Level 5 analysis), the unit of analysis can be composed of many sentences. Since it is the narrative as a whole that is being analyzed, multiple units (or narratives) are necessary for estimating a child's level of development and for setting goals of

BOX 12-13 Longitudinal Summary of Content/Form Goals, Phases 1–8

Child's Name <u>Bill</u>   Dates Included <u>Samples 1–4</u>

CONTENT	PHASE							
	1	2	3	4	5	6	7	8
Existence								
single words	P1							
rel. + subst.		G2-P3						
(+attrib.)			(G3)-P4					
+recurr.				G4				
+possess.				P4				
a				G4				
what Q				P4				
+ copula					P4-G4			
who Q					P4			
Nonexistence								
single words	G1, 2-P3							
neg. + C		G2-P3						
can't					P4			
didn't					P4			
not					P4			
Recurrence								
single words	G1, 2-NR3							
rel. + subst.		P3						
Rejection								
single words	P1							
neg. + C				P3				
don't					G4			
Denial								
single words	(G1, 2)-P3							
neg. + C					P4			
not					P4			
Attribution								
(single words)	(G2)-NR3							
(adj. + N)		P3						
Possession								
(single words)	(G2)-NR3							
(N or Pn + N)		P-3						
-s					G4			
Action								
single words	G1-P2							
2 constit.		G2-P3						
3 constit.			P3					
+attrib.				G3-P4				
+place				G3-G4				
+nonexist.				G3-P4				
+recurr.				G3-X4 ↗				
+vol./int.				G3-P4				
-ing				G3-P4				
irreg. past				G3-P4				
+poss.					P4			
+reject.					P4			
+Multiple Coordinations					G4		P4	
+wh Q								

(continued)

BOX 12-13 Content/Form Summary (*continued*)

CONTENT	1	2	3	4	5	6	7	8
Locative Action	G1-P2							
single words		G2-P3						
2 constit.			P3					
3 constit.								
+vol./int.				G3-P4				
3rd person -s				G3-P4				
V + prep.					P4			
+poss.					P4			
(+nonexist.)					XG4			
-ing					P4			
+attrib.						G4		
(+recurr.)						(G4)		
Locative State								
2–3 constit.			G3-P4					
in, on				P4				
where Q				P4				
State								
2–3 constit.			G3-P4					
V−c+VP				P4				
(+attrib.)					P4 ↗			
(+recurr.)					P4 ↗			
V+*to*+VP					P4			
+poss.						P4		
V+NP−c+VP							G4	
can							P4	
V+NP+*to*+VP								——
should								——
Quantity								
(-s, #s)			X3-P4					
some, many, all					P4			
Notice Perception								
2–3 constit.				G3-P4				
V−c+NP+VP							P4	
V+c+NP+VP								P4
Epistemic								
V+c+NP+VP								
V=know						G4+c		
V−c+NP+VP								
V=think							P4	
Temporal								
Tense								
reg. past							P4	
aux.							——	
now						P3		
VP+/−c+VP						P4		
c=and						G4		
c=then							(G4)	
c=when							——	
when Q								X
(will)								——
Additive								
VP+/−c+VP					P4			
NP+/−c+NP					P4			
Dative								
N+N					G4			
+prep.						——		
Causal								
VP−c+VP					P4			
VP+c+VP								
objective						G4		
subjective						——		
why Q							P4	

(*continued*)

CONTENT	PHASE							
	1	2	3	4	5	6	7	8
BOX 12-13 Content/Form Summary (*continued*)								
Specification								
dem+N					P3			
the						G4		
(dem+[is]+c+VP)							G4	
(VP+c+VP)							G4	
(VP+c+rl. cl.)							___	
Adversative								
VP+c+NP+VP							P4	
Communication								
(V+c+NP+VP)							___	

Key for filling in Summary Sheet

G = goal	P = productive	# = date or sample
X = partial evidence	NR = not relevant	↗ = increase frequency

Key to Content Column

rel. = relational	irreg. = irregular	dem. = demonstrative
subst. = substantive	V = verb	rl. cl. = relative clause
Q = question	prep. = preposition	Pn = pronoun
neg. = negative	c = connective	+ = plus
C = content word	VP = verb phrase	− = minus
adj. = adjective	NP = noun phrase	/ = or
N = noun	reg. = regular	( ) = optional goal
constit. = constituents	aux. = auxiliary	

intervention. Furthermore, multiple examples of different types of narratives should be obtained (e.g., recounting a personal experience versus making up a story), and different contexts of presentation should be sampled (e.g., a listener who has shared the experience versus one who has not, or a peer versus an adult listener). When differences occur among contexts, intervention goals need to be set relative to each of the contexts and narrative types.

The analysis suggested here is based on a set of questions that relates to goals after Phase 8 as set forth in Chapter 11. Before beginning the analysis, Chapter 11 should be reread so as to become familiar with the sequence of intervention goals. In most cases, an estimate of narrative level and of goals of intervention can be made using the questions on the worksheet, and a sentence-by-sentence categorization is not necessary.

Analysis 1: Content/Form

The first analysis is involved with the content/form interactions expressed in the narrative. It focuses on the logical/temporal structure, or the coherence of the narrative. The first procedure is to determine if the narrative is an additive chain, a temporal chain, a causal chain, or a multiple causal chain. By answering the questions in Part I of the worksheet illustrated in Box 12-16, you should be able to make such a determination, as well as determine which subtype of additive, causal, or multiple causal chain best describes the narrative. When a number of narratives have been analyzed in this manner, goals for level of narrative development can be determined. For example, if a child is producing mostly additive chains with only

BOX 12-14   Longitudinal Summary of Use, Phases 1–8

CHILD'S NAME <u>Bill</u>   Dates Included <u>Samples 1–4</u>

	Phases			
	Prelin-guistic	1–3	4–5	6–8

FUNCTION

Indicative	<u>NR</u>			
Comment				
Interactive		<u>P1</u>		
Noninteractive		<u>P1</u>		
Label		<u>P1</u>		
Regulate	<u>P1</u>	<u>G1, 2-P3</u>		
Focus atten.	<u>NR</u>	<u>P1</u>		
Obtain obj.	<u>NR</u>	<u>X1-P3</u>		
Obtain action	<u>NR</u>	<u>X1-P3</u>		
Obtain response	<u>NR</u>	<u>P1</u>		
Obtain information			<u>P3</u>	
Routine	<u>NR</u>	<u>P1</u>		
Protest	<u>NR</u>	<u>P1</u>		
Respond	<u>NR</u>	<u>P1</u>		
Inform				<u>P4</u>

CONTEXT

Nonlinguistic

Perceptual support				
+here and now		<u>P1</u>		
Some immed. past			<u>G3-P4, G4</u>	
−here and now				<u>P4, G4</u>
Talk about				
Actions of self		<u>P1</u>		
Actions of others			<u>G3-P4</u>	
Listener needs				
Repair—phonetic		<u>P3</u>		
Repair—deletion			<u>?</u>	
Repair—substitution				<u>?</u>
Deitic forms				<u>P4</u>
Politeness markers				<u>P4</u>
Attention getters				<u>P3</u>
Explicit information				<u>?</u>

Linguistic

Adjacent utterances				
Most frequent		<u>1</u>		
Nonadjac. more frequent				<u>4</u>
Contingent on another utterance				
By context		<u>1</u>		
Add info-words		<u>P2</u>		
Add info-clause				<u>P4</u>
Recode			<u>P3</u>	

(continued)

BOX 12-14 Summary of Use (*continued*)	Prelin-guistic	1–3	4–5	6–8
			FUNCTION	
Contingent on another utterance (continued)				
Repeat/add			P3	
Repeat/recode/add				P4
Request confirmation			P3	
Other query				P3
Little imitation				1
Contingent on own utterance				
Few			P3	
More				P4
Anaphoric ellipsis				X4

Key:
NR = not relevant   ? = not enough information
P = Productive   X = partial evidence
G = Goal   1-4 = sample number

one or two temporal or causal chains, the goal would be to increase the number of temporal chains. If the child is producing abbreviated or automatic causal chains, the goal of intervention might be to work on developing causal chains that include goals of an animate being (see Chapter 11).

When causal chains are common, it is helpful to look at some of the internal structure of the causal chain to see if facilitating the inclusion of any subcategories (see Part II Box 12-16) of these might improve the quality of the child's narratives. Subcategories of causal chains are examined in Part II. To illustrate such an analysis, the narrative in Box 12-15 is analyzed on the Narrative Assessment Worksheet presented in Box 12-16. The answers given on the worksheet relate to a sample narrative presented in Box 12-15; when numbers are included to support an answer, they refer to the numbered segments of that narrative.

Analysis 2: Use Interacting with Content/Form

The second analysis of narratives investigates the child's ability to take into account the listener and the linguistic context. Part III of the Worksheet concerns adaptations that make a narrative interesting and help the listener "get the point." The questions in Part IV examine the child's skills at forming a cohesive narrative. The answers to questions in both of these sections need to be placed in a developmental framework, such as is presented in Chapter 11, in order to derive goals of intervention.

In the comment sections, further descriptions can be included. Some of these may not directly relate to goals as presented in Chapter 11 (although new develop-

---

BOX 12-15   Sample Narrative Elicited by an Unfamiliar Adult Asking the Child to "Tell Me a Story Either Real or Imaginary"

1. One time when we were camping, m-me, my dad, and my friends and th-my dad's friends.
2. my-we were going on the to ride on the— in a boat
3. that my dad made.
4. and my dad's friend was waterskiing
5. and my dad was driving
6. and we went and me -n- my friend were in the back
7. and we started driving real fast
8. and then, um, something hit the bottom of our boat
9. and we started sinking
10. and my dad didn't know
11. until me and Quinn, my friend, told him
12. that we started going under
13. so then my dad, he threw out these cushions
14. these big cushions that can float
15. and then, so we all jumped on them
16. and I jumped on one of those
17. cause I didn't know how to swim
18. so then I was just floatin'
19. and then my friend, when it crashed,
20. he was on the tip
21. and he dived off onto another cushion.
22. and then this other guy came in a big boat with a giant motor
23. and he he picked up all of our stuff
24. and he got all the cushions and stuff
25. and he brought us back
26. That's all.

Note: From Lahey and Launer, 1986.

---

mental information may enable you to expand those goals). However, further descriptions sometimes help in understanding the problem with, or the strength of, a particular narrative and why one narrative may seem different from others that have been observed.

When the narrative assessment worksheet has been completed for a number of narratives, the results can be placed on a summary sheet from which goals of intervention can be derived. An example of such a worksheet can be found in Table 12-1, which illustrates summary information and indicates the behaviors that could be expected next and are thus the goals of intervention.

One consideration in evaluating the narratives of a child is the style of narration that is evident in the child's culture: the home, neighborhood, etc. If the child's narrative is not complex in terms of the goals of intervention specified here, but is well formed in terms of the child's culture, we have a language difference and not a language disorder. Should the decision be made to teach the child another style of narration, it must be clear to the child and the educators that one style is not

BOX 12-16 Level 5—Narrative Assessment Worksheet

NAME Joe _____ CONTEXT "tell me a story" _____

EVALUATOR _____ DATE _____ SAMPLE NUMBER _____

LOGICAL-TEMPORAL STRUCTURE—Content/Form

PART I. *OVERALL LEVEL*

A. Were the propositions in the text essentially independent so that they could be moved about within the text without changing the meaning? If so, this narrative falls in Level 1 as an *additive chain* and only the following subquestions of A need be answered.   no _____
   1. Was there more than a listing?   _____
   2. Were there any actions?   _____
   3. Was there a theme such as repetition of action, person, or place?   _____
   4. Did the propositions describe a person or place?   _____

B. Were some of the propositions sequentially related (that is, rearrangement of them would change the order of events that occurred), yet there was no cause-or-effect relation among them? If so, this narrative falls in Level 2 as a *temporal chain*.   no _____

C. Was a problem or some disequilibrium described to which other propositions were causally related (by enabling or causing other states or events)? If so, the questions below should be answered. If only one such unit, or episode, is included, this narrative falls in Level 3 as a *causal chain* and D need not be answered.   yes _____
   1. Was this basically a statement of a problem and some aspect of consequence with much information omitted (e.g., plans, goals, and perhaps even resolution)?   no _____
   2. Was the causal chain automatic and not related to goals or plans of another?   no _____
   3. Was the causal chain free of an obstacle between complication and resolution?   yes _____
   4. Did an obstacle intervene in the process of trying to reach the goal?   no _____

D. Was there more than one causal chain or episode? If so, the narrative falls in Level 4 as a *multiple causal chain* and the subquestions below should be answered.   no _____
   1. Were the two episodes related in an additive or temporal fashion and not causally linked?   _____
   2. Did any of the episodes provide the cause, effect, or motivation for another episode?   _____

OVERALL LEVEL ASSIGNMENT <u>Causal—Obstacle</u>

(If the narrative is an additive chain or a temporal chain, omit Part II. Move to Part III.)

(continued)

BOX 12-16   Level 5 (*continued*)

PART II. *SUBCATEGORIES OF CAUSAL CHAINS*

A. INITIATING EVENT OR COMPLICATION: Was there some change in the environment that served as a complicating event or problem of some sort?   yes—#8, 9

B. SETTING: Was information presented that allowed the initiating event to occur and set expectations and conditions for what followed?   yes—#2, 5, 6

C. REACTIONS: Were the events that followed the initiating event causally related to that event?   yes

If so, were they related to the planning or goals of a person rather than to automatic or unplanned results?   yes

(If not, skip D and E and move to F, Consequences.)

D. INTERNAL RESPONSE: If a person was involved:
  1. Were the changes of state and thoughts of the person described?   no
  2. Were the goals of the person described or easily inferred?   yes—#13, 15, 21
  3. Were the plans of the person described or easily inferred?   yes—#13, 15, 21

E. ATTEMPTS: Were the attempts to resolve the problem specified or easily inferred?   yes—#13, 15, 21

F. CONSEQUENCE OR RESOLUTION:
  1. Was the complication resolved in some way?   yes—#22–25
  2. If there were goals, were you told if they were achieved?   yes—#18, 25
  3. Were you told how the experience ended?   only—#25

COMMENTS ON SUBCATEGORY ANALYSIS (including strengths and weaknesses)

All components were present, but internal responses had to be inferred; it was not clear if the pickup by another boat was in any way the result of a plan, or attempts, or was a reaction. We never know what happened to the boat. The story could have been expanded into two episodes if the rescue segment had been developed.

PART III. *TAKING ACCOUNT OF THE LISTENER CONTEXT—Form/Use*

A. OVERALL—Was the narrative presented in a way that was interesting and easy to follow?   moderately so

B. ORIENTATION:
  1. Did the initial orientation give you enough information to understand what had happened?   yes
  2. Did you understand who was involved and where and when the event took place?   enough
  3. Did you know enough about the people and places to feel that you understood the point of the narrative?   yes

C. BEGINNING:
  1. Did the narrator start with some attention getter or stylized beginning so that you knew that a narrative was to take place?   yes
  2. Did the narrator present an abstract of the narrative before giving details?   no

(continued)

BOX 12-16   Level 5 (*continued*)

D. ENDING:
1. Did the narrator let you know that the narrative was
   over?   yes—#26
2. Did the narrator inform you of any long-range
   consequences of the events?   no

E. EVALUATIONS:
1. Do you know how the narrator felt about the
   complicating event?   no
2. Did the narrator provide suspense during the   yes—#10,
   narration by stopping the sequence of action at the   11, 12, 14,
   high point and elaborating?   17, 20
3. Did the narrator use a variety of techniques to
   evaluate the events?   a few

COMMENTS ON PRESENTATION RELATIVE TO LISTENER CONTEXT (You
might comment on the possible role of listener interaction in the presentation,
the role of the child's apparent involvement in the narration, and the effect of
the flow of presentation (e.g., false starts, self-corrections) on ease of following
the narrative.)

*Some indication of feelings would have heightened interest, but generally Joe's
narrative was interesting and easy to follow.*

Part IV. *TAKING ACCOUNT OF LINGUISTIC CONTEXT AND LISTENER
           (COHESION): Form/Use*

A. Did the child use reference?   yes
   If so:
1. Was the original referent easily retrievable?   yes
2. Was the referent usually retrieved:
   a. From the context (exophoric)?   no
   b. From prior text (anaphoric)?   yes—e.g.,
                                                              2-"we"
           15-"them," 25-"us," 19-"it," 23-"he," 16-"those"
   c. By shared culture?   no
   d. By bridging?   no
B. Did the child use ellipsis?   yes—e.g., 5,
                                                              6, 10, 20

   If so:
1. Was appropriate information assumed and omitted?   yes
2. Could presupposed information be easily retrieved?   yes
C. Did the child use conjunction?   yes
   If so:
1. Were linked clauses semantically related?   yes
2. Were appropriate conjunctions used to express the
   relations?   yes
3. Were conjunctions other than *and* and *and then* used? yes,
                                                              17-"cause,"
           11-"until," 13, 18-"so then," 15-"so," 1, 19-"when"
                                                              (*continued*)

BOX 12-16   Level 5 (*continued*)

D. If the child used lexical cohesion or reference,
   1. Were many different referents tied or thematized   "boat," _____
      with these devices?   "friends," _____
                                                              "cushions," "Dad,"
   2. Were they tied frequently throughout the narrative?   yes, e.g., _____
                                                              "Dad"- _____
                                      2, 3, 4, 5, 10, 13, and see below
   3. Was there ever more than a one- or two-clause   yes: "boat"-
      distance between original mention and remention?   2, 8; _____
           "friend"-1, 4, 6, 11; "cushion"-13, 15, 16, 21, 24; "Dad"—above
   4. Were rementioned referents members of different
      grammatical categories from the original mention and
      from each other?   no _____
E. Did the child use Parallel Structures?   yes _____
   If so:
   1. Was the lexical content and structure of the entire   no _____
      clause the same (global parallelism)?
   2. Was the lexical content and structure the same for   no _____
      verb phrase only (lexical parallelism)?
   3. Was verb phrase structure similar, but lexical content sometimes _____
      different (structural parallelism)?   (e.g. 4 & 5)

COMMENTS ON USE OF COHESIVE TIES: (Note that types of lexical cohesion are not included above because there is little information on developmental changes in its use. You may want to comment on whether cohesion was evident primarily in repetition of the same word or in use of related words. Various types of reference were not included for the same reason, but you might want to describe whether most were pronouns, demonstratives, or comparatives.)

Most referents were pronouns, and there was quite a variety. Adaptation to the listener is evident in self-corrections (e.g., change of "the" to "a" in line 2 and identification before (or right after) use of a pronoun (e.g., 1, 13, 19, 22). The only confusion was in the appearance of "friend" in the back and on the front of the boat; though in line 1 he said "friends," this could have been clarified by "another friend." The frequency of and could have been reduced. Lexical cohesion was primarily achieved by repetition.

ADDITIONAL COMMENTS NOT DIRECTLY RELATED TO GOALS (Include frequency of subordinating clauses used throughout, problems with tense markings or shifts, etc.)

Past tense used throughout with past progressive for orientation. Most structures were coordinated; relative clauses in lines 3, 14; subordinate clauses in lines 1, 17, and 19 and changed to one in 15; and a complement in line 1.

SUMMARY: *Narrative would have been improved if the following had been incorporated: internal response including plans and goals; further information on what happened to the boat and any consequences; evaluations that included feelings of the narrator; and decreased use of coordinate structure. The rescue operation could have been expanded to another episode. Strengths lay in the use of cohesive devices, orientations, and the building of some suspense with evaluations.*

TABLE 12-1 Narrative Assessment Summary Sheet

Name <u>Joe</u>   Contexts of Samples <u>1 & 2, tell story; 3–5 prompts in a conversational</u>
<u>setting; all told to an unfamiliar listener in a school setting</u>

	Narrative Sample				
	1	**2**	**3**	**4**	**5**
Form/Content Interactions					
Additive Chain					
Listing					
Concatenated actions					
Theme					
Description					
Temporal Chain				X	
Causal Chain					
Abbreviated					
Automatic			X		
Goal − obstacle	X	X			X
Goal + obstacle					
Multiple Causal Chain					
Additive or temporal					
Causal					
Subcategories of Causal Chains					
Setting	X	X	X		X
Complication	X	X	X		X
Internal response:					
Plans and goals	I	I	0		I
Attempts	X	X	0		X
Resolution	N	X	X		N
Form/Use Interactions					
Beginning			0		
Stylized	X	X		X	X
Abstract					
Orientations					
Limited					
Full information	X	X	X	X	X
Evaluations					
Implied			X	0	
Stated	X	X			X
Variety	L	L	L		L
Endings					
Stylized	X	X	X	X	X
Consequences					
Reference					
Exophoric					
Anaphoric	X	X	X	X	X
Other					
Conjunctions					
and, then		X	X	X	
Other	X				X

(continued)

TABLE 12-1 Narrative Assessment Summary Sheet (continued)

	Narrative Sample				
	1	**2**	**3**	**4**	**5**
Ellipsis					
Given information	X	0	X	X	X
Anaphoric	X	0	X	X	X
Rementioned					
Referents					
Freq. of diff. ref.	4	3	6	5	4
Freq. of repetition	F	F	F	F	F
Grammatical cat.	same	same	same	same	same

OTHER COMMENTS: (e.g., possible cultural patterns of narratives)

GOALS OF INTERVENTION:
    Causal chains with obstacle, and multiple causal chains
    Further development of specification of plans and goals
    Further development of evaluations, particularly internal states of characters
    Further development of conjunctions other than *and* and *then*

KEY
X = evidence of this behavior   N = needs further work
I = inferred   L = little
0 = no occurrence   F = frequent

replacing the other, but is an alternative style that may be useful with different listeners. A summary of procedures for Level 5 analysis is presented in Box 12-17.

Alternative Procedures and Further Comments

As mentioned in Chapter 8, there are a number of alternative plans for language learning based on developmental information. Not all the plans have specific procedures for analyzing a language sample. Those marked with * in Box 8-1 include some procedural instructions for determining which goals of intervention are relevant to a particular child. A comparison of the goals derived from some of these procedures on the basis of analyzing one language sample can be found in Bloom and Lahey (1978) and in J. Miller (1981). In addition, there are some computerized programs for analyzing the form of language samples (e.g., SALT and *Linquest I*). Such programs are efficient means of determining lexical diversity and the presence or absence of various forms, such as grammatical morphemes. So far as I know, none have placed these analyses into a developmental framework (or any framework) that directly leads to goals of intervention. Nor, to my knowledge, have any yet attempted to analyze content or use.

    Procedures, and indeed the plans themselves, are only guidelines, to be varied according to the preferences of the user. Procedures are most helpful when first

---

BOX 12-17   Procedures for Level 5 Analysis

1. Collect a number of narratives in different contexts and about different topics.
2. Transcribe and number clauses.

ANALYSIS 1: CONTENT/FORM

1. Determine type of chain as well as subtype (if relevant) for each narrative (i.e., complete Part I of the worksheet in Box 12-16).
2. For narratives with causal chains, examine the subcategories (i.e., Part II of the worksheet).
3. Place results on the Narrative Assessment Summary Sheet (see Table 12-1).
4. Compare all narratives and determine content/form goals of intervention given a developmental framework (e.g., Chapter 11).

ANALYSIS 2: USE INTERACTING WITH CONTENT/FORM

1. Consider the child's adaptation to listener interest and ease of understanding in each narrative (i.e., Part III of the worksheet).
2. Comment on the possible role of listener interaction, context, etc., on the above results.
3. Analyze the cohesiveness of each narrative (i.e., Part IV of the worksheet).
4. Make any comments that would help understand the findings on cohesion.
5. Place findings on the Summary Sheet (Table 12-1) and determine general trends and patterns.
6. Determine goals of intervention given a developmental framework (e.g., as found in Chapter 11).

---

using a plan; they are often revised and shortened when the evaluator is comfortable with a plan and with analyzing language samples in general. Suggesting procedures is a risk; some may assume that if they follow the procedures, no further thinking or analysis is necessary. This is rarely the case. The procedures help you to make a first pass at the data and present the data in a format that may enable you to examine the information more closely. One should always look at the results with the idea that some further analysis may be helpful. The comments sections on each worksheet can be used to record other thoughts about the data.

Some have suggested that the errors children make should be categorized (e.g., Kretschmer & Kretschmer, 1978). For children whose language productions are unlike those of normal language-learning children at any point in development, this may help in understanding the inductions that a child has made. From such understanding, it may be easier to develop procedures that will foster development of different inductions. A categorization of errors can, however, lead to a focus on the elimination of errors in intervention, at the expense of facilitating developmentally appropriate content/form/use interactions. For example, at one time, the presence of frequent imitations became a focus of intervention, with the goal of extinguishing the behavior. More recently it has become clear that imitation decreases as the child learns more of the content/form/use interactions in language (e.g., regarding non-language-impaired children, see Bloom, Rocissano, & Hood, 1976; regarding language-impaired children, see Howlin, 1982; Shapiro, Chiarandini, & Fish, 1974) and may serve some communicative function for autistic children (see Prizant & Duchan, 1981). It would appear that goals of intervention should concentrate on facilitating developmentally appropriate content/form/use interactions rather than on extinguishing errors or communicative behaviors judged to be inappropriate.

Summary

This chapter considers the use of information obtained from low-structure observations in determining goals of language learning. A number of general issues are discussed, including consideration of context, length of observation, and means of recording the language observed. A variety of contexts is recommended, and some suggestions are made for designing contexts according to the behaviors to be observed. Suggested methods of recording are, in order of preference: videotaping, audiotaping, and hand recording. Five levels of analysis are discussed: Level 1, Co-occurring and precursory nonlinguistic behaviors; Level 2, Early coding of object and relational knowledge with single-word utterances; Level 3, Coding of relations between objects with early syntactic utterances; Level 4, Coding of event relations with multiverb utterances, or early complex sentences; and Level 5, Coding relations among events with narratives. A checklist is suggested for the Level 1 analysis of behaviors that are precursory to language learning. Worksheets illustrate the analysis of content/form/use interactions when a child is producing primarily single-word utterances, early syntactic utterances, or complex sentences (i.e., Levels 2–4). A questionnaire is introduced for the Level 5 analysis of narratives. Finally, summary tables are presented for indicating, on the basis of repeated samples, which behaviors are productive and which will be goals of intervention. Further examples of some of these analyses are presented in Appendix G and blank forms can be found in Appendix H. The procedures suggested here are not a clinical panacea; the thinking clinician must evaluate the results and summaries, probe for further information, and tailor goals and intervention procedures to the individual needs, interests, and cultural background of the child. The next chapter discusses probes for eliciting further information.

Suggested Readings

Read some of the Alternative Plans summarized in Appendix C.

13

Determining Goals of Language Learning From Elicited Information

Information about what a child does with language is best obtained in contexts that are both representative of the child's everyday life and relatively free of observer-imposed constraints, or what was referred to in Chapter 6 as direct observation in a low-structure naturalistic context. Other information is, however, often needed to supplement the language sample that has been obtained in a relaxed structure. Certain content/form/use interactions that were expected to occur given the child's other behaviors may not appear in spontaneous speech because there was no reason for them to be used. For example, it is quite possible that a child might not talk about negation or possession in a clinical language sample. An evaluator may wish to design contexts that will elicit such content/form/use interactions and add the child's responses to the data obtained in the language sample. In other situations, such as when a child is unintelligible or is relatively quiet during the low-structure observation, elicited samples of the child's language may need to serve as the primary source of information for determining goals of intervention.

Two types of elicited information can be utilized; that which has been elicited from others who are familiar with the child (reported observation) and that which has been elicited directly from the child (direct observation). Both types (reported and direct) will be discussed in this chapter as means of obtaining evidence for planning goals of intervention.

Elicited Reported Observations

Those who are in continual contact with the child are a rich source of information about a child's behavior in naturalistic settings. Useful information can often be successfully elicited by asking *specific* questions on a questionnaire or in an interview.

In a pilot study,[*] information obtained from parents of three language-impaired children by means of a questionnaire was strikingly similar to information obtained by analyzing a tape-recorded sample of the children's speech. The questions to the parents specified the content/form interactions at each phase on the C/F/U Goal Plan of Language Learning outlined in Chapter 8 and were in the following format:

Does your child talk about actions on objects:

1. By using one word such as "hit," "eat," and the like?
2. By using two words such as "hit ball," "eat cookie," "me hit," or "mommy eat"?

These questionnaires were long, and obviously not all parents would be willing to complete them. However, the success with which these parents were able to provide information when asked in such a remote fashion (i.e., without direct interview) supports the potential usefulness of questionnaires with at least some parents.

In practice, parents need only be asked about areas where further information is desired and not about each goal. This could have been done in an interview (following direct observation) or with a short questionnaire that is sent home with the parent and returned at a later time. Supplementing an interview with a take-home questionnaire allows parents to observe the child at home with particular behaviors in mind. Teachers, custodians, nurses, and others in constant contact with the child can also describe interactions that will help in determining goals of language intervention. Those who are in charge of a large number of children, such as teachers, may, however, have difficulty in giving specific examples of a child's speech, particularly if the child talks in long utterances. Limiting questions to one or two content/form/use interactions should make the task easier.

When children first begin talking, their linguistic utterances can be widely separated in time, thus making direct observation of these early words difficult. In a 1- or 2-hour observation, an observer may not hear the child say any words. Diaries have often been used to supplement direct observations of children who are just beginning to use single-word utterances (e.g., Bloom, 1984; Flax, 1986; Longtin, 1984; K. Nelson, 1973). In Bloom's data, parents reported the use of first words at least a month before first words were observed in the laboratory context. She hypothesized that these early words were bound to the contexts of their home and everyday activities and were, therefore, more likely to occur in those contexts.

---

[*] L. Green and L. Recca, Montclair State College, 1975.

In contrast, Longtin's diary reports of children in the single-word-utterance period tended not to include words that she had observed the children saying in their homes. All of these unreported words were relational words (e.g., *more, this, that*), which parents had not considered as "real words." Parents' written descriptions are an important means of obtaining information about a child's early use of language, but such data need to be considered in conjunction with data obtained from direct observation and parental interview. Formats for diary data can be found in Braunwald and Brislin (1979), Longtin (1984), J. Miller (1981), and Snyder, Bates, and Bretherton (1981).

If data obtained from direct low-structure observations and from reported observations are not sufficient to determine which content/form/use interactions are reasonable goals of intervention, the next step in assessment is to elicit responses from the child. Elicitation tasks vary in degree of structure and include standardized elicitations and nonstandardized elicitations.

Using Standardized Elicitations

As noted in Chapters 6 and 7, standardized elicitations are generally norm-referenced and are most applicable to identifying a problem (i.e., for comparing one child with other children). Items on most norm-referenced instruments are selected in order to differentiate among individuals in terms of responses within a general domain of behavior; their purpose is not to measure competence on certain aspects of that domain. Thus, the results of standardized elicitations can suggest how a child compares with other children on some aspect of language (such as vocabulary comprehension, syntactic comprehension, or syntactic production), but they do not give us information from which we can infer the child's rule system for particular content/form/use interactions.

The use of standardized tests to infer particular language knowledge has often underestimated the establishment of certain content/form interactions in a child's language system (Blau et al., 1984; Dever, 1972; Prutting et al., 1975). In a comparison of children's responses to the *Northwestern Syntax Screening Test* (Lee, 1971) with their production of the same forms during a language sample, Prutting and her associates found that 30% of the forms that were omitted or incorrectly produced in response to testing were correctly produced by the children in their spontaneous speech 50% of the time. Similarly, language-impaired children made significantly more errors on the *Carrow Elicited Language Inventory* (CELI) (Carrow, 1974) than on comparable scoring of a free speech sample (Blau et al., 1984); differences between performance on the two tasks tended to be greater for the children with the lower MLU. Many of the errors on the CELI occurred on structures or lexical items that the child did not produce in spontaneous speech (e.g., perfect tense or reflexive pronouns); the structural complexity of the stimuli in which other items were embedded on the test was greater than that found in the children's language samples. But some errors were made on lexical items and structures that were produced correctly in spontaneous speech. In addition, some items that were not observed in free speech and had never been used at home (according to parent report) were imitated correctly. Thus, the responses to the CELI both overestimated and underestimated the behaviors observed in low-structure settings; goals of intervention derived from the two sets of data were different.

In constructing tests that are to be appropriate for differentiating language skills of children from 3 to 8 years-old, the range of syntactic structures and lexical items must be considerable. Items will be included that are appropriate to the older normal child, but not the younger, and vice versa. This is not a problem if scores are used as intended, that is, to see how a particular child ranks with age peers; but it is a problem if responses to items are used as the basis for describing what a child does when generating a content/form/use interaction.

Another factor influencing differential performance on standardized versus low-structure observations is the context. Language tests usually elicit responses in a manner that is not representative of normal language use. In order to test the comprehension of a grammatical structure, for example, sentences are devised without semantic and syntactic redundancy and are presented in contexts that do not cue their meaning. Thus, to test certain verb inflections, nouns that are not inflected are used. Sentences designed to test the third person singular −*s* verb inflection, for example, might contrast "the deer run home" with "the deer runs home". Without redundant coding of semantic-syntactic relations, such as is common to both adult and child speech, emphasis is placed on the specific syntactic structure or morphological inflection being tested; this is not representative of the child's normal mode of processing. In production tasks children are asked to say things they do not mean (or perhaps even understand) to people they do not want to say them to. Language topic is constantly changing, and the listener's response is artificial and generally unrelated to the message of the child's utterance. The child is often being asked to manipulate language apart from the meaning it conveys, and thus these tasks often tap metalinguistic skills more than communicative skills. No wonder we find differences between responses to tests and utterances in naturalistic contexts!

An important limitation of standardized observations is the lack of information that can be obtained about the *use* of language through such techniques. Natural settings still appear to be the best means of finding out how a child uses language as a means of communicating ideas and desires, and to determine the purposes for which the child uses language. (Supplemental nonstandardized elicitations may be helpful in determining what the child can do.)

Thus, standardized elicitations are currently not very helpful in planning the goals of intervention for a number of reasons. They do not provide enough examples of each behavior; they do not give information about use; and they are so designed that responses may not be representative of behaviors in the child's natural environment. A preferable alternative when elicited information is necessary in order to plan goals of intervention is nonstandardized elicitations.

Using Nonstandardized Elicitations

Standardized observations are those that have structured tasks with specific instructions, norms, and reliability and validity data (Lyman, 1986). Somewhere between this type of highly structured normed observation and naturalistic observations fall a variety of measures of elicitation that can be referred to as nonstandardized elicitations (see also Leonard, Prutting, Perozzi, & Berkley, 1978).

A few published instruments are currently available that provide structure for describing children's language but reduce some of the problems with standardized observations. One of the earliest nonstandardized elicitation instruments that was published, *Environmental Language Inventory* (ELI) (MacDonald & Blott, 1974; MacDonald & Nickols, 1974) was designed to elicit two-word responses that code the content categories of action, locative action, locative state, recurrence, possession, attribution, negation (rejection and denial), and existence. These interactions are comparable to the content/form interactions presented in Chapters 8 and 9 as Phase 2 goals (with the exception of locative state, which is a Phase 3 goal, and negation, where rejection is a Phase 4 goal and denial a Phase 5 goal). To elicit these interactions, the child is asked to describe an action that the examiner performs (such as throwing a ball), and then to imitate the examiner's utterance (e.g., "say, 'throw ball' "). In all instances the event or object is present in the context. Although specific activities are listed, the authors suggest that other nonlinguistic contexts can be used as well, thus allowing flexibility and the opportunity to take advantage of the child's interests. Additionally, MacDonald and Nickols (1974) suggested recording examples of these same content/form interactions while the child interacts in a free-play setting, thereby combining elicitation with observation in a low-structure setting.

Another nonstandardized elicitation instrument is the *Oral Language Sentence Imitation Diagnostic Inventory* (OLSIDI) (Zachman, Huisingh, Jorgensen, & Barrett, 1977) which elicits multiple examples of particular forms (primarily morphological inflections such as *-ing*) within sentence contexts; the child is asked to imitate these sentences without supporting context. For normal language learners, the authors report high correlations between productions of the elicited forms and production of these forms in free speech samples.

But the use of nonstandardized elicitation techniques is not usually based on published instruments; rather, clinicians tailor techniques based on the information needed for an individual child. Often they adapt tasks that were devised for research purposes, or they use their own ingenuity in devising tasks. Before looking at the techniques to elicit language behaviors, it is important to determine which behaviors need to be elicited for a given child. If a low-structure observation precedes elicitation, it is not usually necessary to elicit a wide range of content/form/use interactions.

What to Elicit

The behaviors elicited are those for which insufficient evidence exists for determining the productivity of a content/form/use interaction that is expected, given the presence of other productive interactions. In analyzing language samples, you may find many content/form/use interactions established at a particular phase with no, or few, examples of utterances coding other interactions in phases adjacent to, within, or below this phase. The absence of examples may not mean that the child cannot or does not produce these interactions; rather, it may be that the situation did not call for such productions.

The purpose of assessment at this point is to make hypotheses about what the

---

BOX 13-1 Examples of Types of Nonstandardized Tasks That Can Be Used for Modeled *or* Nonmodeled Elicitation of Content/Form/Use Interactions

1. Story recall
2. Questions
3. Patterning
4. Role playing
5. Sentence completion
6. Story completion
7. Interview
8. Manipulation of context
9. Communication games
10. Description of actions or pictures

---

child is most likely to learn next, that is, to plan the goals of intervention. If a child is productive with Phase 2 and Phase 3 content/form interactions, you would not elicit Phase 8 interactions just because they did not occur. Following a developmental model, the content/form/use interactions to elicit are those in phases near those that were productive in the free speech sample.

Techniques of Elicitation

To elicit responses from a child about a particular content/form/use interaction, the evaluator must design situations that the child will be willing to respond to and situations that will require the desired response. In certain tasks the stimuli that the evaluator wishes to elicit (i.e., the targets) are spoken in the eliciting stimuli. That is, the target content/form/use interaction is modeled for the child as in an imitation task. In other tasks the situation is designed to elicit responses without modeling the target behavior. Each type of elicitation, modeled and nonmodeled, is discussed below and presented in Box 13-1.

Modeled Elicitations. The most direct form of modeled elicitation is an imitation task. Many clinicians and researchers elicit language behaviors by asking the child to repeat an utterance produced by the evaluator (e.g., "Say, 'the boy put the cake in the pan' ").

Imitation is a frequently used elicitation technique; it is relatively easy to administer, and the evaluator knows what output is obligatory. It has been assumed that the child uses grammatical knowledge to repeat sentences in which the number of words exceeds memory span. While systematic relationships between imitation and spontaneous speech have been reported for language-impaired children (e.g., Blau et al., 1984; Connell & Myles-Zitter, 1982; Lackner, 1968; Lahey et al., 1983; Zachman et al., 1977), it does not follow that content/form interactions produced incorrectly in imitation are necessarily incorrect or not productive in self-generated utterances (or vice versa).

Some evidence suggests that imitation tasks underestimate production in a free speech context. When young normal children are asked to imitate some of their own spontaneous utterances, their imitations are often less complex than the original utterance (Bloom, 1974; Hood & Lightbown, 1978; Slobin & Welsh, 1973). Language-impaired children reportedly make more errors in both immediate and delayed imitative responses than in spontaneous speech (Blau et al., 1984; Lahey et al., 1983; L. K. Nelson & Weber-Olsen, 1980; Prutting et al., 1975). It has been suggested that factors such as nonlinguistic context, MLU, age, and auditory memory may influence a child's responses to elicited imitation tasks.

Nonlinguistic representations of the stimuli (such as the child's own behavior and communicative intent, and the presence of objects and activities represented in the stimulus) are some of the factors that differentiate spontaneous language productions from many elicitation tasks, but in particular from imitation tasks. A number of studies have attempted to sort out the influence of context as well as the influence of age, MLU, and specific language behaviors on the responses to such tasks. Age has been correlated with the number of correct responses in preschool children (e.g., Keller-Cohen, 1974; L. K. Nelson & Weber-Olsen, 1980); younger children make more errors than older children. No effect of age was found in language-impaired children in the study by Lahey et al., 1983; however, over one-third of their subjects were over 5 years of age. It may be that age is an important factor only when the child is very young child or when stimuli are complex for the age of the child. In the Lahey et al. study, differential effects of MLU were not found either, but the complexity of stimuli was controlled and was appropriate for the children's MLU range.

Data on the influence of context have been conflicting; some researchers have reported that contextual support reduced errors on imitations (Hanif & Siegel, 1981; L. K. Nelson & Weber-Olsen, 1980), while others have found that context had little effect (Connell & Myles-Zitzer, 1982; Hood & Lightbown, 1978; Lahey et al., 1983). The addition of a contrived communicative context (an aspect of use) did not improve productions elicited by imitation, nor did it improve the correlation of scores of imitative responses with those based on a language sample in one pilot study (Launer, Schiff, & Lahey, 1979). Three types of contexts that illustrated the content/form interactions in the stimuli were explored by Connell and Myles-Zitzer (1982). Children did not respond differently to the three different conditions (enactment of events, static posed objects displaying an event, and line drawings) or to no context at all. Using pictures as well as actions as a means of contextual support for content/form interactions in stimuli, Lahey et al., (1983) reported few differential effects of context, and the direction of the small differences that were found varied with language behavior (see Figure 13-1). Differences in findings relative to the influence of contextual support may be related to the level of complexity of the stimuli in relation to the language level of the child. In studies reporting little effect of contextual support, stimuli were more in line with the child's language level than in studies where contextual support had an effect.

Another factor influencing the validity of imitation as a predictor of spontaneous speech productions is the content/form interaction in question. Even when stimuli complexity and lexicon are within those expected for the child's language level, imitation is a better predictor of the spontaneous productions of some behaviors than others (Lahey et al., 1983; also see Figure 13-1). For example, imitation of plural s predicts quite accurately the use of this morpheme in sponta-

FIGURE 13-1 Proportion of Correct Responses to Three Conditions: Imitation Minus Contextual Support, Imitation Plus Contextual Support, and Language Samples (from Lahey, Launer, and Schif-Myers, 1983)

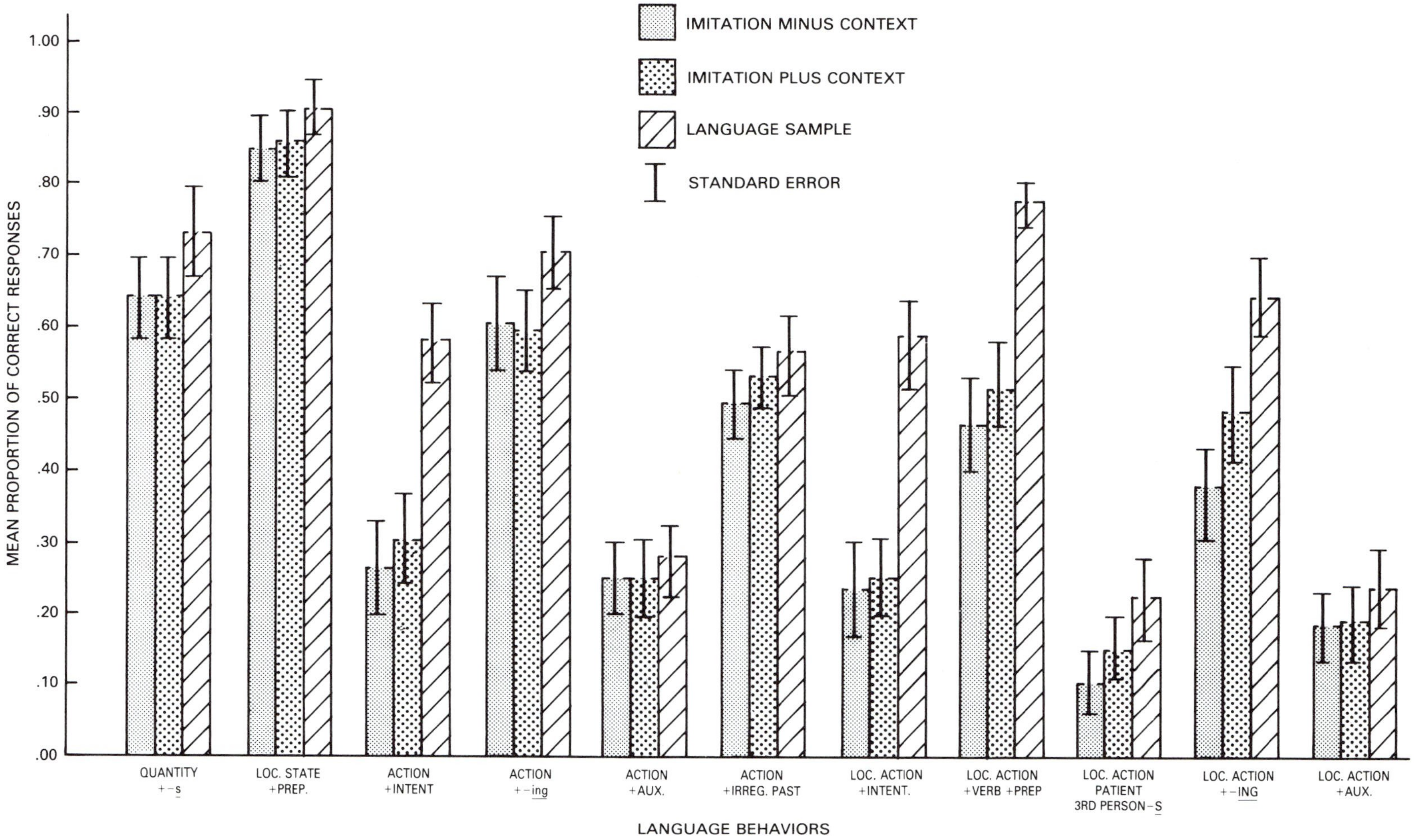

neous speech; imitation of the modal verb *gonna* was not a good predictor of its spontaneous production.

Responses to imitation tasks are often scored in terms of the presence or absence of the forms presented in the model. Exact repetition of a form allows you to infer something about knowledge of form, but it does not allow you to infer the establishment of a content/form interaction in a child's language. Speakers can imitate utterances that are longer than memory span without knowledge of content/form interactions if they are familiar with the form. The recoding of an utterance, so that meaning is essentially the same but the form is different, is, however, stronger evidence that a content/form interaction is established. For example, if in response to a stimulus such as "the boy can't open the door" the child responds with utterances such as "no open it," the evaluator can feel confident that the child knows something about negating two-constituent action utterances. An alternative means of scoring imitation tasks would consider such paraphases and analyze the content/form interactions within them.

This is often the way that children's retelling of stories is scored. Asking a child to recall a story after presentation by an adult is a common means of assessing a child's narrative skills (e.g., Graybeal, 1981; Johnston, 1982b). Recall is generally measured in terms of the propositions recalled and the appropriateness of the forms used rather than verbatim presentation. Story recall is influenced by a number of factors other than the child's narrative skills, however, including the listener, the child's familiarity with the topic of the story, previous stories just heard, and the density of causal chains within the story (e.g., Johnston, 1982b; Page & Stewart, 1985; Trabasso et al., 1984).

Other less direct means of modeling elicitation tasks are available. One technique is to ask questions in which the target form is embedded. In an attempt to elicit higher-level syntactic forms, Lee (1974) recommends that evaluators model such forms in their interactive speech with questions such as "What will he do now?" to elicit modals or "What did the mother say?" to encourage past tense productions.

An example of a questioning technique designed to elicit locative-action utterances is illustrated below in an interaction with a 9½-year-old language-impaired child. The child and clinician are talking about how one bakes a cake, an activity that was familiar to the child. (Note that the situation was designed around a nonpresent, yet familiar, event. Such a context should only be used for assessment if the child has demonstrated the ability to talk about familiar events that are not in the here and now.)

Do you add anything else? Do you put in more things?	milk
Anything else?	put in pan
Put what in pan?	put cake in pan/ in oven
Put cake in oven?	cake oven/ cook/ eat

In this interaction, the evaluator produced three *locative-action* utterances, each in the form of a question. Two of the questions asked for specification of the object (e.g., "Put *what* in pan?"). One could also ask for specification of place, for example, "Put cake where?" or of agent, "Who puts the cake in the oven?" This type of modeled elicitation presents the target content/form interaction in a question and requests a replacement of a *wh* word or pronoun. The problem with the questioning technique, however, is that the child need only fill in the missing element and answer the questions with one word, and so the desired multiword utterances will not be elicited. In addition, the child must be able to understand the question. With young normal children, talking about a content category (such as locative action) generally precedes answering questions about the category (such as *where*) (e.g., Hood & Bloom, 1979 make this point relative to causal questions). Thus, questions may not be a valid way to elicit productions of categories that the child has just begun to talk about unless the evaluator is sure that comprehension is considerably in advance of production for a given child.

In another type of modeling the child is presented with the desired content/form/use interaction but is required to change it in some way. For example, the child can be directed to ask a doll, puppet, or other person questions such as "Ask the doll where she put it," or "Ask Billy why he won't come with us" (see J. Miller, 1981, for further examples of this technique). The task can be embedded in a natural context (e.g., when Billy won't come) or in a formal context when the questions are probably without communicative intent and no doubt will not be answered. Little evidence exists to indicate which might be more predictive of the child's nonelicited productions.

In a similar type of task, the adult sets a pattern by modeling a statement and the desired response to the statement. Such techniques are described in Slobin (1967, and reported by N. J. Lund & Duchan, 1983, and J. Miller, 1981). Negation can be elicited by asking the child to say the opposite of what the adult said. First, the desired response pattern is modeled with instructions such as "I'll say, you can fly the plane, and you say, you can't fly the plane." Any number of variations on this theme can be devised to elicit different forms. Such tasks assume that the child will pick out the pattern and, as with most elicitation tasks, that the child can handle language apart from the child's communicative intent.

Pictures can be used with the above patterning; this contextual support may lighten the cognitive load and decrease the need for pattern induction (but research is needed to support this conjecture). Pictures could illustrate the contrasts to the patterns provided (such as a boy pointing to his shoes for "these are my shoes," and then in the next picture the boy pointing to a girl's shoes for "these are her shoes"). The evaluator would label both pictures for a few examples and then label only one and indicate that the child is to label the second picture. A variation of this has been used on a standardized test, the *Northwestern Syntax Screening Test* (Lee, 1971), where two pictures are presented and labeled by the evaluator (e.g., the baby is sleeping; the baby is not sleeping) and then the child is told to label one. This test is closer to an imitation task than the patterning talked about here. When tasks like this are not embedded in a natural context, they involve some metalinguistic skill and are probably more appropriate for complex language skills of children who have well-developed metalinguistic ability.

Finally, role playing can provide a context for modeled elicitations. Again this may not be a task for the very young child, but it can be useful for those who are willing to play the game. Role playing seems particularly appropriate for negation (see also Schmidt, 1981) where the evaluator can model a recalcitrant child talking with mom; everything mom suggests is negated by the child (e.g., "wash your hands," "no, I won't wash my hands"). Or, as suggested by Schmidt, the mother can be mad at the child and negate everything the child asks to do (e.g., "I want to go out," "no, you can't go out"). The context is modeled and then the child is asked to play the role of the negative person while the evaluator makes the different requests. In any of these latter modeled conditions, where the child must generate the desired form in a new utterance rather than repeat the modeled one, it would seem the production of utterance types is better evidence of rule knowledge. However, it may not tell whether the child does, in fact, produce these content/form/use interactions in spontaneous speech when a model is not present.

Modeled elicitations are intuitively pleasing to the new clinician, because they are an efficient and easy means of eliciting language behaviors and they focus on particular behaviors. Unfortunately, there is little evidence about how the responses to these tasks relate to spontaneous speech production. Even when a child produces a content/form interaction after modeling, it is not clear that the content/form interaction should *not* be a goal of intervention. Interactions that are produced after modeling, but are not produced without a model, may be behaviors the child is just learning [in line with Vygotsky's (1978) zone of proximal development] and be good targets for intervention. Again, research in this area is needed to answer this question. However, in order to follow a plan that is based on what children usually do, such as the one that was presented in Chapter 8, the most relevant data for supplementing a language sample would be interactions produced without a model. Further validation of these techniques is needed.

Nonmodeled Elicitations.   A nonmodeled elicitation differs from those mentioned above in that the desired response is not presented by the evaluator just before the child's utterance. Again, a number of different techniques can be used.

A nonmodeled elicitation situation based on a questioning technique is illustrated in the following interaction with Karen. This interaction preceded the illustration of modeled questions presented in the previous section and was also designed to elicit locative-action utterances.

Do you know how to make a cake, Karen?	**Yeah/ I know**
Can you tell me the steps, the things you must do to make a cake?	**yeah/ first cake in box**
Then what?	**put in bowl**
Then what do you do?	**put egg**
The whole egg, shell too?	**no/ break egg/ put in bowl/ mix up**
Mix them up?	**yeah/ I mix them up**

As noted before, making a cake was a familiar activity for Karen, and this no doubt helped her to communicate about the absent objects and to present the events in sequence. In this part of the interaction, locative-action utterances are elicited by questions that do not contain a model of coding locative action. (Karen's final utterance was a repetition + addition of the clinician's question, but it was of action, not locative action.) Generally, questions by the evaluator were designed to encourage responses about a topic that might demand coding of locative action.

Another means of eliciting without a model is to ask the child to describe an

---

BOX 13-2 Instructions to the Child: "I'll Make the Dog Do Some Things, and You Tell Me About Them".

Situation	Question	Possible Responses
Time plus action		
A dog runs and then stops	"Now, tell me, what?"	"He ran"/ "he stopped"
A dog runs and continues to run	"Now what?"	"He's running"
Quantity plus action		
A boy pets two dogs	"Tell me what's going on?"	"The boy pets the dogs"
One dog barks and stops	"Tell me what's going on?"	"The dog barked"
Two dogs bark and stop	"And now?"	"Two dogs barked"

Note that the target response, in the first situations (time plus action) and in the second situations (quantity plus action), was not coded by the evaluator. The *-ing* form was avoided in the questioning about *time* but was used in the question when *quantity* was the target. Thus, the responses would be considered nonmodeled elicitations.

---

action performed by the child or the adult. Such activities can illustrate relations of time, quantity, dative, recurrence, action, locative action, locative state, causality, temporal sequence, and so forth. Descriptions of enactments have frequently been used for elicitations of tense and aspect (e.g., Bronkart & Sinclair, 1973; Feintuck, 1985). Some examples of situations can be found in Box 13-2.

The objects and the contexts of elicitation tasks can vary according to the age and interest of the child. These are not standardized tasks; the purpose is to elicit coding of certain content categories and not particular topics. The technique is to devise a situation where the content/form interactions illustrated are relevant to the information needed and are obvious to the child, and then to encourage the child to play the "game" of describing.

Sentence completion is another means of eliciting particular content/form/use interactions. The evaluator sets a scene that can be enacted with dolls, puppets, or other objects. It has been used to elicit questions (Marks, Frye-Osler, Reichle, & Schwimmer-Gluck, 1981) by presenting two to four sentences; the final sentence either is incomplete (e.g., "Daddy's driving the car. He's going someplace. Mommy asks _____?") or ends unresolved with the hope the child will question the solution (e.g., in the context of a half-hidden animal present, the evaluator says "It's not a cat. It's not a dog," with the aim of eliciting "What is it?").

To elicit the child's production and comprehension of articles from preschool children, Maratsos (1974) enacted short stories and followed them with a question. Stories were designed to make contexts for definite and indefinite reference obligatory. For example, "Billy's mother said he could buy one pet animal. When he went shopping, he found three cats and one dog. What pet do you think the child bought?" A linguistic response demands either "the dog" (since there was but one) or "a cat" since there was more than one. (Note that articles are not modeled in the story presented above.) The evaluator would probably need to remove or cover the animals (if objects were used) before asking the question, or the child would most likely point and say "that one."

Some content categories need rather complex situations to elicit descriptions of the desired content/form interactions (e.g., state, notice, epistemic, recurrence). For some of these it may be easier to engage the child in activities and attempt to create obligatory (or facilitating) contexts for the language behavior desired. One might hide, or not have visible, certain objects that are needed in order to complete an activity. For example, in painting a picture, perhaps only one color is available and you hope the child will ask for more colors using state ("I need X"), nonexistence ("no red"), or recurrence ("more color"). To elicit denial, you can present the child with an unfamiliar object and identify it as "milk" (or the name of some other familiar object). This may elicit denial utterances such as "no milk" or "that's not milk." If a familiar item such as a penny is identified as milk, the response will most likely be "that's a penny" or the nonsyntactic coding of denial, "no, penny" (Belkin, 1975). Rejection might be elicited by doing or proposing something that the child would most likely not like and would, it is hoped, reject.

Narratives can also be elicited without modeling. One technique is to ask the child to "tell a story" (e.g., Sutton-Smith, 1981). Children without language-learning problems will make some attempt at a story as young as 3 years old. Alternatively, topic can be suggested in a number of ways. A beginning stem can be presented and the child asked to complete the story (e.g., Lahey, 1986; Stein, 1986), or the child can be asked to tell a story about visual stimuli such as a movie or pictures (e.g., Liles, 1985; Martin, 1983). In probably the most naturalistic method, questions about personal experiences can be asked in the process of conversation. Applying the interview technique developed by Labov (1972), C. Peterson and McCabe (1983) elicited personal-experience narratives from children 4 to 9 years of age. The researchers related a short personal experience (e.g., about a trip, a car accident, a pet) as they and the child were occupied with a manual task. Then the researcher would ask the child if he or she had had any similar experience (e.g., "Did you ever go on a trip?" "Have you ever seen a car accident?" "Do you have a pet?"). If the answer was affirmative, they would say, "Tell me about it." Since topic has a major influence on both the length and the structure of a narrative, it is important to give the child an opportunity to talk about a number of topics (C. Peterson & McCabe, 1983; Stein, 1986).

A combination of creativity and experience on the part of the evaluator will make it easier to devise situations that are of interest to a child with topics that are appropriate to the child's age level and that encourage the production of particular language behaviors. Some clinicians find it helpful to keep an index-card file of the various activities that can be used to elicit particular behaviors. The file could be organized by content category, function, linguistic contexts, or other content/form/use interactions, and different colors could be used for modeled versus non-modeled tasks. As you read different studies that have used elicitation techniques or as you create some tasks yourself, note them on cards and file them. The box can be very useful in those moments during assessment when creativity seems to have left you.

Flexibility is important when designing elicitation tasks. Some children enjoy talking through puppets, while others do not. For some, motivation is increased if they give instructions to another person, that is, if there is a listener to whom they can convey not already obvious information, while for others this may make the task more difficult. With some children, token rewards may be necessary as a means of motivating responses. However, with most children, accomplishment of some purpose or social praise of efforts and a relaxed atmosphere are generally all that is needed.

Elicitation of language *use* can also be carried out in an attempt to observe language productions in contexts and for functions that were not available in the low-structure observations. In order to observe how the child talks about the "there and then," the child can be asked open-ended questions about routine events at home or at school, about events that have taken place at school on a previous day, and about future events that the child plans to participate in during the coming weeks.

To observe a child's adaptation to a listener's perspective, a communication game can be played (see Glucksberg, Krauss, & Higgens, 1975, for a review of this literature). The child is seated at a table across from another child or adult, and identical objects or pictures are given to each. A barrier is placed between the two so they cannot see each other's objects or pictures, and the child is asked to describe actions on objects or to describe pictures so the other person can identify or replicate what is being described. Stimuli are designed so that the child must take into account the listener's needs if the task is to be successful. For example, multiple objects may be presented which differ only in some attribute (e.g., color or size) so that the listener will need to be given the attributive information in order to select the appropriate one.°

To observe the child's ability to take the perspective of another, the child can be asked to tell a story from pictures to someone who cannot see the pictures in order to elicit coding of new and old information (see Warden, 1976, for examples of this technique to elicit the use of articles). Alternatively a child can be asked to explain a game to one who is blindfolded to determine the specificity of information that will be provided or the child can be asked to relate an incident to someone who has not shared the experience (see Maratsos, 1973; Menig-Peterson, 1975). Each of these situations provides information that must be further analyzed in much the same way as a language sample for appropriate adjustments of form (as deictic terms or antecedent referents for pronouns) and content (as the inclusion of attribution). (See Geller, in press, and in preparation, for a review of perspective-taking tasks.)

You can also create situations that elicit the use of language for different functions. To elicit comments the child can be asked to describe ongoing activities. The use of novel objects, games, and activities very often elicits requests for information. Demand utterances can be encouraged by withholding some object that is

---

° This also provides a means of eliciting certain content categories, as attribution, but under difficult conditions. If the child does not code the attribute, it cannot be concluded that the child does not use attribution in less complex circumstances.

necessary to complete an activity (e.g., a piece of the puzzle or the block necessary to finish the bridge). Each of these may be coordinated with tasks for eliciting content/form interactions. Requests for repairs (e.g., "what?") might be elicited by mumbling some information that is essential to or was requested by the child. (For further ideas about eliciting aspects of use see Roth and Spekman, 1984b.)

Using the Information from Elicited Tasks

The examples that are elicited without models are added to the information from the language sample—if there are now enough examples to consider the content/form/use interaction productive, the interaction is no longer an immediate goal. Reported observations can be used to add to direct observation, but should not be the sole source of information about productivity. When low-structure and reported observations plus nonmodeled elicitations do not provide enough evidence to infer the child's knowledge of certain interactions, the language behaviors that are expected to develop earlier or at the same time as most of the child's productive language behaviors are listed as goals. Responses to models (e.g., imitations) are not used as evidence to determine productivity. Interactions that can only be produced in imitation may be behaviors that the child does not use at all or those that the child is in the process of learning, but are not well established. If they are established, they will probably emerge readily in the context of intervention and new goals will be set. To err in the direction of setting goals that are already achieved is better than to err in the direction of setting goals that are way beyond the child's current level of functioning. Early success, even if only apparent (since the behaviors were already established), sets a better climate for learning than long-term frustration. Goals of intervention are hypotheses about what the child is most ready to learn—they do not mark the child for life (as may be the case with certain diagnostic labels); goals of intervention are constantly reassessed and changed when necessary.

The situations designed for nonmodeled elicitations in initial assessment are also useful for reassessment if the context and situations are different from those used in the intervention setting. Topics that are different from those employed in teaching are necessary to be assured that the child has generalized the rule as a means of coding content/form/use interactions and has not just memorized certain topic-related utterances.

Summary

This chapter is concerned with eliciting language behaviors directly from children or eliciting descriptions of behaviors from those who know the child well. The elicitation tasks are categorized as modeled elicitations, responses to tasks where the utterance type was presented to the child before the response (the most extreme case being elicited imitations), and nonmodeled elicitations, responses to tasks where the utterance type was not presented to the child before the response. It is suggested that nonmodeled elicitations can be used to supplement or replace direct, low-structure observations, but that responses following modeling provide weaker evidence that content/form/use interactions are productive. Reported observations can also be used to supplement direct observations, but should not serve as the only evidence to decide that a content/form/use interaction need not be a goal.

It is still not clear how evidence from different elicitation techniques relates to evidence from other techniques or to that from a low-structure observation. Further validation studies are needed. Since the sequence of goals suggested in Chapters 8 through 11 is based on language observed in low-structure context, language samples obtained in such contexts should probably serve as the primary source of information when possible.

Suggested Readings

Lahey, M., Launer, P., & Schiff-Myers, N. (1983). Prediction of production: Elicited imitation and spontaneous speech productions of language-disordered children. *Applied Psycholinguistics, 4,* 319–343.

Leonard, L., Prutting, C. A., Perozzi, J. A., & Berkley, R. K. (1978). Nonstandardized approaches to the assessment of language behaviors. *Asha, 20,* 371–379.

Miller, J. (Ed.). (1981). *Assessing language production in children: Experimental procedures.* Baltimore: University Park Press.

Roth, F., & Spekman, N. (1984). Assessing the pragmatic abilities of children: Part 2. Guidelines, considerations, and specific evaluation procedures. *Journal of Speech and Hearing Disorders, 49,* 12–17.

14

General Considerations
of Language Intervention

Language intervention involves modifying a child's environment in a manner that will enhance the child's induction of interactions among language content, form, and use. Certain of these modifications are specific to the contexts in which the goals of language will be facilitated; other modifications are more general in that they may apply to many contexts or need to be considered before, or concurrent with, planning specific contextual modifications. Such general considerations include (1) factors that may be maintaining difficulty with language learning, (2) the context in which language will be facilitated, and (3) the child's response behaviors, such as the techniques of eliciting and maintaining these behaviors, the sense modality to be used, and the relative emphasis on comprehension versus production. Each of these will be discussed in this chapter, while the next chapter will deal with facilitating the induction of content/form/use interactions.

Attempting to facilitate language learning in language-impaired children is both a rewarding and a humbling experience. Little empirical data exist to guide us in our choices of *how* to facilitate language learning; there is little information to suggest that one procedure works better than another for any particular child. Research on intervention rarely includes follow-up over long periods of time, and thus the ultimate influence of a procedure is not known. Practices of intervention are, for the most part, guided by theoretical assumptions about language learning even though individual clinicians and educators may not have made their own views of such assumptions explicit. Obviously, we all begin with the assumption that intervention of some kind can facilitate language learning more rapidly than lack of intervention (see also Fey, 1986). Anyone who is attempting to facilitate language learning and is not simply following a "cookbook" of procedures must be operating with certain other assumptions—about the nature of language, what factors enhance language learning, and what factors may interfere with language learning. Making our current assumptions explicit may aid us in our ability to consider new assumptions or to see how new procedures fit in with or differ from our current assumptions (see also Johnston, 1983).

Given a historical perspective of the field, we can see that our assumptions have changed in many ways (see Aram & Nation, 1982; Launer & Lahey, 1981; and J. E. McLean, 1983, for summaries of historical perspectives). For example, in the 1950s we assumed that categorical placement of a child was essential for intervention (see Chapters 3 and 4); procedures for intervention primarily entailed increasing language input (generalized language stimulation) and increasing the need for expressive language (i.e., motivation for using language). In the 1960s some professionals assumed that remediating deficits in cognitive processing would lead to improved language skills (see Chapters 3 and 5); others assumed that language itself needed to be taught. Within the latter group, different assumptions motivated the procedures for intervention. On the assumption that language learning was similar to other aspects of learning, a number of professionals turned to principles of behavior modification for techniques (to be discussed later in this chapter). The model of language that influenced goals of intervention for many of these clinicians and educators was the adult model; it was assumed that complete sentences should be taught regardless of the child's level of language. In contrast, others argued that language could not be taught by behavioral procedures because it was generated from a system of abstract rules similar to those described by Chomsky (1965); the child needed to learn certain kernel sentences plus a set of transformations. In the mid-1970s assumptions about language evolved from a consideration of aspects of form (in this case, syntax) to a concern for aspects of content (semantics), and later in the 1970s, the emphasis was on use (pragmatics). Furthermore, by the 1970s the prevalent assumption was that normal developmental sequences of language learning provided more appropriate goals than complete adult sentences chosen by adult intuition. Intervention was motivated by the assumption that the induction of the rules of language (i.e., rules governing the interaction of content, form, and use) was best facilitated in naturalistic contexts involving communicative interactions (more specifics are included in this and the next chapter). While some professionals maintained the assumptions about behavioral principles, they utilized more naturalistic contexts and reinforcers. In the 1980s assumptions about the importance of language use and of interactional contexts in the teaching of language have had an increasing impact; assumptions about the utilization of normal development as a best first hypothesis for sequencing language intervention goals have been enriched with new developmental data.

The view of language presented throughout this book (as well as in Bloom & Lahey, 1978) is based on two assumptions. The first assumption is that language is a means for representing information in messages—form cannot be considered apart from the meaning it represents, and children with language disorders need to learn how linguistic forms encode aspects of content that have to do with knowledge of objects and events in the world. The second assumption is that language is a social act and is used to obtain, maintain, and regulate contact with other persons and that language is learned in such contexts. Language form and content always relate to language use. Further assumptions about language intervention that have been discussed in earlier chapters are that the most reasonable and practical hypotheses on which to base intervention goals are to be derived from what is know about normal language development; that goals of intervention should very specifically state what behaviors the child is to manifest; that, since more is known about the sequence of production than comprehension, the sequence of goals is better written in terms of production behaviors; and that, if language learning is the goal of intervention, language and communication should be the focus of intervention (i.e., remediating some presumed etiology may also take place but should not replace direct facilitation of language learning). Other assumptions will be addressed as relevant in this and the next chapter.

Reducing Maintaining Factors

The first assumption to be considered is that certain factors may be currently interfering with language learning, and if such factors are changed, the child will learn language more rapidly. These factors are referred to as *maintaining factors*. A maintaining factor may or may not have been a *precipitating* factor (or an original reason why language was not learned). For example, profound hearing loss from birth can be considered both a precipitating factor (a reason why auditory-vocal language was not learned originally) and a maintaining factor (a factor that is presently inhibiting future language learning); adverse parental reaction to a child who is not talking by the age of 3 years may not have been a precipitating factor but may inhibit future language learning and thus be a maintaining factor; severe illness in the second year of life may have been a precipitating factor but not a maintaining factor for a 5-year-old who is having difficulty learning language. Maintaining factors, either physical or environmental, that are amenable to change are most important in planning intervention.

Maintaining Factors Amenable to Change: Physical

Hearing loss is certainly a factor that can interfere with language learning and is a factor that is often amenable to improvement (i.e., usually the effect of the loss, but sometimes the loss itself). Auditory sensitivity should be routinely checked in all children with a language disorder. Children are first referred to the audiologist, who may then make recommendations about further testing, medical referrals, or the use of amplification. In addition to hearing loss, poor general health can affect any learning, including language learning, and it should be considered as a possible maintaining factor. Most schools demand periodic medical examinations, and clinics often have such medical examinations as a routine part of assessment. When this is not the case, medical referrals should be made if poor health or poor nutrition is suspected. Occasionally medication prescribed for some other condition (e.g., seizures or hyperactivity) can interfere with learning. If you, or those familiar with the child, notice adverse affects on learning that co-ocur with the use of some medication, the child's physician should be consulted.

Maintaining Factors Amenable to Change: Environmental

What aspects of the environment could possibly maintain a language disorder? One hypothesis is that children are delayed in talking because they have no need to talk—either everyone talks for them or no one listens to them. Little evidence supports this hypothesis, although increasing the amount of talking (i.e., content/form/use productions) that a child does, seems to enhance language learning (e.g., Hart & Risley, 1980). Parental demand for a word or sentence before satisfying a child's obvious need is, however, not the solution; such a procedure does not reward communication and usually ends up in tears and frustration. More appropriate techniques for eliciting language are discussed later in this chapter, but having someone willing to listen and respond is always helpful and has been related to language growth in non-language-impaired children (e.g., Olson, Bayles, & Bates, 1986). Other aspects of the environment implicated in maintaining a language disorder are parental interactional patterns and linguistic input.

While there is little doubt that a child must have linguistic input in order to learn a language, there is some controversy over how much and what kind of input makes a difference. Correlational data have linked particular types of parental input with language learning in non-language-impaired children (e.g., Cross, 1978; K. E. Nelson, Carskadden, & Bonvillian, 1973; Newport, Gleitman, & Gleitman, 1977). In addition to the linguistic input, the interactional style of caregivers with NLI children has been implicated in the speed of language learning (e.g., K. Nelson, 1973; Olson et al., 1986), and early experiences and attachments have been associated with how well a child can display competence (e.g., Belsky, Garduque, & Hrncir, 1984). Because of these implications, some have assumed that caregiver–child interactions may be a factor maintaining a language disorder, and training programs often aim at modifying parental interactions and input. To support this assumption, considerable research has focused on the interactions of caregivers and language-impaired children and compared them with those of caregivers and NLI children.

A number of researchers have reported that interactions between mothers and their language-disordered children are different from the interactions between mothers and children of the same age who are learning language normally (e.g., Buium, Rynders, & Turnure, 1974; C. Cunningham, Siegel, van der Spuy, Clark, & Bow, 1985; Goldfarb, Goldfarb, & Scholl, 1966; Goldfarb, Levy, & Meyers,

1972; Goss, 1970; Wulbert, Inglis, Kriegsman, & Mills, 1975). Buium et al. noted differences in the grammatical complexity of input to Down's syndrome children; Goldfarb and his associates reported that mothers of schizophrenic children had inferior speech and language patterns and communicated less clearly with their children; Wulbert et al. noted that mothers of language-delayed children interacted less *with* their children, talked less positively *about* their children, and used shouting, spanking, or threats more often as a means of restricting or punishing their children. Differences reported in interactional patterns of parents and their specific-language-impaired (SLI) children have included fewer questions, lower MLU, more directives, and fewer interactions (e.g., Bondurant et al., 1983; Cramblit & Siegel, 1977; C. Cunningham et al., 1985), and these differences were greatest for younger children with lower comprehension scores (C. Cunningham et al., 1985). When deaf children and their hearing mothers were compared with NLI children and their mothers, differences were found in the responsivity of child and mother to each other (lower for the deaf children), while no overall differences were found in the quantity of mother-child interactions or in the control strategies of the mothers (Wolchik, 1983).

Since these studies matched children according to chronological age, not language skills, it is possible that some of the differences reported were actually characteristic of normal parent-child interactions at an earlier point in development. In fact, many of the differences described (e.g., number of questions, low MLU, more directives) are similar to differences found in the speech of adults to younger versus older children. To explore the possibility that reported differences were actually a reflection of the language-disordered children's lower level of language sophistication, a number of researchers have compared language-disordered children with NLI children whose language skills are similar (usually as indicated by MLU). Fewer differences were reported when language level was controlled with mentally retarded children (Rondal, 1978) and with SLI children (e.g., Conti-Ramsden & Friel-Patti, 1983; B. D. Johnson, 1985; Lasky & Klopp, 1982). When comparing mother-child dyads of SLI children with age-matched and language-level-matched NLI children, Johnson found considerable differences between age-matched and SLI dyads but few differences between MLU-matched and SLI dyads. For example, directives were more frequent for the SLI and language-matched dyads than for the age-matched dyads. Furthermore, when strangers interacted with the same children, the strangers behaved much as the mothers had to each of the children. Johnson concluded that the child's language level influenced the discourse and functional aspects of mother-child speech.

However, even when caregiver interactions with language-impaired children have been compared with those involving NLI children with similar MLUs, some differences have been reported. In a study by Schodorf and Edwards (1983) parents of language-disordered children used fewer expansions and more corrections than parents of NLI children. Differences in the number of semantically related responses to SLI children's utterances have also been reported by Millet and Newhoff (1978). In the dyads studied by Johnson, mothers of SLI children produced as many semantically related responses as the mothers of NLI children and as the strangers who talked with both. However, the mothers of the SLI children did not provide as many utterances about the attentional focus of their children as did the strangers talking with the same children or as the mothers of

NLI children. This finding appeared to be a result of two mothers' unsuccessful attempts to distract their children from persistent play with one toy. A second difference was in the number of nonresponses to the child's utterances; some mothers of SLI children responded much less frequently to the utterances of their child than other dyads. (Interestingly, the nonresponse was often followed by these children's production of sequential topic-related utterances; the mothers may have been, unconsciously, using nonresponse as a device to encourage their children to talk more.) Differences have also been reported when Down's syndrome children and their mothers were compared with language-matched (MLU) NLI children and their mothers (Weistuch, manuscript); mothers of the Down's syndrome children were more controlling with their children (e.g., they used more commands), and they less frequently expanded or extended their children's utterances. However, the children themselves were less responsive, and Weistuck suggested that differences in control may be related to the child's responsivity.

Differences that are not captured by measures of mean length of utterance may account for the interactional patterns. Two examples were given above: differences in the mothers' control strategies might be related to responsivity (Weistuch, manuscript); differences in the number of utterances related to the child's focus of attention might be related to persistent play with one object (B. D. Johnson, 1985). In the study by Conti-Ramsden & Friel-Patti (1983), the SLI children were less likely to initiate dialogue than the normal-language-learning children, and the few differences found in the maternal input to the SLI children were interpreted to be the mothers' adjustments to the children's different interactional patterns.

Matching language-disordered children with non-language-disordered children is complex. The usual means of matching language level has been MLU. However, MLU is but a gross index of language development relative to form (and even this is limited as noted by many, including Bloom & Lahey, 1978; Garman, 1979; Lahey et al., 1983). Mean length of utterance does not describe development or differences in use, such as the number of utterances that are initiated by the child or the child's responsivity to others (see, for example, Gerber, 1987; Wollner, 1983), nor does it describe differences in comprehension which may affect input (Cross, 1978; Van Kleeck & Carpenter, 1980). More careful matching may result in fewer differences between caregivers' interactions with language-disordered children in comparison with non-language-disordered children, but it is not yet clear how to match children. For example, two SLI children matched on all traditional variables (e.g., MLU, age, parent education, size of spoken vocabulary, as well as test scores of vocabulary comprehension, perceptual and motor development, and IQ) were found to differ markedly in their interactions with their mothers and also in their eventual rate of language learning (Constable & Lahey, 1984). Such differences were not evident in an analysis of the mothers' utterance types, but only by a more sociolinguistic analysis of the interactions. It may be that more in-depth analysis of a few children's interactions with caregivers will lead to a better understanding of what factors influence these interactions.

We are not ready to answer many questions concerning the similarity of input to language-disordered children and to non-language-disordered children. When MLU is used as a means of matching the two groups, the differences reported have not been replicated by all researchers (e.g., differences in semantically related responses) or have been related to nonlinguistic variation among the children (e.g., responsivity). Regardless of the similarities, certain interactional behaviors could interfere with the language learning of some language-disordered children. Input that includes aberrant speech or language behaviors, lack of clarity in communicating, topics that are not the child's focus of attention, or lack of responsiveness to the child's attempts to communicate is certainly not designed to enhance language learning. However, such patterns may be amenable to change through counseling and instruction.

With the normal language learner, ideal input may not be necessary for learning basic language skills; for example, Schiff (1979) found that the hearing children of deaf parents had little difficulty learning early language behaviors despite the limited oral language skills of their parents. But what may be an effective linguistic environment for the child learning language without difficulty may not be effective enough to facilitate language learning in the language-disordered child. Thus, even though input to language-disordered children is similar to that received by normal language learners, linguistic input and interactional style could still be factors that maintain a language disorder. This subtle distinction is an important one when working with parents. To assume that certain environmental interactional patterns may be a maintaining factor is not to assume that they caused the problem. There is no evidence that different types of parental input can be a precipitating factor in a child's language-learning problems (see, e.g., Cantwell, Baker, & Rutter, 1977; Leonard, in press). If one attempts to change parental interactions as a means of eliminating a maintaining factor, it should be clear to parents that their interactions have not been "wrong," nor are they the "cause" of the child's problem. However, it can be pointed out that some changes in their interactional style may increase the rate of language learning for this child at this time. In effect we are enlisting their aid as a language facilitator.

If we do enlist the aid of parents in this fashion, we are assuming that a change in the home environment may facilitate the speed of language learning in a particular child. Is there any evidence to support this assumption? Is there any evidence to suggest that *changing* parents' interactions or input facilitates language learning? This question will be discussed in the section on facilitators that follows.

Facilitators

The speech-language pathologist will be responsible for planning goals of intervention, ongoing assessment, and general advisement, but other persons will, it is hoped, be assisting in the language-learning process. Whenever possible, persons who live with the child or who spend considerable time with the child are recruited and trained to help. In general, programs using caregivers as facilitators have reported positive results.

A parent-assisted treatment program where parents were given a 7-week training program (in designing nonlinguistic contexts, in modeling linguistic input, and in providing feedback to the child concerning the appropriateness of his or her responses) was described by MacDonald, Blott, Gordon, Spiegel, and Hartmann (1974). Pretesting and posttesting of three children involved in this program for 4 to 5 months indicated considerable language growth (as measured by MLU) when compared with children who served as controls. In another study, mothers of hearing-impaired children were trained to increase their child's exposure to words, both those words presented in language therapy and other words that the parents wished the child to learn (Cullatta & Horn, 1981). The exposure procedure was effective in increasing the frequency with which the targeted words were produced. In addition, there was an increase in the production of other words that were not targeted when the exposure program went into effect. Parents reported pleasure at having an influence on their child's language learning and found it easiest to carry out the exposure procedures during regular daily activities.

After only brief home-based programs, some researchers have reported gains in the use of linguistic skills that autistic children already possessed (Howlin, 1981). Progress made in another program that taught parents of autistic children operant procedures for language acquisition was maintained 1 year after follow-up, but no further gains had been made once the program ceased (Harris, Wolchik, & Weitz, 1981). In some parent programs, home visits are included so that techniques can be incorporated into the home environment. Behavior management techniques and counseling are often a part of such programs. Parents who participate in these programs often report that they feel more confident in working with their children, have a better understanding of how to help their children, and are able to see improvements in their children (Helm & Kozloff, 1986). Thus, some success is generally reported in all programs that utilize parents as facilitators.

The long-range effect of parent programs has not been well documented; most are carried out for short periods of time, and limited follow-up data are reported. One could speculate that the manner in which parents are involved may well be a factor in long-term success. We might predict more application of the new strategies in interacting with the child, if parents are incorporated into the decision making regarding what is to be done and how, rather than being told what to do and treated as assistants. If the rationale for various strategies is clear to parents, they may be better able to make adaptations when needed. There is some danger in dictating how a parent should interact with a child—particularly when it appears that certain of the parents' interactional patterns may be the result of the child's behaviors (e.g., see the previous section, and Lieven, 1978). The interactional patterns that we as clinicians and educators can maintain with a child for the relatively short periods of time that we see that child are not always easy to maintain when the child lives with you daily. However, if the parents understand the motivation for changing certain interactional patterns, if the method and time of change are worked out with them, and if the changed interactional patterns are, at first, scheduled for very short time periods, continued use and appropriate adaptations may be more likely. (See Fey, 1986, and Hubbell, 1981, for a more complete review of parents as facilitators.)

Other potential facilitators include teachers, teacher's aides, houseparents in institutions, nurses or nurse's aides, and even peers (see Warren & Rogers-Warren, 1985). Most of these people have other responsibilities, and it is imperative that the speech-language pathologist plan, with those involved, methods of incorporating language facilitation techniques into the routines of these potential facilitators. The speech-language pathologist can spend time in the classroom, ward, or housing unit, demonstrating how activities such as mealtime, dressing, exercise, gym, playground, and the like can be adapted to facilitate language learning.

Likewise, the goals of other professionals may be incorporated into the language intervention sessions (e.g., sitting postures, math concepts). Cooperative efforts make it more likely that the child will progress in many different areas and generalize learning to more settings.

Within the past decade a new type of facilitator has emerged—the computer. A number of programs have been designed to teach vocabulary and syntax to language-disordered children. The computer has many advantages: it appears to provide a source of motivation to many children; it can be employed independently without constant attention from a professional; it can store responses and provide a cumulative record of responses; it can provide linguistic input to the child; it can graphically provide contexts (e.g., exemplars of objects and actions); and it can be programmed to adapt to the child's speed of learning (see, e.g., M. S. Wilson & Fox, 1983). It is, therefore, appealing as a potential facilitator.

As with anything that sounds so perfect, there are other factors to consider that dampen our enthusiasm; a number of disadvantages outweigh the advantages for many children. Computer programs for early language intervention, as now designed, are better for facilitating comprehension of content/form interactions than for eliciting the production of these interactions; they are weakest for inductions and elicitation regarding the component of language use. Most are drill-oriented and do not teach language as a tool for communication. Furthermore, they are not, at the early levels of language development, interactive. Evidence suggests that responsive partners enhance children's learning of language (e.g., Olson et al., 1986) and that speaking enhances language learning (e.g., Hart, 1985). If you assume that language is learned most efficiently when the child participates in dialogue, then the computer may not be the best choice as a facilitator unless it is accompanied with a human interactor. While interactive computer programs can be written, they usually require that the child be able to read. To my knowledge, none are presently written that respond to a young child or language-disordered child's variable and frequently distorted pronunciation. However, all is not lost. While the computer cannot take over the role of a facilitator, many programs and games currently available can have a place for some children. They provide the kind of highly structured contexts that some children need as a beginning in language learning and can be used as a setting for interactions with others (e.g., J. Miller & Marriner, 1986; Schiff-Myers, 1987). More about the computer as a setting is discussed below.

The Setting

Intervention can take place in a variety of surroundings that vary from the child's own home, playground, or classroom to the clinic room, teaching booth, or specially designed classroom. Important factors in the choice of setting include the degree of structure considered necessary and the number and type of goals that have been set.

Degree of Structure

The degree of structure that is most conducive to learning varies with children. For most children, language facilitation should be carried out in contexts that are representative of the child's daily life so that generalization of that learning to contexts other than intervention will be easier. Many have suggested contexts in which the child is allowed to take the lead (e.g., Hubbell, 1977), with the rationale that such contexts facilitate more talking and allow for initiation of comments. However, certain children appear to benefit from more constrained and controlling contexts, at least at some points in development. For example, 10 autistic children studied by Clark and Rutter (1981) were more responsive and less resistant when interpersonal demands were high during a model-building task; they were more aggressive and had more ritualistic behaviors in a less demanding context (see also Donnellan, Anderson, & Mesaros, 1984). For other children, familiar routines may provide the needed structure in which language intervention may begin. Experimenting with tasks and structure can help educators and clinicians find the most facilitating setting for individual children.

It has long been felt that certain children learn best when the amount of stimuli presented to them is somehow constrained (e.g., Cruickshank, Bentsen, Retzburg, & Tannhauser, 1961; Hewett, 1965; Straus & Lehtinen, 1947). These children are often described as having poor attention span, being hyperactive, and being easily distracted. Teaching booths or small classrooms with plain walls, sound treatment, and restraining furniture have been used to reduce background stimuli; the task presented has been highlighted by exaggeration of color, size, and texture. Depressing all sensory input other than that related to the demonstration of the task decreases the child's need to sort out relevant stimuli in both linguistic and nonlinguistic context. Such highlighting of relevant stimuli may increase the ease with which some children can induce content/form interactions. The computer could be a tool for such presentations; graphics can help highlight stimuli, or televised events may be used, and feedback can be immediate. It can be used in conjunction with a teaching booth, or it may provide enough inherent motivation that a teaching booth is not necessary.

One serious drawback of highly structured settings is the limited variety of contextual situations that can occur. The demonstration of many semantic relations may be difficult or very stilted. However, computer simulation and television demonstration may alleviate some of this difficulty if the computer itself is not overstimulating to the child. A more important limitation of all highly structured contexts is the difficulty of providing situations in which the child can use language in meaningful communicative interactions. When these problems can be surmounted either within the setting or by supplementing the setting with more natural contexts, the highly structured teaching situation may be a feasible recommendation for particular children—children who appear to learn only when the amount and variety of input stimuli are limited.

One criterion for determining the appropriate degree of structure for intervention is the child's attention to tasks, and, ultimately, the learning that takes place. The categorical classification of a child (i.e., neurologically impaired, mentally retarded, emotionally disturbed, or even hyperactive) does not itself suggest high- or low-structured intervention. If a child will focus on a preferred activity when other stimuli (people or sounds) are present, isolation from stimuli may not be necessary or advisable. Hyperactivity and short attention span are behaviors that are influenced by the tasks at hand; the child who is hyperactive or distractible in one setting may well be lethargic or perseverative in another. Often hyperactivity appears in settings that are beyond the child's capabilities; considerable reduction in hyperactive behavior may occur when the child is involved with tasks that are within motor, cognitive, social, and linguistic capacities. If hyperactivity is influenced in this way, planning language facilitation around activities that a child can accomplish or those that the child selects and enjoys will reduce or eliminate the need for severe reduction of stimuli. Gradual modification of these tasks in the direction of new and different activities may then help the child to increase attention in a variety of situations.

Language intervention in a highly structured setting that is isolated from real-life experience is not recommended unless it is impossible to get a child to attend to relevant stimuli without such isolation. Such a decision would be based on observations, both direct and reported, that the child could not focus on any stimuli without the reduction of all competing stimuli and, in addition, that such reduction did in fact aid both in focusing attention and in facilitating inductions of content/form/use interactions. Even if isolation or high structure is necessary, intervention must eventually include situations that are representative of a child's life, so that *use* of language can also be learned.

In contrast to the highly structured setting, a low-structure setting generally revolves around a child's everyday activities and may take place in group play situations, perhaps in a nursery school or in a classroom, or it may take place in a one-to-one situation, when the child plays, eats, dresses, or is engaged in other daily activities. In such settings the child's interest or daily routine determines the topics and activities; the facilitator provides the relevant linguistic input that codes these ongoing activities and related states, and may at times encourage or demand similar relevant verbalizations from the child. Situations demonstrating various content categories and uses of language readily occur in these contexts and do not have to be artificially created. A major advantage of low-structured settings is the incorporation of language into the child's daily life, so there is not a problem of *carryover* of skills from artificial contexts. (See also Hart, 1985; Spradlin & Siegel, 1982.)

The computer can also be used in such low-structure contexts. Programs written for purposes other than language intervention may serve as motivating stimuli. Some software provides contexts that illustrate many of the concepts that are a part of language intervention (see J. Miller & Marriner, 1986, for a listing) and are probably more interesting than the static pictures so often utilized in intervention. Furthermore, the computer has now become a part of the lives of many children both at school and at home, so it can provide a very naturalistic context in which to facilitate the inductions of content, form, and use if clinicians and educators use the context creatively.

To facilitate language learning in settings that are a part of the child's everyday life may mean changing the traditional role of the speech-language pathologist by moving the clinician from the clinic or office room to the child's environment. In a school setting it may mean that the speech-language pathologist will spend a good part of a day on the playground, lunchroom, or classroom in order to facilitate language learning directly as well as to make suggestions about how the teacher or parent can facilitate language learning during the rest of the day. Even when highly structured contexts are recommended, they must be followed by language learning in other, more natural environments. The current role of the speech-language pathologist, as viewed by many administrators and speech-language pathologists themselves, needs to be changed in order to adapt to current ideas about the teaching of early language skills. One cannot be isolated in a room apart from the child's life, see children 1 or 2 hours a week, and expect them to learn early content/form/use interactions that will generalize to other aspects of their lives.

Number of Goals

It is possible to work on only one particular language goal at a time (e.g., the goal of coding action relations with two constituents as comments on self actions); or work on a number of goals for different content categories (e.g., to code possession, recurrence, action, and existence with word order as comments on objects and activities that are present in the environment); or to include all goals within a phase level (as all content/form/use interactions for Phase 2). The settings in which facilitation will take place and the choice of persons who will be facilitating language learning influence both the number of goals and the specificity of the goals set. In an informal setting, it is easy to include a number of goals, because the child's day will involve many opportunities for coding the various content categories (action, state, recurrence, possession, temporal, etc.). In a more formal setting, where context must be created to demonstrate semantic relations, it is often easier to focus on only one or two particular content categories (such as action or possession). Thus facilitation in a more structured setting may lead to a focus on one or two goals at a time; facilitation in a less structured setting may lead to the inclusion of a greater number of goals across many content categories. This relationship of number of goals to structure of setting usually coincides with a child's learning styles, since the choice of setting should be partially determined by the child's ability to handle a variety of input. The child who learns best with reduced sensory stimuli may also learn best when the focus of a session is one content/form interaction for one use.

But even to focus on one goal in a session does not limit the number of goals that can be worked on in a period of time. One could cycle goals over a number of sessions—say, three different goals with one covered per session for three sessions and then back to goal 1 again, then goal 2, etc. (Fey, 1986). The advantage of having multiple goals is captured by the old saying "Don't put all your eggs in one basket." Our selection of goals is always a hypothesis and liable to error. Furthermore, there is no reason to believe that children can learn only one content/form/use interaction at a time; it is quite possible that working on more than one at a time facilitates the learning of each.

The Child's Language Behaviors

Although it is possible to learn something about language without demonstrating that learning, it is only through observing children's behaviors that the clinician has evidence of learning and is able to plan future modifications. The production of language behaviors also enables children to test hypotheses about their inductions of content, form, and use, and thus become more active in the learning process. But what behaviors are most appropriate and how can they be encouraged or elicited? Some questions to be considered in planning the language behaviors that are expected from the child are: "How can behaviors be elicited and maintained?" "What sense modality should be used?" "Should comprehension or production of the code be the major focus?"

Techniques for Eliciting Language Behaviors

Eliciting a language behavior is not necessarily the same as facilitating inductions of content/form/use interactions; one can elicit form alone. In this section we focus on techniques that can be used to elicit language behaviors; some are more useful than others in terms of inducing interactions among content, form, and use. Some techniques that elicit language behaviors for assessment purposes were discussed in Chapter 13; the application of these and other techniques for the purpose of intervention is discussed here. The techniques include asking the child to imitate the behavior, modeling the desired behavior, providing considerable input either through particular content/form/use interactions or through generalized stimulation, manipulating context so that the behavior is more likely to appear, delaying response to the child, or interacting in a nondirective manner with the child (Fey, 1986; Hart, 1985; Hubbell, 1977; Leonard, 1981).

One of the most direct techniques for eliciting a behavior is to ask the child to imitate the utterances or actions of the clinician, and when the imitations are appropriate, the child is reinforced. Such procedures are outlined in detail by Lovaas, Berberich, Perloff, and Schaeffer (1966), who stressed the production of linguistic forms alone, and by Risley and Wolf (1967), who stressed the production of forms in relation to limited contexts. In essence, the procedure is to teach an imitative set, gradually shape production to approximate the word, and then bring the production under the control of contexts other than the clinician's model utterance. This latter step is done by introducing the object or event that the utterance codes (such as ball) during imitation tasks and then gradually fading the model's utterances. The same techniques can be used to obtain comprehension responses—motor behaviors such as pointing or jumping can be modeled and, when imitated, can be connected to a linguistic stimulus such as "Show me _____" or "Jump." Eliciting language through imitation has been central to the studies of language learning that apply behaviorist principles—the child must produce the behavior in order to be reinforced. These studies have clearly demonstrated the effectiveness of this technique (imitation and reinforcement) in establishing behaviors that were not in the child's repertoire before training. The extent of establishment beyond the original training situation is not clear, because it has rarely been studied. It appears in many cases, however, that the child has learned the task at hand but has not induced a rule about the relationship of form to content and use, since the experimenters are often able to reverse the "learning" with short periods of reinforcement for the wrong response. It may be, as discussed by Levine and Fasnacht (1974), that the child has learned more about earning rewards than about language.

A modification of this technique (imitation and reinforcement) has been suggested by Bandura and Harris (1966). They used a *third person* to model the language behavior that the child was to produce. The *model* was rewarded for appropriate language behaviors, but not for errors; errors were occasionally included to increase discriminability of behavior that was to be learned. The *child* was then asked to try the same task and was reinforced for appropriate responses, but not for errors. Thus, there is a component of imitation, but it is delayed and may not be exact imitation, since the child's task may involve topics that differ from those of the model. Using such a procedure, Bandura and Harris (1966) successfully modified the syntactic style of a group of normal second-grade children to include passive sentence construction in response to pictures. Odom, Liebert, and Fernandez (1969) increased the use of prepositional phrases in a group of retarded children using a similar procedure and found that the increase was still retained 3 weeks after initial training, but, again, the follow-up was in the experimental setting. Certainly the modeling technique approaches the normal conditions of language learning more closely than the elicited imitation procedure and thus has more intuitive appeal. The use of a model seems to demand more active problem solving or rule induction on the part of the child than does immediate imitation and reinforcement.

A number of studies have compared the effects of modeling in contrast to imitation. In a study by Whitehurst & Novak (1973), imitation plus reinforcement was more effective for increasing the use of different phrase types than modeling; modeling was effective for only some children and some phrase types. In contrast, Courtright and Courtright (1976, 1979) reported that modeling was more effective than imitation whether or not they used reinforcement. However, the findings of Courtright and Courtright (1976) were not replicated by Connell, Gardner-Gletty, Dejewski, & Parks-Reinick (1981). No difference between the two techniques was reported by Haynes and Haynes (1980), who suggested that imitation may be best for initially establishing the form and then modeling might be the more effective technique for increasing the use of the form. The relative effectiveness of either technique may well vary with the level of language skill being learned, with the knowledge the child has about content/form/use interactions, and with the learning and communicative styles of the child. Certainly it is not clear at this time that one or the other should be used exclusively. (For further discussion, see the following section on comprehension versus production training.)

Another direct method of eliciting behaviors is through commands such as "Do this" or questions such as "What is this?" coupled with gestures and occasionally the direction to "Say, '_____ .' " Such direct elicitations are generally clinician-oriented, in that the target is selected by the clinician without necessarily being relevant to the child at any particular moment—see Fey (1986) for a discussion of clinician- versus child-oriented approaches.

In many direct elicitations (e.g., imitation) the child is presented with the forms but not the contexts that exemplify content and use. If the assumption is that the child needs only to practice form, then such presentation may be relevant. If the assumption is that the child needs to make an induction about how forms interact with content and use, then such presentation is inappropriate and other contexts must be included (e.g., forms presented in contexts that clearly demonstrate relations and functions to be coded). This can be done with a direct approach by including a third party who takes the child's role and cues the child with the appropriate response. In this way a model of the form is provided in an appropriate context (see, e.g., Swisher & Matkin, 1984). If it is assumed that these inductions are more likely to occur when they are relevant to the child, and more likely to be used when they are learned in ecologically sound environments, then the contexts in which language is elicited should reflect this. For example, if a child is trying to get another child to return a toy, the clinician can direct the child to request the toy by saying "Tell X, 'Give me my _____ .' " In this way the direct approach becomes more ecologically valid and provides input relative to the child's current thoughts and state of mind (see Constable, 1983, for more ideas on establishing contexts, and see the next chapter for more information relative to inductions).

In contrast to these direct attempts to elicit language productions, a more indirect approach has been advocated by others. On the basis of a review of the literature as well as direct experience, Hubbell (1977) concluded that directive interactions with children actually constrain spontaneous talking. He suggests that talking is facilitated by using an approach that follows the child's lead, as, for example, commenting on the child's activities or using parallel talk (rather than using commands), joining in the child's play (rather than directing the play activities), using praise (rather than correction), and waiting for a response (rather than demanding one or asking questions). Delay in responding to a child by looking questioningly and expectantly has also been found effective in eliciting language productions (Hart, 1985). The delay approach usually follows techniques aimed at facilitating the induction of the appropriate content/form interactions or is used to elicit behaviors that the clinician or educator knows are a part of the child's repertoire.

Another indirect approach involves manipulating the environment to increase the likelihood that the child will produce an utterance. For example, after various routines have been established in the intervention sessions, one or two aspects of the routine can be deliberately violated (such as starting to pour juice before passing out the cups) with the intent of eliciting comments from the child or children. In other instances the traditional use of an object (known to the child) can be violated (e.g., trying to get a drink of water from a strainer, or combing hair with a paintbrush). (See Constable, 1983, 1986; Fey, 1986; and Lucas, 1980, for further examples.)

Each of these indirect approaches provides the child with opportunities to practice in appropriate contexts. But most do not help the child make initial inductions about particular content/form/use interactions since they do not provide the child with exemplars in relation to meaning and use; their usefulness is for eliciting productions of content/form/use inductions that have already been made but may need to be practiced, or for producing particular content/form interactions for different functions.

To make inductions about content/form/use interactions, the child must be exposed to forms in appropriate contexts. Some indirect approaches appear to provide contexts in which inductions can be made as well as contexts that tend to elicit language productions. These techniques provide multiple exemplars of input. While they do not request a linguistic response, many have claimed that children do tend to produce these same forms after considerable input. The techniques include training comprehension, and simply providing input in certain contexts. Comprehension training is not often child-oriented and is actually directive in that a response is required. The response is usually manual and not linguistic. For example, the child might be shown two or three pictures and upon hearing a linguistic input is required to indicate which picture has been named. Given feedback, the child eventually pairs form with an exemplar of content and induces the relationship. According to Winitz (1973), this type of training leads to spontaneous production of these forms. This is discussed further in a later section of this chapter.

Alternatively, the child may be presented with multiple examples of forms in contexts that highlight the content and use of that form; no response is requested or required. When such input focuses on particular content/form/use interactions, it has been referred to as *focused stimulation* (Fey, 1986; Leonard, 1981). In one type of focused stimulation, the input is about the child's activities. For example, in one intervention session when a young boy decided he was leaving, the clinician sat in front of the door, and as the boy and the clinician tried to open the blocked door, the clinician kept saying "can't open it" or "it's stuck." Although the child was not asked to respond in any way, he began to say "n open . . . tuk" at first after the clinician and later without a prior utterance from her. Eventually, during the same session he produced the same utterance when a desk drawer would not open (for devious reasons). Children frequently do produce content/form/use interactions after such stimulation if the stimuli are at the appropriate developmental level. The input does not need to focus on the child's activities (i.e., it could focus on pictures or on the clinician's actions), if the facilitator is sure that the input codes what is in the child's consciousness at the moment.

In another type of focused stimulation, the clinician expands the child's utterance, by adding some appropriate lexical item or inflection, or recasts the child's utterance into a different syntactic form (e.g., a statement to a question). In expanding and recasting a child utterance the chances are good that you will be coding what is in the child's mind as well as providing a model for a different means of coding that idea. Since there is a tendency for children to repeat adult repetitions of the child's own utterances (Folger & Chapman, 1978), these techniques are also likely to elicit further language behaviors.

Thus we have both direct and indirect approaches to eliciting language behaviors. Some are more appropriate for giving the child practice in producing behaviors where inductions of content/form/use interactions have been at least partially established. Others are more appropriate for helping the child make such inductions. Furthermore, some are more ecologically valid than others and, therefore, appear better suited for generalization to the child's everyday life. Decisions about which techniques to apply will vary with the child and with the goals of intervention.

Techniques for Maintaining Language Behaviors

When appropriate language behaviors have been elicited, the goal is usually to increase and maintain the productions and to generalize the productions to many contexts. One means of accomplishing this has been by providing feedback to the child. The term *feedback* as used here refers to a means of letting the child know how closely a response approximates the response desired or expected by the language facilitator. Feedback can be provided in a number of ways. For one, the facilitator can follow each response of the child with a statement such as, "Yes, you said X right," or "No, listen, not Y, but X" (where X is the desired response and Y is an inappropriate response). In this manner the child is promptly informed about the correctness of the response and is given a correct model. Although this type of feedback is used by many clinicians and teachers, Muma (1971) suggested that it is ineffective in language learning if it focuses on errors of form.

Feedback in some language training programs has often been supplemented or replaced by a formal schedule of extrinsic reinforcement. In using reinforcement, a correct response by the child is followed by some consequence designed to increase the frequency of that response; undesired or incorrect responses from the child are either ignored or followed by consequences designed to decrease their frequency. What decreases responses from one child may well increase responses from another child; for example, spinning in a chair may be a desired activity for one but a frightening activity for another. Thus, those using reinforcement must determine what consequences can be used.

A variety of consequences can be considered as potential positive reinforcers. These include listener attention, successful communication, social interaction, participation in favorite activities, desired objects, or food. The likelihood that the language behaviors will not only increase but be maintained and generalize to many contexts is greatest when the reinforcers chosen are natural reinforcers that will be found in the child's everyday environment. Perhaps the most natural reinforcers of language are those that approximate the desired effect of language in most environments—listener attention, successful communication, and social interaction. For example, if the child is attempting to manipulate the environment through language and is successful, the success will most likely reinforce this behavior in similar situations. If a child says "want cookie" or "want ball" and obtains the cookie or ball in these contexts, the child is probably more likely to say these same utterances again when these objects are desired than if the child says "want cookie" or "want ball" and someone offers a different object or ignores the vocalizations. In addition, one would expect a relevant response to a comment might be more positively reinforcing than an irrelevant response or no response. For example, if a child says, while riding a bike, "I ride bike," one might expect that the response "And that's a big bike" would be more likely to increase the frequency of meaningful language than the response "Where's daddy?" or "Let's read a book." Unfortunately, little research has been done on the reinforcing effect of related versus unrelated responses to children's utterances. For many children, appropriate response to their attempts at language may be the only reinforcement needed. For other children, supporting social interaction (praise, smiles, or hugs) may also be needed.

There are children for whom social reinforcers are not at first effective but for whom manipulation of some object as a consequence of an appropriate response is enough to increase that response. For others, preferred activities (watching cartoons, being twirled in the air, sliding down a slide) act as positive reinforcement. Since participation in such activities can be disruptive unless tied directly to the teaching of a content/form/use interaction, many clinicians distribute chips or tokens after a correct response and allow the child to *buy* particular objects with these tokens at specified times. The tokens can be cashed in for some object or event the child desires and thus take on reinforcing properties and act to increase the frequency of the correct responses. A last alternative for children who respond to none of the above types of consequences as a positive reinforcer is the use of food. Most children who have not eaten for a period of time will find food positively reinforcing. Small quantities of well-liked, easily consumed food (e.g., ice cream, Fruit Loops, peanuts, or M&Ms) are given or fed to the child following desired responses. These, too, can interrupt verbalizing and eventually lose reinforcing value if the child becomes satiated; they are, indeed, a last resort.

The utilization of reinforcements as a means of increasing, maintaining, and generalizing a response has been extensively written about in a number of sources and will not be discussed further here. Instead, refer to the works of others such as Hart and Rogers-Warren (1978), Hughes (1985), Keller (1965), Lovaas et al. (1966), Mower (1984), Risley and Wolf (1967), and Sloane and McCauley (1968). These readings present the theory behind reinforcement in learning as well as specific procedures in using reinforcement to aid in language learning. However, extrinsic reinforcement should be used with caution. At least one study indicated that extrinsic reinforcements did not improve language performance (Courtright & Courtright, 1979). A number of studies have shown a decrease in the desired behavior as a result of extrinsic reinforcement when these behaviors had some intrinsic satisfaction before the issuing of reinforcers (e.g., Levine & Fasnacht, 1974). Although the desired behavior remained at a high level during the application of a token-type reinforcement by Levine and Fasnacht, it dropped below pre-reinforcement levels when the reinforcements were withdrawn without complicated schedules designed to eliminate extinction. Unless one is willing to follow such extinction procedures, reinforcements that are not a part of the child's natural environment should probably not be utilized. In any case, natural reinforcers are more effective in facilitating generalization of behaviors to the child's everyday life (see, for example, Goetz, Schuler, & Sailor, 1979; Hughes, 1985).

In summary, if we assume that language is a social act that is used as a means of making and maintaining social contact and as a means of manipulating one's environment, then it follows that language should be learned in such social contexts and reinforcements should come from these contexts. Thus, except in the most extreme cases of social withdrawal or rejection, reinforcement should come from naturally occurring reinforcers such as attention, recognition, and satisfaction of desires.

Sense Modality of Linguistic Behaviors

Goals of intervention include a description of the behaviors expected from the child. In Chapters 8–11, goals were presented for the production of linguistic units. The forms described are the forms used in the auditory-vocal language, but the content and use are also relevant in a visual-motor language. Speech is the preferred linguistic response because it is the most common means of communication, but alternative systems must be considered for some children—children for whom intelligible speech appears virtually impossible, at least in the immediate future (e.g., children with paralysis of the articulatory tract musculature). Possible alternatives to speech as a linguistic response are sign language, typewriters, communication boards, and aids with TV display, printed output or synthesized speech. Unfortunately, children who have severe difficulty with speech because of poor muscle control often have poor control of other musculature as well, so that sign language and typewriters are not viable alternatives. When this is so, the communication board (or an aid which utilizes a board arrangement) can become the mode of linguistic response for the child. (See Harris & Vanderheiden, 1980, for a discussion of techniques for these "nonvocal" children.)

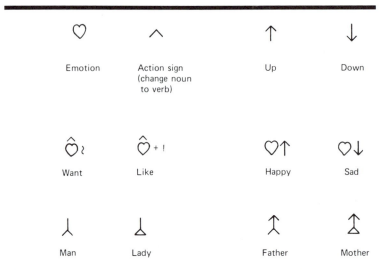

These examples illustrate how symbols can be combined.

FIGURE 14-1 Examples of Bliss Symbols (adapted from Vanderheiden & Harris-Vanderheiden, 1976; and Clark & Woodcock, 1976)

A communication board usually consists of a lap board that is set across the arms of a wheelchair or attached to a bed or a desk and has affixed to it a means of representing objects, actions, and states that are important to the communicator. These representations are most commonly pictures (e.g., a toilet, a glass of water, a bed, mother, and someone eating) and written words—particularly common are the words *yes* and *no.* A few boards have been designed with more abstract symbolic representation, using geometric configurations paired with a written word. The use of these abstract configurations instead of pictures increases the possibilities for combinations of symbols and thus broadens the applicability of the communication board. Any communication board is, however, more limiting than an auditory-vocal system, not only in the number of combinations that are ultimately possible, but also in the speed with which communication can take place.

A pilot implementation of an abstract system has been reported by D. Vanderheiden, Brown, MacKenzie, Reinen, and Scheibel (1975). They used the Bliss symbols (*Bliss Semantography*, Australia: Semantography Publications, as referenced by D. Vanderheiden et al., 1975) instead of pictures because they felt that pictures limited the generalization of a concept and tied it to a specific object or action; for example, the concept "eat" might be tied to the particular food pictured in the eating process (see Figure 14-1 for examples of these symbols). Vanderheiden et al. used the Bliss symbols instead of words because they felt the symbols were less complex than actual words. However, they printed the words under each symbol on the communication board so that persons communicating with the child would not have to learn the geometric symbols. Spoken language was used by the teacher and was presented with the symbolic representation on the board. Thus objects and people in the environment were labeled with the appropriate spoken words, printed words, and Bliss symbols, and the child's response was to point to the symbols on the board. Theoretically then, the child understood speech but produced language through visual symbols.

More efficient communication boards are needed; information about normal language development may be applicable both in the choice of concepts represented and in the organization of the symbols on the board. For example, relational words, which are used frequently in the single-word-utterance period (Bloom, 1973), can be used to refer to many objects and events, and the pro-verbs used most frequently in early sentences are verbs such as *do, get, make,* and *go,* which can be used in more different events than other verbs such as *catch, brush,* and *fill.* (See, e.g., Blau, 1983; Fristoe & Lloyd, 1980). Symbols to represent these words may be more efficient than symbols that represent more specific objects or event relations and may be included on first boards and given prominence in other boards. Finally, the categories of content that have evolved from the study of child language (action, state, etc.) may provide a means of organizing symbols that has more relevance to the child first learning language than, for example, traditional parts of speech such as noun and verb. Unquestionably, further refinements in communication boards—refinements in their operation (computer or other electronic controls), in their makeup (the forms and the content coded), and in the organization of the symbols—will make them more efficient.

Alternative modalities for communication have been attempted recently for a number of children with a language disorder—not so much because the child is unable to produce the speech signal but, instead, because the child seems unable to learn content/form/use interactions when the form is the speech signal. These difficulties seem to be more related to processing the linguistic input than to producing the linguistic signal and are discussed in the next chapter.

Comprehension Versus Production

One question asked by those responsible for facilitating language learning is "What should be the relative importance and sequence of training in comprehension versus production of language?" The question probably arises because so many studies and tests have been directed to either one or the other as evidence of language knowledge. Many studies and language programs have stressed the imitative production of linguistic forms as a first step in language learning for the nonverbal child (Buddenhagen, 1971; Guess, Rutherford, & Twichell, 1969; Hewett, 1965; Lovaas, Berberich, Perloff, & Schaeffer, 1966; McGinnis, Kleffner, & Goldstein, 1956; Sherman, 1965). Based on the concepts that children learn to speak by imitating and that a behavior needs to be produced in order to be reinforced, it was felt that imitative responses would be the "most beneficial and practical starting point for building speech" (Lovaas et al. 1966, p. 706). When an imitative repertoire was established, contexts (such as objects), which eventually were to elicit these responses, were associated with the response and the model utterance was dropped—thus an aspect of meaning was established (Brawley, Harris, Allen, Fleming, & Peterson, 1969; Hewett, 1965; Risley & Wolf, 1967; J. Stark, Giddan, & Meisel, 1968).

Most studies measured the learning of content/form interactions by the degree of generalization of the new behavior to new contexts (such as the production of plurals when shown objects known to the child but not used in training the morpheme). Garcia (1974) trained two profoundly retarded adolescents, speaking in single-word utterances, to "converse" through imitation. They were trained to ask "What is that?" when shown a picture, to label the picture when asked, and to respond "Yes, I do," when asked if they wanted the picture. She noted poor generalization of the same tasks when a different experimenter was used. Most studies have measured generalization within the same setting and with the same person who did the training; few studies have searched for generalizations in the child's natural environment. In one exception, Gray and Ryan (1973) reported that forms taught in formal instruction were used in the classroom "show and tell" discussions with about the same accuracy as in the training program. Furthermore, children were using the same form plus new forms not taught in the program in the home environment. From these observations they concluded:

> Apparently, it is not necessary to build an extensive receptive language repertoire using a non-verbal response (pointing, for example) before teaching expressive language. A child may successfully be asked to emit a verbal response early in the teaching sequence. It is possible that the development of an expressive repertoire may actually enhance the learning of a receptive repertoire [as pointed out by Guess (1969)]. Gray and Ryan (1973, p. 171)

An opposite view is held by D. Johnson and Myklebust (1967) and by Winitz (1973, 1976), who recommended extensive training in comprehension before training or even encouraging productions of forms. "Our task should be to functionalize the environment so that language and thought can be paired . . . not . . . that of forcing production in order to achieve syntactically correct sentences" (Winitz, 1976, p. 404). Winitz suggested problem-solving situations in which the child would induce rules by listening to forms spoken by the clinician and would be rewarded for selecting the picture appropriate to the meaning of the form. He cited one anecdote where the child spontaneously produced a form that was trained in comprehension only. Winitz based his suggestions on experiences with second language learning (German) by college students.

In a later publication, Winitz (1983) described comprehension training more in terms of listening within a communicative environment than in terms of providing evidence of comprehension by responding to input. In this interpretation, comprehension training seems closer to the focused stimulation discussed above. Although D. Johnson and Myklebust (1967) stressed training in comprehension before production (and also noted that spontaneous verbal expression improved with comprehension), they pointed out that using newly learned words can strengthen comprehension.

Few studies have reported training of comprehension only. In one, Striefel and Wetherby (1973) taught an 11-year-old nonlinguistic boy to follow two- to four-word commands that involved actions on objects, occasionally with an instrument ("push car," "rub cheek with washcloth"), but they found no generalization to untrained combinations of actions and objects. Although the child was trained to respond correctly to "point to ear," "point to nose," and "brush hair," he did not correctly respond to "point to hair" but, instead, responded to the action usually associated with the object (i.e., the brushing). In contrast, Baer and Guess (1973),

Guess (1969), and Guess and Baer (1973) reported generalization of responses to morphological inflections (the child pointed to two objects in response to the name of the object plus the plural morpheme -s when presented with words and objects not used in training). The more difficult task of measuring generalization of this comprehension in natural environments has not been carried out.

The interdependence of comprehension and production has been studied using the plural morpheme, lexical items, and word order. Focusing on the plural morpheme, Guess (1969) and Guess and Baer (1973) supported a view of independence between the tasks in at least some children. Using four subjects, Guess and Baer (1973) found mixed results. No generalization was found in one subject, only slight generalization in two subjects, and strong generalization in the fourth subject. In a later study reported by Siegel and Vogt (1984), mixed results were again reported; one child generalized the plural morpheme from production training to comprehension, another generalized from comprehension training to production, and two children did not generalize at all although they were given similar training. Although Siegel and Vogt found no advantage for training in comprehension or production, the children found the comprehension training less interesting than the production training. Finally, training the plural in two retarded adolescents, Holdgrapher (1981) found independence between the comprehension and production training. Thus, training in comprehension did not always lead to correct production, and training in production did not always lead to correct comprehension. The differences among the children are not readily explainable at this time.

Similar results were reported by Ruder, Smith, and Hermann (1974) when examining the effect of imitation and comprehension training on the production of foreign words for familiar objects. They concluded that neither comprehension training alone nor imitation training alone can be used to achieve production of lexical items, but, instead, "the data argue in favor of a training program for lexical items that contains both imitation and comprehension training . . ." (p. 27). In another study, Connell and McReynolds (1981) taught children two different names for objects—one in comprehension training and one in production training. They also found variability among the children: some kept two separate names for each mode, others consistently used the name taught in the first mode of training, and others had variable use of the two names. Children learned to change names better in production training than in comprehension training and were more likely to generalize to comprehension from production training. Since both studies involved learning to change the name of an object and not learning one new name, the results cannot be easily generalized to first language learning. The above studies, in combination with the studies on plural s, suggest that experiences in both comprehension and production may be necessary for lexical learning and for the learning of morphological inflections.

However, one further study on acquisition of lexical items indicated that normal language learners and children with specific language impairment learned to comprehend and produce a number of words based on a focused stimulation approach where no response was required during the training (Leonard, Schwartz, et al., 1982). While the children comprehended more of these words than they produced, they produced some newly learned words during production probes that they did not give evidence of comprehending during comprehension probes. The results suggest that children can learn to both comprehend and produce new words on the basis of input alone but that there is some independence between comprehension and production responses in lexical learning. This independence has also been found in normal language learners—that is, the first words that children comprehend are not always the ones that they produce and vice versa (see Bloom & Lahey, 1978, and Leonard, Schwartz, et al., 1982, for a review of such studies). Before concluding that production practice is not necessary, it is important to note that although production was not required of the children in the Leonard, Schwartz, et al. study, a number of them did spontaneously imitate and spontaneously produce many of these words. Words that were spontaneously imitated and produced during the sessions were more likely to be produced on the production probes at the end of the training (but not more likely to be comprehended), suggesting that unsolicited imitations and productions may facilitate elicited production responses (R. Schwartz & Leonard, 1985) and that such productions may not need to be elicited.

Normal language-learning children can apparently make rapid inductions about form and content when the stimuli are presented in a meaningful context although this induction is often context-bound (see the fast mapping studies by Dollaghan, 1985, and Streim & Chapman, 1986). These inductions enable the children to identify the words but not necessarily to produce the words. While 90% of the children could identify words after one exposure in the Dollaghan study, less than half could label the words after two exposures. In a later study, Dollaghan (1987) found that language-disordered children could also identify words after only one exposure, but they had more difficulty than normals in producing the new words. Naming a word requires a more complete phonetic representation than identification; phonetic representations may become more complete through practice with production (as suggested by R. Brown & McNeill, 1966).

Two further studies related to the issue of comprehension versus production in language learning were carried out by Courtright and Courtright (1976, 1979). These authors compared training procedures that varied in the amount of production required. In one study the target was correct use of the pronoun *they*, and in the second it was the use of a dummy auxiliary form. The procedure that demanded immediate imitation was less successful than the procedure that demanded listening to the correct production of 20 utterances before responding. The authors concluded "that an abstract rule (for example, a language rule) is best learned by passive observation" (p. 661); quoting Zimmerman and Bell's (1972) "interference hypothesis," they questioned the use of imitation approaches.

Replication of such findings (an attempt by Connell et al., 1981) was unsuccessful, and an expansion of such findings to different content/form/use interactions and different populations is necessary before conclusions can be drawn. A number of questions remain unanswered. For example, do differences among children reflect styles of learning, developmental levels, or difficulties with cognitive processing? Would the results differ if the contexts were more ecologically valid (i.e., the interactions taught were immediately relevant to the child)? Would some combination of input and production be more efficient with the same children? Is it possible that there would be greater interdependence between training in comprehension and training in production if the content/form interaction that was taught was developmentally close to the child's present language skills? Finally, does the influence of one type of training (comprehension or production) vary with the type of form (i.e., lexical item or morphological or syntactic rule), the content category, or the interaction?

A recent training study suggests that the answer to the last question may be yes—the content/form interaction being learned may well influence the effectiveness of the type of training. In the training of word order to code semantic-syntactic relations, production training was found effective for learning production, but not comprehension, while comprehension training was not effective for learning comprehension or production responses (Connell, 1986). Six children with specific language impairment were given comprehension and production training on a set of three pictures. (The children were producing only single-word utterances at the time and were giving chance responses to subject-verb-object stimuli with reversible subjects and objects, such as "frog kiss worm"). Production training involved imitation and then labeling of picture pairs (e.g., "worm kiss frog" and "frog kiss worm"), while comprehension training involved pointing to the appropriate picture pair (with assistance at first) when the researcher produced the appropriate sentence. Generalization was measured using 10 additional pictures and analysis of spontaneous conversations. Training in production generalized to the 10 pictures and resulted in an increase in the coding of these semantic-syntactic relations in spontaneous speech, but did not affect comprehension responses. Comprehension training did not result in improved comprehension or production responses for any of the children.

In contrast to similar studies on lexical learning and on morphological inflections, this study suggests that comprehension training is not an effective means of facilitating content/form interactions involving word-order rules. Similarities with normal language learning are again apparent; children use word order in their spontaneous speech before they utilize it to respond to comprehension tasks. But responding to comprehension tasks is a strange and unnatural phenomenon. Any student who has taken a multiple-choice exam can attest to the problem with foils. While you thought you knew the answer to the question, the foil can confuse you. In addition, the attentional (or processing) capacity needed for comprehension responses given the usual testing format is probably greater than that required for production (Bloom, 1974; Connell, 1986). The child must process the sentence produced, as well as the relations expressed in both pictures. Again, further research is needed to verify these findings and to explore other means of measuring comprehension. It appears, however, that tasks for measuring responses to comprehension and production may not be equivalent.

The question about developmental readiness for a form has not been experimentally addressed; however, an analysis of some of the studies suggests that the children may not have had the prerequisite language experience to handle the interactions presented.* Thus, task-specific learning (in contrast to rule induction) may not be unexpected. For example, if the children taught the plural morpheme had language skills comparable to those of the normal child who is first productive with this morpheme, would they have learned the rule in both comprehension and production tasks? Is it possible that differences in language skills could account for

---

* In one study children were more likely to generalize forms that were about the same complexity as those found in their free speech than forms that were longer and more complex (Warren & Kaiser, 1986).

the differences in generalization that did occur among the children in the study by Guess and Baer (1973)?

Certainly the lack of generalization to commands within the comprehension task reported by Striefel and Wetherby (1973) might well be explained by the level of task compared with the level of language skill brought to the task. The children were reportedly nonverbal, but could produce a few names of objects and could imitate. The generalization task demanded knowledge of verb-object to code action-object relations, and some demanded further knowledge of instrument relations as coded by prepositional phrases. It is not surprising then that on generalization probes, the children responded to only one word in the sentence and produced the action that had previously been associated with that object. Similarly, the lack of generalization to another experimenter reported by Garcia (1974) may be related to the unrealistic level of task—the use of discourse—expected from children who know only a few words.

Gray and Ryan (1973) taught content/form interactions through imitation of forms in relation to pictures (a production approach), and reported generalization to the classroom and home. However, they may have been teaching forms that the children were ready to learn (and perhaps forms they already comprehended to some extent). Ruder, Smith, and Hermann (1974) reported a lack of generalization from training in imitation to comprehension of content/form interactions, which is not surprising since the content was never presented when children were asked to imitate forms. They also reported lack of generalization from training in comprehension to production, which is less easy to account for since the children were presented with pictures. The children were certainly developmentally ready for the simple nouns taught, since their language level was reportedly 3.5 years. However, in order to control for prior experience, Spanish words were used for objects that the children probably already had English names for, and this may have accounted for the lack of generalizations.

Thus, it may be, as Winitz (1976) and D. Johnson and Myklebust (1967) have suggested, that there is no need to force production if the child is exposed to forms in the context of objects and events that code their meaning and use. Production may well follow naturally, but this may be true *only* if the input is at a level that the child is ready to accept—a level that allows the child to build on present knowledge of language to learn new interactions. The evidence does not support the view that comprehension tasks (identifying, acting out, etc.) need to precede such production tasks as imitation or vice versa.

In view of this inconclusive evidence, the clinician or educator has two choices. One choice is to elicit both types of responses, that is, to teach each goal with elicited responses that provide evidence of both comprehension and production. Such an approach is counter to the developmental interaction between comprehension and production found in young children learning language without difficulty. While, for example, the receptive vocabulary of normal language learners is larger than their spoken vocabulary, recall that the first words understood are not the same as the first words spoken (see Bloom, 1974; Goldin-Meadow et al., 1976). Furthermore, demonstration of grammatical understanding through comprehension tasks often comes much later than consistent production of the same forms (e.g., Brown, 1973; Chapman & Miller, 1975; and see Bloom & Lahey, 1978, for further discussion of the developmental relationship between comprehension and production). Thus, equivalent responses in both modes are not found in the young language learner. Should we expect them in the language-disordered child? If this choice is selected, then the assumptions are that children will best learn to comprehend content/form/use interactions by having multiple experiences giving direct evidence of that comprehension (e.g., pointing) and that production will be best learned through elicited productions of content/form/use interactions.

The second choice takes into account the findings of most of these studies and the importance of input as well as practice in producing content/form interactions; it exposes the child to naturalistic contexts that illustrate content/form/use interactions (a focused stimulation approach) commensurate with the child's level of development (as determined by methods suggested earlier in this book) and the child's consciousness at the moment. Input is provided from which the child can induce interactions among content/form/and use—an induction necessary for both comprehension and production. If production does not follow after repeated presentations, production can be elicited in similar contexts using the elicitation techniques discussed earlier. In this manner, input would precede output as an intervention strategy, but neither production nor comprehension is considered apart from *use* or apart from each other. The assumptions of this second choice include (1) that the child must be exposed to exemplars of linguistic form in contexts that make obvious the content that the form codes as well as the functions that it can serve; (2) that the child's production of forms facilitates language learning when it takes place in contexts where both coding the content and communicating a function are appropriate; and (3) that the child's pointing to contrastive stimuli based on morphological inflections or syntactic cues is not necessary at the early stages of language learning and need not be a part of an intervention program geared to early language learning.

Summary

Before planning the specific techniques that can lead to induction of content/form/use interactions, a number of more general factors must be considered along with the assumptions about language learning that underlie them. First there are factors that may be maintaining the child's difficulty with language learning and may be amenable to change, such as hearing loss, poor health, or parent-child interactional patterns. Second, there are some considerations that relate to the setting of intervention. Children may differ in the amount of structure that they need in order to induce content/form/use interactions. Observation of the child's attentional patterns in different contexts is the best means of deciding the degree of structure needed. Whenever possible, the context of learning should resemble the natural environment and the caregivers should be involved in the process.

The last general consideration concerns the behaviors that the child is expected to produce. A variety of techniques are available for eliciting and maintaining behavioral responses (e.g., modeling, imitation, reinforcement). Some are more relevant for facilitating the induction of content/form/use interactions, while others are more relevant for practicing and increasing the use of inductions that have already been made. For children who are unable to produce the speech signal, an alternative modality of response is necessary and must be considered.

The nature of this alternative modality will influence techniques used to facilitate language goals. Finally, the relative emphasis that should be placed on comprehension versus production in language intervention is discussed.

Suggested Readings

Fey, M. (1986). *Language intervention with young children.* San Diego: College-Hill Press.

Leonard, L. (1981). An invited article: Facilitating linguistic skills in children with specific language impairment. *Applied Psycholinguistics, 2,* 89–118.

Miller, J., Yoder, D., & Schiefelbusch, R. (Eds.) (1983). *Contemporary issues in language intervention.* ASHA Reports, Rockville, MD: American Speech-Language-Hearing Association.

Warren, S., & Rogers-Warren, A. (1985). *Teaching functional language.* Baltimore: University Park Press.

15

Facilitating the Induction of Content/Form/Use Interactions

Learning language is a process of inducing relationships among regularities the child has perceived in the nonlinguistic world (the concepts that are the content of language), the linguistic signal (the arbitrary units that are the conventional forms of a language), and social interactions (the contexts that affect the use of language as a means of communication). These inductions are necessary for learning language, regardless of age. They are the inductions the normal 2-year-old child is forming spontaneously, but they are also the inductions the 5- or 10-year-old child with a language disorder must make.

If language learning is an induction, how can it be taught? One cannot, in fact, teach a child early language skills, if teaching means imparting information or knowledge. The rules of language cannot be written out, described, or otherwise given to the language learner. One cannot use language to talk about language to a child who is only just learning language. The rules of language must be induced by the learner from tangible experiences with objects and events, linguistic forms, and interpersonal interactions.

The person who intervenes in a child's life to aid in the language-learning process is not, then, a teacher in the traditional sense (i.e., one who gives information or trains in skills) but, instead, one who manipulates these tangible aspects of a child's environment in a way that facilitates the formation of these inductions. To stress this important difference, the term *facilitator* will be used to refer to the person directly responsible for intervention procedures (Taenzer, Bass, & Kise, 1974). The role of the facilitator is to arrange external events in the child's life in a manner that will make it easier for the child to induce the relationships among content, form, and use.

Language intervention can be viewed in terms of the tangible external events available to the facilitator. Figure 15-1 illustrates the factors that are external and, thus, available for manipulation, and the inductions that are the internal desired results of intervention. The linguistic forms that are presented to the child are both external and manipulable. The facilitator may choose from among different lexical items and linguistic structures and, in order to increase their salience, may vary the manner and frequency of their presentation. The nonlinguistic context is also manipulable; the facilitator may present certain objects and manipulate, or have the child manipulate, these objects in relationship to each other and to the child in order to demonstrate the many concepts that language codes. Finally, the facilitator can vary the social context in order to model, reinforce, or create the need for interpersonal communication or to interact in ways appropriate to the child's meanings. These three manipulable factors are represented as external to the child. The induction of the regularities within each of these factors and the relationship among them are internal.

The term *intervention* is used here to refer to changes that are made in a child's environment for the purpose of facilitating the learning of language.

Decisions about the context in which intervention is to take place will influence who will manipulate the environment and how artificial the manipulation might be. As described in Chapter 14, naturalistic contexts with natural reinforcers are preferable; whenever possible, people who are an important part of the child's life should be included. These naturalistic contexts also adapt well to coding ideas that are in the child's consciousness.

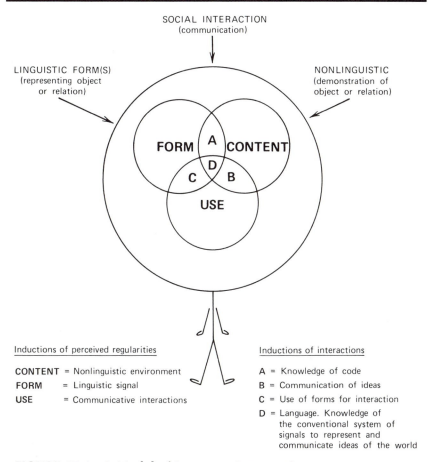

FIGURE 15-1   A Model of Language Intervention

Language intervention involves seeing the child's view and utilizing this view for facilitation of inductions about content/form/use interactions. In order to induce the interaction of content with form, the relationship to be coded (i.e., an exemplar of the content) must be in the child's immediate attention when the form is processed. For example, facilitating inductions about the expression of a particular intention, such as getting attention, is best done when the child shows evidence of attention-getting behavior (no matter how idiosyncratic that attempt may be). Similarly, facilitating inductions of content/form interactions is best done when the child's thoughts appear to be about that content (such as action when the child is acting on an object). It is probably not helpful to present a model that codes possession while the child is focusing on tying a bow in a shoe, trying to put a shoe on, or filling a shoe with beans. In these situations, action or locative-action relations might be more relevant to the child's attentional focus. Thus, regardless of how well an intervention session may be planned, the facilitator must be constantly sensitive to the child's thoughts and intentions.

Following the child's lead (i.e., talking about what the child is doing or saying) is one way of coding what the child is currently thinking about. However, one does not always have to follow the lead of the child; events can often be structured that encourage certain intents or thoughts on the part of the child. One alternative is to utilize familiar routines where the child knows what to expect—familiar routines also have the advantage of a certain amount of automaticity, thus freeing attentional capacity for processing form and for making inductions about content/form/use interactions (see Case, 1985; K. Nelson, 1986; Shatz, 1977). (For example, when children are devoting most of their attentional capacity to tying a knot, they may be unable to focus on linguistic input or make inductions; when such behavior becomes more automatic, or at least less difficult, the context may be an ideal one for facilitating inductions.) However, sensitivity to the child's state of mind is always needed to ensure that the anticipated thoughts and intents have been obtained.

Some operate under the assumption that the functions of language serve as the primary force in language learning and, therefore, should be the primary focus of intervention (e.g., Duchan, 1986). In this view, intervention is involved in inputing an intention to communicative acts and reacting to that intention—goals are to provide more conventional means of expressing the intention, and techniques focus on creating contexts that encourage the expression of many different intentions. Goals of content/form interactions are secondary to the function that they serve. Assessment is geared to an analysis of communicative intents expressed and to the flexibility with which they are expressed, as well as to how language is used to maintain and regulate conversation.

Others vary the primacy of use with the apparent needs of the child. If the language problems of a child are primarily concerned with using the code that they already know, then the focus of intervention is on aspects of language use, such as expressing intentions in various ways or choosing alternative forms according to changes in context. However, other children communicate many functions with a limited code and adapt this limited code to differing contexts quite readily and without facilitative efforts. For these children, the primary goals of intervention relate to content/form interactions (e.g., Lucas, 1980).

Despite unresolved differences in the importance placed on the functions of language as a *motivating* force in language learning, it is generally agreed that the language code is always learned in some context and for some function, and, therefore, *use* is an important consideration in language intervention. For example, it is widely accepted now that intervention should take place in natural and familiar contexts, involve reciprocal interactions with others in contrast to only responses or drill interactions, be meaningful and functional for the child, and utilize the natural consequences of language (as maintaining or getting attention) rather than extrinsic reinforcements (such as tokens or "good talking") (e.g., Bloom & Lahey, 1978; P. Cole, 1982; Constable, 1986; Craig, 1983; Duchan, 1986; Fey, 1986; Hart & Rogers-Warren, 1978; Lucas, 1980; Muma, 1978; Snow, Midkiff-Borunda, Small, & Proctor, 1984). Whether or not the immediate primary goals of intervention involve goals of use or goals of content/form, the interaction of content, form, and use is the ultimate goal of intervention. Facilitating aspects of use may facilitate content/form interactions, and the learning of content/form interactions may facilitate use.

Chapter 14 considered adaptations based on the child's abilities and styles and discussed the setting of intervention. This chapter considers modifications that can be made in a child's environment when facilitating language learning. Aspects of the environment that can be manipulated to relate to the goals of content/form/use interactions presented in Chapters 8–11 include the linguistic input, the nonlinguistic demonstration of relations, and social interactions. The principles discussed in the following section on use are relevant to language intervention for all children—those who are having difficulty learning content/form interactions as well as those who are having difficulty communicating their intentions or choosing among alternative content/form interactions in varying contexts.

Facilitating Inductions about Language Use

Before facilitating the use of content/form interactions, precursory goals of use should be assessed (see Chapter 9). For example, we expect a child to intentionally communicate a number of functions (such as getting attention, requesting actions and objects, pointing out interesting events and objects) using nonlinguistic means before conventional words are used for these functions. In addition, we expect a child to interact with others using interpersonal gaze, showing and giving objects, participating in routines with reciprocal roles, and focusing attention on objects that others are gazing at or pointing out. If such behaviors are not directly observed or reported, then intervention should focus on facilitating such interactions.

Communicating Interpersonal Intentions

Certainly a primary function of language is interpersonal communication. Interpersonal functions that children communicate include establishing contact with others and regulating (e.g., by manipulating another's actions, attempting to obtain desired objects, or getting information). These communicative functions are important considerations in language intervention.

To facilitate the expression of these functions, the child can be placed in many situations where interpersonal interactions are important, such as situations where making contact with another, requesting an object, manipulating another's actions, and obtaining information might make a difference to the child. With children who seem uninterested in interpersonal interactions, other means must be devised. One way to make contact with very severely disturbed children is to imitate the child's actions. For example, Tiegerman and Primavera (1984) reported that imitation of an autistic child's actions resulted in an increase in the frequency and duration of interpersonal gaze. The alert facilitator tunes in carefully to the communicative needs of the child even though they may be expressed in idiosyncratic ways. For example, Prizant and Duchan (1981) noted that echolalia often serves a communicative function (see Belkin, 1983, for examples of sensitivity to a child's interests and attempts to communicate).

For most children, however, communicative intents are varied and not difficult to interpret. Attempts at communication are rewarded by responding to the child's intent and perhaps by providing a more conventional means of expressing that intent. But the initial goal is for the child to communicate intents in any fashion. When a variety of intents are communicated frequently, the goal shifts to the means by which these same intents are expressed. Thus, we might at first be happy for the child to simply reach for an object as a request, but later we want accompanying eye gaze and vocalization and eventually the use of content/form interactions appropriate to the listener. The child's attempts to use the desired means of expression are quickly rewarded by an appropriate response to the intent—*not* by shrieks of joy or phrases like "Good talking!" Taking advantage of the child's sincere communicative desires often supplies considerable motivation and reinforcement for learning.

As noted earlier, to make the code useful to the child means careful observation and a sensitivity that enables one to see a situation from the child's point of view. (See Box 15-1). It means a constant awareness of the function and content that will have the most utility for the child. The forms of expression are selected according to the child's level of development.

Modeling is one technique for facilitating inductions of use with content and form or with other forms of expression. When the child, or other visible person, is clearly trying to communicate a function, the facilitator provides the appropriate forms. For some children, modeling of successful communication by a third party (as discussed by Bandura & Harris, 1966) may help in facilitating the use of language. Another child, or an adult who is engaged in similar activities as the child, can produce the content/form interaction appropriate to both their needs. The utterance by the model is quickly rewarded and perhaps repeated by the facilitator. The modeled situation would need to be timed to coincide with the child's attention to the model and to the child's communicative need. Repeated examples may help some children induce the content/form/use interactions. For example, attention-getting behavior could be modeled in a group context when children are painting; as each child says "see my picture!" the teacher quickly goes to look at and comment on the child's picture. In a clinical setting, an extra person could be included who would model an attention-getting device after completing a puzzle, or some other task, and the clinician would quickly attend and react. Alternatively, the child could be asked to imitate words that communicate an intent, and the imitation could be responded to or the child could simply be provided with the appropriate forms without requesting a response.

Some examples of different techniques that might be attempted in order to facilitate the use of conventional forms for calling attention to objects and for obtaining objects are described below.

Calling Attention to Objects.   A child has completed a high block tower and looks and smiles at the adult and looks back at the tower. The adult might say, "Look! Look at that big tower!" while looking at the tower and then at the child and pointing to the tower. In time, the adult might further suggest that the child "tell X to look! Look at the tower." Thus, a conventional expression of the intent to call attention to the tower is modeled and an attempt is made to elicit the response in a meaningful context if it is felt the child can carry out such a suggestion. Further modeling might be done by others in a group—where each completes some project like a painting, tower, or puzzle and calls attention to the completed

---

BOX 15-1   Facilitating Language Use

On the fourth day of this next experiment I succeeded to my heart's content, and I heard Victor pronounce distinctly, though rather uncouthly it is true, the word lait, *and he repeated it almost immediately. It was the first time that an articulate sound left his mouth and I did not hear it without the most intense satisfaction.*

Nevertheless I made a reflection which in my eyes much diminished the advantage of this first success. It was not until the moment when, despairing of success, I came to pour the milk into the cup which he gave me, that the word lait *escaped him with great demonstrations of pleasure; and it was only after I had poured it again as a reward that he pronounced it a second time. It can be seen why this result was far from fulfilling my intentions. The word pronounced instead of being the sign of his need was, relative to the time when it had been articulated, merely an exclamation of pleasure. If this word had been uttered before the thing which he desired had been granted, success was ours, the real use of speech was grasped by Victor, a point of communication established between him and me, and the most rapid progress would spring from this first triumph. Instead of all this, I had just obtained a mere expression, insignificant to him and useless to us, of the pleasure which he felt. Strictly speaking, it was certainly a vocal sign, the sign of possession. But this sign, I repeat, did not establish any relation between us. It had soon to be neglected because it was useless to the needs of the individual and was swamped by a multitude of irrelevancies, like the ephemeral and variable sentiment for which it had become the sign. The subsequent results of this misuse of the word have been such as I feared.*

It was generally only during the enjoyment of the beverage that the word lait *was heard. Sometimes he happened to pronounce it before and at other times a little after but always without purpose.*

Note: From Itard, 1962, pp. 31 and 32.

This description by Itard of the facilitation of language with Victor, "the wild boy of Averyon," dramatically pictures Itard's sensitivity to the importance of the pragmatic context of language, but an inflexibility that came from his narrow definition of language use. He was particularly insensitive to the intensity of Victor's recognition and pleasure in this more intrapersonal use of his *first word.* Children's early use of language is often intrapersonal in just this way.

---

project by calling the teacher or another child using some conventional means of calling attention.

Obtaining Objects.   A child strains and reaches for a train that is out of reach, whimpers, and looks at the adult. The adult might say: "Train/ Train/ You want the train?" looking back and forth between the child and the train and then pausing for a moment to give the child the opportunity to respond. The child is given the train perhaps with the utterance "you can have the train." A third party can be used to model the appropriate response. For example, other children or adults can be shown some toys, which are then placed out of sight in a bag. The children or adults are asked individually what they want to play with, and they respond with an appropriate level of content/form interaction. Thus, the pragmatic context is appropriate for request; the affective intensity may not be so great as above, allowing more resources for language production; and the appropriate response has been modeled repeatedly (see Constable, 1983, for examples). Such situations can be routines for classroom or intervention sessions.

Other.   Situations can be devised that increase the need for communication. Important, necessary, or favorite objects can be temporarily misplaced, encouraging the child to ask for information ("where X?") or to request an object. Novel or unusual objects can be brought in and placed just out of reach, encouraging similar functions. Objects that are hard to operate, open, or fix may encourage requests for help. Objects can be inappropriately used or routines broken to encourage protests (see Constable, 1983, 1986, and Lucas, 1980, for examples). Eventually the facilitator can delay a response to the child's typical expression of an intent and present a puzzled look in the attempt to elicit a more conventional or sophisticated expression.

However, one cannot divorce the child's expression of content/form interactions from procedures for inducing content/form/*use* interactions anymore than one could separate these factors in setting goals. Unless a particular use can only be expressed with a particular form, it is unlikely that a new function will emerge with a new content/form interaction (or vice versa). As has been reported for form in relation to *content* (Bloom, 1970; Slobin, 1973), new communicative functions are usually expressed with old forms (Gerber, 1987). Thus, when facilitating the expression of new functions, it would be wise to use familiar content/form interactions. New learning builds on old knowledge in small increments, not in giant steps.

Using Language for Intrapersonal Functions

Children and adults use language at times when no interpersonal communicative intent is obvious. The child says "up" while climbing up, "down" while climbing down, "stop" while stopping the truck, and "doll fall" after the doll has fallen. In many instances, there does not seem to be an attempt to direct the utterance to anyone, nor does there seem to be any observable benefit derived from speaking. In other instances the utterances appear to be directed, or interactive, but require no response (Gerber, 1987). Bloom (1970) referred to such utterances as "comments," and Halliday (1975) suggested that such comments may serve a mathetic function; that is, they may serve to direct the child's activities or aid in concept formation (Rees, 1973a). Although it may never be clear what the exact function of such comments is for the child, they are abundant in the speech of the normal child first learning language.

Clinical observation suggests that comments are less frequent with language-disordered children at the same level of linguistic development. The reasons for this could be many, including age, but the implications are clear. Children who talk about what they see and do certainly have considerable opportunity to practice content/form interaction and to obtain feedback from the environment about how appropriate or accurate some form is in relation to content. It may also be that these comments help the child to stabilize the concepts, and they may eventually lead to the use of language as a means of self-regulation. For all of these reasons, language-disordered children should be encouraged to talk about their own actions and states. In order to facilitate content/form interaction, the clinician will be talking about what the child is doing. If, *after* much such input, the child does not spontaneously begin to talk about these actions or imitate the utterances of the facilitator, imitation of utterances that code the child's actions might be encouraged.

In the later stages of language learning (e.g., in Phase 8, when the child's MLU has been over 3.0 for awhile), the child might be helped to use language as a means of pretending. Language used to pretend about events necessarily follows language used to talk of events that are present in the context. Language can first be used to code pretend play as it happens. For example, while standing at a play sink with dishes but no water, the child may pretend to wash the dishes, and this activity can be coded. More fantasy can later be introduced, as with role-playing: "You be the mommy, and I'll be the baby." One would not encourage fantasy until the child could carry out the more literal pretend.

A last intrapersonal use of language that can be facilitated in later stages of development is the expression of emotions—later stages, because to learn content/form interactions about emotional states is not easy. A child must hear the forms while experiencing the state (or observe another's experience of the state and relate that to the child's own experiences of that state). The child must understand that the forms refer to the internal emotions instead of to the physical manifestations of emotions, such as crying (sad), hitting (anger), or smiling (happiness) (see Lahey & Bloom, 1977).

Intrapersonal functions of language, then, include commenting about ongoing events (particularly one's own actions and states or intended actions); pretend or fantasy; and expression of emotion. Certainly there are many other functions that have not been covered. As more is learned about how normal children use language, the implications of these uses for the language-disordered child can be hypothesized and eventually tested—at least on a child-by-child basis. If the child appears to use language for additional functions—such as humor—they too should be encouraged.

Learning to Use Language in Various Contexts

Although the early use of language is about the "here and now," children eventually learn to talk about the "there and then." Talking about objects and events that are not perceptually present means that the child must call to mind from memory representations of these objects and events. This recall, of representations both of the ideas to be talked about and of the content/form interactions to be produced, places an added load on the processing system (e.g., Bloom, 1974; Bloom & Lahey, 1978; K. Nelson, 1986; Shatz, 1977). Some language-disordered children with advanced cognitive skills may have no difficulty recalling past experiences, and thus talking of past events may add little load; such children may use language much earlier than the normal child to talk of past events. But if the language-disordered child does not talk much about nonpresent events by the time content/

form interactions are comparable to those presented in Phases 6 to 8 (Chapter 10), talking about the "there and then" should become a goal of use.

Experience using content/form interactions without the additional load of recalling nonpresent events should be helpful in reaching the eventual goal of talking about such events. In talking about the here and now, the child may develop some automaticity in content/form recall and expression. If we view the child as a limited capacity processor, any automaticity in the production of content/form interactions should allow more processing space (or attentional capacity) for the recall of nonpresent objects and events.

Similarly, any situations that make recall of nonpresent objects and events easier should facilitate recall of content/form interactions and thus talking about objects and events that are not in the here and now. One technique is to use objects in the context that are similar to nonpresent objects with which the child is familiar. Such objects may help cue the recall of the nonpresent object (e.g., the doll in school that is similar to the doll at home, or the puppet in the clinic that is similar to the one on the child's favorite TV show) and be a way of beginning talk about objects and actions not perceptually present. One might also talk about objects that have just been present and events that have just taken place (e.g., food that has just been eaten, or the just completed activity of making cookies). No doubt, familiar activities are easier for children to call to mind than activities experienced only a few times. Such familiar events provide opportunities to talk about past events as well as to predict future happenings within those events. Each of these contexts also provides opportunities for inducing content/form interactions about temporal relations and for facilitating narrative productions (French & Nelson, 1982).

In addition to talking about nonpresent context, the language-disordered child must learn to choose among alternative means of expressing ideas in different contexts and to different listeners. Some forms, such as deictic terms, shift with the context and demand perspective taking on the part of the child (see Geller, in press, and in preparation, for a review of perspective taking and language). What is "here" can be "there" and "bringing" can be "taking," depending on the spatial location of persons and objects. Modeling correct forms must be done in a way that clearly distinguishes between the contexts. For example, group modeling could be used where children take turns placing objects next to themselves while saying "this goes *here*" and placing another object at a distant point while saying "this goes *there*." In a one-to-one session, a model could share the same space as the child in order to model the appropriate "here" versus "there" form.

Using language that takes into account the perspective of another person (i.e., the listener) seems to be more difficult and is a later development for normal language learners. In fact, it probably would not be a goal of intervention until after Phase 8 goals of content/form interaction have been accomplished. Some of the activities that have been traditionally employed to facilitate this use of language have involved situations, often games, where particular forms are needed for the listener to carry out an activity. For example, if the child is giving instructions to a listener who is visually separated from the child, then the child must be more elaborate in descriptions than when the referents are shared visually; gestures and use of pronouns without previous mention of the reference will not suffice. The difficulty of the task can be varied in a number of ways depending on the level of the child and the goals of intervention. A picture-sorting task can, for example, use pictures that differ only in one dimension such as attributes or agent of an action (see Glucksberg, Krauss, & Higgens, 1975). Such tasks are also useful for creating pragmatically appropriate contexts for the use of various content/form interactions such as attribution and agent of an action.

Goals of language use involving discourse would include both initiation of conversation and contingent responses to the utterances of another. When discourse skills are first learned, it would again be helpful to reduce the processing load by talking about present events (so the child will not have to call to mind nonpresent events) or by talking about familiar activities that can be recalled easily. Moreover, use of familiar content/form interactions might further allow the child to allocate most resources to contingent responses that add information or otherwise help maintain the conversation. The oft-quoted adage about "old forms for new functions" and vice versa (Bloom, 1970; Slobin, 1973) is again relevant, with function here interpreted in the broad sense as meaning any use of language, such as discourse, (see also Gerber, 1987).

Language Disorders Involving Use

Many factors could account for problems using language. Some problems with use seen in language-disordered children may well be a result of prior techniques that were applied by others in an attempt to teach form or content/form interactions in noncommunicative contexts. Such techniques may have included the following: focusing on labeling pictures instead of talking about objects and events in the child's natural environment, having the child "say the whole thing" even though an elliptical response is more appropriate, or making the contingencies for expression extrinsic rewards rather than natural consequences of communication. Some children taught in these ways produce routine responses but rarely generate linguistic utterances for communication; some rarely produce the forms outside of the structured learning environment. In such cases, shifting the contexts of intervention and focusing on use may be quite successful.

Other children who have difficulty with language use are children whose interpersonal interactions are limited in every sense. The child may withdraw from most social contact, and the limited use of language appears to be a reflection of general withdrawal from interpersonal contact. With some of these children, content/form interactions may be well developed, and the language goals need to focus on increasing the use of the code for interpersonal functions. Work with such children should be closely coordinated with a clinical psychologist or a psychiatrist who is responsible for improving overall interpersonal relations. Other children, however, with limited interpersonal contact may be withdrawing from contact because of difficulty in learning language.

In contrast, some children may know content/form interactions in language but not use these interactions as effectively as would be expected because of the difficulty they have in expressing these interactions—difficulties either in accessing the knowledge or in executing the expression of that knowledge. For such children, providing contexts and contingencies for language use may also be necessary, particularly if they have a history of failure in attempts to communicate. However, this alone may not be sufficient. Further work may be needed to help in accessing and expressing content/form interactions.

If a child rarely attempts any type of interpersonal communication, then most attempts by the child to communicate intents (with or without linguistic forms) should be promptly acknowledged. When no conventional forms are expressed or when the forms produced are inappropriate, the facilitator provides the appropriate form at the same time. Thus, facilitating the use of language in many contexts and for many functions involves being sensitive to the communication needs of the child and supplying the content/form interactions that will best serve the child's needs. To facilitate the use of language, the child should experience pleasant interpersonal interactions where language is modeled as a means of communication. All aspects of language are probably learned best when one attends to the child and responds meaningfully to the child's linguistic and nonlinguistic interactions in a warm, accepting atmosphere. Language use should always be kept in mind when facilitating content/form interactions even though the child's use appears commensurate with the level of content/form interactions expressed. Similarly, learning of content/form interactions cannot be ignored in the child with problems of language use. The induction of relations between content and form is discussed in the following section.

Induction of Content/Form Interactions

Facilitation of content/form interactions involves repeated presentations of tangible linguistic and nonlinguistic events. In this section we consider the factors that are important in manipulating the tangible input relevant to content and form: timing and repetition of presented events, the presentation of the linguistic signal, the selection of content/form interactions to be presented, and the presentation of the nonlinguistic input. (Some of these same factors have been discussed by Fey, 1986; D. Johnson and Myklebust, 1967; Leonard, 1981; Lucas, 1980; McCormick & Schiefelbusch, 1984; J. E. McLean & Snyder-McLean, 1978; and others.)

Timing

To induce the relationship between linguistic form and perceived regularities in the nonlinguistic context, the child must hear or see the linguistic forms that represent a concept at the same time that the relationship that is represented in that concept is experienced. To facilitate content/form interaction, then, is to arrange for the child to experience objects and events in the environment at the same time as the linguistic forms that represent such objects and events. It is not yet clear whether the presentation of form should precede, occur with, or follow a nonlinguistic demonstration. The exact timing may vary with the concept being coded, with the extent of the child's participation in the demonstration, and with the child. For example, (1) the mental representation of some actions may best be coded as the child is about to act (as when the child is perched on top of a slide ready to go down) or while the child is acting (as when hammering a nail); (2) the actions of others (sliding or hammering) may best be coded at the same time the action occurs; and (3) the mental representation of an internal state may best be coded simultaneously with the child's experience of that state (as when the child is tired). Considerable research is needed to determine whether these are differences that make a difference and, if so, if they vary with differences among children. In any case, both linguistic form and nonlinguistic demonstration of a concept must occur within the same speech event. The facilitator's task is to provide experiences that clearly demonstrate certain concepts while providing the linguistic forms that code these concepts at a time when the child is attentive to both. Both the concepts and the forms chosen will be based on a careful study of what the child already knows and hypotheses about what the child is ready to learn. (See Chapters 8–11.) In some cases this may mean intervening in the nonlinguistic environment by planning particular activities; in other cases it may mean simply talking to the child, using particular forms, about what the child is about to do, is doing, or has just done, and about what another person is doing or has just done.

Repetition

In everyday life a child may wait for days to experience clear examples of linguistic forms used concurrently with a nonlinguistic event demonstrating a particular conceptual relation. When facilitating language learning, such experiences must occur many, many times within each session or day in order to facilitate inductions about content/form interactions. Thus, if the interaction to be established is coding disappearance with "all gone," the facilitator would say "all gone" each time objects or events cease to exist in the child's view, and would create situations (such as hiding objects) to increase the frequency with which this relationship could be coded. Facilitating language learning, then, involves increasing the frequency of exposure to certain linguistic forms in the context of the meanings (content) they code.

Often children with language disorders need more repetitions than the normal child in order to learn. McReynolds (1966), for example, found that some language-disordered children could learn to make some of the same discriminations in auditory stimuli that normal children could make but that it took them many more trials to learn these discriminations. The key to many children is repetition; form with content over and over again may eventually lead to inductions that have not been learned incidentally.

Considerations Regarding the Form of the Linguistic Signal

The linguistic signal can be varied in many ways to increase its salience and to aid a child in processing and categorizing form. The specific variations and degree of variation will differ from child to child and can best be determined by direct observation of the child in response to differences in the presentation of form. Variations of intensity, frequency, and time of the linguistic signal (prosodic patterns) can be decreased or increased (from dull monotone to exaggerated singsong), and the linguistic signal can be increased or decreased in overall intensity and rate (as compared with normal conversation). For some children the more common, and thus preferred, auditory-vocal modality of form may need to be changed to a visual-motor modality. Finally, the unit of form used as input may vary from meaningful units, such as a word, phrase, or sentence, to nonmeaningful units, such as a phoneme or nonsense syllable. The question is, "What, if any, are the variations that will be best for a particular child?"

Prosody

Prosody includes variations in stress, intonation, pause, and duration of the linguistic signal. Variable stress is a possible means of increasing the salience of particular forms in contrast to other forms. For example, if a child already uses the single word *more* to code recurrence and the goal is to produce two-word utterances to code the same category of recurrence, the linguistic input might be "more X" (X standing for recurring objects or events that would be named), with X receiving greater stress in relation to the word *more*. In fact, the actual lexical items and structures presented to a child may not vary much between one or another of the phases in the acquisition of content/form, although the goals for the child's production may be different and, thus, different forms may be stressed. For example, when talking about an action, such as the child eating a cracker, the input might be "Jim is eating the cracker" at a number of phases of development, but in Phase 1 (single-word utterances) the word *Jim, eat,* or *cracker* might be stressed: "Jim is eating the *cracker.*" In Phase 5, when one is trying to facilitate inductions about *-ing* to code ongoing actions, the stress could change to "Jim is *eating* the cracker." And in Phase 8, when the auxiliary verb is the content/form interaction goal, the stress would be changed again: "Jim *is* eating the cracker." Research supports the use of stress as a means of increasing the probability of imitation (Blasdell & Jensen, 1970), but little is known about its effectiveness in enhancing the learning of content/form interactions.

In addition to stress, some clinicians find that variations in intonation are effective with certain children at certain stages of learning. Teachers of normal preschool children often report that the normal child will attend to story time better if intonational patterns are variable and even exaggerated in contrast to a more flat monotone reading. Lewis (1951) reported that children's first inductions about content/form interactions are based on intonation, not on phonemic elements of the signal. According to Berry (1969), variation in intonation is important for language learning and is an important therapeutic tool.

The effectiveness of variations in prosody as an aid to language learning may, however, vary with the inductions the child is learning. Friedlander (1970), for example, reported that children's early preferences for considerable variation in prosody changed in time to a preference for less variation and more monotonous speech. Furthermore, Lahey (1974) reported that prosodic patterns did not aid 4- and 5-year-olds in comprehending certain complex sentences. On the other hand, LaBelle (1973) found that increasing pause length at the end of clauses aided the comprehension of 3- and 4-year-olds; input studies (e.g., Broen, 1972; Snow, 1974) report that mothers characteristically increase pause time at sentence and phrase boundaries. Unfortunately, no evidence is available on the influence of prosodic variation on language learning for the child with a language disorder. It may be that certain inductions are best made with variations in prosody, while others are best learned without such variation.

Children learning single-word utterances may find variations in prosody more helpful than children learning word order as a means of coding relations between objects. Thus, while "all gone" spoken with higher pitch on "all" and lowered pitch on "gone" may make the form more salient, exaggerated intonational patterns superimposed on "Jim is eating the cracker" may not aid but, instead, may even hinder the learning of word order to code agent-action relations. It may also be that certain types of variation (intonation, pause, stress) are more effective for the learning of particular behaviors; or that the effectiveness of variations in prosody is different for different children independent of what inductions are being made; or that there may be some interaction among child, type of variation, and the structure being learned. Although considerable research is needed to answer these questions, the role of prosodic variation cannot be ignored by the practicing clinician. Careful experimentation should be carried out with each child for each goal before varying the *normal* prosodic patterns of input words and sentences.

Rate

A second type of form variation involves the rate at which the linguistic signal is presented. Considerable research has suggested that at least some children with language problems have extreme difficulty processing rapid auditory signals (see Chapter 5). Although it is not clear that slow speech aids comprehension with these same children, other research suggests that slower speech does improve the comprehension of some children (e.g., N. Nelson, 1976) and that parents speak more slowly to younger children than to older children (e.g., Broen, 1972; Snow, 1974). When first learning a language, increasing the time between words and phrases may help one to segment the sound stream and may provide more time for the processing of each word. Thus, the research available coupled with information on normal language learning suggests that a slow rate should be used with children in the early stages of language learning. The ideal rate for a particular child is determined, however, only by observing the results of varying rates with that child.

Modality

A third type of variation in form is the modality of the linguistic signal. The auditory signal is the usual modality of linguistic *form* in first language learning, but it need not be the only modality considered. A number of professionals have reported using the visual-motor modalities (usually in conjunction with the auditory signal) as a means of facilitating language learning (e.g., Barrera, Lobato-Barrera, & Sulzer-Azaroff, 1980; Bonvillian & Nelson, 1976, 1978; Bricker, 1972; Carrier, 1974a, 1974b; Konstantaveas, 1984; L. P. McClean & McClean, 1974; A. Miller & Miller, 1973; Schaeffer, 1980; Yoder & Calculator, 1981). In some cases, chips (wooden or plastic forms) were used to teach nouns to mentally retarded children (e.g., see Carrier as well as L. P. McClean & McClean). More frequently, motor mediation, in the form of either conventional signs or patterns devised by the researcher, has been used to facilitate content/form interactions (usually in autistic or retarded children without any language), and in some cases the motor mediation has led to the spontaneous use of verbalizations (see, e.g., Bricker, A. Miller & Miller, and Schaeffer). The results of these studies suggest that alternative modalities for linguistic form may be a viable way of improving the communication skills of some children who have been unsuccessful learning auditory-vocal language although they have received considerable help.

It is not clear why such procedures work. Some of these children may be having difficulty processing the auditory signal, developing phonetic representations, or executing motor programs to encode phonetic representations. The immediate success and social interaction resulting from alternative modalities could reward communication and enhance language learning in general (Yoder & Calculator, 1981). Once communication skills and associational skills are somewhat established, more processing space may be available to handle the auditory-vocal modality. The success of alternative modalities for inducing content/form interactions (and demonstrating this knowledge) has, however, been primarily reported at the lexical level (see also Romski & Ruder, 1984). Its effectiveness for facilitating content/form inductions in language-impaired children may be limited to lexical learning and probably varies among children.

While the addition of alternative modalities may be helpful for some children, the *substitution* of alternative modalities for the auditory-vocal modality should be considered as a last resort. Before deciding on such a substitution, repeated and varied efforts to facilitate content/form inductions should have been attempted, and careful assessment of precursory behaviors should be undertaken (see, e.g., Chapman & Miller, 1980, and Shane, 1980, as well as Chapters 9 and 12) to establish that the problem is not in forming concepts (relative to the content of language) or in communicating ideas (relevant to the use of language).

If a nonauditory linguistic system is to be presented, there are a number of decisions to be made and, unfortunately, little empirical evidence as yet to support such decisions. First, one must decide whether to use geometric forms (Figure 15-2) or hand configurations as symbols (Figures 15-3 to 15-5) and then decide which system, based on these symbols, to use. (See Carrier, 1974a, 1974b; and L. P. McClean & McClean, 1974, for information on chips; and Bornstein, 1973, 1974; Kent, 1974; and Wilbur, 1976, for information on signs.) As Mayberry (1976) pointed out, there are a number of systems of sign language with considerable variation among them in their approximation to oral English and in the speed with which they can be used to convey a message. Factors influencing a clinician's decision will include the manual dexterity of the child and the ease with which others in the child's environment (including the clinician) can learn the alternative linguistic system. [It is not clear that one system is easier to learn than another (Bristow & Fristoe, 1984), but further research is needed.] But even then, the decision making is not completed. The clinician must also decide whether to include the auditory signal with the visual signal, teach only the visual, or teach the visual first and then the auditory. Again, without evidence from research, the decision must be made based on experimental teaching with each child.

Unit of Form

The general assumption in most language programs is that the smallest unit of form presented to a child as linguistic input is the word—a content/form interaction. Alternatively, the smallest unit of input could be a phoneme or syllable, a unit of form that does not by itself represent any object, event, or relationship (e.g., the

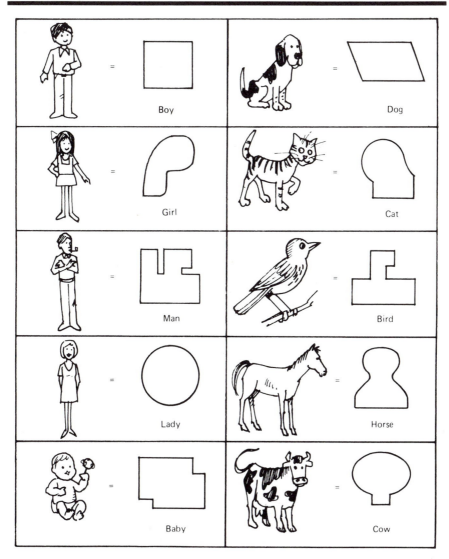

These geometric forms were cut from three-inch squares of masonite. Children were trained to match forms with black line drawings. All symbols were abstract and had no resemblance to the objects pictured.

This is certainly not an efficient means of communication. The placement of forms is a slow process; the child must choose from an array of forms, which takes time, and the number of forms that can be used is limited.

FIGURE 15-2   Geometric Forms Used as Symbols (from Carrier 1974b, p. 513)

GIRL   SISTER

BOY   BROTHER

COME   GO

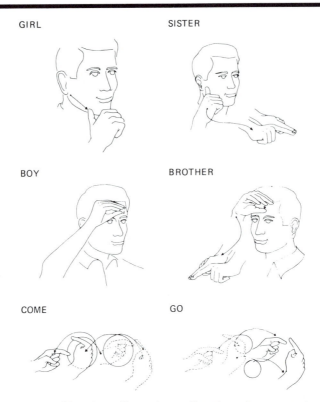

Signs make use of hand configurations, direction of movement, and places where hand moves to and from. Also, signs build on semantically related signs. For example, "sister" and "brother" build from "boy" and "girl," and the same motion is used with each to code the sibling relation. Some relationships are represented in a more abstract form than others (e.g., "come" is less abstract than "brother").

FIGURE 15-3   Sign Language (from A Basic Course in Manual Communication, 1970, pp. 17–18)

phoneme /p/ or the syllable /po/). In a method referred to as the *Association Method* (McGinnis, Kleffner, & Goldstein, 1956; Monsees, 1972), the phoneme is the first unit of form presented. Children are presented with both visual (facial movements) and auditory cues to the phoneme concurrent with a visual representation (the letter) of the sound. Sequences of unconnected phonemes (/m/ /æ/ /t/ or /k/ /æ/ /t/) are heard, produced, and memorized before being "blended" to form words such as *mat* and *cat*. This approach is contrary to normal development and to existing knowledge of speech perception. A. Liberman, Cooper, Shankweiler, and Studdert-Kennedy (1967) pointed out, for example, that stop consonants such as /k/ are not invariable independent acoustic segments but transitions that lead into the following vowel. (See discussion in Chapter 5.) Despite these theoretical arguments against the approach, it has been used, with apparent success, particularly with children described as "aphasic" (i.e., SLI), at the Central

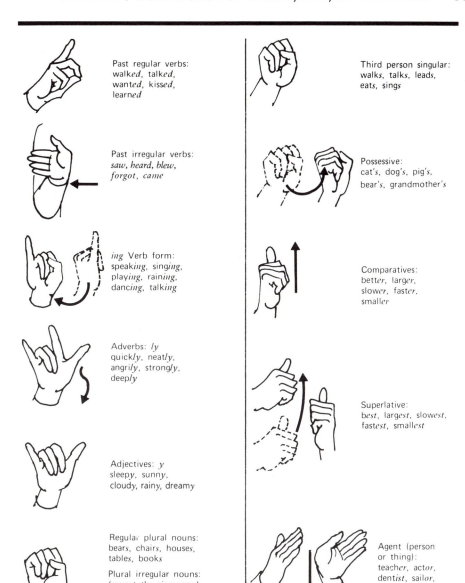

Past regular verbs:
walk*ed*, talk*ed*,
want*ed*, kiss*ed*,
learn*ed*

Past irregular verbs:
saw, heard, blew,
forgot, came

ing Verb form:
speak*ing*, sing*ing*,
play*ing*, rain*ing*,
danc*ing*, talk*ing*

Adverbs: *ly*
quick*ly*, neat*ly*,
angri*ly*, strong*ly*,
deep*ly*

Adjectives: *y*
sleep*y*, sunn*y*,
cloud*y*, rain*y*, dream*y*

Regular plural nouns:
bear*s*, chair*s*, house*s*,
table*s*, book*s*

Plural irregular nouns:
(repeat the sign word
twice)
child*ren*, feet,
sheep, mice, geese

Third person singular:
walk*s*, talk*s*, lead*s*,
eat*s*, sing*s*

Possessive:
cat*'s*, dog*'s*, pig*'s*,
bear*'s*, grandmother*'s*

Comparatives:
bett*er*, larg*er*,
slow*er*, fast*er*,
small*er*

Superlative:
b*est*, larg*est*, slow*est*,
fast*est*, small*est*

Agent (person
or thing):
teach*er*, act*or*,
dent*ist*, sail*or*,
mix*er*, mow*er*

Some systems of sign language parallel spoken English. One of these, "Signed English," has been developed for preschool deaf children and includes sign markers that stand for the morphological inflections of spoken English. These markers are used in combination with signs that represent words.

FIGURE 15-4   Sign Markers (from Bornstein, 1974, p. 334)

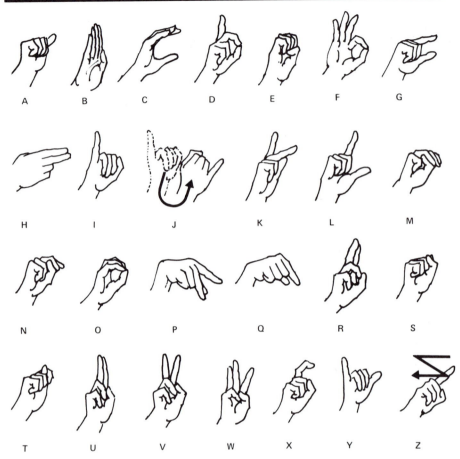

Spelling out words with the manual alphabet is an extremely slow means of communication and is usually used only for uncommon words for which there is no available sign or is used for person and place names.

FIGURE 15-5 The American Manual Alphabet (from Bornstein, 1974, p. 336)

Institute for the Deaf (McGinnis et al., 1956). It is perhaps one of the more extreme distortions of form recommended by any approach and, as with alternative modalities, should be considered only as a last resort.

Considerations in the Selection of Content/Form Interactions as Input

Planning the content/form interactions that will serve as linguistic input is, of course, influenced by the goals for a particular child. The goals do not, however, usually specify the topic, the particular lexical items, or the larger linguistic context in which to embed the syntactic structures that you wish the child to learn. These choices are sometimes made on the spot and are always dependent on the activities and objects involved. But you can talk about the relations between objects in a number of ways. On what bases are lexical items and the larger linguistic context chosen as input?

Selection of Lexical Items

One aspect to be considered in the selection of lexical items is the configurations of the signal that will make up the symbols to be presented and that the child is expected to learn. Again there is no definitive answer to this question: there will be variation among children. At least in the first 50 to 100 words of the child's vocabulary, it is important to consider the phonological preferences of the child. It has been observed that young non-language-impaired children as well as children with specific language impairment tend to prefer words that begin with certain consonants, but the particular consonants preferred vary among the children (see, e.g., Ferguson & Farwell, 1975; R. Schwartz & Leonard, 1982; R. Schwartz, Leonard, Folger, & Wilcox, 1980). This preference influences the words that are learned incidently as well as those that are learned through language intervention. In a study that varied the phonology of words taught to language-impaired children, who had productive vocabularies of 25–75 words, the choice of initial consonant influenced learning (Leonard, Schwartz, et al., 1982). Words that began with consonants that were a part of the child's phonology were more likely to be acquired in production than words beginning with consonants that were not a part of the child's phonology.

Phonological preferences and articulatory constraints may also be important in producing early word combinations (Donahue, 1986a). The presence of phonological selection strategies and a consonant harmony rule (in this case, desire to maintain same place of articulation) appeared to influence which words Donahue's child would produce in combination. Such reports suggest that speech-language pathologists must consider phonological composition of both individual lexical items and combinations of lexical items when selecting targets for intervention.

In addition to the initial consonant, other aspects of phonological composition may be important. Short words of one or two syllables may be easier for the child to reproduce than longer words composed of different syllables (versus repetition of the same syllable). The first words of normal children tend to be monosyllabic, such as *no*, or reduplicated (i.e., repetition of one syllable) such as *dada*. Differences are again found among children, however, in the frequency of their monosyllabic versus multisyllabic productions during the first 50 words (e.g., Fee & Ingram, 1982; Klein, 1981; Lahey, Flax, & Schlisselberg, 1985; R. Schwartz & Leonard, 1983). Shorter words are the words most frequently used by adults (Zipf, 1965), and so may be the words most often heard by the child (R. Brown, 1958). To my knowledge, no one has used syllabic structure as a variable in an intervention study; we do not know how important syllabic structure is in language facilitation, but until data suggest otherwise, it seems any preference for syllabic structure observed in the child should be considered in selecting initial lexical items.

The speech-language pathologist should examine the words already produced by the child before selecting lexical items to be presented in the early stages of vocabulary learning. If the child's utterances are too few to establish a preference, a change in phonological composition might be considered when intervention attempts are not successful with early lexical acquisition or early word combinations. Finally, when considering the phonological structure of words, the clinician might want to select words that are acoustically distinct from each other in order to reduce confusion among the forms presented.

Another consideration in making choices is the efficiency of a lexical item. Certain words, such as *no* or *more*, have broader application to objects and events than other words, such as *cookie* or *car*, and thus may be heard more often and will serve the child more frequently in his or her efforts to communicate. The more frequently a word is heard by a child, the greater is the chance that the child will make inductions about a content/form interaction; the more often the child is able to use a word in daily life, the more opportunity the child will have for practice and reinforcement.

Words used by young children can be dichotomized as substantive words or as relational words. Substantive words refer to particular objects (e.g., person and place names), or refer to categories of objects (e.g., chair and dog). The choice of particular substantive words as input will depend on the child's environment and should include objects that will be frequently encountered. The child's interest directs the choice of objects to be named, but many objects can be referred to by a number of different words (e.g., *nickel, five cents,* or *money; chickadee, bird,* or *animal; apple, fruit,* or *food*), and the clinician must choose which is appropriate. R. Brown (1958) noted that children's vocabulary does not simply build from concrete to abstract; for example, the word *fish* is more abstract than the name of a particular fish and less abstract than the term *vertebrate.* Many concrete words are not learned until one takes science courses or is interested in different makes of cars. According to Brown, adults appear to use two criteria in making decisions about what a "thing" will be called in their speech to children: the object's most common name, and the word that categorizes the object according to its utilization in the child's life. Thus, coins might first be referred to as money and only later as dimes, nickels, and the like, since the young child is not likely to need the differentiation in daily life; fruits will be specifically identified as apple, pear, and so on, since the differentiation is important to daily meals and snacks. It appears that these criteria of selection have relevance to the language facilitator selecting lexical input for the language-disordered child. The words chosen should be commonly used in the child's environment as labels for objects, and the words should categorize the world in ways that relate to the child's cognitive structure and needs.

Relational words are words that refer to a relationship between objects and include parts of speech such as verbs, adjectives, and prepositions. Relational words are less specific than substantive words and may often be used to refer to many or all objects. For example, *no* can be used to reject, deny, or note the disappearance of any object and event. Certain verbs are less object- or event-specific than others. Verbs such as *give, get, make,* and *fall* can refer to more objects than verbs such as *eat* and *throw,* and *eat* and *throw* are less specific than verbs such as *drink* and *tear.* The adjectives *big* and *dirty* can refer to more objects than can the adjectives *orange* and *round.* Thus, in selecting relational words to teach, one might consider first those relational words that are least object-specific and that, therefore, are more likely to be heard, and have the most potential for communication in many different situations because they involve many contexts.

Certain relational words are listed in Table 15-1 according to the content category they code. These particular words have been singled out for two reasons: (1) they are less specific than many other relational words, and (2) they are frequently found in the lexicons of children learning language normally. The listing in Table 15-1 serves as a guideline for choosing relational words that a child may find easiest to learn. Verbs, however, are not frequent early in the single-word-utterance period and should probably not be included in the early goals during Phase 1 (see Chapter 9 for a discussion).

The selection of lexical items continues to be important in the later stages of language learning. For example, we again find preferences among children for different forms in early syntactic utterances. Some children use primarily pronouns in their early word combinations (e.g., "I eat it," "put it there," "my coat"), while others use primarily nouns (e.g., "Gerry eat cookie," "put coat chair," "Gerry hat"). Again, the importance of this preference has not been tested in training studies, but it would seem advisable to follow this preference when selecting lexical items for early syntactic utterances.

A second factor is the familiarity with a lexical item. In normal development, Bloom, Miller, and Hood (1975) reported more frequent use of three constituents

TABLE 15-1   Selection of Lexical Items on the Basis of Content and Form: Relational Words[a]

Content	Form	
Content Category	Relational Words that are not object-specific	Relational Words that are more specific to objects but still relate to many objects
Rejection	no	
Nonexistence or disappearance	no, all gone, away	
Cessation of action	stop, no	
Prohibition of action	no, don't	
Recurrence of objects and actions on objects	more, again, another	
Noting the existence of or identifying objects	this, there, that	
Actions on objects		give, do, make, get, throw, eat, wash, kiss, broke, close, open, fix, push, take, play, find, hold
Actions involved in locating objects or self		put, go, up, down, sit, fall, out, come, away, stand, climb, fit
Attributes or descriptions of objects		big, hot, dirty, heavy
Notice		see, look at

[a] *Note:* Adapted from Lahey and Bloom, 1977.

(subject-verb-complement) when familiar lexical items were used and, correspondingly, a reduction in the number of constituents when new lexical items were used. Even as late as elementary school, familiarity with lexical items and their referents enhances linguistic processing of such complex syntactic constructions as the passive. (See Bransford & Nitsch, 1977, for a discussion of some of these studies.) The use of familiar items may free processing space for processing on more complex syntactic constructions until such operations are more automatic. In any case, such findings suggest using familiar lexical items when first facilitating inductions about complex syntactic structures.

A related third factor concerns verbs. In normal development, a small number of verbs are first produced with verb inflections, questions, and complex sentences (see Chapter 10 for a discussion and listing of verbs). This would imply that verbs are important for such learning although the reasons are not clear. It may relate to amount of processing space, or it may be that some structures (e.g., inflections) are learned by lexical item and then later by rule (see Bloom, Lifter, & Hafitz, 1980). These findings suggest that the variety of verbs expected with the emergence of such constructions be limited and perhaps be selected from the verbs found with these structures in normal development.

Complexity of Linguistic Input

The level of complexity appropriate for linguistic input to a language-disordered child is not well researched. Certainly the complexity of the sentence in which forms to be learned are embedded can influence the salience of those forms. It seems reasonable that new lexical items might best be spoken in isolation or embedded in very simple and familiar constructions. New substantive words might best be introduced as single-word utterances or be placed at the beginning or at the end of short sentences (e.g., "that's an X," "do you want X," or "X can jump") in order to increase their salience.

New structures, combinations of words, or grammatical morphemes might also be presented in isolation or in short, linguistic contexts such as "more X," or embedded in short, simple constructions such as "there is more X," "see more X," or "do you want more X?" In each example, differential stress can be used to accent the words that code the content category of interest (e.g., recurrence in the examples above) and to de-emphasize other words. What is probably least effective for children in the early phases of language learning is to embed key words and two-word combinations in long and complex sentences (e.g., "I thought I saw more X, but now I can't find them at all"). If the child is first learning to code recurrence with two-word utterances, the relevant words will get lost in the excessively long linguistic context.

There are problems, however, with simplifying utterances to too great a degree. First, such input is monotonous, leads to stilted conversational patterns, and has an unnatural prosodic pattern. On the basis of experimental learning conditions with normal language learners, some researchers have concluded that children need a wide variety of input including input that is considerably above the child's current linguistic level (K. E. Nelson & Baker, 1986). They recommend, however, that such input be presented in contexts where the child can compare the more complex form of coding with content/form interactions already established (e.g., recasts, to be discussed later).

The Child's Actions and Utterances

One basis for the selection of particular topics for input is the activities in which the child is engaged. This increases the likelihood that you are coding events that the child is representing mentally. Furthermore, if the topic of linguistic input is about actions that the child performs frequently (such as sliding, banging, or pushing) or that are a part of regular routines, it may well make inductions of content/form an easier task. Activities that are a frequent part of the child's life will provide more opportunities for input and are likely to be more automatized so that less attention is needed for carrying out the activity and more is available for processing the linguistic input.

Another means of determining the topic of input to a child is to base the linguistic input on the child's prior utterance—that is, to provide a semantically contingent response. A number of techniques for facilitating language learning have been based on response to the child's utterance: correction, expansion, expatiation, alternative, use of questions (or "vertical" discourse structure), and recasting (e.g., Baker & Nelson, 1984; Blank, 1973; Fey, 1986; Muma, 1971; R. Schwartz, Chapman, Terrell, Prelock, & Rowan, 1985). The correction technique may be used to correct form (the child says "two book," and the clinician says "not two book, two books") or content (the child looks at an elephant and says "see doggie," and the clinician says "that's an elephant, not a doggie"). Although this technique is frequently used, Muma pointed out that it may be destructive to language *use* when applied to correction of *form*, but may be effective for learning content/form interactions when used to point out errors in meaning. Alternatively, one might respond to a child's utterance by syntactically expanding the utterance. For example, if the child says "there two book," the clinician might respond "yes, there *are* two books," providing the omitted forms. Or expansions can add information to the prior utterance (sometimes referred to as *expatiations*). In this case, the clinician adds new content to the child's utterance. When the child says "there two book," the clinician might reply "yes, there are two big books on the table." Alternatives to the child's utterance provide another view of the context or can point out the logic of the utterance or the situation it codes. For example, if a child is about to wash a wall with a dripping sponge and comments, "lots a water," the clinician might respond "do you need that much water?" Recasts involve repeating the content of the child's utterance and changing one or more components in the sentence to model a content/form interaction that is a goal of intervention. Thus, if the child said, "the boy ate the cake," the clinician might respond "the boy *did* eat the cake, didn't he?" for emphatic *do* and/or tag questions.

Finally, questions about a child's utterance can also be used to facilitate the production of related words in the form of successive single-word utterances from children who are not producing many syntactic utterances. These related words would be in a vertical structure (i.e., related words in separate utterances in contrast to related words that are sequenced within the same utterance in a horizontal structure). For example, the child points to a book and says "book," and the clinician asks "where is the book?" If this question elicits a response such as "table," the clinician joins the two words of the child into a syntactic utterance, "yes, the book is on the table."

Each of these techniques has the advantage of providing input that is most likely related to the child's mental representation and provides this input in a discourse context that is similar to a natural interaction (in fact, many of these techniques have been observed in the language of mothers to non-language-impaired children). Research that utilizes these techniques with language-disordered children has been limited (e.g., R. Schwartz, Chapman, Terrell, Prelock, & Rowan, 1985; Wilcox, 1984) and has not involved comparisons of the various techniques. Thus, again, there is little evidence to support the superiority of one method over another, but familiarity with each allows for flexibility with different children and different goals of intervention.

Considerations in the Presentation of Nonlinguistic Input

It is the task of the language facilitator to arrange external stimuli so the concept to be coded by linguistic form will be illustrated in a way that is clear and salient. Considerations in planning nonlinguistic input involve the type of stimuli to be used, the child's involvement in the demonstration, the variety of different contexts demonstrated, and the actual objects and activities used.

Type of Stimuli

Unfortunately, for those who wish to facilitate language in a formal teaching situation, pictures often do not serve as adequate demonstration of a concept during *early* stages of language learning. Many concepts involve more than the perceptual features of objects available from a picture; they involve functional features that come from acting on the objects as well as perceptual features that can only be extracted from three-dimensional objects. Thus, to learn that the word *ball* refers to a category of objects, the child needs to experience the roundness, bouncing, rolling, and differences in softness, size, and color in order to learn eventually that all of these are part of the concept and that *ball* is not just a red circle on a card. This is true not only when learning vocabulary (single words to refer to a concept) but also when learning to code the relationships among words. If a child is to learn that the person acting is named before the action is named in order to talk about the agent of an action, the child should experience actual demonstrations of persons acting at the same time as the forms that code the demonstration.

Leonard found that children acquired the subject-verb construction more easily when exposed to ongoing events than when exposed to pictures (1975b) or to only form and referents (1975a). Children trained with simultaneous presentation of subject-verb forms with ongoing events could respond to pictures on posttest. However, children exposed to subject-verb forms and pictures did not respond well to *either* ongoing events *or* pictures on posttest. Likewise, children exposed to referents coded by forms but not exposed to a *demonstration* of the referent relationship did not produce subject-verb constructions as often as children exposed to actual events. Leonard concluded that ongoing events demonstrating the relationship coded should be used when facilitating the induction of word order as a means of expressing agent-action relations. It is possible that pictures could be used after an induction has been made to reinforce and practice production or comprehension of the interaction, since the children trained with actual demonstration of events did generalize to pictures in the study by Leonard.

Young children seem more tuned into movement and change than to static objects (see Bloom & Lahey, 1978): young children without language-learning problems first learn to name objects that move (Huttenlocher, 1974) and generally talk about objects as they act upon them (Bloom, 1973). Two studies support the role of action in learning object labels. In one study, object labels were learned better when the objects were presented in an action sequence (such as rolling a ball) rather than in a static pose (Schuler, 1979, as cited by Goetz, Schuler, & Sailor, 1979). In the other, receptive language was more rapidly learned when action on the objects was used as a reinforcer instead of more traditional reinforcements (Jensen & Guess, 1978, as cited in Goetz et al., 1979). However, only two of the four children studied by Olswang, Bain, Dunn, and Cooper (1983) learned words more successfully in an object manipulation condition than in a picture identification condition; one showed no preference, and one was more successful with pictured stimuli. The preferences were related to initial vocabulary size; the two with the smallest expressive vocabularies (six words) were more successful in learning new words when they manipulated objects. The authors suggested that manipulation may be more important for children learning content/form interactions than for children whose problem is mainly learning form.

Thus, activity that illustrates the function of the object appears to be helpful to most children who are first learning the induction of content/form interactions; such manipulations can easily be incorporated into an intervention program aimed at teaching auditory-vocal language. But individual differences exist, and the clinician, as always, must be flexible and willing to try different methods. This is not to say that pictures or books are useless as stimuli—pictures and books can be used to provide additional representations of the stimuli, can be used for practice of inductions already emerging, and themselves provide a social context for language learning (see, e.g., Bruner, 1983). In the initial stages of facilitation, however, real objects and people demonstrating relationships should be used for nonlinguistic input.

The types of objects used may also affect the ease with which a content/form interaction is induced. Sailor and Taman (1972) reported that the locative prepositions *in* and *on* were learned faster by autistic children when each preposition was first trained with an unambiguous object (*containers* for *in* and *supports* for *on*) instead of contrasting the two prepositions using an ambiguous object (such as a hat and a can, which were containers in one position but supports in another). This finding is contrary to the intuitions of many clinicians who felt an ambiguous object was necessary to demonstrate the *difference* between the two prepositions; it is, however, consistent with the nonlinguistic strategies Clark (1973) described for the normal child's comprehension of locative relations.

It should not be surprising that nonlinguistic context influences language learning; there is considerable research demonstrating the effect of nonlinguistic context on the language comprehension and production of normal speakers. Osgood (1971) demonstrated that the nonlinguistic context influenced both the form and content of adults' utterances. By manipulating the sequence of events that were to be described, he influenced the probability that adjectives, articles, negatives, and pronouns would be used. Adjectives were, for example, used more frequently when first describing an object or when similar objects were in the same array. Furthermore, the effect of context on the comprehension of linguistic structure has been consistently demonstrated (e.g., Bransford & Johnson, 1972; Bransford & Nitsch, 1977; Huttenlocher, Eisenberg, & Strauss, 1968; Huttenlocher & Strauss, 1968; Huttenlocher & Weiner, 1971). The effect of similar differences in context has not been described in connection with language learning by the language-disordered child, but it seems possible that they may influence the ease with which a child will learn certain aspects of language. Certainly more research, similar to that by Leonard, by Schuler, and by Sailor and Taman, is needed. In the meantime the evidence from their studies and from normal processing suggests that close attention needs to be given to the nonlinguistic demonstration of objects and relations.

Child Participation and Interest

If you watch a 2- or 3-year-old using language, it will be clear that children first learning language talk most about what they are doing, are about to do, or want others to do. They talk less about states that they are not involved in or about the actions of others that do not involve them. There is no information about the effect of participation in events versus the observation of events on eventual language learning. In the Leonard (1975a, 1975b) studies mentioned above, the children observed a demonstration; the differences he reported did not relate to observation compared with participation but, instead, to difference in what was observed by the children.

Observations of normal children and clinical experience suggest that child participation in the nonlinguistic events that demonstrate the relation being coded may be important in learning early content/form interactions. The importance of the child's participation, however, may vary with the concept being coded. The salience of certain relations may be increased by participation because the sensorimotor experience is an important part of certain concepts. On the other hand, certain actions may so totally involve the child's attentional capacity that the linguistic forms are not attended to. The importance of participation may also vary among children according to conceptual development and attention span. Although future research may help to clarify the role of some of these variables, the clinician must make decisions about how extensively child participation will be intermixed with child observation—decisions based on each child's response.

Certainly planning demonstrations that are of interest to the child is a key to increasing the salience of those demonstrations, whether or not the child is an active participant in the demonstration. Parent interviews as well as unstructured observations are a way of obtaining information about particular interests. For example, if a child likes to bang objects, *bang* may be one of the easiest words for the child to learn.

The important point is not so much who is carrying out the action; rather, it is what the child is thinking about. It does little good to provide demonstrations of relations with relevant linguistic input if the child's thoughts are elsewhere. For the child to induce relations between form and content, it is necessary to coordinate linguistic input (i.e., the forms) with the current mental representations of the child—that is, with the ideas and attitudes about objects and relations among objects that occupy the child's immediate attention.

Variety of Nonlinguistic Demonstrations

Nonlinguistic demonstrations of objects and relations must include more than one example in order for generalization to occur. Even when the lexical items presented refer to specific objects or places (e.g., proper names), the nonlinguistic presentation must involve many contexts that include that specific object (e.g., mommy or a pet). Thus mommy is labeled as she enters the room, hugs the child, is pointed to, leaves the room, or throws the ball, to assure that the induction of content/form is not context-specific (i.e., that the word *mommy* refers to only a picture or that person entering the room, etc.).

Similarly, for the child to understand that certain forms (such as most nouns) refer to not just one object, place, or event, but to a *category*, multiple examples of the concept must be experienced with the forms that represent the concept. Thus, if the child is to learn that *ball* refers to many different objects, the child must experience contact with a number of different balls as the child hears the word as well as contact with balls in different situations. Likewise, to learn that the morphological inflection -*s* can be used to represent plurality, the child must experience demonstrations of *one versus more than one* with many objects (a block and blocks, a truck and trucks, a cat and cats, etc.); to learn subject-verb-object, to express agent-action-object relations, the child must hear the forms at the same time as experiencing a number of different actions as well as the same action with different agents and objects ("mommy eat cake," "doggy eat meat," "mommy wash face," "mommy wash dish," etc.). Thus, all nonlinguistic demonstrations must include a variety of exemplars, because most forms refer to more than one object in one context.

Activities and Contexts

The activities and contexts that best serve to demonstrate the concepts that make up the content of language come from the child's everyday experiences. Situations that consistently arise in life offer opportunities to illustrate the concepts that language codes. Using these situations rather than contrived contexts and activities provides more opportunities for input to the child and more opportunities for the child to receive natural reinforcers when language is eventually used to express these concepts.

Since even the most mundane contexts and activities in a child's life provide demonstrations of many different content categories as well as a number of possible uses of language, the focus of input (e.g., how a child's utterance might be recast) will depend on the content/form/use goals that the speech-language pathologist has set for the child. Those responsible for facilitating language learning should try to tune into the usual activities in the child's life and arrange for stimulation, and possibly elicitation, of different content/form/use interactions.

The basic idea is to select activities with which the child is familiar, which he or she enjoys, and in which he or she can become involved. The aspect of the activity to be focused upon can be emphasized by repetition, exaggeration, gesture, vocal patterns, etc. For example, while grocery shopping, input relative to facilitating the induction of content/form interactions could include such things as comments on locative action ("put in the cart, take off the shelf"), recurrence and quantity ("more X, another one, two cans"), existence (identifying objects in the store), action ("push the cart, open the bag"), attribution (large or small size, dirty or clean, new or old, pretty), nonexistence (when the shelf is empty or as the last one is taken), notice ("look at the X"), and so forth. Likewise, unpacking the groceries at home provides more opportunities for facilitating similar inductions. Taking a bath, getting dressed, preparing and eating meals, cleaning house, working in the yard, going to the park, visiting a friend or relative, reading a book, or playing with the child's toys all provide multiple opportunities for focused stimulation (or modeling) and responses to the child's utterances (such as eliciting vertical discourse structures, or providing expansions, alternatives, or recasts of the child's utterance). When goals of intervention include the coordination of categories, two or three relations found within events become the focus (e.g., "putting the big box in the cart," or "getting more boxes"); and when goals of intervention involve coding of event relations, then the relation between two or three events can become the focus (e.g., "move the cart so we can get the box").

Those activities that occur repeatedly in the child's life are particularly useful. The child no doubt has an event representation of these activities which can be called upon to predict what will happen next. It is likely the child will have in immediate consciousness the event that is just about to occur (such as putting on the shoes right after the socks). The familiarity with such activities may mean the child can partake in them without utilizing much attentional capacity (or processing space) so that attention can be devoted to processing the linguistic input and making inductions (for more information about event representation, or scripts, see K. Nelson, 1986). Moreover, when initial inductions have been made, breaking the routine (such as putting on the shoes before the socks) can be used to elicit the production of certain content/form/use interactions (see Constable, 1983, 1986). Finally, routine events may serve as one of the earliest contexts in which a child may talk about temporally displaced events (K. Nelson, 1986) and about which the child may produce narratives (or descriptions of what happened).

Some typical home and school activities are listed below according to several of the *content* categories presented in the C/F/U Goal Plan for Language Learning discussed in Chapters 8 through 11.

1. *Activities for existence.* After initially pointing out that an object exists, utterances in this category are identification statements. Identification can take place when:
   a. Taking objects out of a container (toy box, grocery bag, drawer, kitchen cabinet, clothes closet, etc.).
   b. Pointing out objects (when shopping in the store, walking in the zoo, walking in the street, taking a drive, looking at pictures or magazines, etc.).

    c. Carrying out a routine (such as reading a favorite book or eating a familiar food, or helping the child dress, etc.). In these cases it may be started with a "what's that (or this)?" question, which, after a pause, is answered by the adult (see Bruner, 1983).

2. *Activities for nonexistence and disappearance.* After identifying an object, the object can be hidden from view, or as the child finishes food or drink, one can comment on its nonexistence or disappearance. Hide-and-seek games provide routine activities for coding both existence and nonexistence. Searches for toys or clothes that are not in their usual location, a common event in many schools and homes, provides further opportunity to talk about nonexistence.

3. *Activities for recurrence.* Nonlinguistic demonstrations of recurrence should involve the reappearance or multiple instances of both objects and events. Again, in a child's normal environment, such situations occur all the time; eating is a continual process of repeated actions ("another cookie," "drink again," etc.). Other situations that lend themselves to the coding of recurrence are:

    a. Playground—slides, seesaws, swings (up and down again).
    b. Shop—bang again, another nail.
    c. Art—another crayon, cut another one.
    d. Blocks and puzzles—another piece or block.
    e. Gym—jump, throw, tumble again.
    f. Looking at a book—another X in the picture, turn another page, turn again.
    g. Sand table—make another one, pour more sand in.
    h. Taking toys out of box, or returning more toys, more trucks.

4. *Activities for possession.* To teach possessor-possessed relationships (mommy's coat, my hat), the demonstration of the concept should include objects the child associates with particular people. R. Brown (1973) reported that objects that could conceivably belong to a number of people (alienable objects) were talked about in terms of possessive relationship before body parts (inalienable objects). It is possible that noting the possessor of a bike or cookie is more important (i.e., less obvious) to code than the owner of a nose or an eye. Thus clothing, art work, personal toys, lunches, and assigned storage spaces, chairs, or desks provide opportunities for nonlinguistic illustration; they are alienable, and they have associations more permanent than the teaching context. To illustrate possessive relationships, it is important that the possessor and possessed object are, in fact, related and not just temporarily assigned for the duration of the lesson.

5. *Activities for action.* Action is a major portion of a child's life, so there should be little problem finding actions in the child's natural environment. Creating them in a clinic room becomes more of a problem. The following are activities that the child can both participate in and observe. The form to be presented can vary from single words to coordinate and subordinate complex sentences, depending on the content/form interaction of interest. For example, in an activity centered around cooking, *pour, open, mix, stir,*

and so on could be presented as single-word utterances or complex causal sentences with *because,* for example, "We can't pour the powder because the box is closed," "Don't touch the pan because it's hot." Thus, particular activities can form the core for learning many content/form interactions. Consider, then, in planning nonlinguistic input for action relations, some of the following inputs and actions.

    a. Playground—slide, run, hop, jump, swing, throw.
    b. Sand table—build, pour, pat, mix, stir, push, spill, make.
    c. Water play—wash, pour, spill, splash, dry.
    d. Cook—mix, bake, stir, pour, cut, make.
    e. Art—cut, draw, color, paint, paste, tear, fold, make.
    f. Shop—hammer, saw, bang, build, turn.
    g. Snack—eat, drink, open, pour, cut, wash, clean, wipe.

6. *Activities for locative action.* Children are often locating objects in their environments. Many opportunities to code such actions occur in the normal classroom and home.

    a. Cleanup time—*putting* many objects in many different places.
    b. Play with trains or trucks and dollhouses also involves much locating activity.
    c. Dressing or undressing—*putting* clothes on and *taking* them off.
    d. Form board and puzzles—*putting* pieces in board.
    e. Telling another or self *where* to hide objects: "Dog goes there" (an example of patient-locative action), "You put it there" (an example of agent-locative action), or "You sit there" (an example of mover-locative action)

7. *Activities for locative state.* Situations referring to the static location of objects are easy to design and certainly are numerous and varied in the child's life. To demonstrate this relationship, it is important to select objects and places that are familiar to the child. One would not choose to use a situation as a microphone on a tape recorder to code locative state if the child has not yet learned about microphones or tape recorders. Static spatial relations follow learning about locative action. Searching activities can incorporate locative state, nonexistence, and *wh* questions about locative state.

8. *Activities for internal state.* It is more difficult to vary external stimuli so that the child will experience an internal state. Ideally, the facilitator will have enough contact with the child to be with him or her when the child experiences and manifests (nonlinguistically) many states that can be coded, such as *tired, scared, sad, mad, hunger, thirsty,* or *happy.* When these situations occur, the linguistic forms can be supplied.

    Wanting is perhaps the easiest state to create and, in fact, the earliest state that normal children learn to code. Desired objects can be made almost available, and if the child reaches for the object, the form can be provided: "You want X." With enough variety of objects and repetition, it is likely the child will induce that the regularity that the form codes has to do with feelings and desires—that is, the child's internal state relative to the object. At first, however, *want* may be used more as an action form similar to *give me.*

Later coding of moods (as volition, intention, obligation) with verbs, such as *want, like, must, go,* or *have,* would involve coding desired, intended, or obligatory actions (such as *eat* or *play*) rather than desired objects. Initially the actions would be those that the child (i.e., subject of the state verb) carries out (e.g., "I'm gonna eat") and, later, those that others who are not the subject of the state verb carry out (e.g., "I want mommy do that"). Intended actions need to be coded as the child is about to do something (e.g., "You're gonna slide down" as the child is perched on top of the slide), or knows someone else is about to do something (as you hold an open milk container tilted over an empty glass, you say, "I'm gonna pour the milk").

9. *Activities for temporal relations.* Early coding of temporal relations appears to involve coding of aspect using verb inflections (see Chapter 10 for a definition of aspect and for further information, and see Box 10-5 for specific verbs on which children first use the different inflections). Thus, *-ing* would be first presented on verbs coding durative noncompletive actions while such activities are ongoing. Some activities could include drawing, painting, or writing; riding a bike; or walking. In contrast, first models of past tense might be presented in contexts that code momentary actions that have an end result, as when something gets broken or gets eaten. Finally, first use of third person *-s* might best be facilitated in contexts of placing objects in their usual location (e.g., a puzzle piece "fits here," or a toy, dollhouse furniture, or a piece of clothing "goes here" when referring to its usual location).

Sequential temporal relations could be facilitated in familiar sequential activities (again using the child's event representation, or script, as a support). Such activities as preparing supper, setting the table, getting dressed, taking a bath, cleaning up, eating a snack, listening at story time, making cookies, going shopping, and so forth all provide temporal sequences. These sequences are familiar to the child and can, at first, be coded as they happen (in a chained manner), and then as they are just about to happen (e.g., as starting to put on socks—"first you put on the socks, and then you put on the shoes"). Simultaneous actions might include such events as the child holding the toy while the adult turns the key, or one child passing the cookies while another passes the napkins, or one sitting while another reads, etc.

Reference to past events can include those events which have just taken place and in which the child has just participated. Again, most success may be found if the event is not a novel event, but one with which the child is familiar. Use of very familiar event sequences may be easier for the child to bring to mind, and they can provide contexts for earliest coding of both past and future tense.

10. *Activities for causal.* Causal relations can be pointed out in everyday events and be incorporated as part of the negotiations between child and adult. For example, prohibitions to the child can be presented with a reason ("don't eat that because it's dirty," "we can't cross the street now because the light is red," "daddy is sleeping so we have to be quiet"), or the child's requests and rejections can be given a reason (e.g., "you want to go so you

can see mommy?''). In addition, more tangible cause-effect relations can be demonstrated and coded during ongoing activities (''I can't see in the box because it's dark,'' ''the truck won't roll because it doesn't have a wheel,'' ''the doll fell in the water so she's all wet''). Familiar routines and the disruption of these routines also provide contexts for presenting cause-effect relations (e.g., ''I'll turn on the water so you can take a bath,'' ''we can't put on your shoes because you don't have your socks on''). Causal utterances can be added to a prior child utterance (e.g., *Child:* ''Don't touch that.'' *Adult:* ''Because it might break?'').

11. *Activities for epistemic.* Coding states of mind about events can be done in contexts where the child demonstrates certainty about an action (such as where puzzle pieces go—''You know where that piece goes''—or how to work a toy—''You know how to make that work'') or uncertainty (as the child looks for a toy—''You don't know where it is?'' ''You think it might be over there?''). It is also possible to code your own state of mind if that state is clear to the child. For example, if the child asks you where something is, you might search around looking puzzled and say, ''I don't know where X is,'' or act enlightened and move toward the shelves saying, ''I think it's over here.''

12. *Activities for adversative.* Contexts that provide contrasts are good opportunities for coding adversative. For example, if one block or puzzle piece won't fit but another one will, the adult might try one and say, ''This one doesn't fit,'' and reach for another and say, ''but this one fits.'' In a routine snack time context the utterance might be: ''You can pour the milk, but not too much,'' or ''Peg has a cup but she has no juice.'' Adversative utterances can also be used to expand the child's utterance (e.g., *Child:* ''I want to play.'' *Adult:* ''But you have to finish dinner first'').

Activities that might be used to facilitate narrative productions follow:

13. *Additive Chains.* To facilitate the use of repeated actions, different objects can be made to perform the same action while the adult is describing what is happening. For example, while putting dolls to bed, the adult might say, ''Mommy goes to bed, daddy goes to bed, baby goes to bed and the girl goes to bed.'' Variation on the object of the action can be facilitated by having the same agent perform the same action on different objects, such as ''Cookie Monster ate the cake, he ate the cookies, and he ate the candy.'' Cleanup time provides opportunity for coding repeated actions, ''This goes here, this goes here,'' etc. Show and tell can be a time for encouraging descriptive sequences as the child shares favorite objects. Encoding and guiding the child's play with animate beings provides models of narratives and can include the internal states (reactions, goals, plans, etc.) of the dolls or animals as well as resolutions. While the child is not yet expected to code the entire scene, such play contexts provide the background for future productions of causal chains by the child (see Sachs, Goldman, & Chaille, 1984).

14. *Temporal Chains.* Activities that usually occur in some sequence are helpful contexts for facilitating temporal chains. Snack time or lunch may be such an activity in some schools or homes: ''First we put the cups out; then we pour the juice,'' or ''We eat our snack, and then we wipe the table and throw the cups away.'' Children can be encouraged to relate familiar se-

quential events such as going out to eat, going to birthday parties, getting on the school bus, etc. If intervention is done within the school, routines within the classroom provide a potential source of action sequences. Again, play can be coded and guided with verbalizations from the adult, and sociodramas can be enacted—at this point the sequential aspects of the play can be stressed (Sachs et al., 1984).

15. *Causal Chains.* Since the essence of the causal chain is some sort of disequilibrium, problems that interfere with the child's usual routines and that have an impact on the child are possible topics for personal experience narratives. Those of us who regularly depend on planes or trains to take us from point A to point B usually have an endless store of personal experiences with problems that we can relate. Many children have either witnessed or experienced accidents or malfunctions with vehicles, disagreements and actual physical fights, problems with pets, or just minor disruptions (such as losing keys to the house or losing mittens, or coming home late for supper) which can be called upon for narration. Furthermore, stories that children have heard and television programs that they have watched provide fantasy scenes that they can adapt, embellish, or simply recall; either most have a villain, or there is some lack (e.g., food, fuel) that provides the disequilibrium (Sutton-Smith, 1981).

Clinicians and educators can create complicating events within the daily routines of clinic and classroom and embellish them to make them interesting enough to relate to others; the lunch boxes can be moved by the janitor (who supposedly forgot to return them after cleaning) before lunchtime, and a search can be organized; or the door to the clinic (or resource) room can be locked when the children and teacher arrive. Such complicating events can then be used to plan attempts to resolve the problem, carry out those attempts, and eventually embed obstacles to the attempts at resolution so that multiple episodes (or causal chains) are enacted and ready to narrate. These experiences can then be discussed immediately after the experiences (along with the child's reactions), and eventually they can be retold to other children or to school and clinic personnel.

Sociodramatic play in which the children take reciprocal roles (such as doctor-patient, mother-child, teacher-student, police officer–robber) provides the child with opportunities to jointly develop narratives that set scenes ("let's pretend we are . . . ," "you be the child, and I'll be the mommy"), including important past events ("you were sick in school today, ok?"), and that have problems ("you have a fever and can't move"), plans ("I'm gonna call the doctor"), and resolutions ("here's your medicine and you're all better") (see Sachs et al., 1984, for information on young children's responses to such play). Encouraging such play may help the child develop an awareness of subcategories of the causal chain (see Chapter 11) and provides opportunity for planning before the enactment and before the retelling.

Encouraging children to dictate stories to a transcribing adult (who might even ask relevant questions to help the child build the story, such as, "and then what happened?") and then having the children enact the dictated stories can be useful both in motivating children to create stories and in increasing the level of narrative productions (McNamee & Harris-

Schmidt, 1985). Repeated exposure to well-developed causal chains has also been suggested as a means of facilitating the child's narrative skills (Van Dongen & Westby, 1986, and see their listing of books). Furthermore, enacting well-structured stories that have been read to the child by the teacher provides the child with an opportunity to understand better the cause-and-effect relations as well as the internal responses and the types of characters depicted; it has resulted in richer retelling of the same stories (Galda, 1984). For further suggestions and information relevant to story comprehension, see, in addition to the above, Page and Stewart, 1985, and Westby, 1984, 1985.

Summary.   In summary, the commonplace activities of the child are useful contexts for facilitating the inductions of content/form and also use interactions. Most contexts provide a variety of relations that can be coded. The task of the facilitator is to select the appropriate relation for each child and to highlight that relation and provide salient forms to code the relation. These contexts occur within the home and school. When you have decided how to use these natural contexts, significant others in the child's life can be called upon to help provide appropriate models and responses to the child's utterances if very specific instructions are provided and limited content/form/use interactions are the focus. Should it be impossible to have access to the child's usual life activities, then activities that simulate natural-occurring events must be devised in the clinical context with information provided by others concerning the types of events the child experiences outside of the clinic.

Language Disorders Involving Content/Form Interactions

Children manifesting difficulty learning *content/form* interactions may have difficulty in conceptualizing the regularities in the linguistic environment (forming word concepts or linguistic categories) or in conceptualizing the regularities in the nonlinguistic environment (forming object and relational concepts that are the content of language). Alternatively, these children may have difficulty in inducing interactions between linguistic and nonlinguistic categories (regularities perceived in the nonlinguistic environment associated with regularities perceived in the linguistic environment). Although each may be a separate problem, the context of intervention may not, in fact, differ drastically.

In all cases the goal is an induction of content/form interaction, which involves *contact* between linguistic and nonlinguistic categories. At first it may appear that a child cannot form inductions about content/form *interaction* until being able to form both linguistic and nonlinguistic categories, and, therefore, each should be worked on separately. However, the presentation of forms concurrent with varied demonstrations of concepts may facilitate the formation of categories of both form and content. The child who has difficulty perceiving regularities or discriminating differences in the acoustic signal (speech) may be aided in that perception by the consistent presentation of that signal (made salient as discussed previously) concurrent with regularly occurring and eventually predictable nonlinguistic events. In this way the child can use his or her concepts of content to aid in building word concepts—strengths the child already has in content can help in learning about form. Furthermore, the ability to see regularities in form may aid in leading a child to discover the regularities in the nonlinguistic environment (R. Brown, 1956). Likewise, the child who has difficulty integrating information from different modalities needs extra repetitions of concurrent linguistic and nonlinguistic presentation. Even when, as a last resort, the visual modality is used to supplement the auditory modality for linguistic forms, both content and form need to be presented concurrently—within the speech event.

In all cases content/form interactions should be facilitated in the contexts of interactive communication. The facilitation of inductions of content/form interactions has been discussed here separately from those of use for the purpose of clarifying the types of contexts that are most facilitative for each, but all input regarding content/form interactions occurs with some use, and all interactions geared toward facilitation of aspects of language use involve *content/form* interactions.

Summary

For a child to learn how linguistic forms can be used to represent ideas of the world, the child must repeatedly experience consistent forms that code the ideas the child is currently holding in consciousness. The task of the facilitator is to arrange stimuli (i.e., to intervene) in the child's environment so that these experiences will be frequent and salient.

Considerations in planning the linguistic input include varying intensity, prosody, and rate to increase the salience of the linguistic signal. In selecting lexical items for initial vocabulary, the facilitator should consider words that are short, compatible with the child's phonological system, nonhomophonous, frequently produced, efficient, and useful to the child. In selecting lexical items to be included within new syntactic structures, the facilitator should consider familiarity of the lexical items, verbs that non-language-disordered children frequently produce when learning these structures, and possible phonological constraints. Finally, the auditory linguistic input should be supplemented with nonlinguistic input that illustrates the meanings to be coded.

Considerations in planning the nonlinguistic input include actual demonstration instead of picture representations of the concepts to be coded, inclusion of different exemplars of a concept, and use of the child's life experiences as core activities to illustrate concepts. Furthermore, consideration should be given to the child's role as a participant in the interactions. Whether the child exhibits problems in categorizing the linguistic input (form), in categorizing the nonlinguistic environment (relevant to content), or in inducing the interactions of form with content, concurrent presentation of content and form should aid in making inductions about the relations between linguistic and nonlinguistic categories.

With some children the task is not so much to aid inductions of form and content, but, instead, to facilitate the use of the code that they are learning or already know. Such facilitation takes into account interpersonal (or social) functions, intrapersonal functions, and the influence of varying contexts. When using alternative forms for various contexts is the goal, then it is important that the differences in context be made salient to the child. When coding of communicative functions is the goal, it is important to know if the child communicates those functions in a nonlinguistic manner. If the child shows no evidence of communicating particular functions in any manner, then the facilitator's task is to devise situations that would encourage such functions; if the goal is to facilitate alternative means of coding particular functions, then the task of the facilitator is to provide appropriate input when the child is ready to express those functions.

In all cases, it is suggested that one important key to the success of language intervention is the facilitator's ability to provide appropriate forms to code the ideas of the world and the communicative intentions that occupy the *child's* immediate attention. To do so requires that the facilitator see the world from the child's perspective. A number of suggestions were made for accomplishing this, including utilizing routines where the child and facilitator can predict what will happen, designing activities that clearly involve the child's attention and that are within the child's processing capacities, following the child's actions, and basing input on the child's utterances (e.g., through recasts).

A second key to success that has been suggested throughout the last two chapters is consideration of the attentional resources that the child can allocate to the tasks at hand. If some new interaction (e.g., some new form for a content/use) is to be induced or practiced, it would seem reasonable, whenever possible, to utilize contexts that do not demand considerable attention to nonlinguistic processing (i.e., to use automatized motor activities, nonstressful social interactions, familiar world knowledge, etc.) or to other aspects of language processing (i.e., to utilize familiar content/use when introducing new forms, or familiar forms when facilitating new form/use, etc.).

Finally, flexibility is as important in intervention procedures as it is in the establishment of goals of intervention or in assessment procedures. As noted in the previous chapter, we have little empirical data to support the exclusive use of one or two techniques. We operate with assumptions that must be open to change, must be implemented with creativity, and must be reevaluated for effectiveness.

Suggested Readings

Baker, N., & Nelson, K. (1984). Recasting and related conversational techniques for triggering syntactic advances by young children. *First Language, 5*, 3–21.

Cole, K., & Dale, P. (1986). Direct language instruction and interactive language instruction with language delayed preschool children: A comparison study. *Journal of Speech and Hearing Research, 29*, 206–217.

Constable, C. (1986). The application of scripts in the organization of language intervention contexts. In K. Nelson (Ed.), *Event Knowledge.* Hillsdale, NJ: Erlbaum.

Duchan, J. (1986). Language intervention through sensemaking and fine tuning. In R. Schiefelbusch (Ed.), *Communicative competence: Assessment and language intervention.* Baltimore: University Park Press.

Fey, M. (1986). *Language intervention with young children.* San Diego: College-Hill Press.

Galda, L. (1984). Narrative competence: Play, storytelling and story comprehension. In A. D. Pellegrin & T. Yawkey (Eds.), *The development of oral and written language in social contexts* (pp. 105–117). Norwood, NJ: Ablex.

Itard, J. (1962). *The wild boy of Aveyron* (pp. 67–86). New York: Appleton-Century-Crofts.

Schwartz, R., Chapman, K., Terrell, B., Prelock, P., & Rowan, L. (1985). Facilitating word combinations in language-impaired children through discourse structure. *Journal of Speech and Hearing Disorders, 50*, 31–39.

APPENDIX A

Conventions for Transcription of Child Language Recordings*

1. All speech by the child and to the child or within the child's hearing is fully transcribed on paper divided by a vertical line. Utterances by the child appear on the right side. Utterances by other speakers appear on the left. The person is identified by an initial (M for mommy, L for Lois, D for daddy, etc.). Information about the situational context also appears on the left and is enclosed in parentheses.

   (M takes cookie from bag; offering it
     to A)
   M: Look what I have/ (A taking
     cookie)   cookie/

2. An action or event that occurs simultaneously with the child utterance appears on the same line with that utterance.

   (E banging blocks together)   crash/

3. When an utterance precedes or follows an action or event, the utterance appears on the preceding or succeeding line.

   (E throws block)

                                          no block/

   (E picks up another block)

                                          more/

4. Note the differential use of verb tenses in describing the situations: progressive for simultaneous action; simple present for actions or events that precede or follow an utterance.

° Prepared by Lois Bloom in collaboration with Lois Hood and Patsy Lightbown.

5. For situational information accompanying utterances by someone other than the child, use the same verb tense conventions, but utterances and description can, of course, succeed one another on different lines since there is rarely enough space to put both on the same line.

(L reaching in bag)
L: Do you know what I have?
(L pulls out truck)
L: I think I'll make the truck go
   under the bridge/

6. Utterances that succeed each other immediately—WITH NO CHANGE IN SITUA-TION—follow each other on the same line.

(G reaching for box of cookies)   more/ more/ cookie

If there is any change in situation, the utterances appear on different lines.

(G reaching for box of cookies;   more/
   taking box off counter;   more/
   reaches in;
   pulling out cookie)   cookie/

When in doubt about the situational context, use separate lines.

Punctuation

7. For utterances of child and other speakers, the usual sign of utterance bound-ary is a slash (/). The boundary is determined by length of pause before the next utterance and by its apparent terminal contour. The judgment is some-times very difficult to make. With older children and adults, the slash may be considered equivalent to a period, but it is important to make each judgment carefully and as objectively as possible.

8. Utterances by adult or child may be followed by an exclamation mark. When a child utterance is exclamatory, it should be followed by *both* an exclamation mark and the usual slash.

(Peter takes tire off car)   there!/ finish/

9. Adult questions are indicated by question marks. For the child utterance, however, there are two different ways of indicating that an utterance has question form. For *wh* questions, a question mark may be used.

(P looking in toy bag)   where's ə car?/

When a child utterance seems to be a question because it has rising intona-tion, it should be followed by a rising arrow (↑) instead of a question mark.

(P shaking empty box)   no more in there ↑/

Even for a "well-formed" yes/no question (i.e., one with subject-verb inver-sion), the arrow to indicate rising intonation is more informative than a simple question mark.

(K meeting L at door)   did you bring the toys today ↑/

In either case, a slash should also be used to mark the utterance boundary clearly.

10. A pause within an utterance is indicated by a dot (·).
    (E trying to fit peg in hole)   put·this one in/

11. A long pause between utterances within the same general situation is indicated by horizontal dots across the center line.

    wheel goes in there/
    (P tries to get wheel on car)

    · · ·
    (P succeeds)

    there!/

12. A long pause between utterances where there is a change in the general situation is marked by three vertical dots on the center line.
    (G trying to stack blocks)   Gia make ə house/
                                         ⋮
    (G running to kitchen)   juice!/ Gia drink juice/

13. A colon is used to indicate that an utterance or word is drawn out.
    (E trying to fit large block inside   no:/
       small one)

14. A curving arrow is used when there is some kind of utterance boundary, but the utterance sounds unfinished, such as when the child is counting or "listing."

    one ↗/
    two ↗/
    three ↗/

15. Stress marks indicate strongly emphasized words.
    L: do you want this one? (L giving G
       a blue disc)   no!/
       (G reaching for red one L is
       holding)   thát one/

Capitalization

16. Names are capitalized. Initial letter of child utterance is not. Initial letter of adult utterance may be.

Other "Punctuation"

17. An utterance may be followed by falling arrow (↓) when it is important to emphasize the fact that the utterance had falling terminal contour.
    (P looking in toy bag;   wheel ↑/
       pulls out tire for car)

                                         wheel ↓/

18. When a child or other speaker suddenly interrupts his or her own utterance —apparently leaving the utterance unfinished—a line (_____) indicates the abrupt stop.

> L: Do you want some _____/
> (E picks up cup and spills juice)

19. When a child or other speaker interrupts his or her own utterance apparently to change or correct it, a "self-correct" symbol (s/c) is used.

> L: Those are your ₅/c my toys/
>
> don't ₅/c ə want toys/

20. An unintelligible utterance or portion of an utterance is indicated by three dashes (– – –). If possible, a phonetic transcription is used instead.

> (E pushing over house of blocks,
>   making loud crash)
>
> no more/– – –/ house/

Abbreviations

21. When a child or other speaker repeats his or her own utterance completely and exactly, an × is used to show the repetition. Any change in the utterance must be indicated, including clear changes in intonation.

> L: Be careful/ ×/
> (P touching tape recorder)
>
> open/ ×/ ×/
> ×!/

22. When an adult repeats a child's utterance, an equal sign (=) is used to show the repetition. When a child repeats an adult utterance, however, the child's utterance is written in full, even if the repetition is exact. An equal sign can never represent a child utterance, although an equal sign may be placed next to the utterance to indicate that it is a repetition of an adult utterance.

> two cookies/
>
> M: =/ I only see one in there/
>
> one in there/=

23. The symbol # may be used to indicate that there is material on the tape that is not transcribed. It can only appear on the left side and usually represents conversations between adults. The symbol is only used when it is reasonable to assume that the child is not attending to or, in fact, does not hear the conversation.

24. (lf) = laugh
    (wh) = whisper
    (cr) = cry   These abbreviations may be useful for behavior that
    (wm) = whimper   occurs fairly frequently. The abbreviation should
    (wn) = whine   appear on the left side of the line.
    (y)   = yell
    (gr) = grunt

Labeling

25. Pages should be numbered front and back, with numbers in upper right corner.

26. In order to make it easier to locate material on the tape, a number should be placed in the right margin every time the counter on the tape recorder registers a multiple of 50.

27. Every time a new tape or a new side of a tape is started, the tape number, side number (1 or 2), and the date and time of the recording session (if different from the previous tape or side) should be indicated.

Some Instruments That Assess Language and Language-Related Behaviors

Adaptive Behavior Scale (ABS). Washington, DC: American Association on Mental Deficiency, 1970.

The Arthur Adaptation of the Leiter International Performance Scale, by G. Arthur. Washington, DC: Psychological Service Center Press, 1952.

Assessment of Children's Language Comprehension, by R. Foster, J. Giddan, & J. Stark. Austin, TX: Learning Concepts, 1969, 1973.

Auditory Discrimination Test, by J. Wepman. Chicago: Language Research Associates, 1958.

Bankson Language Screening Test, by N. W. Bankson. Baltimore: University Park Press, 1977.

Berry-Talbott Exploratory Test of Grammar, by Mildred Berry. Rockford, IL: 1966.

Boehm Test of Basic Concepts, by A. Boehm. New York: Psychological Corp., 1969, 1986.

Boehm Test of Basic Concepts—Preschool Version, by A. Boehm. San Antonio, TX: Psychological Corp., 1986.

Bracken Basic Concept Scale, by B. Bracken. San Antonio, TX: Psychological Corp., 1984.

Elicited Language Inventory, by E. Carrow. Austin, TX: Learning Concepts, 1974.

Children's Drawings as a Measure of Intellectual Maturity: A Revision and Extension of the Goodenough Draw-a-Man Test, by D. B. Harris. New York: Harcourt, Brace & World, 1963.

Clinical Evaluation of Language Functions (CELF), by E. Semel & E. Wiig. San Antonio, TX: Psychological Corp., 1987.

Coloured Progressive Matrices. New York: Psychological Corp., 1962.

Communicative Evaluation Chart from Infancy to Five Years, by R. Anderson, M. Miles, & P. Matheny. Cambridge, MA: Educators' Publishing Service, 1963.

Denver Developmental Screening Test, by W. Frankenburg et al. Denver, CO: LADOCA Project and Publishers Foundation, 1975.

Detroit Test of Learning Aptitude, by H. Baker & B. Leland. Indianapolis: Bobbs-Merrill, 1959.

One-Word Expressive Vocabulary Test, by R. Gardner. Novato, CA: Academic Therapy Publications, 1979.

Fisher-Logeman Test of Articulation Competence, by A. Fisher & J. Logeman. Boston: Houghton-Mifflin, 1971.

The Goldman-Fristoe Test of Articulation, by R. Goldman & M. Fristoe. Circle Pines, MN: American Guidance Service, 1969. 1972, 1986.

The Goldman-Fristoe-Woodcock Test of Auditory Discrimination, by R. Goldman, M. Fristoe, & R. Woodcock. Circle Pines, MN: American Guidance Service, 1972.

The Illinois Test of Psycholinguistic Abilities (rev. ed.). by S. Kirk, J. McCarthy, & W. Kirk. Urbana, IL: University of Illinois Press, 1968.

Interpersonal Language Skills Assessment (ILSA), by C. Blagden & N. L. McConnell. Moline, IL: LingiSystems, 1985.

Kahn-Lewis Phonological Analysis: for Use with the Goldman-Fristoe Test of Articulation, by L. Kahn & N. Lewis. Circle Pines, MN: American Guidance Service, 1986.

Language Processing Test, by G. Richard & M. Hanner. Moline, IL: LinguiSystems, 1985.

Let's Talk Inventory for Children, by C. Bray & E. Wiig. San Antonio, TX: Psychological Corp., 1987.

McCarthy Scales of Children's Abilities, by D. McCarthy. New York: Psychological Corp., 1974.

Miller-Yoder Test of Grammatical Comprehension (M.Y.), by J. Miller & D. Yoder. Madison, WI: Communication Development Group, 1972, 1984.

Northwestern Syntax Screening Test (NSST), by L. Lee. Evanston, IL: Northwestern University Press, 1971.

Peabody Picture Vocabulary Test—Revised, by L. Dunn & L. Dunn. Circle Pines, MN: American Guidance Service, 1981.

Pragmatics Screening Test (PST), by P. Prinz & F. Weiner. San Antonio, TX: Psychological Corp., in press.

Preschool Language Assessment Instrument: The language of learning in practice, by M. Blank, S. Rose, & L. Berlin. New York: Grune & Stratton, 1978.

Preschool Language Scale, by I. L. Zimmerman, V. G. Steiner, & R. Pond. Columbus, OH: Charles Merrill, 1979.

Sequenced Inventory of Communication Development, by D. Hedrick, E. Prather, & A. Tobin. Seattle, WA: University of Washington Press, 1975.

Stanford-Binet Intelligence Scale, by L. Terman & M. Merrill. Boston: Houghton-Mifflin, 1960.

Test for Auditory Comprehension of Language, by E. Carrow. Austin, TX: Learning Concepts, 1973.

Test of Language Competence for Children (TLC-C), by E. Wiig & W. Secord. San Antonio, TX: Psychological Corp., 1987.

Test of Language Development—Intermediate Edition, by D. Hammill & P. Newcomer. San Antonio, TX: Psychological Corp., 1982.

Test of Language Development—Primary Edition, by P. Newcomer & D. Hammill. San Antonio, TX: Psychological Corp., 1982.

Test of Pragmatic Skills—Revised, by B. Shulman. Tucson, AZ: Communication Skill Builders, 1986.

Test of Word Finding, by D. German. Allen, TX: DLM Teaching Resources, 1986.

Wechsler Intelligence Scale for Children—Revised (WISC-R), by D. Wechsler. New York: Psychological Corp., 1974.

Wechsler Preschool and Primary Scale of Intelligence (WPPSI), by D. Wechsler. New York: Psychological Corp., 1967.

Some Alternative Plans for Assessment and Intervention

1. Crystal, D. (1982). *Profiling Linguistic Disability.* London: Arnold.

This includes a revised form of *LARSP* (Crystal, Fletcher, & Garman, 1976) as well as an analysis of phonology, prosody, and semantics. The purpose of the profile analysis is to provide a basis for intervention by identifying linguistic level and suggesting what should be taught. LARSP is the analysis of the form of utterances after separating unintelligible, deviant, incomplete, ambiguous, and stereotypic utterances. Developmental order is broken into seven stages, each analyzed under statements, questions, and commands. Stage 1 concerns single words. In Stage 2, two-element utterances are analyzed by levels of clause and phrase with clausal constituents of subject, verb, object, complement, and adverbial (e.g., SV or VO) and phrasal constituents of adjective, noun, preposition, and verb (e.g., adj. N.). In addition, morphological inflections begin to be coded in Stage 2 and continue to be coded through Stage 5. Transitional between Stages 2 and 3 is the inclusion of phrases into clauses (e.g., the inclusion of articles in utterances with a noun and verb). Stage 3 includes three-element utterances in each category as well as more morphological inflections and the copula and auxiliary. Transitional between Stages 3 and 4 is further inclusion of phrases within clausal utterances. Phase 4 includes longer utterances, and in this stage conjunctions appear. Stages 5 and 6 involve primarily the formation of more complex sentences. Errors are noted if correct production of similar forms is also observed. Moreover, there is an analysis of conversational interaction in terms of stimulus type (question or nonquestion from the adult) and response type (repetition, elliptical, reduced, etc.).

PRISM, the semantic analysis, includes both lexical and grammatical inventories. Lexical items are divided into social and relational use, with social divided into spontaneous, response, and stereotype. Relational items are divided into categories such as prepositional (temporal, spatial, etc.), pronominal, and interrogative. Finally, words are divided into semantic fields. While there is some suggestion that certain fields may precede others in acquisition, the evidence is "only suggestive" (p. 150).

The semantic analysis related to grammar is divided into five stages—four relate to the semantic structure of the clause and one to the semantics of clause sequences. Semantic categories considered include actor, experiencer, dynamic, locative, goal, temporal, and so forth. An utterance can consist of a sequence of semantic "elements" that correspond to the grammatical categories of subject-verb-object, and when an element consists of more than one word, the other words are considered specifications. For example, in *my dog kicked two balls*, the words *my* and *two* would be considered specifications of possession and quantity, while *dog* would be considered an actor, *kicked* a dynamic activity or change of state, and *ball* a goal. Deictic words are coded separately. The number of functions that are expressed within an utterance increases with stage and is coded. This evidence is quantified into the number of elements per clause, the number of specifications per element, and the number of deictics per clause element. Relations between clauses are coded into eight categories (e.g., addition, temporal, contrast, location, purpose, condition), and the presence of connective form is noted, as is the number of semantic elements in each clause. Developmental data are only implied in that sequences grow longer—not that particular categories emerge or are concatenated before others—and that the sequencing of clauses is a later development than sequencing within a clause. No references are given for evidence of developmental data in any of the profiles; it is noted that it comes from the literature.

2. Hubbell, R. D. (1981). *Children's language disorders: An integrated approach.* Englewood Cliffs, NJ: Prentice-Hall.

A language sampling procedure is outlined which is based on the work of Dever (1978) [*TALK: Teaching the American Language to Kids*, Columbus, OH: Merrill] and to some extent Crystal, Fletcher, and Garman (1976). Clause types (e.g., transitive, intransitive, and equative) and clause variations (e.g., imperatives, declaratives, and questions) are identified. In addition, preclausal precursors to clauses are identified (e.g., single words, two-word combinations, and longer preclausal utterances. If a child is using clauses, then noun phrases are analyzed into constituent structure (e.g., determiners, adjectivals, head), and verb phrases into constituents (such as modals, perfective, continuum, passive, head) and past tense, third person, negative, and *do* support. Within the verb phrase analysis, a sequence of development is suggested. Following this, some analysis of complex sentences is suggested. This analysis is one of form. If the child does not use clauses with much frequency, then a preclausal analysis is done and some coding of content is seen here. Preclausal types are analyzed according to certain semantic relations as agent + action, action + object, and locative + X and according to broader function categories as modifier + X, question + X, and negative + X. Suggestions for sequence are limited and, except for verb phrase development, are described as speculative or based on limited data in the literature.

3. Kretschmer, R. R., & Kretschmer, L. W. (1978). *Language development and intervention with the hearing impaired.* Baltimore: University Park Press.

The Kretschmer plan has six parts. The first lists preverbal behaviors related to form and use; the second lists semantic and syntactic descriptions of one- and two-word productions; the third lists semantic and syntactic descriptions of single-proposition productions; the fourth lists syntactic descriptions of complex sentences; the fifth describes aspects of use; and the sixth describes errors or restricted-form types. The analysis was derived for examining written language samples of the hearing impaired but could be used for oral language samples of any population. It incorporates information on content and form (though not the specific interaction between the two) for all but complex sentences; use is described separately with no developmental analysis except for the preverbal period. According to the authors, one of the plan's strengths is the description of deviant structures that are often found in the hearing impaired.

4. Lee, L. (1974). *Developmental sentence analysis.* Evanston, IL: Northwestern University Press.

Lee's book presents two procedures for the analysis of spontaneous speech samples. The developmental sentence scoring (DSS) procedure provides normative data as well as a developmental sequence of eight grammatical forms as used in sentences containing a subject and a predicate: noun modifiers; pronouns, including indefinite and personal pronouns; main verb elaborations, including infinitives and gerunds; secondary verbs; negative forms; conjunctions; interrogative reversals; and *wh*-question forms. The developmental sequence is broken down into eight levels that apply both within and across the eight grammatical features. The sequence of particular features was based on their production in utterances with a subject and a predicate; it is not clear whether the same sequence should be used in less complete sentences. Information on content and use is not included; however, the data on form are sequenced for later stages of language learning than most other plans—they were normed on children 2 through almost 7 years of age.

Developmental sentence type (DST) is an analysis that involves earlier stages of language when utterances do not include a subject and a predicate. It is divided into three levels—single words, two-word combinations, and constructions (utterances over two words that do not include both a subject and a verb). Within these levels there are two subcategories for inclusion of elaborations or modifications such as plural, possessive, conjunction, or question. Utterances at each level are then placed in one of five categories: (1) noun phrase elaborations, including the addition of articles, adjectives, and two nouns; (2) designative utterances, which appear to be primarily identity statements and eventually include the copula; (3) descriptive statements that also eventually include a linking verb; (4) verbal elaborations; and (5) fragments, which need both a subject and a verb to become a sentence. The distribution of utterances within each of these categories is normed on 40 normal children from ages 2 to almost 3 years of age. This was the first procedure to use developmental data for the analysis of language-impaired children's language (Lee, 1966); it does not include information of content or use; developmental information in these areas was not available at that time.

5. Lund, N. J., & Duchan, J. F. (1983). *Assessing children's language in naturalistic contexts.* Englewood Cliffs, NJ: Prentice-Hall.

This book does not present a plan but does present developmental information and suggestions for assessment.

6. McLean, J. E., & Snyder-McLean, L. K. (1978). *A transactional approach to early language training.* Columbus, OH: Merrill.

This book presents data on development and a suggested format for language sample analyses including a semantic analysis for single words up to three-word utterances, a functional analysis, and an analysis of grammatical morphemes.

7. Miller, J. (Ed.). (1981). *Assessing language production in children: Experimental procedures.* Baltimore: University Park Press.

Half-hour samples of free speech are collected and analyzed relative to aspects of form, content, and use. While some interaction of content, form, and use is presented for one- and two-word utterances, the rest of the analysis is of individual components and not their interaction.

Form: Assigning Structural Stage (ASS) is a means of analyzing simple sentences in terms of various grammatical structures, such as noun and verb phrase elaboration, negation, yes/no questions, *wh* questions, and grammatical morphemes. Development of each is related to Brown's MLU stages as have been described in the literature (particularly by Brown and his colleagues). Complex sentences are analyzed by syntactic form and connective form and are also related to MLU stage based on data collected by Paul and presented in the book. When there is much variation in stages across grammatical structures, it is interpreted as evidence of deviance versus delay. The analysis is used to establish "long-range goals for syntactic therapy" (p. 31). Charts are included as are examples of an analysis; exact procedures are not specified.

Content: A semantic analysis is based on vocabulary diversity (using the norms of Templin, 1957; see Box 7-2 in this text) and a listing of semantic categories. Semantic categories found in the single-word-utterance period are specified (based primarily on data from Bloom); taxonomies for other semantic (or content) categories are presented, but they are not related to structural stages.

Use: Use analysis is primarily restricted to function, and this is incorporated into the chart of single-word utterances. A chapter by Chapman, however, summarizes other aspects of use, presenting a number of taxonomies and developmental data (usually by age, not structural stage) as reported in the literature. This summary of use is not, however, set as a plan.

8. Prutting, C. A. (1979). Process /prà/ses/n: The action of moving forward progressively from one point to another on the way to completion. *Journal of Speech and Hearing Disorders, 44,* 3–30.

A general sequence of language behaviors is presented in this article for use, for content, and for form (both syntactic and phonological). For most, the sequence is divided into six periods, including prelinguistic and adult with age equivalencies stated from 9 months to 3+ years. Interactions for specific behaviors are not included, though some description of expected behaviors is given for the different periods.

9. Prutting, C., & Kirchner, D. (1983). Applied pragmatics. In T. Gallagher & C. Prutting (Eds.), *Pragmatic assessment and intervention issues in language.* San Diego: College-Hill Press.

This pragmatic protocol is not developmental but, according to the authors, outlines behaviors that should be used by school-age children and adults. Paralinguistic as well as linguistic modes of expression are included. The taxonomy includes descriptions of the utterance act (e.g., intelligibility, prosody, fluency, physical proximity, eye gaze); the propositional act (e.g., word order, lexical selection, coding of given-new information, articles); and illocutionary and perlocutionary acts (e.g., turn taking, topic). Coding is essentially dichotomous—appropriate or inappropriate.

10. Tyack, D., & Gottsleben, R. (1974). *Language sampling, analysis and training: A handbook for teachers and clinicians.* Palo Alto, CA: Consulting Psychological Press.

The developmental sequence proposed in this procedure was derived from a cross-sectional study of normal language development reported by Morehead and Ingram (1973). Noun phrases and verb phrases are analyzed as well as complex sentences, negation, and questions. There are five levels determined by an average word-morpheme count. Forms and constructions are listed by linguistic level on the analysis forms. A level is passed if forms are used 90% of the time in obligatory contexts (no minimum criterion of productivity is needed). The forms and construction types that are not yet mastered but that are expected at the child's linguistic level (as assigned based on the word-morpheme count in the sample) become the goals of intervention. Directions for analysis are quite explicit with detailed analysis sheets. No developmental information or analysis is included on content or use; developmental information was not available at that time.

11. Waryas, C. L., & Stremel-Campbell, K. (1978). Grammatical training for the language-delayed child. In R. Schiefelbusch (Ed.), *Language intervention strategies.* Baltimore: University Park Press.

This is a revision of the earlier program (Stremel & Waryas, 1974) and is divided into three sections (early, early-intermediate, and late). No plan as such is presented, but the authors follow a child through training and talk of the importance of semantic and pragmatic factors.

APPENDIX D

Rules for Calculating MLU

1. Start with the second page of the transcription unless that page involves a recitation of some kind. In this latter case start with the first recitation-free stretch. Count the first 100 utterances satisfying the following rules.
2. Only fully transcribed utterances are used; none with blanks. Portions of utterances, entered in parentheses to indicate doubtful transcription, are used.°
3. Include all exact utterance repetitions (marked with a plus sign in records).° Stuttering is marked as repeated efforts at a single word; count the word once in the most complete form produced. In the few cases where a word is produced for emphasis or the like (*no, no, no*) count each occurrence.
4. Do not count such fillers as *mm* or *oh*, but do count *no, yeah,* and *hi.*
5. All compound words (two or more free morphemes), proper names, and ritualized reduplications count as single words. Examples: *birthday, rackety-boom, choo-choo, quack-quack, night-night, pocketbook, see saw.* Justification is that no evidence that the constituent morphemes function as such for these children.
6. Count as one morpheme all irregular pasts of the verb (*got, did, went, saw*). Justification is that there is no evidence that the child relates these to present forms.

Note: From R. Brown, 1973, p. 54.

° These two procedures were not followed for the data collected by Bloom and associates (e.g., 1970, 1975, 1982); exact repetitions and doubtful transcriptions were not used. However, in connection with the data analysis for Bloom, Hood, and Lightbown (1974), MLU was calculated both ways—with and without immediate self repetitions—and there were no appreciable differences.

7. Count as one morpheme all diminutives (*doggie, mommie*) because these children at least do not seem to use the suffix productively. Diminutives are the standard forms used by the child.
8. Count as separate morphemes all auxiliaries (*is, have, will, can, must, would*). Also all catenatives: *gonna, wanna, hafta.* These latter counted as single morphemes rather than as going to or want to because evidence is that they function so for the children. Count as separate morphemes all inflections, for example, possessive (s), plural (s), third person singular (s), regular past (d), progressive (ing).

Definitions of Content Categories

Language content refers to the ideas, or propositions, that language codes, or the semantics of language. It has to do with what people know about objects and events in the world and the feelings and attitudes that they have about what they know. Most of the content categories defined here were derived from child data by Bloom and her associates (e.g., 1970, 1974, 1975, 1980) but are similar to those described by other researchers and theoreticians (e.g., Bowerman, 1973; R. Brown, 1973; Fillmore, 1968; Schlesinger, 1971). Children code content categories other than those described here; other categories have not been included in the C/F/U Goal Plan for Language Learning because they have not yet been directly studied, they were not used frequently by the children studied, or they did not exhibit systematic developmental change in the data reported. Alternative categories could be derived, and different names could have (and have) been used for these same categories. The content categories described below are, however, the ones used in the C/F/U Goal Plan for Language Learning presented in this book. For further definition and for examples, see Chapters 8 through 11; for information on how to use the categories in assessment, see Chapters 12 and 13.

Existence Utterances in the existence category refer to objects or persons that exist in the environment. The child may look at, point to, touch, or pick up the object while naming it (e.g., "doggie" or "that a cup") or while pointing out its existence with utterances such as "that," "there," or even the question "what's that?" (Not all utterances that include nouns or demonstrative pronouns are existence utterances; only those that serve to point out the existence of the object or to identify the object are so categorized.) Eventually existence utterances are more clearly identifications and include the copula (e.g., "That's a car"; "these are dogs"), and some nonverb relations may be coordinated with existence (e.g., "That's my car"; "these are big dogs").

Recurrence Utterances in the recurrence category make reference to the reappearance of an object (e.g., "clown again"), or another instance of an object (e.g., "another clown") or event (e.g., "dance again") with or without the original instance still present. In early child language, *more* may be used for all coding of recurrence; later recurrence is coordinated with other categories (e.g., with notice, "I see more cookies"; or with action, "I swing again"). Some relational word that codes recurrence must be included in the utterance in order to place the utterance in this category.

Nonexistence-Disappearance Utterances are placed in the category of nonexistence-disappearance if they make reference to the disappearance of an object (e.g., "milk is all gone") or the nonexistence of an object (e.g., "no wheels" as the child points to the car without wheels) or action ("no open" as the child tries to open the toy box) in a context in which its occurrence might somehow be expected. In early phases, children use terms such as *no*, *all gone*, *no more*, and *away*, but later new forms are included such as *not*, and nonexistence is coordinated with other categories (e.g., with action, "she's not riding her bike"). However, some form of negation must be used to place an utterance in this category.

Rejection If a child opposes an action (e.g., "no bath") or refuses an object (e.g., "no soap") using a form of negation, the utterance is categorized as rejection. In early child language, the negative form is usually *no*, but later, forms such as *don't* are used and rejection is coordinated with

other categories (e.g., with action, "don't touch me").

Denial Utterances are categorized as denial if the child negates the identity, state, or event expressed in a prior utterance, whether it be the utterance of another or the child's own utterance (e.g., mother says "it's time for bed" and child responds "no bed"). Initial coding is with *no*; later utterances may include *not* (e.g., "that's my dad/ no, that's not my dad").

Attribution Utterances placed in the attribution category make reference to properties of objects with respect to (1) an inherent state of the object (e.g., "broken" or "sharp") or (2) specification of an object that distinguishes it from others in its class (e.g., "red," "big," and "party" in "party hat"). Such forms of attribution are eventually coordinated with other categories (e.g., with action, "I rode my new bike"). Another form of coding attribution is to refer to an attribute as a condition of the object with a copula sentence such as "the car is big" or "this is hot." This form of coding attribution is placed in the category of state and called *attributive state*.

Possession Utterances in the possession category indicate that a particular object is associated with a given person. Associations may be permanent (e.g., "my nose") or temporary (e.g., "my chair"), and the possessor may be coded with a noun (e.g., "mommy chair") or with a pronoun (e.g., "his coat"). Inflection of noun forms with *-s* is not essential to placing an utterance within the category. The coding of possession using the order of possessor + possessed-object is later coordinated with other categories (e.g., "I eat my cookies").

As with attribution, there is an alternative form of coding possession: the possessive state of an object can be described with a copula sentence such as "the car is mine." This form of coding is placed in the category of state and called *possessive state*.

Locative Action Utterances in the locative-action category refer to movement where the goal of the movement is a change in location of a person or object. Most locative-action utterances involve an object that is moved and a place or goal of such movement. Three subcategories of locative action can be differentiated by the semantic role of the preverbal consitituent (or the subject of the sentence) whether or not it is expressed; (1) the subject is the *agent* of the action [e.g., "(I) put blocks on table"]; (2) the subject is both the agent of the action and the object moved and can be called the *mover* [e.g., "(You) sit down"]; (3) the subject is the object moved, or *patient*, and the agent is not coded [e.g., "(this) goes here"].

Action Utterances in the action category refer to the movement relationships among people and objects where the goal is not to change location. Action utterances involve a movement or activity engaged in by an agent (animate or inanimate). The movement may or may not affect another person or object (e.g., "I eat cookie" or "I jump"). Frequently used verbs are listed in Chapter 9.

Locative State Utterances in locative-state category refer to static spatial relations (i.e., a person or object and its location) where *no movement* within the context of the speech event (i.e., immediately before, during, or after the child utterance) established the location. Locative-state utterances specify a person or object and its place or location (e.g., "sweater chair," "fish in pond," "mommy's at work," "daddy's lying down").

State Utterances in the state category make reference to states of affairs. A number of subcategories can be described:

1. Internal state codes feelings, attitudes, and emotions of an animate being toward an object, event, or state (e.g., "I like cookies," "I'm hungry," "he's tired"). The attitude of the speaker is often coded by modal-type verbs and includes attitudes such as:
   a. Volition/Intention. Frequent verbs include *want* and *go* (e.g., "I want to go home," "I'm gonna eat now").
   b. Obligation. Frequent verbs include *should, must,* and *have* (e.g., "I have to drink my milk," "you should go to bed").
   c. Possibility. Frequent verbs include *can* (e.g., "I can climb that tree").
2. External state of affairs, such as *darkness* or *cold.*
3. Attributive state referring to the condition or properties of an object (e.g., "it's broken," "my boat is red").
4. Possessive state including a temporary state of ownership (e.g., "I have a pen," "that's mine," "I got a car").

Quantity Utterances are placed within the category of quantity if they designate more than one object or person by use of a number word (e.g., "I have two sheep"), plural *-s* inflection (e.g., "The pens are on the table"), or adjectives such as *many, all,* or *some.*

Notice Utterances are placed in the category of notice if they code attention to a person, object, or event and include a verb of notice (e.g., *see, hear, look, watch, show*). Early utterances code attention to objects or persons (e.g., "I see birdie"), while later utterances code attention to events (e.g., "watch me jump," "I see the bird flying in the sky").

Dative Utterances are placed in the dative category if they designate the recipient of an object or action (i.e., include an indirect object), with or without a preposition (e.g., "give it to me," "open door Lois," "this book for you").

Additive Additive relations involve the joining of two objects, events, or states without a dependency relation between them. For example, when two clauses are joined, each clause is meaningful by itself: the combination of the two clauses does not create a meaning, and the order of clauses could be reversed. This category is used to refer to two objects conjoined intraclausally (e.g., "I got a pen and a knife"), to two events or states joined with or without a conjunction (e.g., "that's a cat/that's a dog" or "I sit here and you sit there"), and to a series of events or states chained together (i.e., the additive chains described in Chapter 11). Sequential events that are coded as the events occur (i.e., the utterances are chained to the actions) are also considered as additive relations (e.g., as child opens box, she says, "I open this" and then while taking out a doll says "and I take out my doll").

Temporal Temporal relations include the coding of aspect (i.e., the tem-poral contour of an event), tense (i.e., the relation between when an event took place and when the event was spoken about), and temporal dependency between and among events such as sequential and simultaneous occurrences. Verb inflections, auxiliary verbs, and adverbs can code tense and aspect (e.g., "I'm playing now," "it broke yesterday"). A dependency between events which involves temporal sequence or simultaneity can be coded by sequenced clauses with or without the use of a connective (e.g., "I get up and then eat breakfast," "I buy food/come home") if at least one of the events was not concurrent with the utterance. Series of utterances that code sequential events are referred to as *temporal chains.* See Chapters 9, 10, and 11 for further information and examples.

Causal Utterances included in the causal category have an implicit or explicit cause-and-effect relationship between states and/or events (i.e., one expressed event or state is dependent on the other for its occurrence). When the relation is between two events or states, two subcategories have been identified (Bloom & Capatides, 1987): objective relations and subjective relations. Objective relations include self-evident relations (i.e., perceptible or imaginable), such as means-end, consequence, or conditional relations (e.g., "I don't have a Christmas tree/because throw it out" or "maybe you could bend him so he can sit"); subjective relations are based on personal, affective, or sociocultural beliefs (e.g., "she put a Band-aid on her shoe and it maked it feel better" or "don't walk/the light is red"). Utterances may or may not include a connective, and the order of clauses (cause-effect or effect-cause) determines the conjunction required. Series of events that include causal relations are referred to as *causal chains* (or plots or episodes) and are discussed with further subcategories in Chapter 11.

Adversative In the adversative category the relation between two events and/or states is one of contrast. Most often one clause negates, qualifies, or somehow limits the other (e.g., "this one big, but this one small" or "the dog barks, but he doesn't bite").

Epistemic Epistemic refers to mental states of affairs (with verbs such as *know, think, remember, wonder*) about an event or state described in the complement (e.g., "know what this is"; "I think I can put him in the house"). As such, it is a type of state, but is here classified separately. Utterances placed in this category are usually complex sentences, but some simple sentences such as "I know her" or those involving ellipsis (e.g., "I don't know") or substitution (e.g., "I know it") may be found; these are often routines in early language development.

Specification Utterances in specification category indicate a particular person, object, or event. Forms coding specification include *contrastive* use of the demonstrative pronouns *this* versus *that* if placed before a noun or produced with contrastive stress (e.g., "this dog is big, but not that one") and the use of the articles *the* versus *a*. (Not all uses of demonstrative pronouns specify particular instances; demonstrative pronouns are used as subjects of copular sentences to code existence and stative relations without contrastive meaning.) Eventually, specification involves the joining of two clauses, one of which specifies or describes an object or person in terms of function, place, or activity (e.g., "that the man who drives the truck," "the couch that goes in the corner," or "it looks like a fishing thing and you fish with it").

Communication Utterances placed in the communication category contain a verb that codes a communicative act, while the complement describes what is to be communicated. Early communication verbs include *say* and *tell* (e.g., "tell mommy I have to finish this" or "mommy said not to do that").

Definitions of Categories of Language Function

Language can serve many functions, most of which involve interactions with other persons; some of the purposes that have been described in child language are described below. Function is determined by looking at the form of the utterance (including prosodic patterns) in relation to aspects of context such as gaze, interactions among people, consequences of utterance, and so forth.

In addition to the functions of language, using language involves varying what we say according to aspects of the nonlinguistic context, such as the listeners, the relationship of the event talked about and the time of the utterance, the relative spatial relationship of objects and persons to the speaker and listener, and the perceptual support available for representation of the objects and events described. Furthermore, we vary what we say according to the linguistic context; to carry on a conversation we must take into account what has been said before and what will follow. Some of the categories suggested in the literature for describing use of children's language relative to context are defined in Chapters 9–12. Below are further definitions of functions. (See also Box 12-4.)

FUNCTIONS

Categories presented here attempt to describe the communicative function that the utterance serves in the context (other terms used to describe functions include illocutionary force, communicative acts, speech acts, etc., although there may be subtle differences implied when different terms are used). Functions have been described in child language by Bates (1976), Bloom (1970), Dore (1977, 1986, and elsewhere), Flax (1986), Gerber (1987), Halliday (1975), Longtin (1984), McShane (1980), Prutting and Kirchner (1983), and others. The descriptions and category names listed below were derived from this body of literature. In some cases more than one function can be described for an utterance (e.g., pretend, direct action).

Comment   Utterances that identify or describe objects, persons, states, or events (including attributes, possessors, location, etc.) with no other apparent function (e.g., to obtain an object or to answer a question) are placed in this category. Utterances may or may not be directed to another person (e.g., climbing up slide, child looks at mother and says "slide down"; or climbing up slide, child pauses and arranges self, saying softly "slide down"). The former may be referred to as interactive (or comment—other), while the latter may be referred to as noninteractive (or comment—self). In early child language, such utterances often accompany the child's actions (e.g., "I ride bike" as the child climbs on the bike; or "truck" as the child takes a truck out of the toy box). Subcategories can be described such as comments on objects versus events or emotions, comments directed to others versus comments to self, or labels that serve to provide the name of something or someone.

Regulate   Some utterances serve to regulate others and require a response, such as the exchange of objects, an action or an utterance by another person, or the attention of another person. Regulatory utterances can be subdivided into categories according to the type of response required:

Focus Attention—The child calls or somehow attempts to draw the attention of another to self, object, or event.

Direct Actions—The child expresses a desire for some action to be carried out by another (such as wanting someone to help the child open a box, or wanting someone to continue to tickle the child).

Obtain an Object—The child expresses a desire for an object that may or may not be in the immediate context.

Obtain Response—The child's utterance obliges a linguistic response from another such as questions for confirmation.

Obtain Information—These are similar to obtaining a response, but here the response must contain information that the child does not already have.

Obtain Participation or Invite—The child's utterance serves to request that the listener participate in some activity with the child (e.g., "wanna play house?").

Other—Any other regulatory utterance that does not fit into the above.

Protest or Rejection   Utterances placed in this category express an objection to or refusal of objects or actions carried out or suggested by another person (e.g., mother tries to wash child's face and child pushes her hand away, whines, and says "don't like soap").

Emote   When the only function of the utterance appears to be the expression of some emotion (e.g., joy, surprise, sadness), the utterance is classified as *emote*.

Routine   This category consists of stereotyped utterances that are used for certain rituals such as exchanging greetings; transferring objects (e.g., "thank you"); talking on the telephone; making noises associated with animals, vehicles, etc.; or reciting memorized pieces (e.g., poems, songs, the alphabet). In addition, the category includes utterances that repeatedly accompany actions (e.g., "this goes here" said over and over when putting toys away) or other utterances that are produced frequently but appear to serve no other function. Finally, sequences of utterances repeated in a playful manner may be categorized as routine after the first exchange (e.g., the child reaches for a toy in front of the clinician and says "I want that," takes it, and smiles, and then repeats the same utterance and action three or four times).

Report or Inform The child talks about objects or events that are not present. This category includes narration of past events, as well as simple mention of nonpresent objects and persons (e.g., child looks at mother's briefcase and looks at clinician and says "mommy").

Pretend The child's utterance may set an imaginary scene ("this is a zoo," said while pointing to a corner of the room), or it may be pretend interactions with animals or dolls (e.g., "the lion says I'm gonna eat you up").

Discourse Utterances that serve to maintain and regulate conversational exchanges are placed within this larger category or one of the subcategories described below.

Respond—Utterances placed in this category serve to provide a response obligated by the utterance of another. They include answers to *wh* and yes/no questions.

Imitate—If an utterance repeats all or part of a preceding utterance and appears to serve no other function, it can be classified as *imitate;* if the imitation serves to affirm, self-direct, or fulfill some other function, it is not classified as imitate.

Affirm or Acknowledge—In response to the utterance of another, the child says "yes" or repeats a part of the utterance in order to indicate agreement.

Negate—In response to the utterance of another, the child indicates disagreement (e.g., "no" or repetition with a negative headshake or other gesture indicating negation).

Feedback (or back channel)—Utterances categorized as feedback serve to let the speaker know that the listener is attending to what the speaker is saying (e.g., "um hum").

Repair—Child responds to request for clarification or to misinterpretation by another. The utterance may be a repetition of a prior utterance (often with some phonological change), or it may be a paraphrase.

Initiate a topic or turn—Child attempts to get the floor or change the topic with an utterance such as "you know what?"

An Illustration of Language Sample Analyses: Levels 2–4[*]

Illustrated in the following tables are analyses of videotape recordings of a 3-year-old boy (whom we will call Bill) obtained in his home or in a studio as he interacted with his mother. Bill is the third child of college-educated parents; he had normal hearing, scored 99 (but did not reach ceiling) on the *Leiter International Performance Scale* (Arthur, 1952), and scored at the 41st percentile on the *Peabody Picture Vocabulary Test* (Dunn, 1965). This illustration is designed to be considered in conjunction with reading Chapter 12.

Level 2 Analyses

The data for the Level 2 analyses were obtained as Bill was videotaped at home with his mother and brother. According to parent report and observations during the session, Bill was using a number of conventional forms to denote adult-like semantic domains. Thus, the major analysis was of his use of conventional forms. Upon completion of this analysis, however, it was evident that few conventional forms were used for requests. Therefore, the transcript was scanned for the use of nonconventional forms associated with requests, and it was found that Bill frequently vocalized the vowel [æ] when requesting. Therefore, the transcript was examined for particular interactions using nonconventional interaction of form with content or use. Although not a content category on the C/F/U Goal Plan, affirmatives were noted because they were used frequently during the session.[°]

On the basis of the analyses illustrated in Table G-1, it appeared that Bill productively coded existence, nonexistence, and rejection with single-word utter-

---

[*]A set of the blank forms that are used in Appendix G are available from the author.

[°] This use of affirmation may be variable among children or may be more frequent in language-impaired children who have good comprehension than in children whose comprehension is closer to their productive skills; appropriate responses to questions require comprehension of the question as well as knowledge of how to code affirmation versus negation.

ances. Action and locative action may have been partially established, but recurrence was not coded. Further information was needed on these three categories; another videotape taken the same day in the home and a third videotaped interaction in a studio during the prior week were available. Scanning these data provided evidence for action (e.g., *woah* for stop and */bu/* for hit). In addition, different nouns were produced (e.g., *bird, ball, daddy, cookies*), and a relational word (*this*) was used in coding existence. However, in these supplemental observations no evidence was found for coding of recurrence, denial, or attribution. No basic changes were made in the goals listed on the worksheet shown in Table G-1.

TABLE G-1

LEVEL 2
Worksheet for Assessment of Single-Word Utterances

Child's Name <u>Bill</u>   Date of Sample <u>Sample 1</u>

Context <u>Play interaction with mother at home</u>   Time <u>45 min</u>

Analysis 1—Content/Form/Use Interactions in Single-Word Utterances

Content	Form		Use		
Category	*Utterance*	*Frequency*	*Linguistic°Context*	*Perceptual Support*	*Function*
Existence					
	I		0	+	Regulate—focus atten.
	I		FSc	+	Discourse—negate
	me	2	0	+	Comment—label
	baby	3	IPU	+	Discourse—acknowledge
	ma	2	0	+	Comment—label
	fish		IPU	+	Comment—label
	fish		0	+	Regulate—focus atten.
Nonexistence					
	no juck		0	−	Comment
	no	3	0	−	Comment
Recurrence	(no examples)				
Rejection					
	no		FQc	+	Discourse—respond
	no	3	0	+	Protest
	no		FSc	+	Discourse—protest
Denial	(no examples)				
Attribution					
	baby/ fish		IPU	+	Comment
					(continued)

° See Box 12-4 for Key to abbreviations.

TABLE G-1   Level 2 *Continued*

Content	Form		Use		
Category	Utterance	Fre-quency	Linguistic° Context	Per-ceptual Support	Function
Possession					
	(no examples)				
Action					
	go	4	IPU	+	Regulate
	open		0	+	Comment
Locative Action					
	down		FSnc	+	Comment
Other					
Quantity					
	1, 2, 3		0	+	Comment
Affirmation or acknowledgment					
	yes	>5	FQc	+	Discourse—acknowledge
	m	>5	FQc	+	Discourse—acknowledge
	okay		FQc	+	Discourse—acknowledge
Context of disappearance					
	fish		0	−	Regulate
	fish		FSc	−	Discourse—affirm
Context of acting on object					
	fish	2	0	+	Comment
Context of getting attention					
	ma	2	0	−	Regulate—focus atten.

Analysis 2—Overextended Conventional Forms (Associated with Sensorimotor Schemes or Chained Associations)

Form	Domains of Reference	Function
None that were observed or reported.		

Analysis 3—Consistent Phonetic Forms (Other than Crying) Associated with Objects, Actions, Affects, or Functions

Form	Frequency	Associated Object, Action, or Affect	Function
[ae]	>5		Request objects and actions

COMMENTS: Bill was very interactive with his mother, producing single vowels or consonants and many gestures; he almost always responded to her statements with some vocalization.

Gesture and vocalization accompanied most requests; vocalization also accompanied many actions.

OBSERVATIONS OF NONLINGUISTIC PLAY BEHAVIOR

Specific play with objects	Yes
Separate object	Not observed
Join objects	Not observed
Search for objects	Yes

(*continued*)

TABLE G-1 Level 2 *Continued*

OBSERVATIONS OF NONLINGUISTIC PLAY BEHAVIOR (*continued*)

Search for objects to join	Not observed
Object-to-object play	Yes (net in water, boat in water, man in boat, etc.)
Use object for creative function	Not observed

COMMENTS: No contexts called the behaviors that were not observed. Given other play behaviors it is assumed that they are a part of his repertoire, but next observation should be designed to attempt to elicit them.

Goals of Intervention:

To code existence with relational words such as *this*

To code recurrence with relational words such as *more*

To code locative action more frequently and with relational words such as *in, out, up, off*

To code nonexistence with relational words such as *all gone, no more*

To code requests with conventional forms (i.e., single words) that are part of his vocabulary

To call attention to objects by using conventional forms (i.e., single words) that are part of his vocabulary

To increase variety of nouns used for commenting when acting upon objects

(Goals were not written for denial, attribution, or possession since they are optional at Phase 1.)

To obtain further information about creative use of objects, search for objects, and joining of objects

---

In terms of use, most functions expected in Phase 1 were present, but requests were primarily coded by means of gesture and nonlinguistic utterances. As expected for Phase 1, utterances generally appeared with the perceptual support of context. Also, as expected, utterances were about the child's own actions rather than the actions of others, and most utterances were comments. In advance of what might be expected given his level of language production, many of Bill's adjacent utterances were contingent, and he had quite a few nonadjacent utterances.

In a 20-minute videotape recorded 4 months later (during which time Bill had attended a preschool class for language-impaired children for 2 months), Bill was coding denial with *no*, and he produced three examples of multiword syntactic utterances—"no room" as a comment on nonexistence, "me want in" as a comment as he located objects, and "me help" as a request that he join an action. Other utterances were still single words similar to the ones above with the exception of some new vocabulary words and the use of the vocative *ma*, preceding some utterances. At this time his mother reported a 50-word vocabulary including action words such as *help, eat, walk, dance,* and *wait.* Locative-action words included *up, down, in, out,* and *off.* In addition, the mother noted Bill's use of social words such as *please* and *sorry* as well as person names and nouns (e.g., *milk, light, juice, apple*) and one attribute, *hot.* Thus, using both reported and direct observations, it was found that denial, action, and locative action had become productive, but recurrence was still nonproductive. The earlier goals could now be rewritten to include Phase 2 behaviors, as follows:

To code action with two constituents

To code locative action with two constituents

To code existence with two-word utterances (e.g., *this boat*, or *a boat*)
To increase coding of nonexistence with two-word utterances (e.g., "no ____ ")

The Phase 1 goals that were now relevant included the following:

To code recurrence with single-word utterances (e.g., "more")
To code nonexistence with single-word utterances such as "all gone"
To increase coding of attribution
To increase lexicon of nouns
To increase the variety of words used for the regulatory function

Thus, based on Sample 2, goals for Bill included Phase 1 and Phase 2 behaviors. The next sample of Bill's language was geared to a Level 3 analysis—that of multiword syntactic utterances.

Level 3

Analysis 1—Verb Relations

To illustrate this level of analysis, a third videotape of Bill was analyzed. This sample was obtained approximately 1 year after the initial sample discussed under Level 2 analysis. Bill had taken part in a preschool program for language-impaired children during this time. Again, the interaction was with his mother, but this time the sample was collected in a studio, rather than in the home. Toys were available in the room at the beginning of the session, and a new set of toys was brought every 10 minutes or so. The major analysis was on the first half-hour of the tape and included over 200 utterances. Following this, further information was obtained by scanning the remaining 30 minutes of the tape.

All utterances that contained two constituents of a verb relation (including object and place in locative utterances) were placed on a worksheet that represented that relation. Only different utterances were recorded on these sheets. If the same utterance was repeated a number of times, it was written once with different comments about use when it differed. The frequency of occurrence (i.e., the number of *tokens*) was stated in parentheses beside the utterance. All available utterances coding verb relations with two constituents were categorized.

To categorize an utterance as an example of *syntactic* coding of a verb relation, at least two of the major constituents of subject-verb-complement (S-V-C) needed to be present.° The term *complement* was used here in its traditional sense and includes any constituents that complete the verb—the object affected by the action (e.g., "eat *cookie*"), the object and place in locative action ("put *book on table*"), and the predicate nominative or adjective (e.g., "here's *Joe*"). Note that locative utterances may have two obligatory constituents within the complement: object and place (e.g., "put *it here*").

To determine the appropriate verb category for each utterance, both the form of the utterance and the context in which it was spoken were used (see Chapters 9,

---

° There is, however, one exception. When the copula *to be* is the main verb in a sentence, the copula subject can be a demonstrative pronoun (e.g., "that's mine, there's daddy"). If the *only* examples of S-V-C produced by the child are demonstrative pronouns as copular subjects, these are not categorized as verb relations, since they are often early-learned routines and are not evidence of knowledge of grammatical relations.

10, and 11 and Appendix E for descriptions and examples of all content categories). For example, if Bill had said "horsie lie down" as he sat the horse, it would have been categorized as locative action; however, the same utterance would be categorized as locative state if he had referred to the fact that a horse was already lying on the floor (a static location and not a locating action). Thus, utterances such as "sit chair," "mommy chair," and "mommy sit" would have been categorized as locative action if they were spoken as mommy was in the process of sitting, but as locative state if they referred to the static location of mommy (i.e., the act of sitting had taken place before the speech event). If the utterance included another content category in addition to the two constituents of a verb relation such as "sit big chair" or "sit my chair" and was spoken in the context of someone sitting, these utterances would also have been categorized as locative action. So far, the categorization discussed has only applied to the semantics of the verb relation in multiword utterances that included two major constituents of a verb relation. Multiword utterances that were simple codings of other categories such as "Bobby car" (possession), "big car" (attribution), "no car" (nonexistence, denial, or rejection), and "two new coats" (attribution and quantity) were categorized separately and will be discussed later.

It is important to note that excessive time was not spent on a few isolated utterances that were difficult to categorize; if in doubt about action versus locative action, the utterance would have been placed on the action sheet and starred to note uncertainty; if in doubt about locative action versus locative state, the utterance would have been placed on the locative-action sheet and starred for uncertainty. All other utterances that fit more than one category would have been called equivocal and listed separately, noting the possible categories in which they might be placed. Any semantically anomalous utterances would have been written on a separate sheet of paper marked undetermined or anomalous. Partially unintelligible utterances would have been included if the intelligible portion contained at least two constituents (e.g., subject-verb, verb-complement). In later coding, it would have been assumed that only two constituents were required so as not to penalize the child for having only two constituents if there was a chance that the unintelligible portion contained the third constituent. Unintelligible portions are generally marked with – – –.

Tables G-2 through G-8 present the utterances in Bill's third language sample that contained at least two major constituents of a verb relation. Each table represents a different verb relation (noted on the top of the sheet as "Content Category"). The utterances were listed in the left column with their number from the transcript. Those utterances obtained from scanning the last 30 minutes of the tape did not have utterance numbers since that part of the tape was not fully transcribed. Instead, they were listed under "Further Information" and identified with a letter to distinguish them from each other. The next four columns, marked "Form Analysis," were used to note the presence or absence of the major constituents (to be discussed below). The information obtained about language form was summarized below the columns in terms of productivity and achievement. The last two columns were used to make comments on use, both the linguistic context of each utterance and the apparent function of the utterance. Coordination of other categories with each verb relation was marked in the middle of each table. Finally, at the bottom third of the table additional utterances that expressed the verb relation, either with one constituent or with mixed word order were noted. Following this, comments were made about content/form/use interactions. The information was summarized by noting which behaviors were productive and which behaviors were goals of intervention.

Productivity and Achievement.   The purpose of this analysis was to ascertain the number of constituents that were included in order to determine whether the verb category was *productive* at Phase 2 or 3, and, if three constituents were productive, to compare the number included in the utterance with the number expected in the model (adult) language in order to determine *achievement*. Last, the particular constituents omitted were noted and described. For example, in Table G-3, the last part of the first utterance, 12 – – *you try it* included the three expected constituents, so a 3 was placed in the column for inclusion of three constituents and in the column for three constituents expected. In contrast, utterance 46, *teach you*, included only two constituents where three were expected. A 2 was placed in the column for inclusion of two constituents and a 3 was placed in the column for three constituents expected. Under comments, it was noted that the subject was omitted.

Each column was totaled to determine the number of constituents productive. Again, using Table G-3 as an example, there were seven examples of action expressed with two constituents and seven examples with three constituents. Certainly Bill was productively using both two- and three-constituent utterances in this sample. Thus, he was productively coding action at Phase 3, and constituent structure would not be a major goal. However, the criterion for achievement was not met for three constituents; when the 7 that included three constituents was divided by the 10 where three were expected, the resulting percentage was 70% and was, therefore, short of the 80%–90% criterion. (Note that for locative state, in Table G-5, achievement was not computed because the use of three constituents was not productive.) The use of three constituents to code action would continue to be checked periodically, and, eventually, the increased use of three constituents might need to become a goal. But at present it seemed that Phase 4 goals were more appropriate.

Coordinated Categories.   Any content beyond the major constituents (e.g., with action other than agent-action-object) was underlined as the utterances were placed on the worksheets. In Bill's sample, examples of coordination with action included the coding of a temporal relations and the inclusion of coding of specification (*that*) in utterance 123 (see Table G-3). The utterance numbers were placed under the appropriate coordinated category in the middle of the worksheet. Some of these coordinations were not a specific goal for action (simply because we do not have information available on when such coordinations become productive). Thus, goals of intervention based on this table were for Phase 4 coordinations with action (e.g., coordination of place, attribution, nonexistence, and volition/intention). These were listed at the bottom of Table G-3. Examples within the content category that did not include two constituents were also listed on Table G-3 if they provided information that was different from what was already on the worksheet. For example, two instances of confused word order were listed here, as well as an example of action + place with one constituent. (Recall that place is not one of the major grammatical constituents for action, only for locative action, and so this utterance has only one constituent, the verb).

Describing Use. In describing use, two factors were considered; the context in which the utterance was spoken and the apparent function of the utterance. As noted in Chapters 1 and 8, this includes the nonlinguistic context (the degree of perceptual support and the adaptation to the listener) as well as linguistic context (how the utterance related to prior utterances). Since few utterances at this level are spoken without perceptual support or use alternative linguistic devices to adapt to the listener, note of any such utterances was made in the Comments section. On the worksheet for verb categories, one column was reserved for linguistic context and one for function. The relation of each utterance to the prior utterances was noted under linguistic context. For example, in Table G-3, the first utterance, number 12, was considered a nonadjacent utterance—that is, the prior utterance seemed too far removed to have been an impetus for the utterance of number 12—so the linguistic context was marked 0. The fourth utterance in Table G-3, number 40, followed a statement of another (FS) but was not contingent (nc) on that statement; utterance 16, however, was contingent (c) on a prior statement. If the prior utterance had been a question, the coding would be FQ for "follows question," as noted in Table G-4 for utterance number 6. When "self" is added, it means that the utterance followed one of the child's own utterances, and its contingency was also noted.

Finally, when a large segment of words from a prior utterance was repeated, the utterance was marked (IPU). Such utterances may have recoded a part of the prior utterance (e.g., changed a noun to a pronoun, or shifted *you* to *I*), in which case they were further marked with an *r* (for recoded). If they added information to the prior utterance with a new word or phrase, they were marked with an *a* (for add). For example, if the utterance *you want a cookie* produced by an adult or other child was followed with *I want a chocolate cookie*, it would be coded IPUra because segments had been included from a prior utterance with recoding of the pronoun *you* and addition of *chocolate*. If IPUa had been frequent, added information would have been further analyzed in terms of whether the addition was a phrase or a clause (the addition of clauses would be expected later in development than the addition of a phrase according to Bloom, Rocissano, & Hood, 1976). When children are highly imitative, further analysis of their imitative utterances may be informative. Utterances that neither recode nor add might be examined in terms of content/form interactions (lexical and syntactic), to see if they are at all related to what the child is learning (see Bloom, Hood, & Lightbown, 1974); in terms of their function, to see if they serve some communicative purpose (see Prizant & Duchan, 1981); and in terms of the utterances that precede them, to see if there are any patterns (see, e.g., Fay & Schuler, 1980; Folger & Chapman, 1978).

In the Function column, judgments of the apparent function that the utterance served were recorded. Definitions of these functions can be found in Appendix F and in Chapters 9–12. Under the Comments section at the bottom of the worksheet, the variety of functions, the variety of forms used for functions, and the child's use of language in linguistic contexts were often further described or summarized. The Comments section was also used for further description of forms included within this content category—particularly the variety of lexical items (with emphasis on verbs), and other information that was not evident from the analysis. Finally, the behaviors from the plan that were productive, based on this analysis, were listed, as were the goals of intervention that followed from the productive behaviors.

TABLE G-2

LEVEL 3
Language Sample Analysis Worksheet—Verb Relations

Content Category <u>Existence</u>   Child's Name <u>Bill</u>   Date <u>S-3</u>

	Form Analysis					*Use Analysis*	
	S-V-C Constituents						
	In-clude		Ex-pect				
Utterances°	2	3	2	3	*Comments*	*Linguistic Context*	*Function*
135 BJ farmer	2			3	−copula	FQnc	comment
Further Information:							
a. horsie · big red	2			3	−copula	0	comment
b. me big red	2			3	−copula	0	comment
Frequency	3	0	0	3	= <u>2</u> constituents productive		
Proportion with		↓		↓			
3 expected		0	÷	3	= <u>0%</u> level of achievement		

Coordinated categories (number of utterances that include 2 constituents plus another category)

Nonexistence	Recurrence	Rejection	Denial	Attribution	Possession	Quantity	Temporal	Specification	Wh-Question	Place	Other

Other examples within category:

c. a big red son	1		1			FQc	comment

COMMENTS: Most utterances coding existence were single-word names of objects coded both on request and as they were picked up. He confused the labels for cow and horse as well as color names. After he named one, he often looked to his mother for confirmation.

PRODUCTIVE AT: Phase ___2___   (infrequent)

GOALS: Phase ___2___   To: Code existence with relational words, such as *a*, *that*, or *this*, plus a substantive word.

Phase ___3___   To: Coordinate attribution with existence (optional goal)

° Numbers in front of utterances refer to number of utterance on the transcript.

TABLE G-3

LEVEL 3
Language Sample Analysis Worksheet—Verb Relations

Content Category <u>Action</u>   Child's Name <u>Bill</u>   Date <u>S-3</u>

	Form Analysis					Use Analysis	
	S-V-C Constituents						
	Include		Expect				
Utterances°	2	3	2	3	Comments	Linguistic Context	Function
12 see·you try it		3		3		0	regulate
16 Luke Ben jump<u>s</u> car		3		3		FSc	comment
25 BJ crash in	2		2			0	comment
40 you try that		3		3		FSnc	regulate
42 me start it		3		3		FSnc	comment
46 teach you	2			3	−subj.	0	comment
58 you make·okay	2		2			0	regulate
105 stop it, pig	2		2		to dolls (high voice)	FSnc	pretend-regulate
123 me get <u>that</u> one		3		3		IPUr	comment
129 tie knot	2		2			0	regulate
168 eat dinner time <u>now</u>	2			3	−subj.	0	comment
170 cut·meat	2			3	−subj.	FSc	comment

Further Observation

Utterances	2	3	2	3	Comments	Linguistic Context	Function
a. you push<u>ed</u> it		3		3		0	comment
b. me play golf <u>now</u>		3		3		0	comment

Frequency   7 7   10 = <u>3</u> constituents productive
Proportion with   ↓   ↓
   3 expected   7 ÷ 10 = <u>70%</u> level of achievement

Coordinated categories (utterances that include 2 constituents plus another category)

Nonexistence	Recurrence	Rejection	Denial	Attribution	Possession	Quantity	Temporal	Specification	Wh-Question	Place	Other
							16 -s 168 now a. ed b. now	123 that			

Other examples within category:

3 BJ Kay							
<u>orange</u> truck ride				3	X word order	0	comment
47 start <u>on there</u>	1		1			FSnc	regulate
173—tea make				3	X word order	0	comment

° Numbers in front of utterances refer to number of utterance on transcript.

(continued)

446

TABLE G-3 *Continued*

LEVEL 3—ACTION

COMMENTS: Quite a few nonadjacent utterances were used. Voice pitch changed when talking for the dolls. Dialogues among dolls were all in this one changed voice (i.e., not different for different dolls). All utterances had perceptual support.

Bill used a wide variety of verbs for action (e.g., *ride, crash, start, stop, get, tie, eat, cut, drive, teach, make*). There may be a slight preference for pronouns; utterances with nouns were less frequent, were said more slowly, and were more likely to have order errors. *Me* was used in subject position, but was not listed as a goal (if necessary, it will, with Phase 6 or 8 behaviors). Although proportional use of three constituents is not yet 80–90%, this will not be a goal until after he is productive with Phase 5 behaviors. Facilitation of coordinated categories may, in itself, lead to greater use of three constituents.

PRODUCTIVE AT: Phase ____3____

GOALS: Phase ____4____   To: Coordinate action with:
                                                Attribution
                                                Place
                                                Recurrence
                                                Intention/volition
                                                Aspect
                                                 -ing
                                                 irregular past

---

TABLE G-4

LEVEL 3
Language Sample Analysis Worksheet—Verb Relations

Content Category <u>Locative Action</u>   Child's Name <u>Bill</u>   Date <u>S-3</u>

	Form Analysis					*Use Analysis*	
	S-V-C Constituents						
	In-clude		Ex-pect				
Utterances°	2	3	2	3	Comments	Linguistic Context	Function
6 on here	2		2			FQc	respond
13 BJ drive truck down		3		3		FSnc	comment
20 cars fall down · down	2		2			0	comment
76 in here	2		2			FQc	respond
83 in barn	2		2			FQc	respond
84 <u>no</u> sheep fit<u>s</u> in		3		3	as move	FSc	comment
85 <u>no</u> him fit in		3		3	as move	FSc self	comment
93 cow fit in · horse		3		3	as move		comment
					s/c	0	comment

(continued)

° Numbers in front of utterances refer to number of utterance on the transcript.

TABLE G-4 *Continued*

Content Category <u>Locative Action</u>   Child's Name <u>Bill</u>   Date <u>S-3</u>

	Form Analysis					Use Analysis	
	S-V-C Constituents						
	Include		Expect				
Utterances°	2	3	2	3	Comments	Linguistic Context	Function
109 dump animals out		3		4	−subj.	0	comment
138—lie down for sleep	2				unintell. to dolls	FSc self	obtain response
140 me in here mom	2			3	as go in	0	comment
218 him fall down	2		2			0	comment
Frequency	7	5		6	= 3 constituents productive		
Proportion with 3 expected		5	÷	6	= 80% level of achievement		

Coordinated categories (utterances that include 2 constituents plus another category)

Nonexistence	Recurrence	Rejection	Denial	Attribution	Possession	Quantity	Temporal	Specification	Wh-Question	Place	Other
84, 85 *no*						20, 109 -*s*	84 -*s*				

Other Examples within Category:

149 lie down <u>*now*</u>	1	1	to dolls	FSc self	pretend regulate

COMMENTS: As in action, Bill is not using the nominative case for the pronoun *I*, but it should not be a goal yet. Utterance 138 appears to be an early example of including two verb relations within one utterance. Some variety of verbs is used within this category (e.g., *fit, lie, fall, dump, drive*). If *put* is not observed in other contexts, it might be considered as a goal.

PRODUCTIVE AT: Phase ___3___,   (high proportional use)

GOALS: Phase ___4___   To: Coordinate locative action with volition/intention

TABLE G-5

LEVEL 3
Language Sample Analysis Worksheet—Verb Relations

Content Category <u>Locative State</u>   Child's Name <u>Bill</u>   Date <u>S-3</u>

	Form Analysis				Use Analysis		
	S-V-C Constituents						
	In-clude		Ex-pect				
Utterances°	2	3	2	3	Comments	Linguistic Context	Function
229 <u>why</u> paper off	2			3	−copula	0	obtain info.
Further Information							
a. <u>where's</u> hammer		3		3	says as finds	0	comment
b. <u>where's</u> pig		3		3		0	obtain info.
Frequency	1	2		3	= <u>2</u> constituents productive		
Proportion with 3 expected			÷		= <u> % </u> level of achievement		

Coordinated categories (utterances that include 2 constituents plus another category)

Nonexistence	Recurrence	Rejection	Denial	Attribution	Possession	Quantity	Temporal	Specification	Wh-Question	Place	Other
									a, b where 229 why		

Other Examples within Category: (none)

COMMENTS: Limited coding of this category was observed, but it may have been due to the context. Two examples of Phase 5 combined with the causal question give three examples of two-constituent coding. Further evidence should be obtained. The "why" question is in advance of the other language skills. While here the contracted copula on *where's* was counted as a constituent, it is most likely that question form *where's* was learned as a unit and does not represent use of the copula.

PRODUCTIVE AT: Phase _____3_____   (Weak evidence)

GOALS:

                        Phase _____3_____   To: Obtain information about
                                                   Phase 3 behaviors
                                                   If not found, goal is use of 2
                                                   or 3 constituents

° Numbers in front of utterances refer to number of utterance on the transcript.

TABLE G-6

LEVEL 3
Language Sample Analysis Worksheet—Verb Relations

Content Category <u>Internal State</u>   Child's Name <u>Bill</u>   Date <u>S-3</u>

	Form Analysis					*Use Analysis*	
	S-V-C Constituents						
	In-clude		Ex-pect			*Linguistic*	
Utterances°	*2*	*3*	*2*	*3*	*Comments*	*Context*	*Function*
Internal State							
97 oh no · want animal out *my* truck	2		2		−subj. doll talk	0	comment
200 want *yellow* one	2			3		FSnc	obtain info.
Further Information							
a. him fraid	2			3	−copula	FSc self	comment
External State							
63 BJ on fire	2			3	−copula	0	comment
90 oops run out gas	2			3	−subj.	0	comment
Possessive State							
125 it BJ McKay	2			3	−copula	FSc	comment
Attributive State							
92 all fill up *now*	2		2			FSc self	comment
134 him crazy	2			3	−copula	FQc	respond
137 mine's dead		3		3	doll talk	FSc self	?
Frequency	8	1		7	= <u>2</u> constituents productive		
Proportion with 3 Expected			÷		= <u> % </u> level of achievement		

Coordinated categories (utterances that include 2 constituents plus another category) =

Nonexistence	Recurrence	Rejection	Denial	Attribution	Possession	Quantity	Temperal	Specification	Wh-Question	Place	Other
				200 yellow 97 my			92 now				

Other examples within category:

199 all picked up *now*	1		3	−copula −subj.	FQc	obtain info.

(continued)

° Number in front of utterances refer to number of utterance on the transcript.

450

LEVEL 3—Verb Relations—Internal State

COMMENTS: Weak evidence of productivity; increase coding internal state with *want*.

PRODUCTIVE AT: Phase _____3_____   (2 constituents)

GOALS:

	Phase _____3_____	To: Increase coding with 2 or 3 constituents for internal state (e.g., *want*)
	_____4_____	To: Volition/intention (*want, go*) + action and/or locative action

---

TABLE G-7

LEVEL 3
Language Sample Analysis Worksheet—Verb Relations

Content Category <u>Notice</u>   Child's Name <u>Bill</u>   Date <u>S-3</u>

	Form Analysis					*Use Analysis*	
	S-V-C Constituents						
	In-clude		Ex-pect			Linguistic	
Utterances°	2	3	2	3	Comments	Context	Function
34 see that	2		2			0	Focus atten.
117 watch this	2		2			FSc	Focus atten.
Frequency	2		2		= ____ constituents productive		
Proportion with 3 expected					= __%__ level of achievement		

Coordinated categories (utterances that include 2 constituents plus another category)

Nonexistence	Recurrence	Rejection	Denial	Attribution	Possession	Quantity	Temporal	Specification	Wh-Question	Place	Other

Other examples within category:

12 see you try it (noted under action)

111 watch– – –	?		0	Focus atten.
118 see	1	1	0	Focus atten.

(continued)

° Numbers in front of utterances on the transcript.

COMMENTS: Limited syntactic coding

PRODUCTIVE AT: Phase _____

GOALS: Phase ___3___   To: Increase coding of notice
                                            with 2 or 3 constituents

TABLE G-8

LEVEL 3
Language Sample Analysis Worksheet—Verb Relations

Content Category Epistemic_____   Child's Name Bill_____   Date S-3_____

	Form Analysis					Use Analysis	
	S-V-C Constituents						
	Include		Expect				
Utterances°	2	3	2	3	Comments	Linguistic Context	Function
31 think so	2			3	−subj.	FQc	respond
119 I *don't* know	2		2		routine	FQc	respond
Further Information							
a. me know *this* pu		3		3		0	comment
b. me know do*ing*		3		3	2nd verb	FSc	comment
c. know what do	2			3	2nd verb	FSc	comment
d. − − −remember that	?			3	unintell.	0	comment
Frequency	3	2		5	= 2 constituents productive		
Proportion with 3 expected			÷		= ___% level of achievement		

Coordinated categories (utterances that include 2 constituents plus another category)

Nonexistence	Recurrence	Rejection	Denial	Attribution	Possession	Quantity	Temperal	Specification	Wh-Question	Place	Other
119. don't							b. ing	a. this			

Other utterances within category:

10 no think (2X)	1		6			FSc	comment

° Numbers in front of utterances refer to number of utterance on the transcript.

452

TABLE G-8   *Continued*

COMMENTS: Bill also used the verb *pretend* as a single-word utterance a number of times. Utterances b and c are further evidence of emergence of utterances with two verbs and provide partial evidence for Phase 7. Most likely, utterances 31 and 119 are routines—119 is the only use of *I* in the sample. Bill is productive with three constituents using epistemic state verbs, but this is not on the plan. No goals at this time.

PRODUCTIVE AT: Phase _____

GOALS: Phase _____   To: (Do not set goals at this time
                                               —coding with sentential
                                               complements will be a later
                                               goal)

Analysis 2: Nonverb Categories

The goal of this analysis was to determine the productivity of the nonverb categories. The worksheet presented in Table G-9 illustrates a nonverb analysis. In the first column the total number of times the nonverb category was found coordinated with all verb relations was entered (e.g., for nonexistence, three examples were found across all verb category analysis worksheets—two in locative action and one in epistemic). A search of the transcript found two more different examples of nonexistence that were syntactic two-word utterances. Since the three coordinated plus the two syntactic utterances were enough evidence to note the productivity of nonexistence at Phase 2, no further search was done. Each new example of two-word utterances was also coded for use.

TABLE G-9

LEVEL 3
Worksheet for Nonverb Category Analysis

Child's Name <u>Bill</u>   Date <u>S-3</u>

Content	Form			Use	
Category	No. of Times Coordinated	Other Examples°	Comments	Linguistic Context	Function
Nonexistence					
	3				
		10 no think (2 times)		FSc	comment
		68 no head		0	comment
		Total Number of Exemplars ___5___			

Types: *no* ___4___ ; *can't* _____ ; *didn't* _____ ; *not* _____ ; other ___1___

       COMMENTS: He talked of nonexistence in relation to action, states, and
             objects.

(continued)

TABLE G-9 Nonverb Analysis *Continued*

Content	Form				Use	
Category	No. of Times Coordinated	Other Examples°	Comments		Linguistic Context	Function

PRODUCTIVE AT: PHASE ____2____

Goals: (see action goals in Table G-3)

Recurrence

____0____

1 more toys		0	regulate
5 white too		FSc	comment
98 you too · horsie	anaph. ellip.	FSc self	comment
151 you too pig	anaph. ellip.	FSc self	comment
206 animals too		FSc	obtain info.

Total Number of Exemplars ____5____

Types: *more* ____1____ ; *another* _____ ; *again* _____ ; *too* ____4____ ; other _____

COMMENTS: Category productive with *too*; need information on use of other forms (e.g., *more, again, another*)

PRODUCTIVE AT: PHASE ____2____

Goals: Increase use of *more* in two-word utterances

Rejection

____0____

237 no more toys	0	comment
124 mom · no	0	protest

Further Information:

a. no peek that	0	regulate

Total Number of Exemplars ____3____ (only 2 syntactic)

Types: *no* ____3____ ; *don't* _____ ; other _____

COMMENTS: Not much coding, but may have been context

PRODUCTIVE AT: PHASE ____1____ (but few examples)

Goals: (None at this time.)

Denial

____0____

30 no · crash	FQc	respond
45 no	FQc	repair
65 no	FQc	repair
94 no was cow	FSc self	repair
185 no · truck	FQc	repair
104 no · this	FQc	repair

Total Number of Exemplars ____6____ (only 1 syntactic)

Types: *no* ____6____ ; *not* _____ ; other _____

(continued)

TABLE G-9 Nonverb Analysis *Continued*

COMMENTS: Denial was frequently used as a part of a repair sequence where mother did not understand what Bill had said and she repeated what she understood with a rising intonation requesting confirmation. When she was wrong, Bill denied with the single word *no* and, he repeated the word usually with a change in pronunciation. Mother repeated her new interpretation and Bill responded with affirmation, or the sequence began again. Only one utterance indicated syntactic coding (number 94).

PRODUCTIVE AT: PHASE ___1___

Goals: None at this time

Attribution

___2___

8 white stripes	FSc	comment
23 big · big size	0	comment
81 nice animals	0	comment self
237 bad cowboys	0	comment self

Total Number of Exemplars ___6___

COMMENTS:

PRODUCTIVE AT: PHASE ___2___

Goals: (see existence)

Possession

___1___

37 my horse– – –	doll talk	self	comment

Further Information

a. Scooby Doo pal		FQc	comment
b. a big red son		FQc	respond
c. my dad	doll talk	FSnc self	comment

Total Number of Exemplars ___5___

Types: Word Order Only ___2___; Pronoun ___3___; -'s _____

COMMENT:

PRODUCTIVE AT: PHASE ___2___

Goals: None at this time unless further evidence indicates that existence is productive through Phase 3.

Quantity

___2___

22 beads	0	label
182 coats	FSnc self	label
225 ghosts	FQc	respond

Total Number of Exemplars ___5___

Types: -s ___5___; number words _____; *some* _____; *many* _____; *all* _____

(continued)

TABLE G-9 Nonverb Analysis *Continued*

Content	Form			Use	
Category	No. of Times Coordinated	Other Examples°	Comments	Linguistic Context	Function

Quantity *(continued)*

COMMENTS: There was no evidence of words spoken in both singular and plural. Many words such as *beads, bombs,* and *cowboys* are normally coded in plural form. Not clear that the distinction is there although marking was often very distinct (e.g., *ghostes* for *ghosts*).

PRODUCTIVE AT: PHASE _____?_____

Goals: Obtain further information about distinction between singular and plural.

Temporal

	3 now				
		149 lie down now		0	comment
	1 -ing				
		151 climbing		FQc	respond
	_2 -ed_				
	1 irreg. past				
	2 third				
	person -s				

Total Number of Exemplars ____11____

Types: -ing ___2___; -irreg. past ___1___; -ed ___2___; -s ___2___; now ___4___; when _____; aux. _____; other _____

COMMENTS:

PRODUCTIVE AT: PHASE ____6____ for *now*

Goals: PHASE ____4____ verb inflections

Dative

_____None_____

Total Number of Exemplars ____0____

Types: Word Order Only _____; *for* _____; *to* _____; other _____

Specification

2 this/that

2 this one   0   obtain info.

Total Number of Exemplars ____3____

Types: *this* ___2___; *that* ___1___; *the* _____; other _____

COMMENTS:

PRODUCTIVE AT: PHASE ____5____ (weak evidence)

Goals: None at this time

° Numbers in front of utterances refer to number of utterance on the transcript.

Comments were made after each nonverb category, and then each was summarized in terms of phase productive and any relevant goals.

Additional Descriptions and Summary of Level 3 Analysis

Below are some comments that summarize the information presented in the preceding tables and describe other aspects of Bill's communicative performance. These additional comments are perhaps most important in terms of use, where taxonomies that are relevant to this level of development are not well established. The comments here may be more extensive than is always possible in a clinical setting, but they serve to illustrate behaviors that can be described.

Play Behavior.   During play, Bill demonstrated object-specific play, symbolic use of objects (e.g., using a ruler as a hose to put out a fire), and sequences of object-to-object play (e.g., pretend food preparation). He searched for objects in order to carry out these sequences and initiated many of the play sequences. In addition, he exchanged roles with his mother (e.g., in hide-and-seek activity) and talked for, and to, the dolls during play sequences.

Use.   In general, Bill's use of language was appropriate to his level of content/form interactions and in some cases was more advanced. For example, many of his utterances were contingent upon those of his mother. Most of his mother's questions (of which there were many with an abundance of yes/no questions) were answered appropriately. More difficult questions such as "How did you know?" were appropriately, but simply, answered (e.g., "easy"). A "why" question from his mother ("why are you beating him up?") was responded to, but it is not clear whether or not the response ("him crazy") was providing a reason for the child's action. Furthermore, on two occasions, Bill used contingent queries ("why") to question what his mother had said.

When Bill was misunderstood, he often made changes in the articulation of the word (phonetic recoding) so that it more closely approximated the adult model. These attempts were generally successful: his mother would request confirmation of her new interpretation, and this was acknowledged by Bill. Thus, a rather complex repair sequence seemed well established. Many of his utterances were difficult to understand even for his mother, so repairs were fairly frequent. Most of Bill's comments were interactive. He often added tags such as "OK?" the function of which was not clear. They may have served as a request for feedback or permission but seemed more likely a means of maintaining the conversation and shifting the "turn" to his mother.

No redundant coding was noticed. Anaphoric ellipsis was appropriately used in answering questions and also in one sequence of utterances where Bill told an animal to lie down and then added "you too, pig." This was the only example of anaphoric ellipsis outside of responses to questions, and it may have been part of a routine. Prosodic patterns appropriately stressed new or contrastive information. In addition, prosody signaled yes/no questions as well as the contrast between certainty and uncertainty. Vocalizations that were a part of play with dolls and were not interactive with other persons were less intelligible and were often spoken in a higher-pitched voice, particularly when he was creating dialogue between dolls or animals.

As might be expected for his level of language productions, Bill talked about the here and now—mainly about what he was doing, was about to do, or wanted others to do. Thus, perceptual support was present. On two occasions, with considerable prompting from his mother, he was able to answer questions about school and about breakfast. He did not talk about the actions of others. A goal of intervention might be to increase the distancing of utterances from events, and to increase the number of utterances about actions of others.

Bill used language to comment, regulate, obtain information, focus attention, and maintain the flow of conversation. These functions did not seem to be restricted to particular forms, given his level of content/form productions. One would expect that utterances intended to obtain information would increase in the near future, but it was a bit early for this to be a goal given his level of content/form development.

Content/Form.   Analysis of Bill's language indicated that content/form interactions were productive through Phase 2, with some behaviors productive at Phase 3 and a few isolated behaviors productive at later phases. Goals of intervention were mainly in Phases 3 and 4 and included the following content/form interactions:

> To increase coding of existence with two constituents including a relational word
> (To code existence coordinated with attribution)
> To code action coordinated with
>> Attribution
>> Place
>> Recurrence
>> Intention/volition
>
> To code locative action coordinated with intention/volition
> To obtain more information about the coding of locative state with two or three constituents
> To increase coding of notice with two or three constituents
> To increase the use of *more* in two-word utterances coding recurrence
> To increase the use of verb inflections (*-ing, -s,* irregular past) to code aspect.

As always, all content/form goals would be incorporated into communicative situations that included the variety of functions and linguistic contexts used with his present productions. New content/form interactions would not be expected to occur in contexts that were not familiar; for example, Bill would be expected to use new content/form interactions only in the context of perceptual support.

Bill's use of the objective case for personal pronouns in the subject position (e.g., *me/I*) was frequent and called attention to his speech as different; such usage was unusual for his age. However, these errors are found in some non-language-impaired children at this level of language development. Despite possible pressure from parents and teachers, it is probably more efficient (and more in keeping with a focus on communication) to work on other behaviors at this time and hold the teaching of appropriate case distinctions in pronouns until a later time—at least until Phase 6 or 7 behaviors are productive, and perhaps even later. Unfortunately, the developmental point at which such confusions are usually worked out is not well documented in the literature.

Reassessment

To reassess Bill's progress in reaching the goals outlined above (based on the third sample) another videotaped sample, which was obtained 6 months later, was scanned for the relevant behaviors. This sample was obtained in the same context as the last one; Bill interacted with his mother in a studio that was set up like a play room, and the same toys were periodically brought into the room. He was 4½ years old at the time and had continued in a preschool class for language-impaired children. Bill had made considerable progress since the first sample (1½ years earlier); he had achieved many of the goals set in Sample 3. Sample 4 contained many multiverb relations that are expected in Phases 5–8, and these needed to be analyzed. However, before the multiverb analysis (i.e., a Level 4 analysis) was undertaken, the data were scanned to determine if some of the goals set in the last Level 3 analysis had been reached and to check on other later interactions that are a part of the Level 3 analysis (since they do not involve relations between verbs). The results of this reassessment are presented in Table G-10.

TABLE G-10

REASSESSMENT OF PROGRESS
Bill, Sample 4

CONTENT/FORM

Existence Productive: Copula (but not achieved); *wh* questions, *what* and *who*; + possession; + attribution

Examples:
These are tree*s*; yes, they are; *who* is gramma; these *your* animal*s*; *what's that* sound; these are *his* friends; this zoo; that's you mommy; this *little* kid *now*; he *my best* friend; *what's* in *that* box; *this* one *easy* puzzle; a kitchen; a bed

GOALS: To coordinate Existence + recurrence
To use article *a*
To increase use of copula

Action Productive: 3 constituents; + attribution; + nonexistence; + volition/intention; + possession; + rejection; + *wh* Q; + recurrence

Examples:
don't wet it; I *can't* do it; no eat it; *what* you doin*g*; I do *one* side; hit *giraffe* leg; I grab *my* knife; *don't* do that; take *the big* giraffe; I hit *pink* one *and yellow* one; tiger drink *his* water; I *wanna* go *first*; I go *again*; *why* they *always* take *my animal* dolls; I crash in *right here*; *what* you *want* me do *now*; one a zebra's · *broke another* ear off; *what* happen*ing* in *little* TV, mom.

GOALS: To Coordinate Action + place
[See time goals for inflections]

Locative Action Productive: + Volition/intention; V + prep.; + possession

(continued)

° Parentheses under Goals indicates optional goal at this time.

Examples:

I *wanna* put *his* shoes back on now; *didn't* go *on* rug; *where* this go; I fall*ing in* pit; *this* guy jump *on* him; *where* it come from; he div*ed* in water; I *gonna* put zebra on *dark* one; this *can't* fit in; I stand *my* guy*s* up.

GOALS: To coordinate Locative action + attribution
(To increase coding with + nonexistence)°
(To increase coding with + recurrence)

Temporal   Productive (but not achieved): *-ing;* irregular past; regular past; third person singular *-s* (see also multiverb relation analysis)

Examples:

you hold*ing* it; maybe goe*s* in here; I do*ing* it right; I gett*ing* truck; I hope it go*es* in here; you *took* them out; maybe I *did*; he *fell*; how he kiss*ed*; he *went* wild; he div*ed* in water; I *saw* you; I crash*ed* you; pretend he *grew* up; you do*ing* it; yes, he do*es*; sett*ing* up this; him sleep*ing* over here; pretend him climb*ing* up; digg*ing* up; *when* I play with animal*s;*

GOALS: To increase frequency of verb inflections in obligatory contexts—particularly *-ing.* [See also multiverb relations.]

State   Productive: 2–3 constituents; + attribution (weak evidence but optional goal); + recurrence (weak evidence but optional goal); + possession; *can;* See also multiverb relation analysis.

Examples:

he have *his king* thing; *this* guy have *bad* fight; he have *him* nail; her have *different* camera; Sue have *this* puzzle; he *can* play with giraffe; little ones *can,* not big ones; I know I *can* do mom; *my* tummy empty.

GOALS: [See Level 4 analysis—relations between verbs.]

Locative State   Productive: 2–3 constituents; *in* and *on; where* Q.

Examples:

he got *another* one in *his* foot; he have nail in *his* foot; *where her* head; *where her* stove; *where his* hat; I *know* tiger is at home; *his* underwear on; but him have pants on.

GOALS: None

Possession   Still not productive with '*s.*

GOALS: To code possession using '*s*

Nonexistence   Productive: Using forms such as *can't, didn't,* and *not.*

Examples:

I *can't* do it; this *can't* fit in; her can't; lion is*n't;* giraffe is*n't;* not this kind; not whole bunch; *this* hose *didn't* match with this; *didn't* go on rug.

GOALS: None

(continued)

TABLE G-10 REASSESSMENT   *Continued*

Rejection   Limited use of *don't*

Examples: _don't_ put it back ok; _don't_ oops do that; no want play with– – –;

GOALS: To increase frequency of coding rejection with *don't*

Denial   Productive: Relational word + substantive word
Examples:
no he is_n't_; both them _not_ belong; no blue

GOALS: To increase coding of denial with *not*

Dative   Not productive
Examples:
Joe give me– – –; for me.

GOALS: To code dative with noun + noun

Notice   Productive: 2–3 constituents. See next analysis for examples. Notice was usually coded as a multiverb relation (e.g., "see how it rolls down")

GOALS: [See multiverb relations]

Quantity   Plurality is well established. Plural -*s* is used in most obligatory contexts, and plural pronouns are used (e.g., *these, those, them, they, us/we*). *Some* and *all* are used, but not *many*.

GOALS: None at this time

Specification   Still not productive with *the*.

GOALS: To code given referent with *the*. [See also multiverb relations analysis]

USE

Function   Bill continued to use functions observed in previous samples and increased the number of utterances that were imaginative. He frequently set up scenes and often used the term *pretend* to describe them. No goals at this time.

Nonlinguistic Context   Utterances conveying information that was not redundant with the context inreased; a few utterances were about nonpresent events. For example, he described a dream, an incident that had happened in the past (both of these are analyzed in the last section of this chapter under narratives), and he mentioned objects that were at school and that were outside in the car.

GOAL: To increase utterances about nonpresent events.

Some utterances referred to the actions of others, but usually in terms of how they affected Bill himself.

GOAL: To increase reference to the actions of others.

(continued)

Other than the use of the deictic terms *this* and *that*, there was little evidence of linguistic adaptation to listener needs. However, since mother and child share so much information and since most utterances are about the "here and now," there was little opportunity to observe adaptations to the listener.

GOAL: To observe interactions with different listeners.

Linguistic Context Utterances continued to be contingent on those of his mother and, in this sample, were more likely to add information. Bill's mother requested fewer repairs, since his articulation was clearer, but he responded to the one request with a rephrased utterance. A marked increased was observed in the number of utterances that were nonadjacent to his mother's but were adjacent to his own prior utterances. That is, he was more likely to produce a number of topically related utterances in succession.

GOALS: None at this time

Level 4

The fourth and last videotaped sample of Bill was used to illustrate a Level 4 analysis. This is the same sample that was used for the reassessment of early syntactic goals discussed in the previous section; in the present analysis, only those utterances with more than one verb relation were included.

The worksheet designed for this analysis separates verb relations by recording each one on a separate line (see Table G-11). The meaning relation, or content, that exists between each of the verb relations (now represented by separate lines) was determined, and under the appropriate content column a notation was made regarding whether or not a connective form was included. When in doubt about the content category a question mark (?) was placed in the column under the content category that seemed most likely; however, such utterances could not be used as the only evidence of productivity for that category. For example, in utterance *d* it was assumed that the giraffe went wild *because* he was hit, but it could have been a temporal sequence without causal connection. Because it was unclear, a question mark was placed in the column that appeared most appropriate, the causal column. If no connective form was included in an obligatory context, a 0 was placed in the content column; if no connective was used, and a connective was not required, an X was noted; if a connective form was used, the actual form (e.g., the word *and*) was written in the column. Utterance numbers are included for the first 30 minutes of the tape; the last 30 minutes were scanned for additional examples, and these were marked with a letter to distinguish one from another.

Since some utterances contained more than two verb relations (e.g., in utterances 264–265 in Table G-11, there were three related verbs, *fell*, *walk*, and the

TABLE G-11

LEVEL 4
Worksheet for Multiverb Relations: Content/Form

Child's Name <u>Bill</u>   Date <u>S-4</u>

Context of Sample _____

Utterance°	V/I	Add.	Temp.	Caus.	Epi.	Spec.	Adv.	Comm.	Not.	Comments
No.										
2 you know / Joe give me– – –					0					
3 I think / it fit up here					X					
4 I wanna / see / this happen	X								0	
6 can't race / 7 this one can							0			
8 no wheels on it / 9 this wheels come off			0							
20 see / how it rolls down									how	
21 I wanna / do something	X									
26 want / play with animals now	0									
49 I know / how do it					how					
54 little ones can / not big ones							0			
62 you do it, mommy / 63 you took them out			X							
70 you try red / 71 I wanna / go first	X					0				

(continued)

° Numbers or letters in front of utterances refer to number or letter of utterance on the transcript.

Key

V/I = Volition/Intention (State)	Adv = Adversative
Add = Additive	Comm = Communication
Temp = Temporal	Not = Notice
Caus = Causal	0 = No connective where obligatory
Epi = Epistemic	X = No connective and not obligatory
Spec = Specification	

TABLE G-11 LEVEL 4 *Continued*
Content

Utterance°	V/I	Add.	Temp.	Caus.	Epi.	Spec.	Adv.	Comm.	Not.	Comments
75 I go				X						
76 who crash on side go again						X				
77 I go again				0						
86 you go then I crashed you			then							
(mother's utterance) 107 but where's ice								but		
108 pretend this					X					
109 he walks and see his ice rips		and							X	
115 it cracks and he jumps		and								
118 sometime him come										
119 him keep him company				0						
121 he wanna eat first	X									
122 he's hungry				X						
131 lion drinks water										
132 him leave			0							
133 tiger drink his water			0							
134 he come back		0								
135 I know tiger is at home					0					
141 us lose King Kong he my best friend							X			
145 – – –have dream							X			
146 bad dream I falling in pit							0			
147 digging up			0							
151 alligators chasing me										
152 I grabbed my knife				0						
153 kill them			0							
159 him have my knife										
160 kill them			0							
175 lion want something eat	0									
176 how he kissed								how		

(continued)

TABLE G-11 LEVEL 4 *Continued*
Content

Utterance°	V/I	Add.	Temp.	Caus.	Epi.	Spec.	Adv.	Comm.	Not.	Comments
192 pretend is fish				X						
195 this guy have bad fight he very mad				?0						
206 I saw you 207 setting up this								X		
(mother's utterance) 210 and me		and								
211 pretend this winter now 213 everybody go bed				X 0						

219 he lay down right
    here
220 and zebra sleep
    under him
		and								

230 pretend him- - -climbing up				X						
234 I did last time not this time 235 I did very nice						X	X			
238 Window & jacket & hat		and								
245 dishes &- - -& cups		and								
247 & room & bed		and								
259 I know 260 I got jelly toast in my car				X						
264 he fell 265 him leg not strong nuff for him walk				0 for						
286 I hope for Betty 287 and Jane		and								
(mother's utterance) 288 but him have pants on							but			
291 he go swimming 292 don't wet it 293 he took pants off	?0			0						
294 I hope so 295 I don't know							0			

(continued)

TABLE G-11 LEVEL 4 *Continued*
Content

Utterance°	V/I	Add.	Temp.	Caus.	Epi.	Spec.	Adv.	Comm.	Not.	Comments
304 pretend					X					
this little kid now										
then he growed up			then							

Utterance and Letter°

Further Information

Utterance°	V/I	Add.	Temp.	Caus.	Epi.	Spec.	Adv.	Comm.	Not.	Comments
a. I saw									X	
you sitting down										
b. lets	X									
go for eat-break										
& coffee break		and								
& soda break		and								
c. (mother's utterance)										
and eat break		and								
d. pretend					X					
this little thing										
hit giraffe leg										
and he went wild				and?						
e. I know					X					
I can do mom										
f. (mother's utterance)								0		
no eat it										
g. I want	0									
play with these										
h. want	0									
see										
i. you holding it									X	
j. I play with it after										
k. don't put it back,				X						
all right										
l. I want	0									
see										
how he knock it down									how	
m. I want graham										
crackers										
no apple juice								0		
n. no want	0									
play catch now										
o. him have	to									
to be at south pole										
p. him have nail										
I took out							0			
q. he got nother one– – –				?0						

(*continued*)

TABLE G-11 LEVEL 4 *Continued*

r. I zoo keeper
sometimes I kill animals   0

s. watch
me hammer really hard   X

t. me like
take off   0

u. both them not belong
(*mother:* "why?")
cuz
(*mother:* "cuz why?")
cuz see not this way   cuz

v. (*mother:* you put on– – –)
no
(*mother:* "why?")
cuz I want– – –   cuz

w. want   0
see
how it race   how

Connective Forms Produced	V/I	Add.	Temp.	Caus.	Epi.	Spec.	Adv.	Comm.	Not.
Totals	14	12	6	17	12	6	9	0	9
−obligatory connective	9	2	4	0	4	2	6	0	1
+connective (list form and frequency of use)	to 1	and 10	then 2	and 1 for 1 cuz 2	how 1	how 1	but 2		how 3

COMMENTS:

Complements:

    Volition/Intention—coded mostly with infinitival complements without use of *to*. The schwa was often used on *want*, but not always (e.g., 26, h, l, n). Verbs include *want*, *have*, *like*, but not *go*. Most of these utterances are Phase 4 with one example at Phase 5 and one at Phase 7 (sentential complement, number 175).

    Epistemic—with verbs *know, pretend, hope* but usually without the connective form needed for *know*.

    Notice—with verbs *see* and *watch* with *see how* used 3 times.

Conjoined (Coordinate and Subordinate):

    Additive—He usually joined phrases and clauses with *and*. In one case a phrase was joined to mother's prior utterance.

    Adversative—the two productions of *but* were used when the utterance was related to his mother's prior utterance. Others were without a connective.

    Temporal—The connective *then* was produced only twice. Other instances were without connectives. All temporal relations were sequential, not simultaneous.

(*continued*)

TABLE G-11 LEVEL 4 *Continued*

Causal—the connectives *for, cuz,* and *and* used, but only one or two times each. The relation was frequently manifest in successive utterances.

Successive Utterances:
Causal—Generally expressed with successive utterances without a connective
Specification—Generally expressed with successive utterances without a connective

Relative Clauses:
None

Comments on Use:
Most utterances were related to a prior utterance of the child and not those of another. A number of utterances were about events that were not ongoing—(e.g., talking of a dream, food in the car, a story about animals, and mother's actions of a few minutes before).

PRODUCTIVE AT: PHASE <u>4</u> Volition/intention, V − c + NP
PHASE <u>5</u> Additive, VP +/− c + VP and NP + c + NP
Temporal, VP − c + VP
Causal, VP − c + VP
PHASE <u>7</u> Notice, V − c + NP + VP and V + c + NP + VP
Epistemic, V − c + NP + VP

GOALS: PHASE <u>5</u> To code volition/intention, V + *to* + VP with increased use of *have* and use of *like* and *go*
PHASE <u>6</u> To code sequential time with VP + c + VP with c = *and*
To code objective causal relations with VP + c + VP with c = *so* and/or *because*

Based on partial evidence within this sample, some of the following Phase 7 goals might also be considered.

PHASE <u>7</u> To code temporal with VP + c + VP with c = *then* for sequential time
To code epistemic with V + c + NP + VP with V + c = *know what* or *know where*
To code adversative with VP + c + NP + VP with c = *and* or *but*
To code subjective causal relations with VP + c + VP with c = *so* and/or *because*

missing copula), a bracket was used to indicate which clauses were related. Let's look at the utterances more closely. The animal in question in utterances 264 and 265 can't walk because his leg is not strong enough, so these two verbs (i.e., the missing copula and "walk") were related and bracketed; he fell because his leg wasn't strong enough to walk so the clause about falling was connected to the bracket joining the verb relations in utterance 265.

If Bill's utterance was related to the prior utterance of another person (e.g., an answer to a "why" question) rather than to a prior clause of his own, this was so noted (see, for example, utterance 288 where Bill's utterance "but him have pants on" was related to his mother's prior statement). When all of the multiverb relations had been entered, the columns were totaled, with subtotals computed for the use of each connective form. A space was left for comments beside each utterance and at the end of the worksheet. This space might have been used to note other behaviors in the utterance that are of relevance to other goals. For example, the presence or absence of morphological inflections might be noted after a child is productive and the goal is to increase the proportional use, or a notation might be made about syntactic structure (e.g., whether utterances were successive, complements, etc.). Finally, the content/form interactions that were productive were noted, and then the goals for content/form interactions were listed.

Most of the multiverb relations were spoken as comments; however, a few were used to regulate (e.g., utterances 62, 75, b, j) and to establish imaginative scenes (e.g., utterances 211, 304). Most utterances were related to the child's own prior utterance; three were related to the mother's prior utterance. On two occasions there were short narratives (or a sequence of related utterances about events not presently occurring). One was difficult to follow; the other was co-constructed with his mother. Other aspects of use (e.g., the increased frequency of utterances to obtain information, to talk about events not in the here and now, and to seek clarification) were considered under the previous analysis.

APPENDIX H

A Content/Form/Use Goal Plan for Language Development Goals

USE Goal Numbers* Function / Context	PHASE	EXISTENCE	NONEXISTENCE	RECURRENCE	REJECTION	DENIAL	ATTRIBUTION	POSSESSION	ACTION	LOCATIVE ACTION	LOCATIVE STATE	STATE
				(For prelinguistic goals, see Chapter 10)								
1,2 / 10, 3,4 / 11, 5,6 / 12, 7,8,9 / 13, 14	1	sw	sw	sw	sw	(sw)	(sw)	(sw)	sw	sw		
	2	R + S	Neg + C C + Neg	R + S S + R			(Adj + N)	(N or P + N)	2 Constit.	2 Constit. V + Prep. Prep + N		
	3	(+ATTRIB.)					(+EXIST.)		3 Constit.	3 Constit.	2–3 Constit.	2–3 Constit. V = "want"
above plus 15, 16 / 17, 18, 19, 20, 21, 22, 23	4	+RECURR. +POSSESS. "a" What Q	+Action	+EXIST +ACTION	(Neg + C)		+ACTION	+EXIST.	+ATTRIB.* +PLACE +NONEXIST* +RECURR.* +VOL/INT –ing irreg. past	VOL/INT V + s	+Prep "in" "on" Where Q	VOL/INT V – c + VP V = "want" "go"
	5	+Copula Who Q (+LOC. ACT.)	"can't" "didn't" "not"	(+STATE)	"don't" ACTION	Neg + C "not"	(+STATE)	N + s +ACTION +LOC. ACT.	+POSSESSION* +REJECTION* Multiple-Coord.	V + Prep.* +POSSESSION* (+NONEXIST.*) –ing		(+ATTRIB.) (+RECURR.) VOL/INT V + "to" + VP V = "want" "like" "have"
above plus 24, 25, 26 / 27, 28, 29, 30, 31, 32, 33, 34, 35	6			(+LOC. ACT.)			+LOC. ACT.	(+STATE)		+ATTRIB.* (+RECURR.*)		(+POSS.)
	7								"What" "How" Q			VOL/INT V+NP–"to"+VP V="want" POSSIBILITY "can"
	8											VOL/INT V+NP+"to"+VP V="want" OBLIGATION "should"
Chapter 11	8+											

*Numbers refer to number preceding each goal of USE in Chapter 8, pages 192–193.

(Handwritten annotations: "verbs + adj" with arrow pointing to R/S; "objects" with arrow pointing to Inflect; "epithet" near R; "nouns, verbs, adj + adverbs" near C)

KEY

R = Relational word	Inflect = Inflection
S = Substantive word	Dur = Durative
C = Content word	irreg. pst = irregular past
N = Noun	Habit = Habitual
V = Verb	Prep = Preposition
VP = Verb Phrase	Constit = major grammatical constituents
NP = Noun Phrase	(subject-verb-complement)
Dem = Demonstrative	( ) = optional goal–can be postponed
Neg = Negative word	* = first productions may be with two
c = Connective	instead of three constituents
P = Pronoun	+ = plus
sw = single word	Rel Cl = Relative Clause
sent. = sentence	Cx = Context
F = Function	Int = Intention
Vol = Volition	EXIST. = Existence
	LOC.ACT. = Locative Action
	RECURR. = Recurrence
	POSSES. = Possession
	ATTRIB. = Attribution
	Coord. = Coordination

QUANTITY	NOTICE PERCEPTION	TEMPORAL	ADDITIVE	CAUSAL	SPECIFICATION	DATIVE	EPISTEMIC	ADVERSATIVE	COMMUNICATION
	2–3 Constit.	ASPECT V Inflect. +Dur –ing –Dur ireg. pst +Habit. –s							
"some" "many" "all"			VP+/–c+VP NP+/–c+NP c="and"	VP–c+VP	Dem+N Dem="this" vs "that"	N+N			
		"now" SEQUENCE VP+/–c+VP c="and"		OBJECTIVE VP+c+VP c="so""and" "because"	"the"	+Prep "to' "for"			
	V–c+NP+VP V="see""look"	SEQUENCE VP+c+VP c="then" SIMULTANEOUS c="when"	VP+c+VP SEQUENCE c="then"	SUBJECTIVE VP+c+VP c="so""and" "because"	(Dem+(is)+c+VP) c="what" "where" (VP+c+VP) c="and"		V+c+NP+VP V+c="know what" "know where" V–c+NP+VP V–c="think"	VP+c+NP+VP c="and""but"	
	V–c+NP+VP (V–c="watch") ("show") V+c+NP+VP V+c="see what" "see if" "look what"	("When" Q) +TENSE–Aux= "is" "was" ("will") "-ed"		"Why" Q	(VP+c+Rel Cl) c="that"				(V+c+NP+VP) V="tell" "say" "ask"
		(Sent+Sent+++)	Sent+Sent+++	(Sent+Sent+++)					

References

Affolter, F., Brubaker, R., & Bischofberger, W. (1974). Comparative studies between normal and language disturbed children. *Acta Otolaryngology (Suppl.* 323), pp. 1–32.

Akmajian, A., Demers, R., & Harnish, R. (1984). *Linguistics: An introduction to language and communication. Second edition.* Cambridge, MA: MIT Press.

American Psychiatric Association. (1980). *Diagnostic and statistical manual of mental disorders DSM III* (3rd ed.). Washington, DC.

American Psychological Association. (1974). *Standards for educational and psychological tests.* Washington, DC: American Psychological Association.

Amerman, J., Daniloff, R., & Moll, K. (1970). Lip and jaw coarticulation for the phoneme /æ/. *Journal of Speech and Hearing Research, 13,* 147–161.

Ammons, R., & Ammons, H. (1948). *Full range picture vocabulary test,* Missoula, MT: Psychological Test Specialists.

Anastasi, A. (1982). *Psychological testing* (5th ed.). New York: Macmillan.

Anderson, R., Miles, M., & Matheny, P. (1963). *Communicative evaluation chart from infancy to five years.* Cambridge, MA: Educators' Publishing Service.

Antinucci, F., & Miller, R. (1976). How children talk about what happened. *Journal of Child Language, 3,* 169–189.

Applebee, N. (1978). *The child's concept of story.* Chicago: University of Chicago Press.

Aram, D. M., Ekelman, B. L., & Nation, J. E. (1984). Preschoolers with language disorders: Ten years later. *Journal of Speech and Hearing Research, 27,* 232–244.

Aram, D. M., Ekelman, B. L., & Whitaker, H. (1986). Spoken syntax in children with acquired left and right hemisphere lesions. *Brain and Language, 27,* 75–100.

Aram, D. M., & Nation, J. E. (1975). Patterns of language behavior in children with developmental language disorders. *Journal of Speech and Hearing Research, 18,* 229–241.

Aram, D. M., & Nation, J. E. (1980). Preschool language disorders and subsequent language and academic difficulties. *Journal of Communication Disorders, 13,* 159–170.

Aram, D. M., & Nation, J. E. (1982). *Child language disorders.* St. Louis: Mosby.

Arthur, G. (1952). *The Arthur adaptation of the Leiter International Performance Scale.* Washington, DC: Psychological Service Center Press.

Asha (1987, July). Special education on population down for first time; Report finds many violations called minor, 7.

Aten, J. (1974). Auditory memory and auditory sequencing. *Acta Symbolica, 5,* 37–65.

Aten, J., & Davis, J. (1968). Disturbances in the perception of auditory sequence in children with minimal cerebral dysfunction. *Journal of Speech and Hearing Research, 11,* 236–246.

Aurnhammer-Frith, N. (1969). Emphasis and meaning in recall in normal and autistic children. *Language and Speech, 12,* 29–38.

Ayres, A. J. (1975). Sensorimotor foundation of academic ability. In W. Cruickshank & D. Hallahan (Eds.), *Perceptual and learning disabilities in children* (pp. 361–393). Syracuse, NY: Syracuse University Press.

Baer, D. M., & Guess, D. (1973). Teaching productive noun suffixes to severely retarded children. *American Journal of Mental Deficiency, 77,* 498–505.

Baker, N., & Nelson, K. (1984). Recasting and related conversational techniques for triggering syntactic advances by young children. *First Language, 5,* 3–21.

Baltaxe, C. (1977). Pragmatic deficits in the language of autistic adolescents. *Pediatric Psychology, 2*(4), 176–180.

Baltaxe, C. A. M., & Simmons, J. Q. (1975). Language in childhood psychosis: A review. *Journal of Speech and Hearing Disorders, 40,* 439–458.

Bandura, A., & Harris, M. A. (1966). Modification of syntactic style. *Journal of Experimental Child Psychology, 4,* 341–352.

Bangs, T. E. (1982). *Language and learning disorders of the pre-academic child* (2nd ed.). Englewood Cliffs, NJ: Prentice-Hall.

Bankson, N. W. (1977). *Bankson Language Screening Test.* Baltimore: University Park Press.

Barrera, R. D., Lobato-Barrera, D., & Sulzer-Azaroff, B. (1980). A simultaneous treatment comparison of three expressive language training programs with a mute autistic child. *Journal of Autism and Developmental Disabilities, 10,* 21–37.

Barry, H. (1961). *The young aphasic child: Evaluation and training.* Washington, DC: Alexander Graham Bell Association for the Deaf.

Barsch, R. (1967). *Achieving perceptual-motor efficiency: A space-oriented approach to learning.* Seattle, WA: Special Child Publications.

Bartak, L., & Rutter, M. (1976). Differences between mentally retarded and normally intelligent autistic children. *Journal of Autism and Childhood Schizophrenia, 6,* 109–120.

Bartak, L., Rutter, M., & Cox, A. (1975). A comparative study of infantile autism and specific developmental receptive language disorder: I. The children. *British Journal of Psychiatry, 126,* 127–145.

Bartlett, E. (1982). *Anaphoric reference in written narratives of good and poor elementary school writers.* Unpublished manuscript, New York University Medical Center, New York.

Bartolucci, G., & Albers, R. J. (1974). Deictic categories in the language of autistic children. *Journal of Autism and Childhood Schizophrenia, 4,* 131–141.

Bartolucci, G., Pierce, S., Streiner, D., & Eppel, P. T. (1976). Phonological investigation of verbal autistic and mentally retarded subjects. *Journal of Autism and Childhood Schizophrenia, 6,* 303–316.

A basic course in manual communication (1970). Silver Spring, MD: National Association of the Deaf.

Bates, E. (1976). *Language in context.* New York: Academic Press.

Bates, E. (1979). *The emergence of symbols: Communication and cognition in infancy.* New York: Academic Press.

Bates, E., Bretherton, I., & Snyder, L. (in press). *From first words to grammar.* New York: Cambridge University Press.

Bauman, R., & Sherzer, J. (1974). *Explorations in the ethnography of speaking.* London: Cambridge University Press.

Beasley, D. S., Maki, J., & Orchik, D. (1976). Children's perception of time compressed speech on two measures of speech discrimination. *Journal of Speech and Hearing Disorders, 41,* 216–225.

Bedrosian, J. L., & Prutting, C. A. (1978). Communicative performance of mentally retarded adults in four conversational settings. *Journal of Speech and Hearing Research, 21,* 79–95.

Beeghly, M., & Cicchetti, D. (1986). *Early language development in children with Down's syndrome: A longitudinal study.* Paper presented at the Boston University Conference on Language Development, Boston.

Belkin, A. (1975). *Investigation of the functions and forms of children's negative utterances.* Unpublished doctoral dissertation, Teachers College, Columbia University, New York.

Belkin, A. (1983). Facilitating language in emotionally handicapped children. In H. Winitz (Ed.), *Treating language disorders: For clinicians by clinicians.* Baltimore: University Park Press.

Bellugi, U., & Klima, E. (1972). Roots of language in the sign talk of the deaf. *Psychology Today, 6,* 61–64.

Belsky, J., Garduque, L., & Hrncir, E. (1984). Assessing performance, competence, and executional capacity in infant play: Relation to home environment and security of attachment. *Developmental Psychology, 30,* 406–417.

Benedict, H. (1979). Early lexical development: Comprehension and production. *Journal of Child Language, 6,* 183–200.

Bennett-Kastor, T. (1983). Noun phrases and coherence in child narratives. *Journal of Child Language, 10,* 135–149.

Bennett-Kastor, T. (1986). Cohesion and predication in child narrative. *Journal of Child Language, 13,* 353–370.

Benton, A. (1964). Developmental aphasia and brain damage. *Cortex, 1,* 40–50.

Bernstein, D. (1986, September) The development of humor: Implications for assessment and intervention. *Topics in Language Disorders, 6,* 65–72.

Bernstein, L. (1981). Language as a product of dialogue. *Discourse Processes, 4,* 117–147.

Bernstein, L., & Stark, R. (1985). Speech perception development in language-impaired children: A 4-year follow-up study. *Journal of Speech and Hearing Disorders, 50,* 21–30.

Berry, M. (1966). *Berry-Talbott Exploratory Test of Grammar.* Rockford, IL.

Berry, M. (1969). *Language disorders of children: The bases and diagnoses.* New York: Appleton-Century-Croft.

Bersoff, D. (1971). Current functioning myth: An overlooked fallacy in psychological assessment. *Journal of Consulting and Clinical Psychology, 37,* 319–393.

Bettelheim, B. (1967). *The empty fortress: Infantile autism and the birth of self.* New York: Free Press.

Bever, T. G. (1970). The cognitive basis for linguistic structures. In J. Hayes (Ed.), *Cognition and the development of language.* New York: Wiley.

Birch, H. G. (1964). *Brain damage in children.* Baltimore: Williams & Wilkins.

Blagden, C. M., & McConnell, N. L. (1985). *Interpersonal Language Skills Assessment (ILSA).* Moline, IL: LinguiSystems.

Blank, M. (1973). *Teaching learning in the preschool: A dialogue approach.* Columbus, OH: Merrill.

Blank, M., Gessner, M., & Esposito, A. (1979). Language without communication: A case study. *Journal of Child Language, 6,* 329–352.

Blank, M., Rose, S., & Berlin, L. (1978). *Preschool Language Assessment Instrument: The language of learning in practice.* New York: Grune & Stratton.

Blanton, R. (1968). Language learning and performance in the deaf. In J. Rosenberg & J. Koplin (Eds.), *Developments in applied psycholinguistics research.* New York: Macmillan.

Blasdell, R., & Jensen, P. (1970). Stress and word position determinants of imitation in first language learners. *Journal of Speech and Hearing Research, 13,* 193–202.

Blau, A. (1983). Vocabulary selection in augmentative communication: Where do we begin? In H. Winitz (Ed.), *Treating language disorders: For clinicians by clinicians.* Baltimore: University Park Press.

Blau, A., Lahey, M., & Oleksiuk-Velez, A. (1984). Planning goals for intervention: Can a language test serve as an alternative to a language sample? *Journal of Childhood Communicative Disorders, 7,* 27–37.

Beitchman, J., Nair, R., Clegg, M., & Patel, P. (1986). Prevalence of speech and language disorders in 5-year-old kindergarten children in the Ottawa-Carleton region. *Journal of Speech and Hearing Disorders, 51,* 98–109.

Bloom, B., Hastings, J., & Madaus, G. (1971). *Handbook on formative and summative evaluation of student learning.* New York: McGraw-Hill.

Bloom, L. (1970). *Language development: Form and function in emerging grammars.* Cambridge, MA: M.I.T. Press.

Bloom, L. (1973). *One word at a time: The use of single-word utterances before syntax.* The Hague: Mouton.

Bloom, L. (1974). Talking understanding and thinking: Developmental relationship between receptive and expressive language. In R. L. Schiefelbusch & L. Lloyd (Eds.), *Language perspectives—Acquisition, retardation, and intervention* (pp. 285–312). Baltimore: University Park Press.

Bloom, L. (1976). An interactive perspective on language development. *Papers and Reports on Child Language Development,* Stanford University, Palo Alto, CA.

Bloom, L. (1980). Language development, language disorders, and learning disabilities: LD3. *Bulletin of the Orton Society, 30,* 115–133.

Bloom, L. (1981, January 16). *The importance of language for language development: Linguistic determinism in the 1980's.* Paper presented to the New York Academy of Sciences Conference on Native Language and Foreign Language Acquisition.

Bloom, L. (1984, December). *The transition to language: Contributions from cognition, affect, and intentionality.* Paper presented to the New York Academy of Sciences.

Bloom, L. (1987, July). *Language development is in the mind and action of the child.* Plenary address from The International Congress for the Study of Child Language. Lund, Sweden.

Bloom, L. (in press). Development in expression: Affect and speech. In *The Proceedings on the psychological and biological development of emotions, University of Chicago, 1986.*

Bloom, L., & Beckwith, R. (1986). *Intentionality and language development.* Unpublished manuscript, Teachers College, Columbia University, New York.

Bloom, L., & Capatides, J. (1983). *The language of cause and the causes of language.* Unpublished manuscript, Teachers College, Columbia University, New York.

Bloom, L., & Capatides, J. (in press a) Sources of meaning in the acquisition of complex syntax: The sample case of causality. *Journal of Experimental Child Psychology.*

Bloom, L., & Capatides, J. (in press b), Expression of affect and the emergence of language. *Child Development.*

Bloom, L., Hood, L., & Lightbown, P. (1974). Imitation in language development: If, when and why. *Cognitive Psychology, 6,* 380–420.

Bloom, L., & Lahey, M. (1978). *Language development and language disorders.* New York: Wiley.

Bloom, L., Lahey, M., Hood, L., Lifter, K., & Fiess, K. (1980). Complex sentences: Acquisition of syntactic connectives and the semantic relations they encode. *Journal of Child Language, 7,* 235–261.

Bloom, L., Lifter, K., & Broughton, J. (1985). The convergence of early cognition and language in the second year of life: Problems in conceptualization and measurement. In M. Barrett (Ed.), *Single word speech.* New York: Wiley.

Bloom, L., Lifter, K., & Hafitz, J. (1980). Semantics of verbs and the development of verb inflection in child language. *Language, 56,* 386–412.

Bloom, L., Lightbown, P., & Hood, L. (1975). Structure and variation in child language. *Monographs of the Society for Research in Child Development, 40* (Serial No. 160).

Bloom, L., Merkin, S., & Wooten, J. (1982). Wh-questions: Linguistic factors that contribute to the sequence of acquisition. *Child Development, 53,* 1084–1092.

Bloom, L., Miller, P., & Hood, L. (1975). Variation and reduction as aspects of competence in language development. In A. Pick (Ed.), *Minnesota symposia on child psychology* (Vol. 9). Minneapolis: University of Minnesota Press.

Bloom, L., Rispoli, M., Gartner, B., & Hafitz, J. (1987). *Acquisition of complementation.* Unpublished manuscript, Teachers College, Columbia University, New York.

Bloom, L., Rocissano, L., & Hood, L. (1976). Adult-child discourse: Developmental interaction between information processing and linguistic knowledge. *Cognitive Psychology, 8,* 521–552.

Bloom, L., Tackeff, J., & Lahey, M. (1983). Learning *to* in complement constructions. *Journal of Child Language, 10,* 391–406.

Bloomfield, L. (1933). *Language.* New York: Holt, Rinehart and Winston.

Boehm, A. (1969, 1986). *Boehm Test of Basic Concepts.* New York: Psychological Corp.

Bondurant, J. L., Romeo, D. J., & Kretschmer, R. (1983). Language behaviors of mothers of children with normal and delayed language. *Language, Speech and Hearing Services in the Schools, 14,* 233–242.

Bonvillian, J. D., & Nelson, K. E. (1976). Sign language acquisition in a mute autistic boy. *Journal of Speech and Hearing Disorders, 41,* 339–347.

Bonvillian, J. D., & Nelson, K. E. (1978). Development of sign language in autistic children and other handicapped individuals. In P. Siple (Ed.), *Understanding language through sign language research.* New York: Academic Press.

Bonvillian, J. D., Raeburn, V. P., & Horan, E. A. (1979). Talking to children: The effect of rate, intonation, and length on children's sentence imitation. *Journal of Child Language, 6,* 459–467.

Bornstein, H. (1973). A description of some current sign systems designed to represent English. *American Annals of the Deaf, 118,* 454–463.

Bornstein, H. (1974). Signed English: A manual approach to English language. *Journal of Speech and Hearing Disorders, 39,* 330–343.

Bortner, M. (1971). Phrenology, localization, and learning disabilities. *Journal of Special Education, 5,* 23–29.

Botvin, G. J., & Sutton-Smith, B. (1977). The development of structural complexity in children's fantasy narratives. *Developmental Psychology, 13,* 377–388.

Bowerman, M. (1973). *Early syntactic development: A cross-linguistic study with special reference to Finnish.* London: Cambridge University Press.

Bowerman, M. (1978). Systematizing semantic knowledge: Changes over time in the child's organization of word meaning. *Child Development, 49,* 977–987.

Bowerman, M. (1979). The acquisition of complex sentences. In P. Fletcher & M. Garman (Eds.), *Language acquisition.* London: Cambridge University Press.

Bowerman, M. (1982). Reorganizational processes in lexical and syntactic development. In E. Wanner & L. Gleitman (Eds.), *Language acquisition: The state of the art.* (pp. 319–346). London: Cambridge University Press.

Brannon, J. (1968). Linguistic word classes in the spoken language of normal, hard-of-hearing and deaf children. *Journal of Speech and Hearing Research, 11,* 279–287.

Bransford, J., & Johnson, M. (1972). Contextual prerequisites for understanding: Some investigations of comprehension and recall. *Journal of Verbal Learning and Verbal Behavior, 11,* 717–726.

Bransford, J., & Nitsch, K. (1977). How can we come to understand things that we did not previously understand? In J. Kavanagh & P. Strange (Eds.), *Language and speech in the laboratory, school and clinic.* Cambridge, MA: M.I.T. Press.

Braunwald, S., & Brislin, R. (1979). The diary method updated. In E. Ochs & B. Schieffelin (Eds.), *Developmental pragmatics*. New York: Academic Press.

Brawley, E. R., Harris, F. R., Allen, K. E., Fleming, R. S., & Peterson, R. F. (1969). Behavior modification of an autistic child. *Behavioral Science, 14,* 87–97.

Bray, C., & Wiig, E. (1987). *Let's talk inventory for children.* San Antonio, TX: Psychological Corp.

Brenner, R. (1940). An experimental investigation of memory span. *Journal of Experimental Psychology, 26,* 467–482.

Bretherton, I., & Beeghly, M. (1982). Talking about internal states: The acquisition of an explicit theory of mind. *Developmental Psychology, 18,* 906–921.

Bricker, D. (1972). Imitative sign training as a facilitator of word-object association with low-functioning children. *American Journal of Mental Deficiency, 76,* 509–516.

Bricker, W. A., & Bricker, D. D. (1974). An early language training strategy. In R. Schiefelbusch & L. Lloyd (Eds.), *Language perspectives—Acquisition, retardation, and intervention.* Baltimore: University Park Press.

Bricker, D. & Carlson, L. (1980). The relationship of object and prelinguistic social-communicative schemes to the acquisition of early linguistic skills in developmentally delayed infants. Paper presented at the Conference on Handicapped and At-Risk Infants. Monterey, CA.

Brinton, B., & Fujiki, M. (1982). A comparison of request-response sequences in the discourse of normal and language-disordered children. *Journal of Speech and Hearing Disorders, 47,* 57–63.

Brinton, B., Fujiki, M., Winkler, E., & Loeb, D. (1986). Responses to requests for clarification in linguistically normal and language-impaired children, *Journal of Speech and Hearing Disorders, 51,* 370–377.

Bristow, D., & Fristoe, M. (1984). Learning of Blissymbols and manual signs. *Journal of Speech and Hearing Disorders, 49,* 145–151.

Broen, P. (1972). The verbal environment of the language learning child. *ASHA Monographs* (No. 17). Rockville, MD: American Speech-Language Hearing Association.

Bronckart, J. P., & Sinclair, H. (1973). Time, tense, and aspect. *Cognition, 2,* 107–130.

Brown, J. B., Redmond, A., Bass, K., Liebergott, J., & Swope, S. (1975). *Symbolic play in normal and language-impaired children.* Paper presented at the 50th Convention of the American Speech and Hearing Association, Washington, DC.

Brown, R. (1956). Language and categories. Appendix to J. S. Bruner, J. J. Goodnow, & G. A. Austin, *A study in thinking.* New York: Wiley.

Brown, R. (1958). How shall a thing be called? *Psychological Review, 65,* 14–21.

Brown, R. (1968). The development of wh questions in child speech. *Journal of Verbal Learning and Verbal Behavior, 7,* 279–290.

Brown, R. (1973). *A first language, the early stages.* Cambridge, MA: Harvard University Press.

Brown, R., & McNeill, D. (1966). The tip of the tongue phenomena. *Journal of Verbal Learning and Verbal Behavior, 5,* 1–11.

Bruner, J. (1983). *Child's talk: Learning to use language.* New York: Norton.

Buddenhagen, R. (1971). *Establishing vocalizations in mute mongoloid children.* Champaign, IL: Research Press.

Buium, N., Rynders, J., & Turnure, J. (1974). Early maternal linguistic environment of normal and Down's syndrome language-learning children. *American Journal of Mental Deficiency, 79,* 52–58.

Burgener, G. W., & Mouw, J. T. (1982). Minimal hearing loss' effect on academic/intellectual performance of children. *Hearing Instruments, 33,* 3.

Bzoch, K., & League, R. (1971). *Assessing language skills in infancy: A handbook for the multidimensional analysis of emergent language.* Baltimore: University Park Press.

Campbell, M., Geller, B., Small, A., Petti, T., & Ferris, S. (1978). Minor physical anomalies in young psychotic children. *American Journal of Psychiatry, 135,* 573–575.

Campbell, M., Hardesty, A., Breuer, H., & Polevoy, N. (1978). Childhood psychosis in perspective. *Journal of the American Academy of Child Psychiatry, 17,* 14–28.

Campbell, T. F., & McNeil, M. R. (1985). Effects of presentation rate and divided attention on auditory comprehension in children with an acquired language disorder. *Journal of Speech and Hearing Research, 28,* 513–520.

Cantwell, D. P., Baker, L., & Rutter, M. (1977). Families of autistic and dysphasic children II: Mother's speech to the children. *Journal of Autism and Childhood Schizophrenia, 7,* 313–327.

Cantwell, D. P., Baker, L., & Rutter, M. (1978). A comparative study of infantile autism and specific developmental receptive language disorder. IV. Analysis of syntax and language function. *Journal of Child Psychology and Psychiatry, 19,* 351–362.

Carrier, J. (1974a). Application of functional analysis and a non-speech response mode to teaching language. In L. McReynolds (Ed.), *Developing systematic procedures for training children's language. ASHA Monographs* (No. 18).

Carrier, J. (1974b). Nonspeech noun usage training with severely and profoundly retarded children. *Journal of Speech and Hearing Research, 17,* 510–518.

Carrow, E. (1972). Assessment of speech and language in children. In J. E. McLean, D. E., Yoder, & R. L. Schiefelbusch (Eds.), *Language intervention with the retarded.* Baltimore: University Park Press.

Carrow, E. (1973). *Test for auditory comprehension of language.* Austin, TX: Learning Concepts.

Carrow, E. (1974). *Elicited language inventory.* Austin, TX: Learning Concepts.

Carrow-Woolfolk, E., & Lynch, J. (1982). *An integrative approach to language disorders in children.* New York: Grune & Stratton.

Carter, A. (1979). Prespeech meaning relations: An outline of one infant's sensorimotor morpheme development. In P. Fletcher & M. Garman (Eds.), *Language acquisition.* Cambridge: Cambridge University Press.

Casby, M. W., & Ruder, K. F. (1983). Symbolic play and early language development in normal and mentally retarded children. *Journal of Speech and Hearing Research, 26,* 404–412.

Case, R. (1978). Intellectual development from birth to adulthood: A neo-Piagetian interpretation. In A. Siegler (Ed.). *Children's thinking: what develops* Hillsdale, NJ: Erlbaum.

Case, R. (1985). *Intellectual development: Birth to adulthood.* New York: Academic Press.

Case, R., Kurland, M., & Goldberg, J. (1982). Operational efficiency and the growth of short term memory span. *Journal of Experimental Child Psychology, 33,* 386–404.

Cattell, P. (1947). *The measurement of intelligence of infants and young children.* New York: Psychological Corp.

Cazden, C. (1970). The neglected situation in child language research and education. In F. Williams (Ed.), *Language and poverty, perspectives on a theme.* Chicago: Markham.

Ceci, S. (Ed.) (1986). *Handbook of cognitive, social, and neuropsychological aspects of learning disabilities Volume 1.* Hillsdale, NJ: Erlbaum.

Chafe, W. (1971). *Meaning and the structure of language.* Chicago: University of Chicago Press.

Chapman, R. (1977). Comprehension strategies in children. In J. Kavanagh & P. Strange (Eds.), *Language and speech in the laboratory, school and clinic.* Cambridge, MA: M.I.T. Press.

Chapman, R. (1981). Exploring children's communicative intents. In J. Miller (Ed.), *Assessing language production in children.* Baltimore: University Park Press.

Chapman, R., & Miller, J. (1975). Word order in early two and three word sentences. *Journal of Speech and Hearing Research, 18,* 355–371.

Chapman, R., & Miller, J. (1980). Analyzing language and communication in the child. In R. Schiefelbusch (Ed.), *Nonspeech language and communication: Analysis and intervention.* Baltimore: University Park Press.

Cherry, C. (1957). *On human communication: A review, a survey, and a criticism.* Cambridge, MA: M.I.T. Press.

Chi, M. T. H. (1978). Knowledge structures and memory development. In R. Siegler (Ed.), *Children's thinking: What develops?* Hillsdale, NJ: Erlbaum.

Chi, M. T. H. (Ed.). (1983). *Trends in memory development research.* New York: Karger.

Chomsky, N. (1965). *Aspects of the theory of syntax.* Cambridge, MA: M.I.T. Press.

Chomsky, N. (1966). *Cartesian linguistics: A chapter in the history of rationalist thought.* New York: Harper & Row.

Chomsky, N. (1972). *Language and mind.* New York: Harcourt Brace Jovanovich.

Clark, C. R., & Woodcock, R. W. (1976). Graphic systems of communication. In L. Lloyd (Ed.), *Communication assessment and intervention strategies.* Baltimore: University Park Press.

Clark, E. (1973). Non-linguistic strategies and the acquisition of word meanings. *Cognition, 2,* 161–182.

Clark, E., & Andersen, E. (1979). Spontaneous repairs: Awareness in the process of acquiring language. *Papers and Reports in Child Language Development,* Stanford University, Palo Alto, CA. *16,* 1–12.

Clark, P., & Rutter, M. (1981). Autistic children's responses to structure and to interpersonal demands. *Journal of Autism and Developmental Disabilities, 11,* 201–217.

Coggins, T. (1979). Relational meaning encoded in the two-word utterances of stage I Down's syndrome children. *Journal of Speech and Hearing Research, 22,* 166–178.

Coggins, T., Olswang, L., & Guthrie, J. (1987). Assessing communicative intents in young children: Low structured observation or elicitation tasks? *Journal of Speech and Hearing Disorders, 52,* 44–49.

Cohen, A. (1973). Smallest space analysis of the Revised Illinois Test of Psycholinguistic Abilities. *Psychology in the Schools, 10,* 107–110.

Cole, K., & Dale, P. (1986). Direct language instruction and interactive language instruction with language delayed preschool children: A comparison study. *Journal of Speech and Hearing Research, 29,* 206–217.

Cole, L., & Campbell-Calloway, M. (1983). Resource guide to mulitcultural tests and materials supplement I. *Asha, 21,* 37–41.

Cole, P. (1982). *Language disorders in preschool children.* Englewood-Cliffs, NJ: Prentice-Hall.

Coleman, M. (1980). An overview of Down's syndrome. *Seminars in Speech and Language, 1,* 1–8.

Connell, P. (1986). Acquisition of semantic role by language-disordered children: Differences between production and comprehension. *Journal of Speech and Hearing Research, 29,* 366–374.

Connell, P., Gardner-Gletty, D., Dejewski, J., & Parks-Reinick, L. (1981). Response to Courtright and Courtright. *Journal of Speech and Hearing Research, 46,* 146–148.

Connell, P., & McReynolds, L. (1981). An experimental analysis of children's generalization during lexical learning: Comprehension and production. *Applied Psycholinguistics, 2,* 309–332.

Connell, P., & Myles-Zitzer, C. (1982). An analysis of elicited imitation as a language evaluation procedure. *Journal of Speech and Hearing Disorders, 47,* 390–396.

Connelly, R. (1974). *The effect of knowledge of linguistic codes on auditory sequential memory.* Unpublished manuscript, Montclair State College, NJ.

Constable, C. (1983). Creating communicative context. In H. Winitz (Ed.), *Treating language disorders: For clinicians by clinicians.* Baltimore: University Park Press.

Constable, C. (1986). The application of scripts in the organization of language intervention contexts. In K. Nelson (Ed.), *Event knowledge.* Hillsdale, NJ: Erlbaum.

Constable, C., & Lahey, M. (1984). *Analyzing interactional episodes: Does the method make a difference?* Paper presented at the Symposium on Research in Child Language Disorders, Madison, WI.

Conti-Ramsden, G., & Friel-Patti, S. (1983). Mothers' discourse adjustments to language-impaired and non-language-impaired children. *Journal of Speech and Hearing Disorders, 48,* 360–367.

Cooper, J. M., & Griffiths, P. (1978). Treatment and prognosis. In M. Wyke (Ed.), *Developmental dysphasia.* London: Academic Press.

Coplan, J. (1983). *Early Language Milestone Scale,* Tulsa, OK: Modern Education Corp.

Corman, H., & Escalona, S. (1969). Stages of sensorimotor development: A replication study. *Merrill-Palmer Quarterly, 15,* 351–361.

Courtright, J. A., & Courtright, I. C. (1976). Imitative modeling as a theoretical base for instructing language-disordered children. *Journal of Speech and Hearing Research, 19,* 655–663.

Courtright, J. A., & Courtright, I. C. (1979). Imitative modeling as a language intervention strategy: The effects of two mediating variables. *Journal of Speech and Hearing Research, 22,* 389–402.

Courtright, J. A., & Courtright, I. C. (1983). The perception of nonverbal vocal cues of emotional meaning by language-disordered and normal children. *Journal of Speech and Hearing Research, 26,* 412–418.

Cox, A., Rutter, M., Newman, S., & Bartak, L. (1975). A comparative study of infantile autism and specific developmental receptive language disorder II: Parental characteristics. *British Journal of Psychiatry, 126,* 146–159.

Crabtree, N. (1958). *The Houston Test of Language Development.* Houston: Houston Test Co.

Craig, H. (1983). Applications of pragmatic language models for intervention. In T. Gallagher & C. Prutting (Eds.), *Pragmatic assessment and intervention issues in language.* San Diego: College-Hill Press.

Craig, H., & Gallagher, T. (1986). Interactive play: The frequency of related verbal responses. *Journal of Speech and Hearing Research, 29,* 375–383.

Crais, E., & Chapman, R. (1987). Story recall and inferencing skills in language/learning-disabled children. *Journal of Speech and Hearing Disorders, 52,* 50–55.

Cramblit, N. S., & Siegel, G. M. (1977). The verbal environment of a language-impaired child. *Journal of Speech and Hearing Disorders, 42,* 474–482.

Creak, M., & Committee. (1961). Schizophrenic syndrome in childhood. *Cerebral Palsy Bulletin, 3,* 501–504.

Cromer, R. F. (1978). The basis of childhood dysphasia: A linguistic approach. In M. A. Wyke (Ed.), *Developmental dysphasia* (pp. 104–105). New York: Academic Press.

Cromer, R. (1986, October). *Case studies of dissociations between language and cognition.* Paper presented at the 11th Annual Boston University Conference on Language Development, Boston.

Cronbach, L. (1984). *Essentials of psychological testing, fourth edition,* New York: Harper & Row.

Cross, T. (1978). Mothers' speech and its association with rate of linguistic development in young children. In N. Waterson & C. E. Snow (Eds.), *The development of communication.* New York: Wiley.

Cruickshank, W. M., Bentsen, F. A., Retzburg, F. H., & Tannhauser, M. T. (1961). *A teaching method for brain injured and hyperactive children.* Syracuse, NY: Syracuse University Press.

Crystal, D. (1982). *Profiling linguistic disability.* London: Arnold.

Crystal, D., Fletcher, P., & Garman, M. (1976). *The grammatical analysis of language disability: A procedure for assessment and remediation*. London: Arnold.

Cullata, B., & Horn, D. (1981). Systematic modification of parental input to train language symbols. *Language, Speech, and Hearing Services in the Schools, 12*, 4–13.

Cunningham, C., Siegel, L., van der Spuy, H., Clark, M., & Bow, S. (1985). The behavioral and linguistic interactions of specifically language-delayed and normal boys and their mothers. *Child Development, 56*, 1389–1403.

Cunningham, M. (1968). A comparison of the language of psychotic and non-psychotic children who are mentally retarded. *Journal of Child Psychology and Psychiatry, 9*, 229–244.

Curtiss, S. (1981). Dissociations between language and cognition: Cases and implications. *Journal of Autism and Developmental Disorders, 11*, 15–31.

Curtiss, S., Prutting, C. A., & Lowell, E. L. (1979). Pragmatic and semantic development in young children with impaired hearing. *Journal of Speech and Hearing Research, 22*, 534–552.

Damasio, A. R., & Mauer, R. G. (1978). A neurological model for childhood autism. *Archives of Neurology, 35*, 777–786.

Damasio, H., Mauer, R., Damasio, A., & Chui, H. (1980). Computerized tomographic scan findings in patients with autistic behavior. *Archives of Neurology, 37*, 504–510.

Danwitz, M. W. (1981). Formal versus informal assessment: Fragmentation versus holism. *Topics in Language Disorders, 1*, 95–106.

Darley, F. L. (1979). *Evaluation of appraisal techniques in speech and language pathology*. Reading, MA: Addison-Wesley.

Darley, F. L., & Moll, K. (1960). Reliability of language measures and size of language sample. *Journal of Speech and Hearing Research, 3*, 166–173.

Das, J. P., Dirby, J. R., & Jarman, R. F. (1975). Simultaneous and successive syntheses: An alternative model for cognitive abilities. *Psychological Bulletin, 82*, 87–103.

Davis, J., Elfenbein, J., Schum, R., & Bentler, R. (1986). Effects of mild and moderate hearing impairments on language, educational, and psychosocial behavior of children. *Journal of Speech and Hearing Disorders, 51*, 53–62.

Davis, J., Shepard, N., Stelmachowicz, P., & Gorga, M. (1981). Characteristics of hearing-impaired children in the public schools: Part II, psychoeducational data. *Journal of Speech and Hearing Disorders, 46*, 130–137.

Deal, V., & Yan, M. (1985). Resource guide to multicultural tests and materials: Supplement II. *Asha, 27*, 43–49.

deBaryshe, B., Whitehurst, G., & Fischel, J. (1986). *Referential and expressive speech styles in children with delayed productive language*. Poster paper at the Boston University Conference on Language Development, Boston.

deHirsch, K., & Jansky, J. (1977). Patterning and organizational deficits in children with language and learning disabilities. *Bulletin of the Orton Society, 27*, 88–101.

Delacato, C. H. (1963). *The diagnosis and treatment of speech and reading problems*. Springfield, IL: Thomas.

Dempster, F. (1981). Memory span: Source of individual and developmental differences. *Psychological Bulletin, 89*, 63–100.

De Meyer, M. K., Hingtgen, J. N., & Jackson, R. D. (1981). Infantile autism reviewed: A decade of research. *Schizophrenia Bulletin, 7*, 388–443.

Denkla, M. (1985). Motor coordination in dyslexic children: Theoretical and clinical implications. In F. Duffy & N. Geshwind (Eds.), *Dyslexia: A neuroscientific approach to clinical evaluation*. Boston: Little, Brown.

Denkla, M. (1986). New diagnostic criteria for autism or related behavioral disorder—Guidelines for research protocols. *Journal of the American Academy of Child Psychiatry, 25*, 221–224.

Denkla, M., & Rudel, R. (1976a). Naming of object-drawings by dyslexic and other learning disabled children. *Brain and Language, 3,* 1–15.

Denkla, M., & Rudel, R. (1976b). Rapid "automatized" naming (RAN): Dyslexia differentiated from other learning disabilities. *Neuropsychologia, 14,* 471–478.

Denkla, M., Rudel, R., & Broman, M. (1981). Tests that discriminate between dyslexic and other learning-disabled boys. *Brain and Language, 13,* 118–129.

Dever, R. (1972). A comparison of the results of a revised version of Berko's test of morphology with the free speech of mentally retarded children. *Journal of Speech and Hearing Research, 15,* 169–178.

Dever, R. (1978). *TALK: Teaching American language to kids,* Columbus, OH: C. Merrill.

Dever, R., & Bauman, P. (1974). Scale of children's clausal development. In T. Longhurst (Ed.), *Linguistic analysis of children's speech.* New York: M.S.S. Information Corp.

de Villiers, J., & de Villiers, P. (1973). A cross-sectional study of the acquisition of grammatical morphemes. *Journal of Psycholinguistic Research, 2,* 267–278.

de Villiers, P., & de Villiers, J. (1986). *Parallels and divergences in the acquisition of oral English by deaf and hearing children: Evidence for structural constraints.* Paper presented at the Boston University Conference on Language Development, Boston.

Diamond, S. (1979). *Short term memory as a function of familiarity with a linguistic code.* Unpublished master's thesis, Hunter College of the City University of New York.

Doll, E. A. (1965). *Vineland Social Maturity Scale.* Minneapolis: American Guidance Service.

Dollaghan, C. (1985). Child meets word: "Fast mapping" in preschool children. *Journal of Speech and Hearing Research, 28,* 449–454.

Dollaghan, C. (1987). Fast mapping in normal and language-impaired children. *Journal of Speech and Hearing Disorders, 52,* 218–222.

Dollaghan, C., & Miller, J. (1986). Observational methods in the study of communicative competence. In R. Schiefelbusch (Ed.), *Language competence: Assessment and intervention.* San Diego: College-Hill Press.

Donahue, M. (1986a). Phonological constraints on the emergence of two-word utterances. *Journal of Child Language, 13,* 209–218.

Donahue, M. (1986b). Linguistic and communicative development in learning-disabled children. In C. Ceci (Ed.), *Handbook of cognitive, social, and neuropsychological aspects of learning disabilities* (Vol. 1). New York: Erlbaum.

Donahue, M., Pearl, R., & Bryan, T. (1980). Learning disabled children's conversational competence: Responses to inadequate messages. *Applied Psycholinguistics, 1,* 387–404.

Donahue, M., Pearl, P., & Bryan, T. (1982). Learning disabled children's syntactic proficiency on a communicative task. *Journal of Speech and Hearing Disorders, 47,* 397–403.

Donnellan, A. M., Anderson, J. L., & Mesaros, R. A. (1984). An observational study of stereotypic behavior and proximity related to the occurrence of autistic child and family member interactions. *Journal of Autism and Developmental Disabilities, 14,* 205–210.

Dore, J. (1975). Holophrases, speech acts, and language universals. *Journal of Child Language, 2,* 21–40.

Dore, J. (1977). Children's illocutionary acts. In R. O. Freedle (Ed.), *Discourse processes: Advances in research and theory: Vol. 1. Discourse production and comprehension.* Norwood, NJ: Ablex.

Dore, J. (1986). The development of communicative competence. In R. Schiefelbusch (Ed.), *Language competence: Assessment and intervention.* San Diego: College-Hill Press.

Dore, J., Franklin, M., Miller, R., & Ramer, A. (1976). Transitional phenomena in early language acquisition. *Journal of Child Language, 3,* 13–28.

Downs, M. (1983). Audiologist's overview of sequelae of early otitis media. *Pediatrics, 71,* 643–644.

Duchan, J. (1982). The elephant is soft and mushy: Problems in assessing children's language. In N. Lass, L. McReynolds, J. Northern, & D. Yoder (Eds.), *Speech, language, and hearing.* Philadelphia: Saunders.

Duchan, J. (1986). Language intervention through sensemaking and fine tuning. In R. Schiefelbusch (Ed.), *Communicative competence: Assessment and language intervention.* Baltimore: University Park Press.

Duchan, J., & Erickson, J. G. (1976). Normal and retarded children's understanding of semantic relations in different verbal contexts. *Journal of Speech and Hearing Research, 19,* 767–777.

Dunn, L. (1965). *Peabody Picture Vocabulary Test.* Circle Pines, MN: American Guidance Service.

Dunn, L., & Dunn, L. (1981). *Peabody Picture Vocabulary Test—Revised.* Circle Pines, MN: American Guidance Service.

Dunn, L., Padilla, E., Lugo, D., & Dunn, L. (1986). *Test de Vocabulario en Imagenes Peabody: Adaptacion Hispanoamericana.* Circle Pines, MN: American Guidance Service.

Eckelman, B. L., & Aram, D. M. (1983). Syntactic findings in developmental verbal apraxia. *Journal of Communication Disorders, 16,* 237–250.

Efron, R. (1963). Temporal perception, aphasia, and deja vu. *Brain, 86,* 403–424.

Eisenberg, L. (1967). Psychotic disorder in childhood. In L. D. Eron (Ed.), *The classification of behavior disorders.* Chicago: Aldine.

Eisenson, J. (1968). Developmental aphasia: A speculative view with therapeutic implications. *Journal of Speech and Hearing Disorders, 33,* 3–13.

Eisenson, J. (1972). *Aphasia in children.* New York: Harper & Row.

Eisenson, J., & Ingram, D. (1972). Childhood aphasia—An updated concept based on recent research. *Acta Symbolica, 3,* 108–116.

Elkins, J. (1972). *Some psycholinguistic aspects of the differential diagnosis of reading disability in grades I and II.* Doctoral dissertation, University of Queensland.

Emerick, L., & Hatten, J. (1974). *Diagnosis and evaluation in speech pathology.* Englewood Cliffs, NJ: Prentice-Hall.

Emerick, L., & Haynes, W. (1986). *Diagnosis and evaluation in speech pathology. Third edition.* Englewood Cliffs, NJ: Prentice-Hall.

Engler, L., Hannah, E., & Longhurst, T. (1973). Linguistic analysis of speech samples: A practical guide for clinicians. *Journal of Speech and Hearing Disorders, 38,* 192–204.

Ervin-Tripp, S., & Gordon, D. (1986). The development of requests. In R. Schiefelbusch (Ed.), *Language competence assessment and intervention.* San Diego: College-Hill Press.

Evans, D., & Hampson, M. (1968). The language of mongols. *British Journal of Disorders of Communication, 3,* 171–181.

Fay, W. H. (1969). On the basis of autistic echolalia. *Journal of Communication Disorders, 2,* 38–47.

Fay, W. H., & Schuler, A. L. (Eds.). (1980). *Emerging language in autistic children.* Baltimore: University Park Press.

Fee, J., & Ingram, D. (1982). Reduplication as a strategy of phonological development. *Journal of Child Language, 9,* 41–54.

Feintuck, F. (1985). *A cross-sectional study of the development of verb inflections in child language.* Unpublished doctoral dissertation, City University of New York.

Ferguson, C., & Farwell, C. B. (1975). Words and sounds in early language acquisition. *Language, 51,* 419–439.

Ferguson, C., Peizer, D., & Weeks, T. (1973). Model-and-replica phonological grammar of a child's first words. *Lingua, 31,* 35–39.

Fey, M. (1986). *Language intervention with young children.* San Diego: College-Hill Press.

Fey, M., Leonard, L., & Wilcox, K. (1981). Speech style modifications of language impaired children. *Journal of Speech and Hearing Disorders, 46,* 91–96.

Fillmore, C. (1968). The case for case. In E. Bach & R. T. Harms (Eds.), *Universals in linguistic theory.* New York: Holt, Rinehart and Winston.

Flax, J. (1986). *Functional intonation in the prelinguistic and early linguistic child.* Unpublished doctoral dissertation, City University of New York.

Fletcher, J., & Morris, R. (1986). Classification of disabled learners: Beyond exclusionary definitions. In S. Ceci (Ed.), *Handbook of cognitive, social, and neuropsychological aspects of learning disabilities.* Hillsdale, NJ: Erlbaum.

Flores d'Arcais, G. (1978). The acquisition of the subordinate constructions in children's language. In R. Campbell & P. Smith (Eds.), *Recent advances in the psychology of language.* Plenum Press.

Fodor, J., Bever, T. G., & Garrett, M. F. (1974). *The psychology of language.* New York: McGraw Hill.

Folger, J. P., & Chapman, R. S. (1978). A pragmatic analysis of spontaneous imitations. *Journal of Child Language, 5,* 25–38.

Folstein, S., & Rutter, M. (1977). Genetic influences and infantile autism. *Nature, 265,* 726–728.

Forster, K. (1976). Accessing the mental lexicon. In M. Wales & E. Walker, *New approaches to language mechanisms.* New York: Elsevier.

Foster, R., Giddan, J., & Stark, J. (1973). *Assessment of children's language comprehension.* Austin, TX: Learning Concepts.

Fowler, A. (1986). *Maturational determinants and constraints in rate of language growth in children with Down's syndrome.* Paper presented at the Boston University Conference on Language Development, Boston.

Fowler, A. (in press). The development of language structure in children with Down syndrome. In D. Cicchetti and M. Beeghly (Eds.), *Down Syndrome: The developmental perspective.* New York: Cambridge University Press.

Fowler, A., Gelman, R., & Gleitman, L. (1980). *A comparison of normal and retardate language equated on MLU.* Paper presented at the Boston University Conference on Language Development, Boston.

Fowles, B., & Glanz, M. E. (1977). Competence and talent in verbal riddle comprehension. *Journal of Child Language, 4,* 433–452.

Fraiberg, S. (1977). *Insights from the blind.* London: Souvenir Press.

Frankenburg, W., & Dodd, J. (1969). *Denver developmental screening test.* Denver, CO: University of Colorado Medical Center.

Frankenburg, W., et al. (1975). *Denver developmental screening test.* Denver, CO: LADOCA Project and Publishers Foundation.

Freedman, P. P., & Carpenter, R. L. (1976). Semantic relations used by normal and language-impaired children at stage 1. *Journal of Speech and Hearing Research, 19,* 784–795.

Freidus, E. (1964). Methodology for the classroom teacher. In J. Hellmuth (Ed.), *The special child in century 21.* Seattle, WA: Special Child Publications of the Seguin School.

French, L. A., & Nelson, K. (1982). Taking away the supportive context: Preschoolers' talk about the "then and there." *The Quarterly Newsletter of the Laboratory of Comparative Human Cognition, 4,* 1–6.

Friedlander, B. S. (1970). Receptive language development in infancy. *Merrill-Palmer Quarterly, 16,* 7–51.

Fristoe, M., & Lloyd, L. (1980). Planning an initial expressive sign lexicon for persons with severe communication impairment. *Journal of Speech and Hearing Disorders, 45,* 170–180.

Furth, H. (1966). *Thinking without language: Psychological implications of deafness.* New York: Free Press.

Gaines, B. H., & Prutting, C. A. (1982). *Non-social and social tool use abilities of Down's syndrome and normal infants.* Unpublished paper.

Galda, L. (1984). Narrative competence: Play, storytelling, and story comprehension. In

A. D. Pellegrin & T. Yawkey (Eds.), *The development of oral and written language in social contexts* (pp. 105–117). Norwood, NJ: Ablex.

Gall, F. L. (1835). *Organology* (W. Lewis, Trans.; Vol. 5). Boston: Marsh, Cappen & Lyon.

Gallagher, T. (1977). Revision behaviors in the speech of normal children developing language. *Journal of Speech and Hearing Research, 20,* 303–318.

Gallagher, T. (1981). Contingent query sentences within adult-child discourse. *Journal of Child Language, 8,* 51–62.

Gallagher, T. (1983). Pre-assessment: A procedure for accommodating language use variability. In T. Gallagher & C. Prutting (Eds.), *Assessment and intervention issues in language.* San Diego: College-Hill Press.

Gallagher, T., & Darnton, B. (1978). Conversational aspects of the speech of language disordered children: Revision behaviors. *Journal of Speech and Hearing Research, 21,* 118–135.

Garcia, E. (1974). The training and generalization of a conversational speech form in non-verbal retardates. *Journal of Applied Behavior Analysis, 7,* 137–149.

Gardner, R. (1979). *One-word Expressive Vocabulary Test.* Novato, CA: Academic Therapy Publications.

Garman, M. (1979). Early grammatical development. In P. Fletcher & M. Garman (Eds.), *Language acquisition.* London: Cambridge University Press.

Garrard, K. R., & Clark, B. S. (1985). Otitis media: The role of the speech-language pathologist. *Asha, 27,* 35–39.

Gat, I., & Keith, R. (1979). An effect of linguistic experience on auditory word discrimination by native and non-native speakers of English. *Audiology, 17,* 339–345.

Gee, J., & Savasir, I. (1985). On the use of WILL and GONNA: Towards a description of activity types for child language. *Discourse Processes, 8,* 143–175.

Geers, A., & Moog, J. (1987). Predicting spoken language acquisition of profoundly hearing-impaired children. *Journal of Speech and Hearing Disorders, 52,* 84–94.

Geers, A., Moog, J., & Schick, B. (1984). Acquisition of spoken and signed English by profoundly deaf children. *Journal of Speech and Hearing Disorders, 49,* 378–388.

Geller, E. (in press). The assessment of perspective taking skill. In A. Luce (Ed.), *Seminars in speech and language.*

Geller, E. (in preparation). *The interplay between social and linguistic knowledge in perspective taking by autistic children.* Doctoral dissertation in progress, City University of New York.

Geller, E., & Wollner, S. (1976). *A preliminary investigation of the communicative competence of three linguistically impaired children.* Paper presented to New York State Speech and Hearing Association.

Gerber, S. (1987). *Form and function in early language development.* Unpublished doctoral dissertation, City University of New York.

Gerkin, K. P. (1984). The high risk register for deafness. *Asha, 26*(3), 17–23.

German, D. (1986). *Test of Word Finding.* Allen, TX: DLM Teaching Resources.

Gibson, J. J. (1966). *The senses considered as perceptual systems.* Boston: Houghton Mifflin.

Glaser, R., & Nitko, A. (1971). Measurement in learning and instruction. In R. Thorndike (Ed.), *Educational measurement.* (pp. 625–670). Washington, DC: American Council on Education.

Gleitman, L. (1986). *Discussant. Theoretical issues in the acquisition of grammar: Evidence from children with sensory, cognitive or neurological deficits.* Boston University Conference on Language Development, Boston.

Glucksberg, S., Krauss, R., & Higgens, E. T. (1975). The development of referential communication skills. In F. Horowitz (Ed.), *Review of child development research* (Vol. 4). Chicago: University of Chicago Press.

Goda, S., & Griffith, B. C. (1962). The spoken language of adolescent retardates and its relation to intelligence, age, and anxiety. *Child Development, 33,* 489–498.

Goetz, L., Schuler, A., & Sailor, W. (1979). Teaching functional speech to the severely handicapped: Current issues. *Journal of Autism and Developmental Disorders, 9,* 325–343.

Goldin-Meadow, S., Seligman, M., & Gelman, R. (1976). Language in the two-year-old: Receptive and productive stages. *Cognition, 4,* 189–202.

Goldfarb, W., Goldfarb, N., & Scholl, H. (1966). The speech of mothers of schizophrenic children. *American Journal of Psychiatry, 122,* 1220–1227.

Goldfarb, W., Levy, D., & Meyers, D. (1972). The mother speaks to her schizophrenic child: Language in childhood schizophrenia. *Psychiatry, 35,* 217–226.

Goldman, R., Fristoe, M., & Woodcock, R. W. (1969, 1972). *The Goldman-Fristoe-Woodcock Test of Auditory Discrimination.* Circle-Pines, MN: American Guidance Service.

Goldman, R., Fristoe, M., & Woodcock, R. W. (1974). *The Goldman, Fristoe, Woodcock Auditory Skills Battery.* Circle Pines, MN: American Guidance Service.

Goldstein, R., Landau, W., & Kleffner, F. (1958). Neurologic assessment of some deaf and aphasic children. *Annals of Otology, Rhinology and Laryngology, 67,* 468–479.

Golinkoff, R., & Markessini, J. (1980). "Mommy sock:" The child's understanding of possession as expressed in two-noun phrases. *Journal of Child Language, 7,* 119–136.

Goorell, S. (1971). *An investigation of the social interactions occurring among comparable groups of normal hearing and hearing impaired children using an interaction scale.* Unpublished master's thesis, University of Cincinnati, Cincinnati, OH.

Gopnik, A. (1981). The development of non-nominal expressions: Why the first words are not about things. In D. Ingram & P. Dale (Eds.), *Child language: An international perspective.* Baltimore: University Park Press.

Gorth, W., & Hambleton, R. (1972). Measurement considerations for criterion-referenced testing and special education. *Journal of Special Education, 6,* 303–314.

Goss, R. (1970, March). Language used by mothers of deaf children and mothers of hearing children. *American Annals of the Deaf,* pp. 93–95.

Graham, N. C. (1968). Short-term memory and syntactic structure in educationally subnormal children. *Language and Speech, 11,* 209–219.

Gray, B. B., & Ryan, B. (1973). *A language training program for the non-language child.* Champaign, IL: Research Press.

Graybeal, C. M. (1981). Memory for stories in language-impaired children. *Applied Psycholinguistics, 2,* 169–283.

Greenfield, P., & Smith, J. (1976). *The structure of communication in early language development.* New York: Academic Press.

Greenwald, C. A., & Leonard, L. (1979). Communicative and sensorimotor development of Down's syndrome children. *American Journal of Mental Deficiency, 84,* 296–303.

Griffiths, R. (1970). *The abilities of young children.* London: Child Development Research Centre.

Grossman, H. J. (1973). *Manual on terminology and classification in mental retardation* (Special Publication Series No. 2). Washington, DC: American Association for Mental Deficiency.

Guess, D. (1969). A functional analysis of receptive language and productive speech: Acquisition of the plural morpheme. *Journal of Applied Behavior Analysis, 2,* 55–64.

Guess, D., & Baer, D. M. (1973). An analysis of individual differences in generalization between receptive and productive language in retarded children. *Journal of Applied Behavior Analysis, 6,* 311–329.

Guess, D., Rutherford, G., & Twichell, A. (1969). Speech acquisition in a mute, visually impaired adolescent. *New Outlook for the Blind, 63,* 8–13.

Guralnick, M., & Paul-Brown, D. (1986). Communicative interactions of mildly delayed and normally developing preschool children: Effects of listener's developmental age. *Journal of Speech and Hearing Research, 29,* 2–10.

Hafitz, J., Gartner, B., & Bloom, L. (1980). *Giving complements when you're two: The acquisition of complement structures in child language.* Paper presented at the Boston University Conference on Language Development, Boston.

Hall, P., & Tomblin, J. (1978). A follow-up study of children with articulation and language disorders. *Journal of Speech and Hearing Disorders, 43*, 227–241.

Halliday, M. A. K. (1973). *Explorations in the functions of language.* London: Edward Arnold.

Halliday, M. A. K. (1975). *Learning how to mean—Explorations in the development of language.* London: Arnold.

Halliday, M. A. K., & Hasan, R. (1975). *Cohesion in English.* London: Longman.

Hammill, D., Brown, B. S., Larsen, S. C., & Wiederholt, J. (1980). *Test of Adolescent Language.* Austin, TX: Pro-Ed.

Hammill, D., & Larsen, S. C. (1974). The effectiveness of psycholinguistic training. *Exceptional Children, 40*, 5–13.

Hammill, D., Leigh, J. E., McNutt, G., & Larsen, S. C. (1981). A new definition of learning disabilities. *Learning Disability Quarterly, 4*, 336–342.

Hammill, D., Newcomer, P. (1982). *Test of Language Development: Intermediate Edition.* San Antonio, TX: Psychological Corp.

Hanif, M. H., & Siegel, G. M. (1981). The effect of context on verbal elicited imitation. *Journal of Speech and Hearing Disorders, 46*, 27–30.

Hardy, W. G. (1965). On language disorders in young children: A reorganization of thinking. *Journal of Speech and Hearing Disorders, 30*, 3–16.

Harris, D. B. (1963). *Children's drawings as a measure of intellectual maturity. A revision and extension of the Goodenough Draw-A-Man Test.* New York: Harcourt, Brace and World.

Harris, D., & Vanderheiden, G. (1980). Augmentative communication techniques. In R. Schiefelbusch (Ed.), *Nonspeech language and communication: Analysis and intervention.* Baltimore: University Park Press.

Harris, S., Wolchik, S., & Weitz, S. (1981). The acquisition of language skill by autistic children: Can parents do the job? *Journal of Autism and Developmental Disabilities,* 373–384.

Hart, B. (1985). Naturalistic language training techniques. In S. Warren and A. Rogers-Warren (Eds.), *Teaching functional language.* Baltimore: University Park Press.

Hart, B., & Risley, T. (1968). Establishing the use of descriptive adjectives in the spontaneous speech of disadvantaged preschool children. *Journal of Applied Behavior Analysis, 1*, 109–120.

Hart, B., & Risley, T. (1980). In vivo language intervention: Unanticipated general effects. *Journal of Applied Behavior Analysis, 13*, 407–432.

Hart, B., & Rogers-Warren, A. (1978). A milieu approach to language teaching. In R. L. Schiefelbusch (Ed.), *Language intervention strategies.* Baltimore: University Park Press.

Haynes, W., & Haynes, M. (1980). A comparison of nonimitative modeling and mimicry procedures for training the singular copula in black preschool children. *Journal of Communication Disorders, 13*, 277–288.

Heath, S. B. (1986, December). Taking a cross-cultural look at narratives. *Topics in Language Disorders, 7*, 84–95.

Hecaen, H. (1983). Acquired aphasia in children: Revisited. *Neuropsychologia, 21*, 581–587.

Hedrick, D., Prather, E., & Tobin, A. (1975). *Sequenced Inventory of Communication Development.* Seattle, WA: University of Washington Press.

Heider, F. K., & Heider, G. M. (1940). A comparison of sentence structure of deaf and hearing children. *Psychological Monographs, 52*, 42–103.

Hejna, R. (1959). *Developmental Articulation Test.* Ann Arbor, MI: Speech Materials.

Helm, D., & Kozloff, M. (1986). Research on parent training: Shortcomings and remedies. *Journal of Autism and Developmental Disabilities, 16*, 1–22.

Henderson, K. B. (1961). Uses of subject matter. In B. O. Smith & R. H. Ennis (Eds.), *Language and concepts in education* (pp. 43–58). Chicago: Rand McNally.

Henig, R. M. (1986, May). The problem with learning problems. *Psychology Today*, pp. 74–75.

Hermelin, B., & Frith, U. (1971). Psychological studies of childhood autism: Can autistic children make sense of what they see and hear? *Journal of Special Education, 5,* 107–116.

Hess, L. (1972). *The development of transformational structures in a deaf and a normally hearing child over a period of five months.* Unpublished master's thesis, University of Cincinnati, Cincinnati, OH.

Hewett, F. M. (1965). Teaching speech to an autistic child through operant conditioning. *American Journal of Orthopsychiatry, 35,* 927–936.

Hively, W. (1974). Domain referenced testing: Symposium. *Educational Technology, 14,* 5–64.

Holdgrapher, G. (1981). Mode relations in language learning by language deficient retarded subjects. *Perceptual and Motor Skills, 53,* 520–522.

Holland, A. (1984). *Language disorders in children.* San Diego: College-Hill Press.

Holm, V. A., & Kunze, L. H. (1969). Effect of chronic otitis media on language and speech development. *Pediatrics, 43,* 833–839.

Hood, L., & Bloom, L. (1979). What, when, and how about why: A longitudinal study of early expressions of causality. *Monographs of the Society for Research in Child Development, 44,* (Serial No. 6).

Hood, L., & Lightbown, P. (1978). What children do when asked to "Say what I say;" Does elicited imitation measure linguistic knowledge? *Allied Health, 1,* 195–220.

Howlin, P. (1981). The results of a home based language training program with autistic children. *British Journal of Communication, 16,* 73–88.

Howlin, P. (1982). Echolalic and spontaneous phrase speech in autistic children. *Journal of Child Psychology and Psychiatry, 23,* 281–293.

Hsu, J. R., Cairns, H. S., & Fiengo, R. W. (1985). The development of grammars underlying children's interpretation of complex sentences. *Cognition, 20,* 25–48.

Hubatch, L., Johnson, C., Kistler, D., Burns, W., & Moneka, W. (1985). Early language abilities of high-risk infants. *Journal of Speech and Hearing Disorders, 50,* 195–207.

Hubbell, R. D. (1977). On facilitating spontaneous talking in young children. *Journal of Speech and Hearing Disorders, 42,* 216–231.

Hubbell, R. D. (1981). *Children's language disorders: An integrated approach.* Englewood Cliffs, NJ: Prentice-Hall.

Hughes, D. (1985). *Language treatment and generalization.* San Diego: College-Hill Press.

Hulme, C. (1984). Developmental differences in the effects of acoustic similarity on memory span. *Developmental Psychology, 20,* 650–652.

Hulme, C., Thomson, N., Muir, C., & Lawrence, A. (1984). Speech rate and the development of short-term memory span. *Journal of Experimental Child Psychology, 38,* 241–253.

Hurtig, R., Enarud, S., & Tomblin, J. B. (1982). The communicative function of questions productive in autistic children. *Journal of Autism and Developmental Disabilities, 12,* 57–69.

Huttenlocher, J. (1974). The origins of language comprehension. In R. Solso (Ed.), *Theories in cognitive psychology.* New York: Halsted.

Huttenlocher, J., & Burke, D. (1976). Why does memory span increase with age? *Cognitive Psychology, 8,* 1–31.

Huttenlocher, J., Eisenberg, K., & Strauss, S. (1968). Comprehension: Relation between perceived actor and logical subject. *Journal of Verbal Learning and Verbal Behavior, 7,* 527–530.

Huttenlocher, J., & Strauss, S. (1968). Comprehension and a statement's relation to the situation it describes. *Journal of Verbal Learning and Verbal Behavior, 7,* 300–304.

Huttenlocher, J., & Weiner, S. (1971). Comprehension of instructions in varying contexts. *Cognitive Psychology, 2,* 369–385.

Hynd, G., & Obrzut, J. (Eds.) (1981). *Assessment of school-aged children.* New York: Grune & Stratton.

Ingram, D. (1972a). The acquisition of questions and its relation to cognitive development in normal and linguistically deviant children. *Papers and Reports on Child Language.* Stanford University, Palo Alto, CA.

Ingram, D. (1972b). The acquisition of the English verbal auxiliary and copula in normal and linguistically deviant children. *Papers and Reports on Child Language.* Stanford University, Palo Alto, CA.

Ingram, D. (1976). *Phonological disability in children.* New York: Elsevier.

Inhelder, B. (1976). Observations on the operational and figurative aspects of thought in dysphasic children. In D. M. Morehead & A. E. Morehead (Eds.), *Normal and deficient child language.* Baltimore: University Park Press.

Iran-Nejad, A., Ortony, A., & Rittenhouse, R. (1981). The comprehension of metaphorical uses of English by deaf children. *Journal of Speech and Hearing Research, 24,* 446–454.

Irwin, O. C., & Hammill, D. (1964). Some results with an abstraction test with cerebral palsied children. *Cerebral Palsy Journal, 25,* 10–11.

Irwin, O. C., & Hammill, D. (1965). Effect of type, extent and degree of cerebral palsy on three measures of language. *Cerebral Palsy Journal, 26,* 7–9.

Irwin, J., & Marge, M. (1972). *Principles of childhood language disabilities.* New York: Appleton-Century-Crofts.

Itard, J. (1962). *The wild boy of Aveyron.* New York: Appleton-Century-Crofts.

Jansky, J., & de Hirsch, K. (1972). *Preventing reading failure: Prediction, diagnosis, intervention.* New York: Harper & Row.

Jastak, J. F., & Jastak, S. (1978). *Wide Range Achievement Test.* Los Angeles: Western Psychological Services.

Jensen, C., & Guess, D. (1978). Use of function as a consequence in training receptive labeling to severely and profoundly retarded individuals. *AAESPH Review, 3,* 246–258.

Jerger, J., Burney, P., Mauldin, L., & Crump, B. (1974). Predicting hearing loss from the acoustic reflexes. *Journal of Speech and Hearing Disorders, 39,* 11–22.

Johnson, B. D. (1985). *Adult linguistic interaction with specific language disordered and normally developing children.* Unpublished doctoral dissertation, City University of New York.

Johnson, D., & Myklebust, H. (1967). *Learning disabilities: Educational principles and practices.* New York: Grune & Stratton.

Johnson, W., Darley, F., & Spriestersbach, D. (1963). *Diagnostic methods in speech pathology.* New York: Harper & Row.

Johnston, J. (1982a). Interpreting the Leiter IQ: Performance profiles of young normal and language-disordered children. *Journal of Speech and Hearing Research, 25,* 291–297.

Johnston, J. (1982b). The language disordered child. In N. J. Lass, L. McReynolds, J. Northern, & D. Yoder (Eds.), *Speech, language, and hearing: Vol. 2. Pathologies of speech and language.* Philadelphia: Saunders.

Johnston, J. (1983). Discussion: Part I: What is language intervention? The role of theory. In J. Miller, D. Yoder, & R. Schiefelbusch (Eds.), *Contemporary issues in language intervention* (ASHA Reports 12). Rockville, MD: American Speech-Language-Hearing Association.

Johnston, J., & Kamhi, A. (1980). *The same can be less: Syntactic and semantic aspects of the utterances of language-impaired children.* Paper presented at the Symposium on Research in Child Language Disorders, Madison, WI.

Johnston, J., & Ramsted, V. (1977). *Cognitive development in pre-adolescent language-im-

paired children. Paper presented at the American Speech and Hearing Association, Chicago.

Johnston, J., & Schery, T. (1976). The use of grammatical morphemes by children with communication disorders. In D. M. Morehead & A. E. Morehead (Eds.), *Normal and deficient child language.* Baltimore: University Park Press.

Johnston, J., & Weismer, S. E. (1983). Mental rotation abilities in language disordered children. *Journal of Speech and Hearing Research, 26,* 397–403.

Kahn, L., & Lewis, N. (1986). *Kahn-Lewis phonological analysis: For use with the Goldman-Fristoe Test of Articulation.* Circle Pines, MN: American Guidance Service.

Kail, R., & Leonard, L. B. (1986). Word-finding abilities in language-impaired children. *ASHA Monographs* (No. 25). Rockville, MD: American Speech-Language-Hearing Association.

Kamhi, A. G. (1981). Nonlinguistic symbolic and conceptual abilities of language impaired and normally developing children. *Journal of Speech and Hearing Research, 24,* 446–453.

Kamhi, A., & Catts, H. (1986). Toward an understanding of developmental language and reading disorders. *Journal of Speech and Hearing Disorders, 51,* 337–347.

Kamhi, A., Catts, H., Koenig, L., & Lewis, B. (1984). Hypothesis-testing and nonlinguistic symbolic abilities in language-impaired children. *Journal of Speech and Hearing Disorders, 49,* 169–177.

Kamhi, A., & Johnston, J. (1982). Towards an understanding of retarded children's linguistic deficiencies. *Journal of Speech and Hearing Research, 25,* 435–445.

Kamhi, A., & Koenig, L. (1985). Metalinguistic awareness in normal and language-disordered children. *Language, Speech and Hearing Services in Schools, 16,* 199–210.

Kamhi, A., Lee, R., & Nelson, L. (1985). Word, syllable, and sound awareness in language-disordered children. *Journal of Speech and Hearing Disorders, 50,* 207–212.

Kanner, L. (1943). Autistic disturbances of affective contact. *The Nervous Child, 2,* 217–223.

Kanner, L. (1946). Irrelevant and metaphorical language in early infantile autism. *American Journal of Psychiatry, 103,* 242–266.

Kanner, L. (1973). *Childhood psychosis: Initial studies and new insights.* New York: Wiley.

Kanner, L., & Eisenberg, L. (1956). Early infantile autism. *American Journal of Orthopsychiatry, 26,* 556–564.

Karmiloff-Smith, A. (1979). *A functional approach to child language.* Cambridge: Cambridge University Press.

Karmiloff-Smith, A. (1985). Language and cognitive processes from a developmental perspective. *Language and Cognitive Processes, 1,* 61–85.

Karr, S., & Punch, J. (1984). PL 94-142 state child counts. *Asha, 26,* 33.

Katz, J. (1977). The staggered spondaic word test. In R. W. Keith (Ed.), *Central auditory dysfunction.* New York: Grune & Stratton.

Katz, J. (Ed.) (1978). *Handbook of clinical audiology* (2nd ed.). Baltimore: Williams & Wilkins.

Katz, R., Healy, A., & Shankweiler, D. (1983). Phonetic coding and order memory in relation to reading proficiency: A comparison of short-term memory for temporal and spatial order information. *Applied Psycholinguistics, 4,* 229–250.

Keil, F. C. (1984). Mechanisms of cognitive development and the structure of knowledge. In R. Sternberg (Ed.), *Mechanisms of cognitive development.* New York: Freeman.

Keith, R. (Ed.) (1977). *Central auditory dysfunction.* New York: Grune & Stratton.

Keith, R. (Ed.) (1981). *Central auditory and language disorders.* San Diego: College-Hill Press.

Keith, R. (1984). Central auditory dysfunction: A language disorder? *Topics in Language Disorders, 4,* 48–56.

Keller, F. S. (1965). *Learning: Reinforcement theory.* New York: Random House.

Keller-Cohen, D. (1974). *Elicited imitation in lexical development; Evidence from a study of temporal reference.* A revised version of a portion of the author's doctoral dissertation, Department of Linguistics at SUNY, Buffalo, NY.

Kennett, K. F. (1976). Adaptive behavior and its assessment. In P. Mittler (Ed.), *Research and practice in mental retardation*, (Vol. II). Baltimore: University Park Press.

Kent, L. (1974). *Language acquisition program for the retarded or multiply impaired.* Champaign, IL: Research Press.

Kephart, N. C. (1960). *The slow learner in the classroom.* Columbus, OH: Merrill.

Kernan, K. (1977). Semantic and expressive elaborations in children's narratives. In S. Ervin-Tripp & C. Mitchell-Kernan (Eds.), *Child discourse.* New York: Academic Press.

Kessler, J. (1966). *Psychopathology of childhood.* Englewood Cliffs, NJ: Prentice-Hall.

King, R. R., Jones, C., & Lasky, E. (1982). In retrospect: A fifteen-year follow-up report of speech-language disordered children. *Language, Speech and Hearing Services in the Schools, 13*, 24–32.

Kintsch, W. (1974). *The representation of meaning in memory.* Hillsdale, NJ: Erlbaum.

Kirk, S., & Chalfant, S. (1984). *Academic development and learning disabilities.* Denver, CO: Lowe Publishing Co.

Kirk, S., & Kirk, W. (1971). *Psycholinguistic learning disabilities.* Urbana, IL: University of Illinois Press.

Kirk, S., & Kirk, W. (1978). Uses and abuses of the ITPA. *Journal of Speech and Hearing Disorders, 43*, 58–75.

Kirk, S., & McCarthy, J. (1961). *The Illinois Test of Psycholinguistic Abilities*—An approach to differential diagnosis. *American Journal of Mental Deficiency, 66*, 399–412.

Kirk, S., McCarthy, J., & Kirk, W. (1968). *The Illinois Test of Psycholinguistic Abilities* (rev. ed.). Urbana, IL: University of Illinois Press.

Klecaen-Adler, J., & Hedrick, D. (1985). A study of the syntactic language skills of normal school-age children. *Language, Speech and Hearing Services in the Schools, 16*, 187–198.

Kleffner, F. (1973). *Language disorders in children.* New York: Bobbs-Merrill.

Kleffner, F. R. (1975). The direct teaching approach for children with auditory processing and learning disabilities. *Acta Symbolica, 4*, 65–93.

Klein, H. (1981). Productive strategies for the pronunciation of early polysyllabic lexical items. *Journal of Speech and Hearing Research, 24*, 389–406.

Konstantaveas, M. M. (1984). Sign language as a communication prosthesis with language-impaired children. *Journal of Autism and Developmental Disabilities, 14*, 9–25.

Kracke, I. (1975). Perception of rhythmic sequences by receptive aphasic and deaf children. *British Journal of Disorders of Communication, 10*, 43–51.

Krashen, D. S. (1975). The critical period for language acquisition and its possible bases. In D. Aaronson & R. W. Rieber (Eds.), Developmental psycholinguistics and communication disorders. *Annals of the New York Academy of Sciences*, No. 263.

Kretschmer, R. R., & Kretschmer, L. W. (1978). *Language development and intervention with the hearing impaired.* Baltimore: University Park Press.

Kuhl, P. K., & Meltzoff, A. N. (1982). The bimodal perception of speech in infancy. *Science, 218*, 1138–1144.

LaBelle, J. L. (1973). Sentence comprehension in two age groups of children as related to pause position or the absence of pauses. *Journal of Speech and Hearing Research, 6*, 231–237.

Labov, W. (1970). The logic of nonstandard English. In F. Williams (Ed.), *Language and poverty: Perspectives on a theme.* Chicago: Markham.

Labov, W. (1972). *Language in the inner city.* Philadelphia: University of Pennsylvania Press.

Labov, W., & Labov, T. (1977). Learning the syntax of questions. In Campbell, R., & Smith, P. (Eds.), *Recent advances in the psychology of language.* New York: Plenum Press.

Labov, W., & Waletzky, J. (1967). Narrative analysis: Oral versions of personal experience. In J. Helm (Ed.), *Essays on the verbal and visual arts.* Seattle, WA: American Ethological Society.

Lackner, J. R. (1968). A developmental study of language behavior in retarded children. *Neuropsychologia, 6,* 301–320.

Lahey, M. (1974). Use of prosody and syntactic markers in children's comprehension of spoken sentences. *Journal of Speech and Hearing Research, 17,* 656–668.

Lahey, M. (1978). Disruptions in the development and integration of form, content and use in language development. In J. Kavanagh & W. Strange (Eds.), *Language and speech in the laboratory, school, and clinic.* Cambridge, MA: M.I.T. Press.

Lahey, M. (1981). Learning disabilities: A puzzle without a cover picture. *Preliminary Proceedings of an Interdisciplinary Conference, Symposium on Language, Learning and Reading: A new decade.* New York: Queens College.

Lahey, M. (1984). The dissolution of text in written language. *Discourse Processes, 7,* 419–445.

Lahey, M. (1986). *Many ways to tell a tale.* Paper presented at the Emerson College Institute for Learning Disabilities, Boston.

Lahey, M., & Bloom, L. (1977). Planning a first lexicon: Which words to teach first. *Journal of Speech and Hearing Disorders, 42,* 340–350.

Lahey, M., & Edwards, J. (in preparation). Forming and executing phonetic representations: A comparison of language impaired and non-language impaired children. Emerson College.

Lahey, M., Flax, J., & Schlisselberg, G. (1985). A preliminary investigation of reduplication in children with specific language impairment. *Journal of Speech and Hearing Disorders, 50,* 186–194.

Lahey, M., & Launer, P. (1986). *Unraveled yarns: Narrative development in children.* Paper presented at the California Speech, Language, Hearing Association. Monterey.

Lahey, M., Launer, P., & Schiff-Myers, N. (1983). Prediction of production: Elicited imitation and spontaneous speech productions of language-disordered children. *Applied Psycholinguistics, 4,* 319–343.

Landau, B., & Gleitman, L. (1985). *Language and experience: Evidence from the blind child.* Cambridge, MA: Harvard University Press.

Landau, W. M., Goldstein, R., & Kleffner, F. R. (1960). Congenital aphasia: A clinico-pathologic study. *Neurology, 10,* 915–921.

Lasky, E. Z., & Klopp, K. L. (1982). Parent-child interactions in normal and language disordered children. *Journal of Speech and Hearing Disorders, 47,* 7–18.

Lassman, F. M., Fisch, R. O., Vetter, D. K., & LaBenz, E. S. (1980). *Early correlates of speech, language, and hearing.* Littleton, MA: PSG Publishing Co.

Launer, P. (1982). *"A plane" is not "to fly": Acquiring the distinction between related nouns and verbs in American Sign Language.* Unpublished doctoral dissertation, City University of New York.

Launer, P., & Lahey, M. (1981). Passages: From the fifties to the eighties in language assessment. *Topics in Language Disorders, 1,* 11–30.

Launer, P., Schiff, N., & Lahey, M. (1979). Is it so simple to imitate a sample? Paper presented at the American Speech-Language-Hearing Association, Atlanta, GA.

Layton, T., Strawson, L., & Baker, P. (1981). Description of semantic-syntactic relations in an autistic child. *Journal of Autism and Developmental Disabilities, 11,* 385–399.

Leach, G. (1970). *Towards a semantic description of English.* Bloomington, IN: Indiana University Press.

Lee, L. (1966). Developmental sentence types: A method for comparing normal and deviant syntactic development. *Journal of Speech and Hearing Disorders, 31,* 311–330.

Lee, L. (1970). A screening test for syntax development. *Journal of Speech and Hearing Disorders, 35,* 103–112.

Lee, L. (1971). *Northwestern Syntax Screening Test (NSST)*. Evanston, IL: Northwestern University Press.

Lee, L. (1974). *Developmental sentence analysis*. Evanston, IL: Northwestern University Press.

Lee, L., & Canter, S. (1971). Developmental sentence scoring: A clinical procedure for estimating syntactic development in children's spontaneous speech. *Journal of Speech and Hearing Disorders, 36*, 315–341.

Lenneberg, E. (1967). *Biological foundations of language*. New York: Wiley.

Lenneberg, E., Nichols, I., & Rosenberger, E. (1964). Primitive stages of language development in mongolism. In D. Rioch and E. A. Weinstein (Eds.), *Disorders of communication* 119–137 (Research Publications of the Association for Research in Nervous and Mental Disease). Baltimore: Williams & Wilkins.

Leonard, L. (1972). What is deviant language? *Journal of Speech and Hearing Disorders, 37*, 427–447.

Leonard, L. (1975a). Relational meaning and the facilitation of slow-learning children's language. *American Journal of Mental Deficiency, 80*, 180–185.

Leonard, L. (1975b). The role of nonlinguistic stimuli and semantic relations in children's acquisition of grammatical utterances. *Journal of Experimental Child Psychology, 19*, 346–357.

Leonard, L. (1979). Language impairment in children. *Merrill-Palmer Quarterly, 25*, 205–231.

Leonard, L. (1981). An invited article: Facilitating linguistic skills in children with specific language impairment. *Applied Psycholinguistics, 2*, 89–118.

Leonard, L. (1982). Phonological deficits in children with developmental language impairment. *Brain and Language, 16*, 73–86.

Leonard, L. (in press). Is specific language impairment a useful construct? In S. Rosenberg (Ed.), *Advances in applied psycholinguistics: Vol. I. Disorders of first-language development*. New York: Cambridge University Press.

Leonard, L., Bolders, J., & Miller, J. A. (1976). An examination of the semantic relations reflected in the language usage of normal and language-disordered children. *Journal of Speech and Hearing Research, 19*, 371–392.

Leonard, L., Camarata, S., Rowan, L. E., & Chapman, K. (1982). The communicative functions of lexical usage by language impaired children. *Applied Psycholinguistics, 3*, 109–125.

Leonard, L., Nippold, M., Kail, R., & Hale, C. (1983). Picture naming in language-impaired children. *Journal of Speech and Hearing Research, 26*, 609–615.

Leonard, L., Prutting, C. A., Perozzi, J. A., & Berkley, R. K. (1978). Nonstandardized approaches to the assessment of language behaviors. *Asha, 20*, 371–379.

Leonard, L., Sabbadini, L., Leonard, J., & Volterra, V. (1986). *Specific language impairment in children: A cross-linguistic study*. Paper presented at the Stanford Child Language Research Forum, Stanford University, Palo Alto, CA.

Leonard, L., Sabbadini, L., Volterra, V., & Leonard, J. (1986). *Specific language impairment in two languages: Converging evidence*. Paper presented at the Boston University Conference on Language Development, Boston.

Leonard, L., Schwartz, R., Chapman, K., Rowan, L., Prelock, P., Terrell, B., Weiss, A., & Messick, C. (1982). Early lexical acquisition in children with specific language impairment. *Journal of Speech and Hearing Research, 25*, 554–559.

Leonard, L., Steckol, K., & Panther, K. (1983). Returning meaning to semantic relations: Some clinical applications. *Journal of Speech and Hearing Disorders, 47*, 25–35.

Leopold, W. (1939). *Speech development of a bilingual child*. Evanston, IL: Northwestern University Press.

Levine, F., & Fasnacht, G. (1974). Token rewards may lead to token learning. *American Psychologist, 29*, 816–820.

Levitt, H., McGarr, N., & Geffner, D. (1988). *Development of language and communication skills in hearing-impaired children. ASHA Monographs.* (No. 26).

Lewis, M. M. (1938). The beginning and early functions of questions in a child's speech. *British Journal of Educational Psychology, 8,* 150–171.

Lewis, M. M. (1951). *Infant speech, a study of the beginnings of language.* New York: Humanities Press.

Liberman, A. (1970). The grammars of speech and language. *Cognitive Psychology, 1,* 301–323.

Liberman, A., Cooper, F., Shankweiler, D., & Studdert-Kennedy, M. (1967). Perception of the speech code. *Psychological Review, 74,* 431–461.

Liberman, A., Delattre, P., & Cooper, F. (1952). The role of selected stimulus variables in the perception of the unvoiced stop consonants. *American Journal of Psychology, 65,* 497–516.

Liberman, I. (1985). Should so-called modality preferences determine the nature of instruction for children with reading disabilities? In J. Duffy & N. Geshwind (Eds.), *Dyslexia.* Boston: Little, Brown.

Liberman, I., Shankweiler, D., Fischer, F., & Carter, B. (1974). Explicit syllable and phoneme segmentation in the young child. *Journal of Experimental Child Psychology, 18,* 201–212.

Lieven, E. V. M. (1978). Conversations between mothers and young children: Individual differences and their possible implications for the study of language learning. In N. Waterson & C. E. Snow (Eds.), *The development of communication.* New York: Wiley.

Lifter, K. (1982). *Development of object related behavior during the transition from prelinguistic to linguistic communication.* Unpublished doctoral dissertation, Columbia University.

Lifter, K., & Bloom, L. (1986). *Object play and the emergence of language.* Unpublished manuscript, Teachers College, Columbia University.

Liles, B. (1985). Cohesion in the narratives of normal and language disordered children. *Journal of Speech and Hearing Research, 28,* 123–133.

Limber, J. (1973). The genesis of complex sentences. In T. Moore (Ed.), *Cognitive development and the acquisition of language.* New York: Academic Press.

Longhurst, T., & File, J. (1977). *A comparison of developmental sentence scores from Head Start children collected in four conditions.* Unpublished manuscript, Kansas State University, Manhattan, Kansas.

Longhurst, T., & Grubb, S. (1974). A comparison of language samples collected in four situations. *Language, Speech and Hearing Services in the Schools, 5,* 71–78.

Longtin, S. (1984). *The relationship between functional orientation and early lexical development.* Unpublished doctoral dissertation, City University of New York.

Lovaas, O. I., Berberich, J. P., Perloff, B. F., & Schaeffer, B. (1966). Acquisition of imitative speech by schizophrenic children. *Science, 151,* 701–707.

Lovaas, O. I., Schreibman, L., Koegel, R., & Rehm, R. (1971). Selective responding by autistic children to multiple sensory input. *Journal of Abnormal Psychology, 77,* 211–222.

Lovell, K., & Bradbury, B. (1967). The learning of English morphology in educationally subnormal special school children. *American Journal of Mental Deficiency, 71,* 609–615.

Lovell, K., Hoyle, H. W., & Siddall, M. W. (1968). A study of some aspects of the play and language of young children with delayed speech. *Journal of Child Psychology and Psychiatry, 9,* 41–50.

Lowe, A., & Campbell, R. (1965). Temporal discrimination in aphasoid and normal children. *Journal of Speech and Hearing Research, 8,* 313–315.

Lubert, N. (1981). Auditory perceptual impairments in children with specific language disorders: A review of the literature. *Journal of Speech and Hearing Disorders, 46,* 3–9.

Lucas, E. (1980). *Semantic and pragmatic language disorders: Assessment and remediation.* Rockville, MD: Aspen Systems Corp.

Ludlow, C. L., & Cooper, J. (Eds.) (1983). *Genetic aspects of speech and language disorders.* New York: Academic Press.

Lund, K. A., Foster, G. E., & McCall-Perez, F. C. (1978). The effectiveness of psycholinguistic training. *Exceptional Children, 45,* 310–319.

Lund, N. J., & Duchan, J. F. (1983). *Assessing children's language in naturalistic contexts.* Englewood Cliffs, NJ: Prentice-Hall.

Luria, A. R., & Yudovich, F. (1979). *Speech and the development of mental processes in the child.* London: Penguin Press.

Lust, B., & Mervis, C. A. (1980). The development of coordination in the natural speech of young children. *Journal of Child Language, 7,* 279–304.

Lyman, H. (1986). *Test scores and what they mean* (4th ed.). Englewood Cliffs, NJ: Prentice-Hall.

Lyons, J. (1968). *Introduction to theoretical linguistics.* London: Cambridge University Press.

MacGinitie, W. (1964). Ability of deaf children to use different word classes. *Journal of Speech and Hearing Research, 7,* 141–150.

MacDonald, J., & Blott, J. (1974). Environmental language intervention: The rationale for a diagnostic and training strategy through rules, context, and generalization. *Journal of Speech and Hearing Disorders, 39,* 244–257.

MacDonald, J., Blott, J., Gordon, K., Spiegel, B., & Hartmann, M. (1974). An experimental parent-assisted treatment program for preschool language-delayed children. *Journal of Speech and Hearing Disorders, 39,* 395–415.

MacDonald, J., & Nickols, M. (1974). *The environmental language inventory.* Columbus, OH: Nisonger Center, Ohio State University, 1974.

MacGinitie, W. (1964). Ability of deaf children to use different word classes. *Journal of Speech and Hearing Research, 7,* 141–150.

MacWhinney, B., & Bates, E. (1978). Sentential devices for conveying givenness and newness: A cross-sectional developmental study. *Journal of Verbal Learning and Verbal Behavior, 17,* 539–558.

Mahecha, N. (1981). *Effects of stimuli familiarity on short term memory recall skills.* Unpublished master's thesis, Hunter College, the City University of New York.

Mahecha, N., & Lahey, M. (in preparation). The effect of linguistic familiarity on auditory memory span.

Mann, L. (1971). Psychometric phrenology and new faculty psychology: The case against ability assessment and training. *Journal of Special Education, 5,* 3–14.

Mann, V. A. (1986). Why some children encounter reading problems: The contribution of difficulties with language processing and phonological sophistication to early reading disability. In J. Torgesen & B. Wong (Eds.), *Psychological and educational perspectives on learning disabilities.* New York: Academic Press.

Manning, W. H., Johnston, K. L., & Beasley, D. S. (1977). The performance of children with auditory perceptual disorders on a time-compressed speech discrimination measure. *Journal of Speech and Hearing Disorders, 42,* 77–84.

Maratsos, M. (1973). Nonegocentric communication abilities in preschool children. *Child Development, 44,* 697–700.

Maratsos, M. (1974). Preschool children's use of definite and indefinite articles. *Child Development, 45,* 446–455.

Marks, S., Frye-Osler, H., Reichle, J., & Schwimmer-Gluck, S. (1981). Modeling procedure for eliciting Wh-questions. In J. Miller (Ed.), *Assessing language production in children: Experimental procedures.* Baltimore: University Park Press.

Marschark, M., & West, S. (1985). Creative language abilities of deaf children. *Journal of Speech and Hearing Research, 28,* 73–78.

Martin, J. R. (1983). The development of register. In J. Fine & R. Freedle (Eds.), *Developmental issues in discourse.* Norwood, NJ: Ablex.

Masland, M., & Case, L. (1968). Limitation of auditory memory as a factor in delayed language development. *British Journal of Disorders of Communication, 3,* 139–142.

Matkin, N. (1983). *Perspectives on evaluation of central auditory testing.* Paper presented at the American Speech and Hearing Association Convention, Toronto.

Matkin, N., & Hook, P. (1983). A multidisciplinary approach to central auditory testing. In E. Lasky & J. Katz (Eds.), *Central auditory processing disorders.* Baltimore: University Park Press.

Mattes, L., & Omark, D. (1984). *Speech and language assessment of the bilingually handicapped.* San Diego: College-Hill Press.

Mattingly, J. (1978). *Semantic relations and grammatical forms used by language-delayed preschoolers.* Unpublished doctoral dissertation, Columbia University.

Mattis, S., French, J. H., & Rapin, I. (1975). Dsylexia in children and young adults: Three independent neurological syndromes. *Developmental Medicine and Child Neurology, 17,* 150–163.

Maxwell, S., & Wallach, G. (1984). The language-learning disabilities connection: Symptoms of early language disability change over time. In G. Wallach & K. Butler (Eds.), *Language learning disabilities in school-age children.* Baltimore: Williams & Wilkins.

Mayberry, R. (1976). If a chimp can learn language, surely my nonverbal client can too. *Asha, 18,* 223–228.

McCarthy, D. (1930). The language development of the preschool child. *Institute of Child Welfare Monograph* (Series No. 4). Minneapolis: University of Minnesota Press.

McCarthy, D. (1954). Language development in children. In P. Mussen (Ed.), *Carmichael's manual of child psychology.* New York: Wiley.

McCarthy, D. (1974). *McCarthy Scales of Children's Abilities.* New York: Psychological Corp.

McCauley, R., & Swisher, L. (1984a). Psychometric review of language and articulation tests for preschool children. *Journal of Speech and Hearing Disorders, 49,* 34–42.

McCauley, R., & Swisher, L. (1984b). Use and misuse of norm-referenced tests in clinical assessment: A hypothetical case. *Journal of Speech and Hearing Disorders, 49,* 338–348.

McCormick, L., & Schiefelbusch, R. (1984). *Early language intervention.* Columbus, OH: Merrill.

McCune-Nicholich, L. (1981). Toward symbolic functioning: Structure of early pretend games and potential parallels with language. *Child Development, 52,* 785–797.

McDaniel, D., & Cairns, H. (1986). *The child as informant: Eliciting linguistic intuitions from young children.* Unpublished manuscript, Queens College, New York.

McGinnis, M. (1963). *Aphasic children.* Washington, DC: Alexander Graham Bell Association.

McGinnis, M., Kleffner, F., & Goldstein, R. (1956). Teaching aphasic children. *Volta Review, 58,* 239–244.

McGuiness, D. (1985). *When children don't learn: Understanding biology and psychology.* New York: Basic Books.

McLean, J. E. (1983). Historical perspectives on the content of child language programs. In J. Miller, D. Yoder, & R. Schiefelbusch (Eds.), *Contemporary issues in language intervention.* Rockville, MD: American Speech-Language-Hearing Association.

McLean, J. E., & Snyder-McLean, L. K. (1978). *A transactional approach to early language training.* Columbus, OH: Merrill.

McLean, L. P., & McLean, J. E. (1974). A language training program for non-verbal autistic children. *Journal of Speech and Hearing Disorders, 39,* 186–193.

McNamee, G., & Harris-Schmidt, G. (1985). Narration and dramatization as a basis for remediation of language disorders. *Quarterly Newsletter of the Laboratory of Comparative Human Cognition, 7,* 6–15.

McReynolds, L. (1966). Operant conditioning for investigating speech sound discrimination in aphasic children. *Journal of Speech and Hearing Research, 9,* 519–528.

McShane, J. (1980). *Learning to talk.* Cambridge: Cambridge University Press.

Mecham, M. (1955). The development and application of procedures for measuring speech improvement in mentally defective children. *American Journal of Mental Deficiency, 60,* 301–306.

Mecham, M. (1958, 1971). *Verbal Language Development Scale.* Circle Pines, MN: American Guidance Service.

Mecham, M., Joy, J. L., & Jones, J. D. (1967). *Utah Test of Language Development.* Salt Lake City, UT: Communication Research Associates.

Mein, R. (1961). A study of the oral vocabularies of severely sub-normal patients II: Grammatical analysis of speech samples. *Journal of Mental Deficiency Research, 5,* 52–59.

Mein, R., & O'Connor, N. (1960). A study of the oral vocabularies of severely sub-normal patients. *Journal of Mental Deficiency Research, 4,* 130–143.

Menig-Peterson, C. (1975). The modification of communicative behavior in preschool-aged children as a function of the listener's perspective. *Child Development, 46,* 1015–1018.

Menn, L. (1971). Phonotactic rules in beginning speech. *Lingua, 26,* 225–251.

Menolascino, F., & Egger, M. (1978). *Medical dimensions of mental retardation.* Lincoln, NE: University of Nebraska Press.

Menyuk, P. (1964). Comparison of grammar of children with functionally deviant and normal speech. *Journal of Speech and Hearing Research, 7,* 109–121.

Merrill, C. (1982). Update II, Columbus, OH: Merrill.

Merrill, C. (1984). Update IV, Columbus, OH: Merrill.

Michaels, S. (1986). *Hearing the logic in children's oral and written discourse.* Paper presented at the Emerson College Institute on Language Learning Disabilities, Boston.

Miller, A., & Miller, E. E. (1973). Cognitive-developmental training with elevated boards and sign language. *Journal of Autism and Childhood Schizophrenia, 3,* 65–85.

Miller, G., Galanter, E., & Pribram, K. (1960). *Plans and the structure of behavior.* New York: Holt-Dryden.

Miller, J. (Ed.) (1981). *Assessing language production in children: Experimental Procedures.* Baltimore: University Park Press.

Miller, J. (1986). *SALT database project.* Unpublished report. University of Wisconsin, Madison.

Miller, J., Campbell, T., Chapman, R., & Weismer, S. (1984). Language behavior in acquired childhood aphasia. In A. Holland, *Language disorders in children.* San Diego: College-Hill Press.

Miller, J., & Chapman, R. (1981). The relation between age and mean length of utterance in morphemes. *Journal of Speech and Hearing Research, 24,* 154–162.

Miller, J., & Marriner, N. (1986). Language intervention software: Myth or reality. *Child Language Teaching and Therapy, 2,* 85–96.

Miller, J., & Yoder, D. (1974). An ontogenetic language teaching strategy for retarded children. In R. Schiefelbusch & L. Lloyd (Eds.), *Language Perspectives—Acquisition, retardation and intervention.* Baltimore: University Park Press.

Miller, J., & Yoder, D. (1984). *Miller-Yoder Test of Grammatical Comprehension (M.Y.).* Madison, WI: Communication Development Group.

Miller, J., Yoder, D., & Schiefelbusch, R. (Eds.) (1983). *Contemporary issues in language intervention* (Asha Reports). Rockville, MD: American Speech-Language-Hearing Association.

Miller, L. (1978). Pragmatics and early childhood language disorders: Communicative interactions in a half-hour sample. *Journal of Speech and Hearing Disorders, 43,* 419–436.

Millet, A., & Newhoff, M. (1978). *Language disordered children: Language disordered mothers?* Paper presented at the American Speech and Hearing Association, San Francisco.

Mitchell, J. V. (Ed.) (1985). *The ninth mental measurement yearbook.* Lincoln, NE: University of Nebraska Press.

Monsees, E. (1968). Temporal sequence and expressive language disorders. *Exceptional Children, 35,* 141–147.

Monsees, E. (1972). *Structured language for children with special language learning problems.* Washington, DC: Children's Hospital of District of Columbia.

Morehead, D. (1975). The study of linguistically deficient children. In S. Singh (Ed.), *Measurement in hearing, speech and language.* Baltimore: University Park Press.

Morehead, D., & Ingram, D. (1973). The development of base syntax in normal and linguistically deviant children. *Journal of Speech and Hearing Research, 16,* 330–352.

Morley, M. E. (1965). *The development and disorders of speech in childhood* (2nd ed.). Edinburgh: Churchill Livingstone.

Mower, D. E. (1984). Behavioural approaches to treating language disorders. In D. Muller (Ed.), *Remediating children's language.* San Diego: College-Hill Press.

Muma, J. (1971). Language intervention: Ten techniques. *Language, Speech and Hearing Services in the Schools, 2,* 7–17.

Muma, J. (1978). *Language handbook: Concepts, assessment intervention.* Englewood Cliffs, NJ: Prentice-Hall.

Muma, J. (1986). *Language acquisition.* Austin, TX: Pro Ed.

Musiek, F. E., & Geurkink, N. A. (1980). Auditory perceptual problems in children: Considerations for the otolaryngologist and audiologist. *The Laryngoscope, 20,* 962–971.

Musiek, F. E., Geurkink, N. A., & Kietel, S. A. (1982). Test battery assessment of auditory perceptual dysfunction in children. *The Laryngoscope, 22,* 251–257.

Myers, P., & Hammill, D. (1969). *Methods for learning disorders.* New York: Wiley.

Myklebust, H. (1954). *Auditory disorders in children: A manual for differential diagnosis.* New York: Grune & Stratton.

Nadel, L. (1986). *Neuropsychological studies.* Paper presented at the Conference on Autism. University of Arizona, Tucson, AZ.

Naremore, R., & Dever, R. (1975). Language performance of educable mentally retarded and normal children at five age levels. *Journal of Speech and Hearing Research, 18,* 82–95.

National Joint Committee on Learning Disabilities (1987, May). Learning disabilities and the preschool child. *Asha, 29,* 35–38.

Naus, M., & Ornstein, P. (1983). Development of memory strategies: Analysis, questions and issues. In M. Chi (Ed.), *Trends in memory research.* Basel: Karger.

Needleman, H. (1977). Effects of hearing loss on early recurrent otitis media on speech and language development. In B. Jaffe (Ed.), *Hearing loss in children.* Baltimore: University Park Press.

Needleman, R., Ritvo, E. R., & Freeman, B. J. (1980). Objectively defined linguistic parameters in children with autism and other developmental disabilities. *Journal of Autism and Developmental Disorders, 10,* 389–398.

Nelson, K. (1973). Structure and strategy in learning to talk. *Monographs of the Society for Research in Child Development, 38* (Serial No. 149).

Nelson, K. (1975). The nominal shift in semantic-syntactic development. *Cognitive Psychology, 7,* 461–479.

Nelson, K. (Ed.) (1986). *Event knowledge.* Hillsdale, NJ: Erlbaum.

Nelson, K. E., & Baker, N. (1986). *Theoretical and applied implications of experimentally-induced advances in children's language.* Paper presented at the Boston University Conference on Language Development, Boston.

Nelson, K. E., Carskadden, G., & Bonvillian, J. (1973). Syntax acquisition: Impact of experimental variation in adult verbal interaction with the child. *Child Development, 44,* 497–504.

Nelson, L. K., & Weber-Olsen, M. (1980). The elicited language inventory and the influence of contextual cues. *Journal of Speech and Hearing Disorders, 45,* 549–563.

Nelson, N. (1976). Comprehension of spoken language by normal children as a function of speaking rate, sentence difficulty, and listener age and sex. *Child Development, 47,* 299–303.

Newcombe, N., & Zaslow, M. (1981). Do 2½ year olds hint? A study of directive forms in the speech of 2½ year-old children to adults. *Discourse Processes, 4,* 239–252.

Newcomer, P., & Goodman, L. (no date). Effect of modality of instruction on the learning of meaningful and nonmeaningful material by auditory and visual learners. Unpublished manuscript.

Newcomer, P., & Hammill, D. (1977, 1982). *The Test of Language Development.* Austin, TX: Pro Ed.

Newcomer, P., Hare, B., Hammill, D., & McGettigan, J. (1973). *Construct validity of the Illinois Test of Psycholinguistic Abilities.* Tucson, AZ: University of Arizona, LTI-LD Report, Department of Special Education.

Newfield, M., & Schlanger, B. (1968). The acquisition of English morphology by normal and educable mentally retarded children. *Journal of Speech and Hearing Research, 11,* 693–706.

Newport, E., Gleitman, H., & Gleitman, L. (1977). Mother, I'd rather do it myself: Some effects and noneffects of maternal speech style. In C. Snow & C. Ferguson (Eds.), *Talking to children: Language input and acquisition.* New York: Cambridge University Press.

Odom, R. D., Liebert, R. M., & Fernandez, L. (1969). Effects of symbolic modeling on the syntactical productions of retardates. *Psychonomic Science, 17,* 104–105.

Ojemann, G. A. (1983). Brain organization for language from the perspective of electrical stimulation mapping. *The Behavioral and Brain Sciences,* pp. 189–206.

Ojemann, G. A., & Mateer, C. (1979). Human language cortex: Localization of memory, syntax, and sequential motor-phoneme identification systems. *Science, 205,* 1401–1403.

Oller, D. K., Eilers, R. E., Bull, D. H., & Carney, A. E. (1985). Prespeech vocalizations of a deaf infant: A comparison with normal metaphonological development. *Journal of Speech and Hearing Research, 28,* 47–63.

Oller, D. K., Wieman, W., Doyle, J., & Ross, C. (1976). Infant babbling and speech. *Journal of Child Language, 3,* 1–11.

Olson, G. M. (1973). Developmental changes in memory and the acquisition of language. In T. Moore (Ed.), *Cognitive development and the acquisition of language.* New York: Academic Press.

Olson, S., Bayles, K., & Bates, J. (1986). Mother-child interaction and children's speech progress: A longitudinal study of the first two years. *Merrill-Palmer Quarterly, 32,* 1–20.

Olswang, L., Bain, B., Dunn, C., & Cooper, J. (1983). The effects of stimulus variation on lexical learning. *Journal of Speech and Hearing Disorders, 48,* 192–202.

Olswang, L., & Carpenter, R. (1978). Elicitory effects on the language obtained from young language-impaired children. *Journal of Speech and Hearing Disorders, 43,* 76–88.

Osgood, C. E. (1957). Motivational dynamics of language behavior. *Nebraska symposium on motivation.* Lincoln, NE: University of Nebraska Press.

Osgood, C. E. (1971). Where do sentences come from? In D. D. Steinberg & L. H. Jakobovits (Eds.), *Semantics* (pp. 497–529). London: Cambridge University Press.

Page, J., & Stewart, S. (1985, March). Story grammar skills in school-age children. *Topics in Language Disorders,* 16–30.

Palin, M., Mordecai, D., & Palmer, C. (1985). *Lingquest 1: Language sample analysis software.* San Antonio, TX. Psychological Corp.

Panagos, J. M. (1978). Abstract phonology, grammatical reduction and delayed speech development. *Acta Symbolica, 7,* 1–12.

Panagos, J. M., Quine, M., & Klich, R. (1979). Syntactic and phonological influences on children's articulation. *Journal of Speech and Hearing Research, 22,* 841–848.

Paul, R. (1981). Analyzing complex sentence development. In J. Miller (Ed.), *Assessing language production in children: Experimental procedures.* Baltimore: University Park Press.

Paul, R., & Shriberg, L. (1982). Associations between phonology and syntax in speech-delayed children. *Journal of Speech and Hearing Research, 25,* 536–547.

Peterson, A. H., & Marquardt, T. P. (1981). *Appraisal and diagnosis of speech and language disorders.* Englewood Cliffs, NJ: Prentice-Hall.

Peterson, C., & McCabe, A. (1983). *Developmental psycholinguistics: Three ways of looking at a child's narrative.* New York: Plenum Press.

Pettit, J., & Helms, S. (1979). Hemispheric language dominance of language-disordered, articulation-disordered, and normal children. *Journal of Learning Disabilities, 12,* 71–76.

Piaget, J. (1954). *The construction of reality in the child.* New York: Basic Books.

Piaget, J. (1955, originally 1924). *The language and thought of the child.* Cleveland, OH: World.

Piaget, J. (1951, 1962). *Play, dreams and imitation in childhood.* New York: Norton.

Pitcher, E., & Prelinger, E. (1963). *Children tell stories: An analysis of fantasy.* New York: International Universities Press.

Poole, I. (1934). Genetic development of articulation of consonant sounds in speech. *Elementary English Review, 11,* 159–161.

Popham, W. J., & Husek, T. R. (1969). Implications of criterion-referenced measurement. *Journal of Educational Measurement, 6,* 1–9.

Prinz, P., & Ferrier, L. (1983). "Can you give me that one?" the comprehension, production and judgment of directives in language-impaired children. *Journal of Speech and Hearing Disorders, 48,* 44–54.

Prinz, P., & Weiner, F. (in press). *Pragmatics Screening Test (PST).* San Antonio, TX: Psychological Corp.

Prizant, B. M. (1983). Language acquisition and communicative behavior in autism: Toward an understanding of the "whole" of it. *Journal of Speech and Hearing Disorders, 48,* 296–308.

Prizant, B., & Duchan, J. (1981). The functions of immediate echolalia in autistic children. *Journal of Speech and Hearing Disorders, 46,* 241–250.

Prutting, C. (1979). Process \'prä|,ses\n: The action of moving forward progressively from one point to another on the way to completion. *Journal of Speech and Hearing Disorders, 44,* 3–30.

Prutting, C., Gallagher, T., & Mulac, A. (1975). The expressive portion of the N.S.S.T. compared to a spontaneous language sample. *Journal of Speech and Hearing Disorders, 40,* 40–49.

Prutting, C., & Kirchner, D. (1983). Applied pragmatics. In T. Gallagher & C. Prutting (Eds.)., *Pragmatic assessment and intervention issues in language.* San Diego: College-Hill Press.

Prutting, C., & Kirchner, D. (1987). A clinical appraisal of the pragmatic aspects of language. *Journal of Speech and Hearing Disorders, 52,* 105–119.

Quigley, S., Wilbur, R., & Montanelli, D. (1976). Complement structures in the language of deaf students. *Journal of Speech and Hearing Research, 19,* 448–466.

Quigley, S., Wilbur, R., Power, D., Montanelli, D., & Steinkamp, M. (1976). *Syntactic structures in the language of deaf children.* Urbana, IL: University of Illinois, Urbana-Champaign. Final Report Project No. 232175, U.S. Department of Health, Education and Welfare, National Institute of Education.

Randall, D., Rynell, J., & Curwen, M. (1974). A study of language development in a sample of three-year-old children. *British Journal of Disorders of Communication, 9,* 3.

Read, B. K., & Cherry, L. J. (1978). Preschool children's production of directive forms. *Discourse Processes, 1,* 233–246.

Rees, N. (1973a). Noncommunicative functions of language in children. *Journal of Speech and Hearing Disorders, 38,* 98–110.

Rees, N. (1973b). Auditory processing factors in language disorders: The view from Procrustes' bed. *Journal of Speech and Hearing Disorders, 38,* 304–315.

Rees, N. (1981). In R. Keith (Ed.), *Central auditory and language disorders.* San Diego: College-Hill Press.

Reitan, R., & Boll, T. (1973). Neuropsychological correlates of minimal brain dysfunction. *New York Academy of Science,* No. 205, 65–88.

Renfrew, C. (1966). Persistence of the open syllable in defective articulation. *Journal of Speech and Hearing Disorders, 31,* 370–373.

Rescorla, L. (1986, October). *Pretend play in 2-year-olds with expressive language delay.* Poster paper presented at the Boston University Language Development Conference, Boston.

Reynell, J. K. (1969). *Reynell Developmental Language Scales, Experimental Edition.* Windsor: N.F.E.R.

Richard, G., & Hanner, M. (1985). *Language Processing Test.* Moline, IL: LinguiSystems.

Richman, N., & Graham, P. J. (1971). A behavioural screening questionnaire for use with three-year-old children. *Journal of Child Psychology and Psychiatry, 12,* 5.

Ricks, D. M. (1975). Vocal communication in pre-verbal normal and autistic children. In N. O'Connor (Ed.), *Language, cognitive deficits, and retardation.* London: Butterworths.

Rimland, B. (1962). *Infantile autism.* New York: Appleton-Century-Crofts.

Risley, T., & Wolf, M. (1967). Establishing functional speech in echolalic children. *Behavior Research and Therapy, 5,* 73–88.

Ritvo, E. R., & Freeman, B. J. (1978). National Society for Autistic Children's definition of the syndrome of autism. *Journal of the American Academy of Child Psychiatry, 17,* 565–576.

Rocissano, L. (1979). *Object play and its relation to language in early childhood.* Unpublished doctoral dissertation, Columbia University.

Rom, A., & Bliss, L. (1981). A comparison of verbal communicative skills of language-impaired and normal-speaking children. *Journal of Communication Disorders, 14,* 133–140.

Rom, A., & Bliss, L. (1983). The use of nonverbal pragmatic behaviors by language-impaired and normal-speaking children. *Journal of Communication Disorders, 16,* 251–256.

Romski, M., & Ruder, K. (1984). Effects of speech and speech and sign instruction on oral language learning and generalization of action + object combinations by Down's syndrome children. *Journal of Speech and Hearing Disorders, 49,* 293–302.

Rondal, J. (1978). Patterns of correlations for various language measures in mother-child interactions for normal and Down's syndrome children. *Language and Speech, 21,* 242–252.

Rosenberg, S. (Ed.). (in press). *Advances in applied psycholinguistics. Vol. 1: Disorders of first-language development.* New York: Cambridge University Press.

Rosenthal, W. (1972). Auditory and linguistic interaction in developmental aphasia: Evidence from two studies of auditory processing. *Papers and Reports in Child Language Development,* Stanford University, Palo Alto, CA. 4, 19–35.

Rosenthal, W., Eisenson, J., & Luckau, J. (1972). A statistical test of the validity of the diagnostic categories used in childhood language disorders: Implications for assessment procedures. *Papers and Reports in Child Language Development,* Stanford University, Palo Alto, CA. 4, 121–143.

Rosinski-McClendon, M. K., & Newhoff, M. (1987). Conversational responsiveness and assertiveness in language-impaired children. *Language, Speech, and Hearing Services in the Schools, 18,* 53–62.

Roth, F., & Clark, D. (1987). Symbolic play and social participation abilities of language-impaired and normally developing children. *Journal of Speech and Hearing Disorders, 52,* 17–29.

Roth, F., & Spekman, N. (1984a). Assessing the pragmatic abilities of children: Part 1. Organizational framework and assessment parameters. *Journal of Speech and Hearing Disorders, 49,* 2–11.

Roth, F., & Spekman, N. (1984b). Assessing the pragmatic abilities of children: Part 2. Guidelines, considerations, and specific evaluation procedures. *Journal of Speech and Hearing Disorders, 49,* 12–17.

Roth, F., & Spekman, N. (1986). Narrative discourse: Spontaneously generated stories of learning-disabled and normally achieving students. *Journal of Speech and Hearing Disorders, 51,* 8–23.

Rourke, B. P., & Gates, R. D. (1981). Neuropsychological research and school psychology. In G. Hynd & J. Obrzut (Eds.), *Neuropsychological assessment and the school-age child.* New York: Grune & Stratton.

Rowan, L. I., Leonard, L., Chapman, K., & Weiss, A. (1983). Performative and presuppositional skills in language-disordered and normal children. *Journal of Speech and Hearing Research, 26,* 97–106.

Rubin, H., & Liberman, I. (1983). Exploring the oral and written language errors made by language disabled children. *Annals of Dyslexia, 33,* 111–120.

Rudel, R. (1985). The definition of dyslexia: Language and motor deficits. In F. Duffy & N. Geshwind (Eds.), *Dyslexia: A neuroscientific approach to clinical evaluation.* Boston: Little, Brown.

Ruder, K., & Smith, M. D. (1974). Issues in language learning. In R. Schiefelbusch & L. Lloyd (Eds.), *Language perspectives—Acquisition, retardation and intervention.* Baltimore: University Park Press.

Ruder, K., Smith, M. D., & Hermann, P. (1974). Effect of verbal imitation and comprehension on verbal production of lexical items. In L. McReynolds (Ed.), *Developing systematized procedures for training children's language. ASHA Monographs* (No. 18). Rockville, MD: American Speech and Hearing Association.

Rumelhart, D. E. (1975). Notes on a schema for stories. In D. G. Bobrow & A. Collins (Eds.), *Representation and understanding: Studies in cognitive science.* New York: Academic Press.

Rupp, S. K. (1985). *Language tests and minority-language children.* Paper presented at the Second Biennial Conference on Minority Assessment, Tucson, AZ.

Ruttenberg, B., & Wolf, E. (1967). Evaluating the communication of the autistic child. *Journal of Speech and Hearing Disorders, 32,* 314–325.

Rutter, M. (1966). Behavioral and cognitive characteristics. In L. Wing (Ed.), *Early childhood autism: Clinical, educational and social aspects.* Oxford: Pergamon Press.

Rutter, M. (1968). Concepts of autism: A review of research. *Journal of Child Psychology and Psychiatry, 9,* 1–25.

Rutter, M. (1978). Diagnosis and definition. In M. Rutter & E. Schopler (Eds.), *Autism: A reappraisal of concepts and treatment.* New York: Plenum Press.

Rutter, M., Graham, P. J., & Yule, W. (1970). *A neuropsychiatric study in childhood. Clinics in developmental medicine* (No. 35/36). London: S.I.M.P. with Heinemann.

Rutter, M., Tizard, J., & Whitmore, K. (1970). *Education, health and behaviour.* London: Longmans.

Ryan, J. (1977). The silence of stupidity. In J. Morton & J. Marshall (Eds.), *Psycholinguistics: Developmental and pathological.* Ithaca, NY: Cornell University Press.

Ryckman, D., & Wiegerink, R. (1969). The factors of the Illinois test of Psycholinguistic Abilities: A comparison of 18 factor analyses. *Exceptional Children, 36,* 107–115.

Sachs, J. (1983). Talking about the there and then: The emergence of displaced reference in parent-child discourse. In K. E. Nelson (Ed.), *Children's language* (Vol. 4). Hillsdale, NJ: Erlbaum.

Sachs, J., Goldman, J., & Chaille, C. (1984). Planning in pretend play: Using language to coordinate narrative development. In A. D. Pellegrini & T. Yawkey (Eds.), *The development of oral and written language in social contexts.* Norwood, NJ: Ablex.

Sailor, W., & Taman, T. (1972). Stimulus factors in the training of prepositional usage in three autistic children. *Journal of Applied Behavior Analysis, 5,* 183–190.

Salame, P., & Baddeley, A. (1982). Disruption of STM by unattended speech: Implications for the structure of working memory. *Journal of Verbal Learning and Verbal Behavior, 21,* 150–164.

Salvia, J., & Ysseldyke, J. (1981). *Assessment in special and remedial education.* Boston: Houghton-Mifflin.

Sapir, E. (1921). *Language.* New York: Harcourt Brace & World.

Sarachan-Deily, A. (1985). Written narratives of deaf and hearing students: Story recall and inference. *Journal of Speech and Hearing Research, 28,* 151–159.

Satz, P., & Bullard-Bates, C. (1981). Acquired aphasia in children. In M. T. Sarno (Ed.), *Acquired aphasia* (pp. 399–426). New York: Academic Press.

Savich, P. (1984). Anticipatory imagery ability in normal and language-disabled children. *Journal of Speech and Hearing Research, 4,* 494–501.

Schaeffer, B. (1980). Spontaneous language through signed speech. In R. Schiefelbusch (Ed.), *Nonspeech language and communication: Analysis and intervention.* Baltimore: University Park Press.

Schatz, C. (1954). The role of context in the perception of stops. *Language, 30,* 47–56.

Schery, T. (1985). Correlates of language development in language-disordered children. *Journal of Speech and Hearing Disorders, 50,* 73–83.

Schiff, N. (1979). The influence of deviant maternal input on the development of language during the preschool years. *Journal of Speech and Hearing Research, 22,* 581–603.

Schiff-Myers, N. (1987, April). *The micro-computer: Basic operations in client management.* Paper presented at the New York State Speech-Language Hearing Association.

Schlanger, B. (1954). Environmental influences on the verbal output of mentally retarded children. *Journal of Speech and Hearing Disorders, 19,* 339–343.

Schlesinger, I. (1971). Production of utterances and language acquisition. In D. Slobin (Ed.), *The ontogenesis of grammar.* New York: Academic Press.

Schlesinger, I. (1974). Relational concepts underlying language. In R. L. Schiefelbusch & L. Lloyd (Eds.), *Language perspectives—Acquisition, retardation and intervention.* Baltimore: University Park Press.

Schmidt, S. (1981). Eliciting negative structures through role playing. In J. Miller (Ed.), *Assessing language production in children* (pp. 148–149). Baltimore: University Park Press.

Schnur, M. (1971). *Auditory discrimination and temporal ordering by children with normal language and children with language impairments.* Unpublished doctoral dissertation, Teachers College, Columbia University.

Schodorf, J. K., & Edwards, H. T. (1983). Comparative analysis of parent-child interactions with language-disordered and linguistically normal children. *Journal of Communication Disorders, 16,* 71–83.

Schuler, A. L. (1979). *An experimental analysis of conceptual and representational abilities in a mute autistic adolescent: A serial versus a simultaneous mode of processing.* Unpublished doctoral dissertation, University of California at Santa Barbara.

Schuler, A. L. (1980). Aspects of communication. In W. H. Fay & A. L. Schuler (Eds.), *Emerging language in autistic children.* Baltimore: University Park Press.

Schwartz, E. (1974). Characteristics of speech and language development in the child with myelomingocele and hydrocephalus. *Journal of Speech and Hearing Disorders, 39,* 465–468.

Schwartz, R., Chapman, K., Terrell, B., Prelock, P., & Rowan, L. (1985). Facilitating word combinations in language-impaired children through discourse structure. *Journal of Speech and Hearing Disorders, 50,* 31–39.

Schwartz, R., & Leonard, L. (1982). Do children pick and choose? Phonological selection and avoidance in early lexical acquisition. *Journal of Child Language, 9,* 319–336.

Schwartz, R., & Leonard, L. (1983). Some further comments on reduplication in child phonology. *Journal of Child Language, 10,* 441–448.

Schwartz, R., & Leonard, L. (1985). Lexical imitation and acquisition in language-impaired children. *Journal of Speech and Hearing Disorders, 50,* 141–149.

Schwartz, R., Leonard, L., Folger, M., & Wilcox, M. J. (1980). Early phonological behavior in normal-speaking and language disordered children: Evidence for a synergistic view of linguistic disorders. *Journal of Speech and Hearing Disorders, 45,* 357–377.

Scollon, R. (1976). *Conversations with a one year old: A case study of the developmental foundation of syntax.* Honolulu: University Press of Hawaii.

Seller, L. (1981). *The effect of task and familiarity of the stimuli on auditory discrimination.* Unpublished master's thesis, Hunter College, the City University of New York.

Selz, M., & Reitan, R. (1979). Neuropsychological test performance of normal, learning disabled and brain-damaged older children. *Journal of Nervous and Mental Disorders, 167,* 298–302.

Semel, E., & Wiig, E. (1980, 1987). *Clinical Evaluation of Language Functions (CELF).* Columbus, OH: Merrill.

Semel, E., & Wiig, E. (1987). *Clinical Evaluation of Language Functions—Revised (CELF-R).* San Antonio, TX: Psychological Corp.

Shane, H. (1980). Approaches to assessing the communication of non-oral persons. In R. Schiefelbusch (Ed.), *Nonspeech language and communication.* Baltimore: University Park Press.

Shankweiler, D., Liberman, I. Y., Mark, L. S., Fowler, C. A., & Fisher, F. W. (1979). The speech code and learning to read. *Journal of Experimental Psychology: Human Perception and Performance, 5,* 531–545.

Shapiro, T., Chiarandini, I., & Fish, B. (1974). Thirty severely disturbed children: Evaluation of their language development for classification and prognosis. *Archives of General Psychiatry, 30,* 819–825.

Shapiro, T., Roberts, A., & Fish, B. (1970). Imitation and echoing in young schizophrenic children. *Journal of the American Academy of Child Psychiatry, 9,* 421–439.

Shatz, M. (1977). The relationship between cognitive processes and the development of communication skills. In C. B. Keasey (Ed.), *Nebraska symposium on motivation* (Vol. 25). Lincoln, NE: University of Nebraska Press.

Shatz, M., & Gelman, R. (1973). The development of communication skills: Modifications in the speech of young children as a function of listener. *Monographs of the Society for Research in Child Development, 38* (Serial No. 152).

Shea, S., & Raffin, M. (1983). Assessment of the electromagnetic characteristics of Willeford's central auditory processing test battery. *Journal of Speech and Hearing Research,* 18–21.

Shepard, N., Davis, J., Gorga, M., & Stelmachowicz, P. (1981). Characteristics of hearing-impaired children in the public schools: Part I Demographic data. *Journal of Speech and Hearing Disorders, 46,* 123–129.

Sheridan, M. D. (1973). Children of seven years with marked speech defects. *British Journal of Disorders of Communication, 9,* 3.

Sherman, J. A. (1965). Use of reinforcement and imitation to reinstate verbal behavior in mute psychotics. *Journal of Abnormal Psychology, 70,* 155–164.

Shriner, T. H., Holloway, M. S., & Daniloff, R. G. (1969). The relationship between articulatory deficits and syntax in speech defective children. *Journal of Speech and Hearing Research, 12,* 319–325.

Shulman, B. (1986). *Test of Pragmatic Skills—Revised.* Tucson, AZ: Communication Skill Builders.

Siegel, G. M., & Broen, P. (1976). Language assessment. In L. Lloyd (Ed.), *Communication assessment and intervention strategies* (pp. 73–122). Baltimore: University Park Press.

Siegel, G., & Vogt, M. (1984). Pluralization instruction in comprehension and production. *Journal of Speech and Hearing Disorders, 49,* 128–135.

Siegel R. (1982). Reproductive, perinatal, and environmental factors as predictors of the cognitive and language development of preterm and full term infants. *Child Development, 53,* 963–973.

Silliman, E. (in press). Individual differences in the classroom performance of language-impaired students. In D. Ripich (Ed.), *Seminars in speech and language.*

Silliman, E., Campbell, M., & Mitchell, R. (in press). Genetic influences in autism and assessment of metalinguistic performance in siblings of autistic children. In G. Dawson (Ed.), *Autism: Perspectives on nature and treatment.* New York: Guilford Press.

Silva, P. A. (1980). The prevalence, stability and significance of developmental language delay in preschool children. *Developmental Medicine and Child Neurology, 22,* 768–777.

Silverman, S. R. (1971a). The education of deaf children. In L. E. Travis (Ed.), *Handbook of speech pathology and audiology.* New York: Appleton-Century-Crofts.

Silverman, S. R. (1971b). Hard-of-hearing children. In L. E. Travis (Ed.), *Handbook of speech pathology and audiology.* New York: Appleton-Century-Crofts.

Simmons, A. A. (1962). A comparison of the type-token ratio of spoken and written language of deaf and hearing children. *Volta Review, 64,* 417–421.

Simmons, J. Q., & Baltaxe, C. A. M. (1975). Language patterns of adolescent autistics. *Journal of Autism and Childhood Schizophrenia, 5,* 333–351.

Simon, C. (Ed.) (1985). *Communication skills and classroom success: Assessment of language learning disordered students.* San Diego: College-Hill Press.

Sinclair, H. (1970). The transition from sensory-motor behavior to symbolic activity. *Interchange, 1,* 119–126.

Sinclair, H., & Bronckart, J. P. (1972). S.V.O. A linguistic universal? A study in developmental psycholinguistics. *Journal of Experimental Child Psychology, 14,* 329–348.

Skarakis, E. A. (1982). *The development of symbolic play and language in language disordered children.* Unpublished doctoral dissertation, University of California, Santa Barbara.

Skarakis, E. A., & Greenfield, P. M. (1982). The role of new and old information in the verbal expression of language-disordered children. *Journal of Speech and Hearing Research, 25,* 462–468.

Skinner, B. F. (1957). *Verbal behavior.* New York: Appleton-Century-Crofts.

Sleight, C., & Prinz, P. (1985). Use of abstracts, orientations, and codas in narration by language-disordered and nondisordered children. *Journal of Speech and Hearing Disorders, 50,* 361–371.

Sloane, H. N., & McCauley, B. D. (Eds.) (1968). *Operant procedures in remedial speech and language training.* Boston: Houghton Mifflin.

Slobin, D. (Ed.) (1967). *A field manual for cross-cultural study of the acquisition of communicative competence.* Berkeley, CA: University of California Press.

Slobin, D. (1973). Cognitive prerequisites for the development of grammar. In C. Ferguson & D. Slobin (Eds.), *Studies of child language development.* New York: Holt, Rinehart and Winston.

Slobin, D., & Welsh, C. (1973). Elicited imitation as a research tool in developmental psycholinguistics. In C. A. Ferguson & D. Slobin (Eds.), *Studies of child language development.* New York: Holt, Rinehart and Winston.

Smith, B. (1982). Some observations concerning premeaningful vocalizations of hearing-impaired infants. *Journal of Speech and Hearing Disorders, 47,* 439.

Smith, B., & Oller, D. K. (1981). A comparative study of premeaningful vocalizations produced by normal and Down's syndrome infants. *Journal of Speech and Hearing Disorders, 46,* 46–51.

Smith, C. M. (1971). The relationship of reading method and reading achievement to I.T.P.A. sensory modalities. *Journal of Special Education, 4,* 143–149.

Smith, M. E. (1933). The influence of age, sex, and situation on the frequency, form, and function of questions asked by preschool children. *Child Development, 4,* 201–213.

Snow, C. (1972). Mothers' speech to children learning language. *Child Development, 43,* 549–565.

Snow, C. (1974, September). Mother's speech research: An overview. Paper presented at the Conference on Language Input and Acquisition, Boston.

Snow, C., Midkiff-Borunda, S., Small, A., & Proctor, A. (1984, September). Therapy as social interaction: Analyzing the contexts for language remediation. *Topics in Language Disorders, 4,* 72–85.

Snyder, L. (1975). *Pragmatics in language disordered children: Their prelinguistic and early verbal performatives and presuppositions.* Unpublished doctoral dissertation, University of Colorado.

Snyder, L. (1984). Developmental language disorders: Elementary school age. In A. Holland (Ed.), *Language disorders in children.* San Diego: College-Hill Press.

Snyder, L., Bates, E., & Bretherton, I. (1981). Content and context in early lexical development. *Journal of Child Language, 8,* 565–582.

Spradlin, J. E., & Siegel, G. M. (1982). Language training in natural and clinical environments. *Journal of Speech and Hearing Disorders, 47,* 2–7.

Spring, C. (1976). Encoding speed and memory span in dyslexic children. *Journal of Special Education, 10,* 35–40.

Stanton, A. (1986). *Factors underlying sentence interpretation in young children: Word order, real world knowledge, and linguistic structure.* Unpublished doctoral dissertation, City University of New York.

Stark, J., Giddan, J., & Meisel, J. (1968). Increasing verbal behavior in an autistic child. *Journal of Speech and Hearing Disorders, 33,* 42–48.

Stark, J., Poppen, R., & May, M. (1967). Effects of alterations of prosodic features on the sequencing performance of aphasic children. *Journal of Speech and Hearing Research, 10,* 849–855.

Stark, R. (1979). Prespeech segmental feature development. In P. Fletcher & M. Garman (Eds.), *Language acquisition.* Cambridge: Cambridge University Press.

Stark, R., & Bernstein, L. (1984). Evaluating central auditory processing in children. *Topics in Language Disorders, 4,* 57–70.

Stark, R., & Tallal, P. (1975). Speech perception and production errors in dysphasic children. *Journal of the Acoustical Society of America, 57,* 526.

Stark, R., & Tallal, P. (1979). Analysis of stop-consonant production errors in developmentally dysphasic children. *Journal of the Acoustical Society of America, 66,* 1703–1712.

Stark, R., & Tallal, P. (1981). Selection of children with specific language deficit. *Journal of Speech and Hearing Disorders, 46,* 114–122.

Steckol, K. F., & Leonard, L. (1979). The use of grammatical morphemes by normal and language-impaired children. *Journal of Communication Disorders, 12,* 291–301.

Stein, N. (1986, October). *A model of children's storytelling skill.* Paper presented at the Boston University Conference on Language Development, Boston.

Stein, N., & Glenn, C. (1982). Children's concept of time: The development of a story schema. In W. J. Friedman (Ed.), *The developmental psychology of time* (pp. 255–282). New York: Academic Press.

Stein, N., & Policastro, M. (1984). The concept of a story: A comparison between children's and teachers' viewpoints. In H. Mandl, N. Stein, & T. Trabasso (Eds.), *Learning and comprehension of text.* Hillsdale, NJ: Erlbaum.

Stephens, M. I., & Montgomery, A. (1985). A critique of recent relevant standardized tests. *Topics in Language Disorders, 5,* 21–45.

Stern, D. (1977). *The first relationship.* Cambridge, MA: Harvard University Press.

Stevenson, J., & Richman, N. (1976). The prevalence of language delay in a population of three-year-old children and its association with general retardation. *Developmental Medicine Child Neurology, 18,* 431–441.

Strauss, A. A., & Lehtinen, L. E. (1947). *Psychopathology and education of the brain-injured child.* (Vol. I). New York: Grune & Stratton.

Streim, N., & Chapman, R. (1986, October). *A case study of fast mapping of novel action verbs: The roles of event and discourse context.* Paper presented at the Boston University Conference on Language Development, Boston.

Striefel, S., & Wetherby, B. (1973). Instruction-following behavior of a retarded child and its controlling stimuli. *Journal of Applied Behavior Analysis, 6,* 663–670.

Stremel, K., & Waryas, C. (1974). A behavioral psycholinguistic approach to language training. In L. McReynolds (Ed.), *Developing systematic procedures for training children's language.* ASHA Monographs (No. 18).

Sugarman, S. (1973). *A description of communication development in the pre-linguistic child.* Unpublished honors paper, Hampshire College.

Sutton-Smith, B. (1981). *The folkstories of children.* Philadelphia: University of Pennsylvania Press.

Sutton-Smith, B. (1986). The development of fictional narrative performances. *Topics in Language Disorders, 7,* 1–10.

Swisher, L. (1985). Language disorders in children. In J. Darby (Ed.), *Speech and language evaluation in neurology: Childhood disorders* (pp. 33–69). New York: Grune & Stratton.

Swisher, L., & Matkin, A. (1984). Specific language impairment. The method of L. Swisher and A. Matkin. In W. H. Perkins (Ed.), *Current therapy of communication disorders: Language handicaps in children.* New York: Thieme-Stratton.

Swisher, L., & Pinsker, E. J. (1971). The language characteristics of hyperverbal hydrocephalic children. *Developmental Medicine and Child Neurology, 13,* 746–755.

Swisher, L., Reichler, R., & Short, A. (1976). Language development history and change in autistic children. In S. Hirsh, E. Eldredge, I. Hirsh, & S. Silverman (Eds.), *Hearing and Davis: Essays honoring Hallowell Davis.* St. Louis: Washington University Press.

Systematic Analysis of Language Transcripts (SALT). Madison, WI: Waisman Center on Mental Retardation and Human Development.

Taenzer, S., Bass, M., & Kise, L. (1974). The young child—*A language explorer: A Piagetian-based approach to language therapy.* Paper presented at the American Speech and Hearing Association, Las Vegas, NV.

Taenzer, S., Harris, L., & Bass, M. (1975). *Assessment in a natural context.* Paper presented at the American Speech and Hearing Association National Convention, Washington, DC.

Tallal, P. (1976). Rapid auditory processing in normal and disordered language development. *Journal of Speech and Hearing Research, 19,* 561–571.

Tallal, P. (1980). Perceptual requisites for language. In R. Schiefelbusch (Ed.), *Nonspeech language and communication: Analysis and intervention.* Baltimore: University Park Press.

Tallal, P., & Piercy, M. (1973a). Defects of non-verbal auditory perception in children with developmental aphasia. *Nature, 241,* 468–469.

Tallal, P., & Piercy, M. (1973b). Developmental aphasia: Impaired rate of nonverbal processing as a function of sensory modality. *Neuropsychologia, 11,* 389–398.

Tallal, P., & Piercy, M. (1974). Developmental aphasia: Rate of auditory processing and selective impairment of consonant perception. *Neuropsychologia, 12,* 83–93.

Tallal, P., & Piercy, M. (1975). Developmental aphasia: The perception of brief vowels and extended stop consonants. *Neuropsychologia, 13*, 69–74.

Tallal, P., & Piercy, M. (1978). Defects of auditory perception in children with developmental dysphasia. In M. Wyke (Ed.), *Developmental dysphasia.* New York: Academic Press.

Tallal, P., Stark, R., & Curtiss, S. (1976). The relation between speech perception impairment and speech production impairment in children with developmental dysphasia. *Brain and Language, 3*, 305–317.

Tallal, P., Stark, R., Kallman, C., & Mellits, D. (1980). Perceptual constancy for phonemic categories: A developmental study with normal and language impaired children. *Applied Psycholinguistics, 1*, 49–64.

Tallal, P., Stark, R., & Mellits, D. (1985a). The relationship between auditory temporal analysis and receptive language development: Evidence from studies of developmental language disorder. *Neuropsychologia, 23*, 527–534.

Tallal, P., Stark, R., & Mellits, D. (1985b). Identification of language-impaired children on the basis of rapid perception and production skills. *Brain and Language, 25*, 314–322.

Tamari, P. (1978). *Language acquisition of mentally retarded children: The development of form and meaning.* Unpublished doctoral dissertation, Columbia University.

Taylor, L. (1969). *A language analysis of the writing of deaf children.* Unpublished doctoral dissertation, State University of Florida.

Taylor, O. (Ed.) (1986). *Nature of communication disorders in culturally and linguistically diverse populations.* San Diego: College-Hill Press.

Tedeschi, T. J. (1983, June). Children with central auditory disorders, Part II: Therapeutic strategies. *The Hearing Journal,* pp. 19–20.

Templin, M. (1957). *Certain language skills in children.* Minneapolis: University of Minnesota Press.

Templin, M., & Darley, F. (1969). *Templin-Darley Test of Articulation* (2nd ed.). Bureau of Education Research and Services, Iowa City: University of Iowa.

Terman, L., & Merrill, M. (1960). *Stanford-Binet Intelligence Scale.* Boston: Houghton Mifflin.

Terrace, H. (1985). In the beginning was the "Name." *American Psychologist, 9*, 1011–1028.

Terrell, B., Schwartz, R., Prelock, P., & Messick, C. (1984). Symbolic play in normal and language-impaired children. *Journal of Speech and Hearing Research, 27*, 424–430.

Tervoort, B. T. (1967). *Analysis of communicative structure patterns in deaf children* (Final report, Project No. R.D.-467-64-65). Washington, DC: USO HEW, Vocational Rehabilitation Administration.

Tiegerman, E., & Primavera, L. (1984). Imitating the autistic child: Facilitating communicative gaze behavior. *Journal of Autism and Developmental Disabilities, 14*, 27–38.

Tomblin, J. B. (1984). Specific abilities approach: An evaluation and an alternative method. In W. Perkins (Ed.), *Language handicaps in children.* New York: Thieme-Stratton. pp. 27–42.

Tomblin, J. B., & Quinn, M. A. (1983). The contribution of perceptual learning to performance on the repetition task. *Journal of Speech and Hearing Research, 26*, 369–372.

Torgesen, J. K. (1985). Memory processes in reading disabled children. *Journal of Learning Disabilities, 18*, 350–358.

Torgesen, J. K., & Wong, B. Y. (Eds.) (1986). *Psychological and educational perspectives on learning disabilities.* New York: Academic Press.

Trabasso, T., Secco, T., & van den Broek, P. (1984). Causal cohesion and story coherence. In H. Mandl, N. Stein, & T. Trabasso (Eds.), *Learning and comprehension of text.* Hillsdale, NJ: Erlbaum.

Tulving, E. (1972). Episodic and semantic memory. In E. Tulving & W. Donaldson (Eds.), *Organization in memory*. New York: Academic Press.

Tyack, D., & Gottsleben, R. (1974). *Language sampling, analysis and training: A handbook for teachers and clinicians*. Palo Alto, CA: Consulting Psychologists Press.

Tyack, D., & Gottsleben, R. (1986). Acquisition of complex sentences. *Language Speech and Hearing Services in the Schools, 17*, 160–174.

Tyack, D., & Ingram, D. (1977). Children's production and comprehension of questions. *Journal of Child Language, 4*, 211–224.

Umiker-Sebeok, D. J. (1979). Preschool children's intra-conversational narratives. *Journal of Child Language, 9*, 91–109.

Urwin, C. (1976). *Speech development in blind children: Some ways into language*. Paper prepared for Internationales Symposium des Blinden-und-Sehschwachen-Verbandes der DDR.

Urwin, C. (1984, September). Language for absent things: Learning from visually handicapped children. *Topics in Language Disorders, 4*, 24–37.

Uzgiris, I. C., & Hunt, J. M. (1975). *Assessment in infancy*. Urbana, IL: University of Illinois Press.

Vaisse, L. (1866). Des sourds-muets et de certains cas d'aphasie congenitale. *Bulletins de la societe d'Anthropologie de Paris*, pp. 146–150.

Vanderheiden, G., Brown, W., MacKenzie, P., Reinen, S., & Scheibel, C. (1975). Symbol communication for the mentally handicapped. *Mental Retardation, 13*, 34–37.

Vanderheiden, G., & Harris-Vanderheiden, D. (1976). Communication techniques and aids for the nonvocal severely handicapped. In L. Lloyd (Ed.), *Communication assessment and intervention strategies*. Baltimore: University Park Press.

Van Dongen, R., & Westby, C. (1986). Building the narrative mode of thought through children's literature. *Topics in Language Disorders, 7*, 70–83.

Van Kleeck, A. (1984). Metalinguistic skills: Cutting across spoken and written language and problem-solving abilities. In G. Wallach & K. Butler (Eds.), *Language learning disabilities in school-age children*. Baltimore: Williams & Wilkins.

Van Kleeck, A., & Carpenter, R. (1980). The effects of children's language comprehension level on adults' child-directed talk. *Journal of Speech and Hearing Research, 23*, 546–569.

Van Kleeck, A., & Frankel, T. (1981). Discourse devices used by language disordered children. *Journal of Speech and Hearing Disorders, 46*, 250–257.

Vellutino, F. R. (1977). Alternative conceptualizations of dyslexia: Evidence in support of a verbal-deficit hypothesis. *Harvard Educational Review, 47*, 334–354.

Vellutino, F. R. (1979). *Theory and research in dyslexia*. Cambridge, MA: M.I.T. Press.

Vellutino, F. R., Pruzek, R., Steger, J. A., & Meshoulam, U. (1973). Immediate visual recall in poor and normal readers as a function of orthographic-linguistic familiarity. *Cortex, 9*, 368–384.

Ventry, I. M. (1980). Effects of conductive hearing loss: Fact or fiction. *Journal of Speech and Hearing Disorders, 45*, 143–156.

Ventry, I. M. (1983). Research design issues in studies of middle ear effusion. *Pediatrics, 71*, 644.

Vygotsky, L. S. (1978). *Mind in Society: The development of higher psychological processes*. Cambridge, MA: Harvard University Press.

Walker, H., & Birch, H. (1970). Neurointegrative deficiency in schizophrenic children. *Journal of Nervous and Mental Disease, 151*, 104–113.

Wallach, G., & Butler, K. (Eds.) (1984). *Language learning disabilities in school-age children*. Baltimore: Williams & Wilkins.

Wallach, G., & Liebergott, J. (1984). Who shall be called "learning disabled": Some new directions. In G. Wallach & K. Butler (Eds.), *Language learning disabilities in school-age children*. Baltimore: Williams & Wilkins.

Warden, D. (1976). The influence of context on children's use of identifying expressions and references. *British Journal of Psychology, 67,* 101–112.

Warren, S., & Kaiser, A. (1986). Generalization of treatment effects by young language-delayed children: A longitudinal analysis. *Journal of Speech and Hearing Disorders, 51,* 239–251.

Warren, S., & Rogers-Warren, A. (1985). *Teaching functional language.* Baltimore: University Park Press.

Waryas, C. L., & Stremel-Campbell, K. (1978). Grammatical training for the language-delayed child: A new perspective. In R. Schiefelbusch (Ed.), *Language intervention strategies* (pp. 145–192). Baltimore: University Park Press.

Watson, J. B., Sullivan, P., Moeller, M., & Jensen, J. (1982). Nonverbal intelligence and English language ability in deaf children. *Journal of Speech and Hearing Disorders, 47,* 199–203.

Wechsler, D. (1949). *Wechsler Intelligence Scale for Children (WISC).* New York: Psychological Corp.

Wechsler, D. (1974). *Wechsler Intelligence Scale for Children—Revised (WISC-R).* New York: Psychological Corp.

Wechsler, D. (1967). *Wechsler Preschool and Primary Scale of Intelligence (WPPSI).* New York: Psychological Corp.

Weiner, P. (1984). The study of childhood language disorders in the nineteenth century. *Asha, 26,* 35–38.

Weir, R. (1964). *Language in the crib.* The Hague: Mouton.

Weismer, S. (1985). Constructive comprehension abilities exhibited by language-disordered children. *Journal of Speech and Hearing Research, 28,* 175–184.

Weistuch, L. (no date). *A comparison of maternal/child linguistic interchanges when handicapped and non-handicapped children are matched for MLU.* Unpublished manuscript, Rutgers Medical School, NJ.

Wepman, J. (1958). *Auditory Discrimination Test.* Chicago: Language Research Associates.

Wepman, J., Jones, L. V., Bock, R. D., & Van Pelt, D. (1960). Studies in aphasia: Background and theoretical formulations. *Journal of Speech and Hearing Disorders, 25,* 323–332.

Wepman, J., & Morency, A. (1973). *Auditory Memory Span Test.* Chicago: Language Resources Associates.

Westby, C. (1984). Development of narrative language abilities. In G. Wallach & K. Butler (Eds.), *Language learning disabilities in school-age children.* Baltimore: Williams & Wilkins.

Westby, C. E. (1985). Learning to talk—Talking to learn: Oral literate language differences. In C. E. Simon (Ed.), *Communication skills and classroom success: Therapy methodologies for language-learning disabled students* (pp. 181–213). San Diego: College-Hill Press.

Wetherby, A., Koegel, R., & Mendel, M. (1981). Central auditory nervous system dysfunction in echolalic autistic individuals. *Journal of Speech and Hearing Research, 24,* 420–429.

Whitehurst, G. J., & Novak, G. (1973). Modeling, imitation training, and the acquisition of sentence phrases. *Journal of Experimental Child Psychology, 16,* 332–345.

Wiig, E. H., & Secord, W. (1987). *Test of Language Competence for Children (TLC-C).* San Antonio, TX: Psychological Corp.

Wiig, E. H., & Semel, E. M. (1976). *Language disabilities in children and adolescents.* Columbus, OH: Merrill.

Wiig, E. M., Semel, E. M., & Nystrom, L. (1982). Comparison of rapid naming abilities in language-learning disabled and academically achieving eight-year-olds. *Language Speech Hearing Services in the Schools, 13,* 11–22.

Wilbur, R. (1976). The linguistics of manual languages and manual systems. In L. Lloyd

(Ed.), *Communication assessment and intervention strategies.* Baltimore: University Park Press.

Wilcox, M. J. (1984). Developmental language disorders: Preschoolers. In A. Holland (Ed.), *Language disorders in children.* San Diego: College-Hill Press.

Willeford, J. (1977). Assessing central auditory behavior in children: A test battery approach. In R. Keith (Ed.), *Central auditory dysfunction.* New York: Grune & Stratton.

Willeford, J., & Billger, J. (1978). Auditory perception in children with learning disabilities. In J. Katz (Ed.), *Handbook of clinical audiology.* Baltimore: Williams & Wilkins.

Wilson, B., & Risucci, D. (1986). A model for clinical-quantitative classification. Generation I: Application to language-disordered preschool children. *Brain and Language, 27,* 281–309.

Wilson, M. S., & Fox, B. J. (1983). Microcomputers: A clinical aid. In H. Winitz (Ed.), *Treating language disorders: For clinicians by clinicians.* Baltimore: University Park Press.

Wing, L. (1972). What is an autistic child? *Communication, 6,* 5–10.

Wing, L. (1975). A study of language impairment in severely retarded children. In N. O'Connor (Ed.), *Language, cognitive deficits and retardation.* London: Butterworths.

Wing, L. (1981). Language, social, and cognitive impairments in autism and severe mental retardation. *Journal of Autism and Developmental Disorders, 11,* 31–44.

Winitz, H. (1973). Problem solving and the delaying of speech as strategies in the teaching of language. *Asha, 15,* 583–586.

Winitz, H. (1976). Full time experience. *Asha, 18,* 404.

Winitz, H. (Ed.) (1983). *Treating language disorders: For clinicians by clinicians.* Baltimore: University Park Press.

Wolchik, S. (1983). Language patterns of parents of young autistic and normal children. *Journal of Autism and Developmental Disorders, 13,* 167–180.

Wolf, M. (1986). Rapid alternating stimulus naming in the developmental dyslexias. *Brain and Language, 27,* 360–379.

Wolfus, B., Moscovitch, M., & Kinsbourne, M. (1980). Subgroups of developmental language impairment. *Brain and Language, 9,* 152–171.

Wollner, S. (1983, December). Communicating intentions: How well do language-impaired children do? *Topics in Language Disorders,* pp. 1–14.

Woods, B. T., & Carey, S. (1979). Language deficits after apparent clinical recovery from childhood aphasia. *Annals of Neurology, 6,* 405–409.

Wulbert, M., Inglis, S., Kriegsmann, E., & Mills, B. (1975). Language delay and associated mother-child interactions. *Developmental Psychology, 11,* 61–70.

Yoder, D., & Calculator, S. (1981). Some perspectives on intervention strategies for persons with developmental disorders. *Journal of Autism and Developmental Disorders, 11,* 107–124.

Zachman, L., Huisingh, R., Jorgensen, C., & Barrett, M. (1977). *OLSIDI instruction manual.* Moline, IL: LinguiSystems.

Zimmerman, B. J., & Bell, J. A. (1972). Observer verbalization and abstraction in vicarious rule learning, generalization, and retention. *Developmental Psychology, 7,* 227–231.

Zimmerman, I. L., Steiner, V. G., & Evatt, R. (1969). *Preschool Language Scale.* Columbus, OH: Merrill.

Zimmerman, I. L., Steiner, V. G., & Pond, R. (1979). *Preschool Language Scale.* Columbus, OH: Merrill.

Zipf, G. K. (1965). *The psycho-biology of language: An introduction to dynamic philology.* Cambridge, MA: M.I.T. Press.

Author Index

Subject Index